Payne's Handbook of Relaxation Techniques

A PRACTICAL GUIDE FOR THE HEALTH CARE PROFESSIONAL

Payne's Handbook of Relaxation Techniques

A PRACTICAL GUIDE FOR THE HEALTH CARE PROFESSIONAL

Fifth Edition

Edited by

DR. CAROLINE. A. BELCHAMBER

(DPROF, MSC, BSC (HONS), PGCE, HCPCREG, FHEA, RFRSM)

Senior Lecturer in Physiotherapy,
Programme Lead for MSc Physiotherapy (pre-registration),
Visiting Fellow Bournemouth University
School of Rehabilitation, Sport and Psychology,
AECC University College,
Parkwood Campus, Parkwood Road, Brounemouth

ELSEVIER

Content Strategist: Poppy Garraway
Content Development Specialist: Andrae Akeh
Project Manager: Rukmani Krishnan
Design: Renee Duenow
Illustration Manager: Muthukumaran Thangaraj
Marketing Manager: Deborah Watkins

Printed in India
Last digit is the print number: 9 8 7 6 5 4 3 2 1

Working together
to grow libraries in
developing countries

www.elsevier.com • www.bookaid.org

CONTRIBUTORS

DR HELEN BOLDERSTON, (PHD, MSC, BSC, CPSYCHOL)
Clinical Psychologist
Senior Lecturer in Psychology
Department of Psychology, Faculty of Science and Technology
Bournemouth University
Poole House, Fern Barrow, Poole

PROFESSOR TEENA CLOUSTON, (PHD, MBA, DIPRCOT, DIPCOUNS, DIPAROM, CERTHYP, HCPCREG, SFADVHE)
School of Healthcare Sciences, College of Biomedical and Life Sciences
Cardiff University, Wales

DR RUTH T NAYLOR, (BA, MSC, MBA (HONS) USPHS FELLOW, AA (HONS), DIPAT, DIPCBH, PHD, NCPSNRACCRED, CPSYCHOL)
Trustee: British Autogenic Society

FOREWORD

R elaxation is often seen as a panacea for stress. As such, it has given rise to many different approaches designed to cope with everyday stressors.

When people are unwell and/or under pressure at work, stress and tension mount; sleep is affected and other body systems are negatively influenced. Some people with a chronic pattern of stress-related behaviour can find it difficult to unlearn these behaviours and adopt a calmer lifestyle, reducing their quality of life and their ability to cope.

Many relaxation techniques are presented in this book. They have been selected with particular criteria in mind: that they should be easily learned and applied without requiring expensive equipment or specialized expertise. Their transferability is also important in that they can be adopted by small groups as well as individuals, and in a wide variety of settings across different age groups. Certain specialized techniques, such as yoga, are not covered in this book precisely because they require specific training or because, like biofeedback, they rely on special equipment.

An excellent introduction to the topic can be found in this book with its jargon-free style and its readability. Although addressed to both qualified and novice health care professionals, it does not demand particular health care knowledge or specific previous training and therefore has wide applicability. The book takes us through different aspects of relaxation, starting with a discussion on physiological and psychological dimensions of stress, leading into chapters containing different coping techniques to help manage stress. With the increasing number of people living with palliative and supportive care needs, these non–drug-free approaches to improve quality of life are important for the person with complex chronic conditions, as well as their family members and carers. In addition to this, in today's society, back pain is a major cause of absenteeism, where the link between stress, muscle tension and perceptions of illness becomes particularly relevant. Furthermore, with the recent pandemic these relaxation techniques may prove invaluable to support people post COVID and those who have found isolation and shielding stressful. The book then moves through a variety of somatic approaches, including progressive muscle relaxation, breathing re-education, physical activity and passive relaxation. Cognitive approaches include imagery, visualizations, autogenics, meditation and some simple cognitive–behavioural techniques.

A common format running through the chapters makes this book easy to dip in and out of and allows the easy comparison of one technique with another. The final chapters relate to issues around outcome measures, a topic that is essential for any kind of audit. There is also a chapter indicating which conditions are likely to benefit from particular techniques. The book is essentially a practical manual with a step-by-step approach, allowing the reader to feel in touch with the practicality of each technique.

If you are feeling stressed, then this is the book to pick up. Its pages will make you feel both more relaxed and more in control.

Ilora Finlay, FRCP, FRCGP
Baroness Finlay of Llandaff, Professor of
Palliative Medicine, Cardiff University;
President of the Chartered Society of Physiotherapy,
London, UK

PREFACE TO THE FIFTH EDITION

For this fifth edition, the book has moved to a new authorship, Dr. Caroline Belchamber, Senior Lecturer in Physiotherapy at AECC University College and a Chartered Physiotherapist, who has worked in palliative, supportive and end of life care since 2000, delivering non-drug related approaches for symptoms of breathlessness and pain. She is an advocate of rehabilitation in palliative, supportive and end of life care, providing education and training to qualified, as well as undergraduate and postgraduate healthcare professionals. Caroline has undertaken her Masters and Doctoral research in palliative, supportive and end of life care, with evidence-based practice development to improve the quality of palliative care practice and personalised care. This has enabled the introduction of palliative, supportive and end of life care with a fresh comprehensive review of the literature informing the evidence-based practice outlined in this book. In accordance with earlier editions, the aim has been to produce a book containing a broad range of relaxation techniques, which may be found useful by qualified and novice healthcare professionals whose background lie in a wide variety of professional fields.

The book is addressed primarily to qualified and novice healthcare professionals such as nurses, occupational therapists, physiotherapists, social workers and speech and language therapists. General practitioners and psychologists may also find the book useful. It can equally be used by the general public since it is written in a jargon-free style and may be a useful adjunct in managing stress and carer burn out in palliative care, as well as for people in other healthcare and work environments, helping to promote resilience.

The book focuses on relaxation techniques which do not require specialized expertise or elaborate equipment but consists of simpler approaches which can be applied in the stressful situation. The division between somatic and cognitive is, to some extent, an arbitrary one, and one which has no place in the holistic context to which the author subscribes. However, for the purpose of organizing material in the book, such a presentation has been adopted and maintained from previous additions.

In this edition, Caroline has kept the original title of 'Payne's handbook in memory of Rosemary Payne and in honour of the hard work she put into developing the first and preceding editions. This edition of the book has been structured in six parts. Section one sets the scene and has been organised slightly differently by describing states of stress first and then states of relaxation to understand its context and provide guidance on preparing for relaxation. Sections Two and Three guide the reader through 21 somatic and cognitive approaches, each occupying a separate chapter. A new Section four has been added focusing on application in practice, providing three new chapters on long-term conditions, palliative, supportive and end of life care and coronavirus disease (COVID-19), which have been included to reflect the growing number of people living longer with complex conditions and more recently with the effects of COVID-19. Section 5 focuses on working towards best practice and includes an overview of measurement tools, as well as exploring evidence from research for a number of conditions, culminating in a review of combined relaxation techniques that can be successfully applied in practice. Section 6 provides appendices, a glossary of terms and an index, which the author hopes the reader will find useful.

In this edition the chapters have been substantially updated with the addition of three new chapters. The book has also been restructured with key points, aims and objectives included with reflection points to guide the reader through each chapter. To aid understanding of the application of techniques, cases studies have been added to some chapters and expanded in others, standardising this throughout the book. References pertaining to each chapter have been conveniently moved to the end of each chapter rather than at the end of the book. Evidence-based practice throughout the book has been updated and given a new emphasis, but the early work has not been entirely eliminated since it provides a useful historical context for understanding the different approaches. It is hoped readers will find this arrangement helpful.

It is not intended that qualified and novice healthcare professionals should, on the strength of reading this book, consider themselves teachers of Autogenics or the Alexander technique. Such methods require lengthy training. These two methods are, however, included to indicate the importance of their contribution to the field; they are described for interest and for the applicability of their central ideas. For example, images of warmth and heaviness (Autogenics) are relaxing in any context, and postural advice (Alexander technique) helps to promote a sense of wellbeing. Such concepts have universal value.

Like its forebears, this new edition is essentially a practical manual, easy to follow and conveniently sized to carry around.

DR CAROLINE BELCHAMBER 2021

BACKGROUND TO THE FIRST AND PRECEDING EDITIONS

W hen Rosemary Payne, a chartered physiotherapist, qualified psychologist and original author of this book, was giving a talk on relaxation techniques, she was asked by a social worker if the techniques she was describing could all be found in one publication. She said she was unaware of such a book. After this, other health care professionals had, on different occasions, put similar questions to her: Is there a book which focuses on the practical side of relaxation training? Can the detail of the methods be found under one cover?

Rosemary found that many books at the time mentioned relaxation techniques but tended not to present them in any depth, unless the entire work was devoted to a single method. She therefore identified a gap in the market, which needed to be filled. The evidence at the time, which remains true today, confirmed this need, where an estimated 80% of modern diseases were shown to have their beginnings in stress (Powell & Enright 2015). With improved treatments we are also now experiencing a growth of at least 15 million people in England living with one or more long-term conditions, including stress-related symptoms for both the person living with the long-term condition as well as his or her caregivers. This is expected to increase to an estimated 18 million by 2025–2030 (DOH 2012). In addition, while completing this book COVID-19 became a feature of our lives, bringing with it a number of stress-related issues which have yet to unfold in full with the impact unknown at this stage. Furthermore, over the years there has been an increasing interest in non-drug treatments, with research around relaxation techniques growing, especially within the field of long-term conditions, palliative, supportive and end-of-life care. In the future we will also start to see the impact of relaxation techniques in managing post–COVID-19,

as research grows in this area. Therefore the selected audience of health care professionals is fitting to address this book to, and it continues to be written in such away that it will also be easily understood by the general public.

Factors of practicality governed Rosemary's selection of methods for this book. Thus techniques which required expensive equipment or specialized expertise were not included, and the methods chosen were those which lent themselves to presentation in small group settings.

The original book began with a review of some of the theories surrounding stress and relaxation. This was followed by a chapter on general procedure which was applicable to all methods. Chapter 2 discussed stress, beginning with a further passage of theory and moving on to consider a variety of practical coping skills. The following 21 chapters dealt with specific techniques: 12 chapters were, broadly speaking, concerned with physical or muscular techniques and 9 dealt with mental or psychological methods. There followed a chapter concerning 'on-the-spot' techniques for dealing with stressful situations, using skills drawn from earlier lessons. Assessment was also addressed, and the final chapter took a look at a few topics that had not already been discussed: the relation between the approaches themselves, some ways in which they could be combined, and a brief reference to approaches which were not included. Physical and psychiatric disorders were not within the scope of this original work. Rosemary went onto develop and revise the book in the second and third editions. In the fourth edition there was then a move from a single to a dual authorship with the introduction of Marie Donagh, professor of physiotherapy and dean of the School of Health

Sciences at Queen Margaret University in Edinburgh. This brought a new perspective to the book with the introduction of two new chapters, one on mindfulness mediation, which was included to reflect the growing interest and popularity of this approach, and the other on choice of technique for 35 specific conditions.

In the fifth edition the mindfulness mediation chapter has been developed and brought up to date with current practice. Three more specific conditions, chronic obstructive pulmonary disease, dementia and inflammatory bowel disease, have also been added to the 35 original specific conditions, with weight problems re-categorized under eating disorders. This chapter has also been extensively updated with the current evidence base, as research interest in relaxation techniques increases. Furthermore, the fifth edition has been substantially updated with re-structuring of all of the chapters, expanding upon and adding case studies throughout, as well as incorporating learning outcomes at the beginning of each chapter and key

points, reflections and activities situated at the end of each chapter. To complete the update of the new book a summary of all the relaxation techniques, their key points and precautions have been added to give a quick reference guide to the reader. Finally the new author, Dr Caroline Belchamber, brings a whole new outlook to the book with three new chapters added on long-term condition; palliative supportive and end of life care; and COVID-19. With her knowledge of rehabilitation and the non-pharmacological approach to managing a variety of complex symptoms these influencing attributes are a valuable addition to the book, especially in light of the COVID-19 pandemic.

REFERENCES

Department of Health (DOH). (2012). *The National Health Service and Public Health Service in England: Secretary of State's annual report 2011/2012*. London: The Stationary Office Limited.

Powel, T. J., & Enright, S. J. (2015). *Anxiety and stress management* (2nd ed.). Routledge London.

ACKNOWLEDGEMENTS

First of all, I would like to thank Dr Christopher Rowland Payne for inviting me to continue his mother's important work, of which I feel very privileged to have had this opportunity and hope that we have done her book justice. In addition, I would like to thank Professor Teena Clouston, Dr Helen Bolderston and Dr Ruth Naylor for all their knowledge, experience and contributions in the development of the fifth edition of this internationally recognised and well-loved handbook. Their work and contributions in their field of expertise have enhanced this edition enormously, of which I am extremely grateful.

Thanks also goes to my daughter Catherine Belchamber, a Psychology student at the time, who reviewed and provided feedback on the chapters to ensure the book met student requirements and was standardised throughout. Thank you with all my heart for the extra time, commitment and support taken out of an already busy student timetable, it was much appreciated, and I hope that you have learnt from this experience.

I would also like to acknowledge my colleagues, students, friends and family and by no means least my husband, all of who have made huge contributions to my thinking over the years and who have helped me shape my view of health, relaxation, physical activity, and mind–body integration, spirituality, humanisation, as well as palliative, supportive and end of life care.

Finally, a big thank you to our publishers who have supported us throughout this process. It has been a pleasure working with you all.

DR CAROLINE BELCHAMBER

TRIBUTE

Rosemary Payne trained as a Physiotherapist at Cardiff Royal Infirmary and obtained a BSc in Pyschology at the University of Wales, Cardiff running classes in the evening for women with menopausal depression. On her retirement, Rosemary chose to write the first edition of Payne's Relaxation Techniques. This book gained worldwide recognition, a bestseller that was published in five languages. Thanks to Rosemary's sheer determination, self-discipline and enormous reserves of energy she went on to update four editions of this book, completing the 4th edition at the grand age of 81. To her credit this book is still referred to in NHS relaxation advice booklets. Rosemary also published articles in a number of journals and newspaers on subjects such as Cardiff tree protection, travel in Burma and car seat design to aid the prevention of back pain.

Rosemary had many attributes, which included strong convictions with a profound and abiding concern for medical ethics, dignity and independence for individuals. She was activey involved in both the Patients Association, Voluntary Euthanasia Society and in the 1980's took part in the Greenham Common Women's Peace Campaign. Rosemary was also an accomplished clay sculpturess and a pianist. She was knowledgeable about art, furniture, architecture and geology and pasionate about gardening, walking and nature. Rosemary was most content when walking on a windy mountain or along a wooded path, but most beloved was her garden – a beautiful place in all seasons. She was graceful, warm, sensitive and enormously considerate. The feelings of others were never far from the front of her mind.

During the second world war, Rosemary was evacuated to Brillantmont International School, Switzerland. Having attended this school myself in the 1980's I sensed a strong connection with Rosemary and it felt right to continue Rosemary's remarkable work. I hope as a reader you will enjoy this new edition.

(Extracts taken from Rosemary Payne's Obituary, The Guardian, 5th August 2015, with kind permission of Dr Chrisopher Rowland Payne)

CONTENTS

Section 1

SETTING THE SCENE

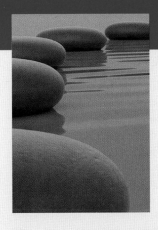

INTRODUCTION

DR CAROLINE BELCHAMBER

CHAPTER CONTENTS

Stress is an important response that occurs when our body is faced with challenging stimuli (stressors), which trigger physiological, behavioural and psychological adjustments to cope with the situation (Esch et al 2002, Cramer et al 2013). When the body becomes unable to adequately cope with the stressor or it is not possible to remove the stressor, the body's coping abilities decline, affecting the person's physical and mental health, as well as impacting their well-being and quality of life; this is known as *chronic stress*. Chronic stress can lead to the development of conditions such as inflammatory bowel disease (Mizrahi et al 2012), heart conditions, circulatory disease, increased blood pressure and pain (Cramer et al 2013). In addition, where there is an inability to cope with social or environmental stressors, depression and anxiety can occur (Andrykowski et al 2008).

Rest is recognized as a basic human need (Maslow 1954), which can be differentiated into physical, mental and spiritual rest – all of which are important in the achievement of a healthy balanced lifestyle (Weinblatt & Avrech-bar 2003). Rest has been described on two levels: (1) a state of relative non-reaction and (2) a state of relaxation (Reber 1992). Relaxation in this case is used in the context of healing or rehabilitation.

Many people find it difficult to relax and feel that time for rest is scarce. This has come about with today's accepted norm of work and leisure activities filling active hours. For many people, leisure activities provide a source of relaxation. As an occupation devoid of deadlines, leisure activities allow the mind to free flow in an unconstrained manner, inducing a sense of inner calm. Leisure activities which give pleasure tend to fall into this category. Some of these require moderate-to-high levels of physiological arousal, such as active non-competitive sport, while others, such as listening to music or watching the waves breaking on a favourite beach, do not. Both, however, are characterized by an absence of stress.

It is when these activities fail to relieve stress that formal relaxation training can play a useful role. Such a training programme can help to lower a stress-induced, high physiological arousal level, thereby protecting the organs from damage. It can also help to make the body's innate healing mechanisms more available. On a cognitive level, relaxation training can calm the mind and allow thinking to become clearer, and on a philosophical level, as practised in some Asian countries, it can bring an increased awareness of the self (Donaghy et al 2008). Therefore relaxation promotes a state of both physiological and mental rest, which can be achieved through relaxation techniques (Mizrahi et al 2012). There are a number of different relaxation techniques available, each of which comprise a method, process or activity that helps the person to relax; reach a state of calm; and reduce levels of anxiety, stress or tension (Dudley-Brown 2002). Thus a general state of relaxation can be induced by using either somatic (relating to the body) or cognitive (relating to the mind) approaches. The relaxation techniques brought together in this unique handbook are categorized into these two areas and are easy to learn requiring few resources.

PURPOSE OF THE BOOK

The book seeks to provide a compendium of different relaxation techniques and to describe them in relation to their underpinning rationales. Their selection has been governed by factors of practicality such as the following, that the method should:

- be easily learned and applied
- not require specialized expertise on the part of the trainer
- not require elaborate equipment
- be portable and capable of being used without attracting attention
- be convenient for use with individuals and small groups
- be suitable for all ages.

It is addressed principally to qualified and novice health care professionals who are not familiar with the topic of relaxation or to those who want to extend their knowledge about relaxation techniques. The book may also be helpful to health care professionals working in palliative, supportive and end-of-life care, as well as family and carers, including people with chronic long-term conditions, such as rheumatoid arthritis, multiple sclerosis, chronic obstructive pulmonary disease, heart failure, cancer or enduring mental health conditions and, more recently, those who are recovering from, and families who are dealing with, the aftermath of COVID-19 who wish to teach themselves relaxation as a personal coping mechanism.

Relaxation training has certain advantages which may make it particularly attractive to some people, such as being non-invasive and giving the person a sense of being in control. Benefits to employers and organizations include its low financial cost, support for mental health and well-being and promoting resilience among staff.

STRUCTURE AND CONTENT

The book commences with an introduction to stress and relaxation and then presents a variety of relaxation methods and techniques, devoting one chapter to each coping strategy. The techniques are drawn from recognized sources and appear in slightly paraphrased versions of the originals with the methods described and organized in a step-by-step manner. Each chapter commences with learning objectives to guide the reader and ends with key points, a case study and a time for reflection to re-inforce new knowledge.

An introduction to the evidence is found at the beginning of each chapter directing the reader to available research, but it is beyond the scope of this book to provide a systematic review of the literature. Where appropriate, the reader is referred to other works such as the narrative review of Kerr (2000) whose paper covered progressive relaxation (see Chapter 5), the Mitchell method (see Chapter 13), massage, the Alexander technique (see Chapter 12), Benson's relaxation response (see Chapter 22) and hatha yoga.

Chapter topics feature somatic and cognitive approaches. The present author writes from a firmly holistic position in keeping with the previous authors, where any kind of division runs counter to their philosophy. However, for descriptive purposes, it was found convenient to separate techniques with a cognitive focus from those with a somatic focus. Such a division is, however, largely artificial.

Somatic approaches presented in this book are:

- breathing awareness
- Jacobson's progressive muscular relaxation
- Bernstein and Borkovec's modified version
- Everly and Rosenfeld's passive relaxation
- Madders' release-only
- Öst's applied relaxation
- Poppen's behavioural relaxation training
- the Mitchell method
- the Alexander technique
- differential relaxation
- stretchings
- exercise.

Cognitive approaches presented here are:

- cognitive–behavioural methods
- self-awareness
- imagery

- goal-directed visualization
- autogenic training
- meditation
- Benson's relaxation response
- mindfulness meditation.

A table summarizing the principles of each relaxation technique and suggesting applications for its use may be found in Appendix 1.

The range of methods is not comprehensive because it does not include those methods which require long training periods, such as hypnosis, yoga and advanced autogenics, or elaborate apparatus, such as biofeedback. However, some of these methods are referred to for interest and background information. In the case of yoga, as taught in the West, the component parts of breathing, stretching and meditation may be found in separate chapters.

Most methods described here are claimed to be relaxation techniques. However, there are a few which induce an indirect relaxation effect by increasing the sense of well-being. The Alexander technique is one of these.

There is a difference between methods which create 'deep' relaxation and those which create 'brief' relaxation (see Chapter 24). *Deep relaxation* refers to procedures which induce an effect of large magnitude and which are carried out in a calm environment with the trainee lying down, for example, progressive relaxation and autogenic training. *Brief relaxation* refers to techniques (often contracted versions of those previously mentioned) which produce immediate effects, and which can be used when the individual is faced with stressful events, the object being the rapid release of excess tension. Thus, whereas deep relaxation refers to a full process of total-body relaxation, brief relaxation applies these procedures in everyday life.

REFERENCES

Andrykowski, M. A., Lykins, E., & Floyd, A. (2008). Psychological health in cancer survivors. *Seminars in Oncology Nursing, 24,* 193–201.

Cramer, H., Lauche, R., Langhorst, J., Dobos, G., & Paul, A. (2013). Characteristics of patients with internal disease who use relaxation techniques as a coping strategy. *Complementary Therapies in Medicine, 21,* 481–486.

Donaghy, M. E. (2008). Cognitive-behavioural approaches in the treatment of alcohol addiction. In M. E. Donaghy, M. Nicol, & E. Davidson (Eds.), *Cognitive-behavioural interventions in physiotherapy and occupational therapy* (pp. 105–120). Edinburgh: Butterworth-Heinemann Elsevier.

Dudley-Brown, S. (2002). Prevention of psychological distress in persons with inflammatory bowel disease. *Issues in Mental Health Nursing, 23,* 403–422.

Esch, T., Stefano, C. B., Fricchione, G. L., & Benson, H. (2002). Stress in cardio-vascular diseases. *Medical Science Monitor, 8*(RA), 93–101.

Kerr, K. M. (2000). Relaxation techniques: a critical review. *Crit. Rev. Phys. Rehabil. Med, 12,* 51–89.

Maslow, A. H. (1954). *Motivation and personality.* New York: Harper & Row.

Mizrahi, M. C., Reicher-Atir, R., Levy, S., Haramati, S., Wengrower, D., Israeli, E., & Goldin, E. (2012). Effects of guided imagery with relaxation training on anxiety and quality of life among patients with inflammatory bowel disease. *Psychology and Health, 27*(12), 1463–1479.

Reber, S. (1992). *Lexicon lemunahey apsychologia [Dictionary of psychology].* Jerusalem: Keter Publication.

Weinblatt, N., & Avrech-bar, M. (2003). Rest: A qualitative exploration of the phenomenon. *Occupational Therapy International, 10*(4), 227–238.

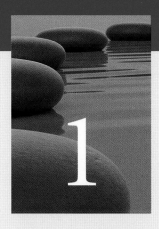

1

STATES OF STRESS

DR CAROLINE BELCHAMBER

LEARNING OBJECTIVES

The aim of this chapter is to draw attention to different states of stress and effects of stressors on the body's physical and mental well-being.

By the end of this chapter you will be able to:

1. Understand stress processes and mechanisms

2. Recognize symptoms and theories of stress

3. Identify ways of measuring stress

4. Differentiate sources of stress

5. Discern personality types and clinical anxiety

This chapter will conclude with key points and time for reflection, providing learning opportunities through case studies.

INTRODUCTION TO STRESS

Stress is described as a state where any stressor (demand our environment makes on us) upsets the natural equilibrium of the body (Mizrahi et al 2012). Stress is experienced when the perceived demands on our environment are greater than the perceived ability to cope. Stress is a commonly experienced emotion closely associated with physical symptoms such as increased heart rate, increased rate of breathing, and sweating. When we are stressed we are likely to experience feelings of anxiety, worry and fear. These are normal emotions (acute stress). However, when stress in our everyday lives becomes unrelenting (chronic stress), it can cause a wide range of illnesses and emotional disturbances (Mizrahi et al 2012) leading to ill health and absenteeism from work. In Europe, stress is now the most common cause of absenteeism, with stress-related illnesses costing Europe €240 billion per year (EASHW 2014).

INTRODUCTION TO EVIDENCE

The term *stress* was first described by Hans Selye in 1936. He viewed stress as the body's attempt to respond by adapting to a stressor. In the short term this was seen as a protective mechanism by the body to manage an acute stressor. In the long term, when a stressor persisted and became chronic, serious damage could occur to the body, causing stress-related illnesses. Hans Selye, whose concern was centred on physiological aspects, viewed stress as the non-specific response of the body to any demand made on it. (By non-specific, he meant that the same response would occur irrespective of the nature of the stimulus.) Forty years later, the psychologists Cox and Mackay (1976) defined stress as 'a perceptual phenomenon arising from a comparison between the demand on the person and their ability to cope. An imbalance gives rise to the experience of stress and to the stress response'. The emphasis here is on the individual's perceptions, on the subjective nature of stress and on its psychological dimension. Hans Selye had ignored the role of psychological processes (Cox 1978).

The topic of stress was developed further by Lazarus and Folkman (1984), who defined stress as an imbalance between the demands of the situation and the self-perceived resources of the individual. The imbalance gives people a subjective feeling of stress because they feel they do not have the capacity to control the demands made on them.

THEORIES OF STRESS

Hans Selye (1950) described the first theory of stress, the General Adaptation Syndrome, which identified a three-stage process that the body goes through to adapt to a stressor (Fig. 1.1):

1. *Alarm reaction:* Exposure to the stressor results in the release of hormones and chemicals whose purpose is to create appropriate physiological changes in preparation for the fight or flight response. The alarm reaction is cancelled as soon as the stressor is withdrawn.
2. *Resistance:* If exposure to the stressor persists, the body will attempt to adapt by developing a resistance to the stressor, which serves it well at the time. Such resistance, however, takes a toll on

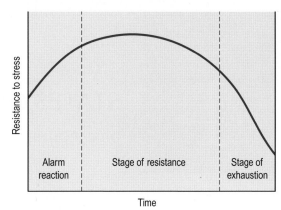

Fig. 1.1 ■ The general adaptation syndrome.

the organism's resources and may cause damage to the heart and blood vessels. Over time, as the stressor becomes chronic, the parasympathetic nervous system is activated to conserve energy for the longer term. This takes the body into the final stage.

3. *Exhaustion:* As the body's resources become depleted, the body's adaptation to the chronic stressor starts to fail and a stage of exhaustion takes over. Sympathetic arousal that was triggered in the alarm reaction is re-experienced by the individual, with sweating and increased blood pressure and heart rate. This may cause damage to the adrenal glands and compromise the immune system, leading to stress-related illness or, as Selye described, the 'disease of adaptation', which included depression, coronary heart disease and raised blood pressure.

Cox and Mackay (1976) described an alternative theory of stress called the Psychological Model of Occupational Stress. This model introduces the idea of perceived coping powers as a factor governing the resulting stress. If an individual perceives his or her ability to cope as weak and sees environmental demands as heavy, the level of stress the individual experiences will be high. If the person's self-perceived coping powers are strong, then those same demands may be readily tolerated and the level of stress experienced will be comparatively low. The environmental demands may, however, be too low, so low that stress arises from boredom. When the individual's perception of environmental demand is matched by his or her perceived coping ability, a state of balance can be said to exist.

It is clearly desirable for the individual to operate in situations where demands and coping skills are balanced. Establishing and maintaining that balance may involve regulating the person's exposure to the stressor. Alternatively individuals could reduce their anxiety levels and increase their coping ability.

This is a model which allows for variation among individuals, as well as for changing perceptions over time in the same person. The ideas enshrined in it have led to the concept of the 'human performance curve', which is based on the relationship between demands placed on the individual and his or her coping ability (Fig. 1.2). Moderate levels of demand are associated with efficient performance. When demands are perceived as too heavy, the overtaxed individual begins to experience fatigue; when they are too low, boredom results from understimulation. Distress is experienced in both events (Looker & Gregson 1991).

At the top of the curve is the zone of high performance. Here individuals operate at levels of demand which match their coping skills. Daily variation may result in one slightly outweighing the other: for example, sometimes they feel that they have more capacity than they are being called on to use, which gives them a feeling of confidence and control; at other times, they may feel that environmental demands are drawing on untapped inner resources, creating the rewarding experience of being pleasantly stretched. These feelings are collectively referred to as 'eustress' or 'good' stress.

Lower down the curve, on either side, the individual's performance gradually declines as the curve runs through transition zones of moderate stress and, ultimately, into zones of deep distress.

Thus, although distress erodes the person's quality of life, eustress enhances it, with the right amount of stress having a positive immune-enhancing effect and benefit to the individual's immunity (Dhabhar 2018). Thus working at levels of arousal that feel comfortable promotes not only the efficiency of the individual's output, but also his or her mental well-being.

Most stress results from a sense of perceived harm or a sense of threat; however, if the individual feels confident to handle the situation, the conditions which give rise to it will appear more as a challenge than as a threat.

SYMPTOMS OF STRESS

Acute stress is associated with physiological symptoms characteristic of sympathetic nervous system activity. These symptoms relate to the fight or flight response (later in this chapter) and are summarized here, together with the psychological symptoms of stress, both the subjective (how a person feels) and the behavioural (how a person acts), although there is considerable overlap in these areas. Chronic stress occurs when the fight or flight response becomes constant (later in this chapter). The physiological components of the response can then cause or exacerbate illness and heighten psychological symptoms (Mizrahi et al 2012).

The symptoms vary among individuals because of the differing sensitivities of organs to the experience of stress.

Physiological Symptoms

Physiological symptoms include the following:

- Raised heart rate
- Increased blood pressure
- Sweating
- Indigestion, constipation, diarrhoea
- Raised blood coagulation rate
- Increased ventilation
- Raised blood glucose level

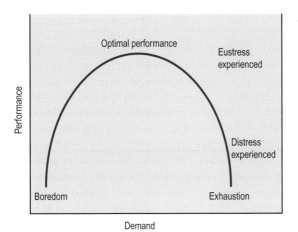

Fig. 1.2 ■ Human performance curve.

Subjective Symptoms

Subjective symptoms include the following:

- Tiredness and/or difficulty in sleeping
- Muscle tension, particularly in neck and shoulder muscles
- Palpitations
- Headache
- Difficulty in concentrating and a tendency to worry
- Impatience; feeling irritable and easily roused to anger

Behavioural Symptoms

Behavioural symptoms include the following:

- Increased consumption of alcohol, tobacco, food, etc.
- Loss of appetite or excessive eating
- Restlessness
- Loss of sexual interest
- A tendency to experience accidents

Chronic Symptoms

Chronic symptoms include the following:

- Distress
- Anxiety
- Depression
- Reduced quality of life and well-being

Anxiety can refer either to an emotional state or to a personality disposition (see Personality Types). The first is called 'state' anxiety, and the second is 'trait' anxiety. State anxiety occurs as a temporary reaction to an event perceived as adverse or threatening; it refers to the experience of apprehension in a precise moment. Such feelings are normal reactions to life circumstances and are often accompanied by worry and physical symptoms such as dry mouth, raised heart rate, sweating and butterflies in the stomach. Trait anxiety, by contrast, is characterized by the individual's tendency to view all neutral events as potentially stressful and to experience state anxiety as a response to them

(Spielberger 1980). State anxiety tends to accompany most disorders and is a natural concomitant of adverse conditions.

MEASURING STRESS

A physiological assessment of stress includes such measurements as heart rate, blood pressure, respiratory rate and skin conductance. Psychological as well as physiological methods have been devised to measure stress. One which has had some influence is the Social Readjustment Rating Scale (SRRS) of Holmes and Rahe (1967). These researchers compiled a table of life events ranging from minor violations of the law to the death of a spouse, rating each one in terms of the mental readjustment it demanded. A high score in any one year was associated with a high risk of developing a stress-related illness. But the SRRS has its critics: Whereas Holmes and Rahe (1967) had proposed that any change in a person's circumstances, positive or negative, contributed to the risk, other researchers (Dohrenwend 2006, Lazarus et al 1980) argued that positive experiences could moderate the effects of negative life events, making them less damaging to the immune system. For example, a broken bone is easier to tolerate if it coincides with the announcement of good exam results.

Another point of discussion raised by the SRRS is whether the stress caused by a series of minor adverse events is more harmful than one major adverse event. Lazarus and colleagues (1980) believe it can be and devised a tool for measuring small, day-to-day problems, calling it the Hassles and Uplifts Scale (Kanner et al 1981). However, after a number of years of research on the Hassles and Uplifts Scale some limitations were identified; for instance, the meaning that an event has for the individual needs to be considered – moving house, for example, can be a pleasant form of stress if you choose to move but a source of deep distress if you are forced to do so. Our interpretation of an event thus determines the nature and intensity of our response (Lazarus 1991). This has led to the scale being updated to the Hassles and Uplifts Questionnaire (DeLongis et al 1988). Further research supported the notion that a major crisis perceived to be solvable and of short-term duration is less harmful than a long-lasting succession of small hassles which the individual feels unable to control (Stevens & Price 2016). In spite of these and other criticisms, the SRRS has been highly influential as a tool for measuring the effects of stress. Changing social values have, however, rendered some of the ratings out of date and created a need for additional items. As a result, the original scale was succeeded by a revised instrument, the Recent Life Changes Questionnaire (Rahe 1975), which has itself been rescaled (Miller & Rahe 1997) (see Appendix 3). It is acknowledged that there are other measures of life events which have been used in more recent research (Artani et al 2017, Picardi et al 2005). However, Miller and Rahe (1997) will be described because of its historical relevance and its accessibility.

In the previously described measures, stress is represented in the form of life events. This is an objective way of viewing stress. Subjective measures also are in common use and consist of questionnaires which have been standardized for validity and reliability. Aspects of mood are itemized and the individual asked to tick the box which best reflects how they are feeling (see Chapter 28).

SOURCES OF STRESS

Stress can arise from a multitude of sources. Broadly speaking, these sources can be categorized as those in the environment and those within the individual (Powell & Enright 2015).

External Stressors

The Work Environment

The work environment is thought to be the main predictor of different health outcomes. The greatest threat to employee well-being is the combination of high job demands and low job control (Giorigi et al 2015).

The individual may be suffering from work overload in the form of unrealistic deadlines, long hours or a feeling that the job is beyond their competence. On the other hand, the job may lack stimulation, causing the person to feel bored, or it may lack opportunity to demonstrate his or her ability. There may be uncertainty as to the boundaries of the person's responsibility, and the work objectives may be inadequately defined. As a consequence the person may be obliged to move to other departments or to other geographical locations. In addition, being declared redundant or forced to retire earlier than planned can cause stress in the working environment (Wickramasinghe 2010). On the other hand, relationships with colleagues and superiors may be strained, with workplace bullying and social exclusion affecting the person's health and well-being over a long period (Einarsen et al 2011). Therefore a supportive social environment at work is an important factor in reducing psychological distress (Giorigi et al 2015).

The Social Environment

Social ties seem to play a large part in determining the way in which we cope with negative events. These ties include partners, relatives, friends and acquaintances and they act as a buffer between the event itself and the person's reaction to it. Among the many researchers to demonstrate this association are Ifeagwazi (2008), who showed the protective and therapeutic value of having a confidante, and in more recent research, Cohen et al 2015, who demonstrated that stress-related illnesses are less likely to occur among people with strong social support, especially where emotional support is provided through hugs – a behavioural sign of emotional support. Social and cultural issues such as isolation, poverty and disability are considered to be major causes of mental stress, as well as chemical stressors, which include additives in food and drink and pollutants in the air and water. These stressors can have an effect on the person's genes, and the individuals' responses to these stressors are linked to their personality type, which is partly under genetic control (Goldberg & Goodyer 2005).

Internal Stressors

Personality Types

Research exploring links between personality, stress and illness commenced in the 1950s. In 1974, Friedman and Rosenman described a personality type particularly associated with coronary heart disease. This type was characterized by a tendency for an individual to drive themselves to achieve goals one after another, to create a programme filled with deadlines and to perform activities in a competitive manner with a constant need for recognition.

People who displayed these tendencies were referred to as 'type A' personalities, while those with the opposite characteristics were described as 'type B' and were found to be almost immune to coronary heart disease. Type A characteristics are seen as negative in so far as they may lead to stress-related illness. However, they also lead to high achievement, which is to be valued. Cooper (1981) suggests emphasizing the need to *manage* type A behaviour rather than extinguish it. This may mean slowing down, resetting goals, regularly taking 5 minutes off and recording the occasions when this is performed. It may also mean seeking alternative ways of gaining rewards.

Kobasa (1982) described what he called the 'hardy' personality. Such people were seen as being relatively resistant to stress by virtue of possessing three qualities: a sense of control over their life; a feeling of being committed to their work, hobby or family; and a sense of challenge in which change was viewed as an opportunity to develop themselves, rather than as a threat to their equilibrium. People who do not possess these qualities are more likely to suffer from stress-related illness than those who do.

Temoshok (1987) described a third personality type, 'type C' or 'people pleasers', who strive to be compliant. These people are often seen as passive, self-sacrificing, with no end of patience, avoiding conflict at all costs. This extreme repression of emotion has been linked with the development of cancer. Dattore and colleagues (1980) also showed a link between type C personalities with cancer, and also depression. On the scale used by the researchers to measure repression of emotions and symptoms of depression the group without a diagnosis of cancer did not repress their emotions and were unlikely to acknowledge they were depressed, whereas the group with cancer reported significantly greater emotional repression and symptoms of depression.

Personality traits are, however, not set in stone. The genetic predispositions we are born with are subject to external influences, particularly in early life, resulting in some traits being emphasized while others are diminished (Cassidy 1999, Goldberg & Goodyer 2005). The findings from longitudinal research studies suggest that by early adulthood personality traits are more or less fixed (Matthews et al 2003). However, others would argue that because our actions are governed less by trait than by contingency (Dawes 2009), the genetic element is less influential than it appears. Stress levels and associated behaviour in the individual can vary, which suggests a view of personality as a shifting entity (Dunlop 2015). The inability always to predict behaviour from personality traits has led to the development of theories around personal causation and self-confidence. These approaches include how effective we feel when predicting achievement in day-to-day activities and how much control we feel we have over our lives.

Self-Efficacy

Self-efficacy is the term used to describe a person's sense of ability to deal with events and situations in their life. It is therefore concerned with confidence. Self-efficacy is the *belief* that a particular task can be successfully achieved. This leads into the area of expectation (Bandura 1977, 1986, Lopez & Snyder 2012).

Bandura (1986) suggests that people's beliefs lead to expectations, which can be classified in two ways: one is the expectation of efficacy and the other is the expectation of outcome. The first relates to the level of confidence people have in being able to carry out a task successfully – that is, whether they think they have the ability; the second concerns beliefs which allow the prediction of results – that is, whether people think their efforts will succeed. Self-efficacy is enhanced by the successful outcome of target behaviours. Increases in self-efficacy, in their turn, make it more likely that future outcomes will be successful because high levels of self-efficacy are related to self-perceptions of control and optimism. When we are successful, we build a sense of personal mastery, which gives us a feeling of being in control of our lives. Being persuaded by other people that we can cope and succeed in difficult circumstances helps intensify this feeling of mastery.

People with low levels of confidence in predicting success can be helped to develop these qualities in three ways by: (1) modelling themselves on others who are successful, (2) the persuasive words of others, and (3) emphasizing any success they may have had in the past.

Self-efficacy, as a concept, originated in the clinical setting as a way of modifying a person's reactions to adverse events, such as those which lead to phobias

(Bandura 1977, 1986, 1997). It has since proved to be a very powerful determinant of health-related behaviour (Schwartzer 1992), known as health locus of control, which is key to self-management of chronic long-term conditions (Bjørkløf et al 2016, Cramer et al 2013).

Health Locus of Control

Health locus of control is a phrase which describes health behaviour as a function of control beliefs, which can be categorized as either internal (health depends on the person's attributes or behaviour) or external (health depends on the behaviour of other people – e.g., fate or luck) (Bjørkløf et al 2016, Cramer et al 2013).

Health locus of control is a feature which has been studied in various contexts, one of which is stress, where low vulnerability to stress seems to be related to internal locus and high vulnerability to external locus. Thus the more influence people believe they have over their environment, the less likely they are to experience stress. Therefore the person's perception of what is stressful is key to his or her overall health and well-being.

Perception of Stress

Each person is thought to perceive stress in a different way; for example, what is deemed a negative stressful event (a threat) to one person may be seen as a positive stressful event (challenge) to another (Roesch et al 2002). Beck (1984) referred to stressors within the person, such as the tendency to interpret events in a consistently negative way. Ellis (1962) also described the maladaptive effect of holding unrealistic belief systems – for instance, believing one has to be right every time to be a worthwhile person (Chapter 2). Dryden (1994) acknowledged that key features of Ellis' original ideas remain current, such as the link among the process of knowing, expression of feelings and behaviour, but adds the dimension of healthy and unhealthy negative emotions. Some of these maladaptive styles include the following:

- Having unclear or unrealistic goals, leading to wasted effort and disappointment
- Failing to make decisions: Unmade decisions can so preoccupy individuals that they cannot get on with their life. The unresolved matter continues

to claim their attention and eventually wears them out
- Bottling up emotions: Anxiety and anger are examples of emotions that people often keep to themselves, allowing the feelings to grow out of proportion
- Having low self-esteem: a feeling that one lacks the rights that are accorded to others. Such people may allow themselves to be overruled on every side.

These unhealthy negative emotions can affect the person's physical and mental health and consequently their overall health and well-being (Roesch et al 2002), such as in clinical anxiety.

CLINICAL ANXIETY

Commonly experienced feelings of stress and anxiety are different from clinically recognized anxiety disorders, in which the anxiety is experienced at greater intensity and for longer duration. Unlike the fleeting periods of anxiety experienced in everyday life, clinical anxiety disorders may be profoundly disabling. If left undiagnosed and untreated, they tend to persist and may become chronic.

The American Psychiatric Association (APA 2013) has described a number of these anxiety disorders, descriptions which remain in use today.

- *Specific phobia*: Significant and persistent anxiety in relation to a specific object or situation. Examples include spiders, storms, blood, injection, injury, tunnels and lifts. Contact leads to an immediate anxiety reaction. The person may rationalize that the fear is greater than it should be but feels powerless to avert the reaction. Situations are avoided for fear of further exposure.
- *Social phobia*: also known as social anxiety. The main feature is fear of one or more social situations where the individual worries that she will act in a way that is judged negatively by those around.
- *Generalized anxiety disorder*: Main features here are significant worry and anxiety on most days, the worries covering a range of events and

activities. The person is likely to experience physical symptoms such as muscle tension, sleep disruption and poor concentration.

- *Panic disorder*: Panic attacks involve an experience of intense fear which includes a range of symptoms such as palpitations, sweating, trembling, chest pain, nausea and fear of losing control. People with this condition experience these symptoms frequently and they worry about having further attacks. Panic disorder may also be associated with agoraphobia and a fear of enclosed spaces such as buses, trains and shops. Typically these situations are avoided.

- *Obsessive compulsive disorder (OCD)*: This disorder consists of unwanted thoughts and images which intrude into a person's everyday life. The most commonly experienced obsessions revolve around fears of contamination, with associated compulsions of frequent handwashing or bathing. Fears about personal safety are also common, with associated compulsions of repeated checking of electrical appliances, door locking, and so on. The compulsive behaviour reduces the anxiety for a short time but has to be repeated.

- *Post-traumatic stress disorder (PTSD)*: Here the person has been exposed to a traumatic event which may be relived over and over again. Intrusive images and upsetting dreams are features of the condition. In an attempt to protect himself or herself, the individual will try and avoid any triggers such as places, thoughts, feelings and conversations relating to the event. Associated symptoms include feeling emotionally distant from others, disturbed sleep, irritability, difficulty concentrating, hypervigilance and heightened startle response.

One of the features of clinical anxiety disorders is co-morbidity with other conditions. Co-occurring depression (Knyazev et al 2016) affects as many as one in six adults (McManus et al 2016), and PTSD is often co-occurring with depression (Rytwinski et al 2013) and substance misuse (Debdell et al 2014). Personality disorders also co-occur with anxiety disorders

(Grant et al 2005). It is important, therefore, for health care professionals to recognize when anxiety symptoms reach the level of clinical disorder, and to make the appropriate referral.

MANAGING STRESS

Because stress is an acknowledged component of many conditions, health care professionals are increasingly being asked to help alleviate it. One way to achieve this is through relaxation techniques, which will be discussed in Chapter 2. This does not mean that relaxation techniques should, in any sense, be seen as a substitute for medical help. Rather, they can be seen as useful adjuncts to other treatments. They also have a preventive role.

KEY POINTS

1. Stress is an imbalance between the demands of the situation and the perceived resources of the person.
2. Stress can arise externally from the environment, in both work and social situations, or internally within the person as a function of their personality or behaviour.
3. The force of the stressor can be ameliorated by social support, which acts as a buffer.

Reflection

Describe your experience(s) of stress.
How did you react to the stressor(s)?
Why did you react / respond in that way?
What did you learn from this / these experience(s)?
What coping mechanism(s) did you put in place? Did they work?
What is your future action plan?

CASE STUDY LEARNING OPPORTUNITIES

The key points and reflection provide the background and knowledge required in relation to the case studies; Matthew (Case Study 1) and Angela (Case Study 2) to help deepen understanding of how stress can affect physical and mental well-being.

CASE STUDY 1

Tension Headache: *Introduction to Matthew*

Matthew works in an office, where he spends most of his time seated at a computer. He likes his job and sets high standards for himself – sometimes impossibly high. He has been there for 15 years and has received promotion at regular intervals. He is married to Deborah, who works in the local supermarket, and they have two children. Matthew's hobbies are building model aircraft and growing orchids; he and Deborah are also enthusiastic ballroom dancers. In the last year or two, however, he has increasingly suffered from discomfort in his neck, and from headaches which make his job difficult and interfere with his ballroom dancing events. The headaches seem to get worse as the day progresses. At first he thought they were brought on by cigarette smoke, but a ban on smoking has been imposed and the headaches have persisted. Sometimes things go wrong in the office, such as people taking advantage of his dedication to the work, and this makes the headaches worse. Also, the newly commissioned seating arrangements at work are not as comfortable as the old ones and seem to aggravate the pain in his neck, which spreads to his shoulders. He has been arriving home exhausted and has to lie down. He worries about the cause; he also worries about his future in the job.

His friends tell him he should consult his general practitioner (GP), so eventually he does, but the GP can find nothing organically wrong. Matthew is advised to start a course of relaxation training because the headaches might be associated with stress. He accepts this diagnosis – after all, many people suffer from stress, nothing to be ashamed of.

CASE STUDY 2

Panic Disorder and Agoraphobia: *Introduction to Angela*

Angela is a professional carer who has looked after a succession of disabled people in the 20 years she has been in the job. She has enjoyed her work most of the time. It took her out and about and she always managed to find herself with people who appreciated her visits. She found the job emotionally rewarding. Bill, her husband, an insurance agent, would pick her up after work in his car and they would drive home together. Bill would settle down to read his paper while she prepared the evening meal. Eighteen months ago, however, Bill died. Angela was devastated. Her life crumbled. No Bill at home. No lifts after work. The whole structure of her life collapsed. At 52 she was left high and dry, with apparently nothing to live for.

Everything seemed to be going wrong. Her job evaporated. Her mortgage payments fell behind. Things rose to crisis point one day when, selecting fruit in her supermarket, she accidentally knocked over a tall stand of tomatoes. She abandoned her trolley and rushed out of the shop.

Since that occasion she has not been back and has become increasingly tied to the house. Not eating properly, she began to feel physically ill. Pressure from friends, neighbours and relatives drove her to look for treatment and she was given antidepressants. The medication made her feel better but only for as long as she took it. If she stopped, her symptoms returned, but she did not want to take antidepressants forever.

ACTIVITY

For each of the case studies:

1. List the stress factors that are contributing to the condition.
2. Write down the impact stress is having from a physical perspective.
3. Write down the impact stress is having from a psychological perspective.
4. Write down the impact stress is having from an emotional perspective.
5. Consider how these impacts are affecting overall quality of life.

Chapter 2 will focus on the state of relaxation and how this may help both Matthew and Angela.

REFERENCES

American Psychiatric Association (APA) (2013). *Diagnostic and statistical manual for mental disorders* (5th edn). DMS-5, Washington, DC 20024-2812.

Artani, A., Bhamani, S., Azam, I., AbdulSultan, M., Khoja, A., & Kamal, A. K. (2017). Adaptation of the Recent Life Changes Questionnaire (RLCQ) to measure stressful life events in adults residing in an urban megapolis in Pakistan. *BMC Psychiatry*, 17, 169.

Bandura, A. (1977). Self-efficacy: Toward a unifying theory of behavioral change. *Psychological Review*, 84(2), 191–215.

Bandura, A. (1986). *Social foundations of thought and action: A social cognitive theory*. Englewood Cliffs, NY: Prentice-Hall.

Bandura, A. (1997). *Self-efficacy: The exercise of control*. San Francisco, CA: WH Freeman.

Beck, A. T. (1984). Cognitive approaches to stress management. In R. L. Woolfolk, & P. M. Lehrer (Eds.), *Principles and practice of stress management*. New York: Guilford Press.

Bjørkløf, G. H., Engedala, K., Selbæka, G., Maiaf, D. B., Coutinhof, E. S. F., & Helvika, A. (2016). Locus of control and coping strategies in older persons with and without depression. *Aging and Mental Health*, 20(8), 831–839.

Cassidy, T. (1999). *Stress, cognition and health*. London: Routledge.

Cohen, S., Janicki-Deverts, D., Turner, R. B., & Doyle, W. J. (2015). Does hugging people provide stress-buffering social support? A study of susceptibility to upper respiratory infection and illness. *Psychological Science*, 26(2), 135–147.

Cooper, C. L. (1981). *The stress check*. Hoboken, NJ: Prentice-Hall.

Cox, T. (1978). *Stress*. London: Macmillan.

Cox, T., & Mackay, C. J. (1976). *A psychological model of occupational stress. Paper presented to: Medical Research Council* London: Mental Health in Industry.

Cramer, H., Lauche, R., Langhorst, J., Dobos, G., & Paul, A. (2013). Characteristics of patients with internal diseases who use relaxation techniques as a coping strategy. *Complementary Therapies in Medicine*, 21, 481–486.

Dattore, P. J., Shontz, F. C., & Coyne, L. (1980). Premorbid personality differentiation of cancer and noncancer groups: A test of the hypothesis of cancer proneness. *Journal of Consulting and Clinical Psychology*, 48, 388–394.

Dawes, R. M. (2009). *House of cards: Psychology and psychotherapy built on myth*. New York: Free Press.

Debdell, F., Fear, N. T., Head, M., et al. (2014). A systematic review of the comorbidity between PTSD and alcohol misuse. *Social Psychiatry and Psychiatric Epidemiology*, 49, 1401–1425.

DeLongis, A., Folkman, S., & Lazarus, R. S. (1988). The impact of daily stress on health and mood: Psychological and social resources as mediators. *Journal of Personality and Social Psychology*, 54(3), 486–495.

Dhabhar, F. S. (2018). The short-term stress response – mother nature's mechanism for enhancing protection and performance under conditions of threat, challenge and opportunity. *Frontiers in Neuroendocrinology*, 49, 175–192.

Dohrenwend, B. (2006). Inventorying stressful life events as risk factors for psychopathology: Toward resolution of the problem of intracategory variability. *Psychological Bulletin*, 132(3), 477–495.

Dryden, W. (1994). Reason and emotion in psychotherapy: Thirty years on. *Journal of Rational-Emotive and Cognitive-Behavior Therapy*, 12(2), 83–99.

Dunlop, W. L. (2015). Contextualized personality, beyond traits. *European Journal of Personality*, 29(3), 310–325.

Einarsen, S., Hoel, H., Zapf, D., & Cooper, C. L. (2011). *Bullying and harassment in the workplace: Development in theory, research and practice* (2nd ed.). London: CRC Press.

Ellis, A. (1962). *Reason and emotion in psychotherapy*. New York: Lyle Stuart.

European Agency for Safety and Health at Work (EASHW). (2014). *Calculating the Cost of Work-Related Stress and Psychosocial Risks: European Risk Observatory Literature Review*. Bilbao, Spain: European Agency for Safety and Health at Work.

Friedman, M., & Rosenman, R. H. (1974). *Type A behaviour and your heart*. New York: Knopf.

Giorigi, G., Shoss, M. K., & Perez-Leon, J. (2015). M. Going beyond workplace stressors: Economic crisis and perceived employability in relation to psychological distress and job dissatisfaction. *Int J Stress Manage*, 22(2), 137–158.

Goldberg, D., & Goodyer, I. (2005). *The origins and course of common mental disorders*. London: Routledge.

Grant, B. F., Hasin, D. S., Stinson, F. S., et al. (2005). Co-occurrence of 12-month mood and anxiety disorders and personality disorders in the U.S.: Results from the National Epidemiologic Survey on Alcohol and Related Conditions. *Journal of Psychiatric Research*, 205(46), 1–5.

Holmes, T. H., & Rahe, R. H. (1967). The social readjustment rating scale. *Journal of Psychosomatic Research*, 11, 213–218.

Ifeagwazi, C. M. (2008). Self-disclosure: A therapeutic process. *Interdisciplinary Journal of Communication Studies*, 8, 231–238.

Kanner, A. D., Coyne, J. C., Schaefer, C., & Lazarus, R. S. (1981). Comparison of two modes of stress management: Daily hassles and uplifts versus major life events. *Journal of Behavioral Medicine*, 4, 1–3.

Kobasa, S. C. (1982). The hardy personality. In G. Sanders, & J. Suls (Eds.), *The Social Psychology of Health and Illness*. New Jersey: Lawrence Erlbaum.

Knyazev, G., Savostyanov, A., Bocharov, A., & Rimareva, J. (2016). Anxiety, depression and oscillatory dynamics in a social interaction model. *Brain Research*, 1644, 62–69.

Lazarus, R. S., Cohen, J. B., Folkman, S., Kanner, A., & Schaefer, C. (1980). Psychological stress and adaptation: Some unresolved issues. In H. Selye (Ed.), *Selye's guide to stress research* (pp. 90–117). (vol. 1). New York: Van Nostrand Reinhold.

Lazarus, R. S., & Folkman, S. (1984). *Stress, appraisal and coping*. New York: Springer.

Lazarus, R. S. (1991). Cognition and motivation in emotion. *American Psychology*, 46, 352–367.

Looker, T., & Gregson, O. (1991). *Stresswise: A practical guide for dealing with stress* (2nd ed.). London: Hodder and Stoughton.

Maddux, J. E. (2012). Self-efficacy: The power of believing you can. In S. Lopez, & C. R. Snyder (Eds.), *The Oxford handbook of positive psychology* (2nd ed.). Oxford: Oxford University Press.

Matthews, G., Deary, I. J., & Whiteman, M. C. (2003). *Personality traits* (2nd ed.). Cambridge, UK: Cambridge University Press.

McManus, S., Bebbington, P., Jenkins, R., & Brugha, T. (Eds.). (2016). *Mental health and wellbeing in England: Adult psychiatric morbidity survey 2014*. Leeds, UK: NHS Digital.

Miller, M. A., & Rahe, R. H. (1997). Life changes scaling for the 1990s. *Journal of Psychosomatic Research*, *43*(3), 279–292.

Mizrahi, M. C., Reicher-Atir, R., Levy, S., et al. (2012). Effects of guided imagery with relaxation training on anxiety and quality of life among patients with inflammatory bowel disease. *Psychology & Health*, *27*(12), 1463–1479.

Picardi, A., Mazzotti, E., Gaetano, P., et al. (2005). Stress, social support, emotional regulation and exacerbation of diffuse plaque psoriasis. *Psychosomatics*, *46*, 556–564.

Powell, T. J., & Enright, S. J. (2015). *Anxiety and stress management*. London: Routledge, Taylor and Francis.

Rahe, R. H. (1975). Epidemiological studies of life change and illness. *The International Journal of Psychiatry in Medicine*, *6*, 133–146.

Selye, H. (1950). Stress and the general adaptation syndrome (GAS). *British Medical Journal*, *17*, 1383–1392.

Roesch, S. C., Wiener, B., & Vaughn, A. A. (2002). Cognitive approaches to stress and coping. *Current Opinions in Psychiatry*, *15*(6), 627–632.

Rytwinski, N. K., Scur, M. D., Feeny, N. C., & Youngstrom, E. A. (2013). The co-occurrence of major depressive disorder among individuals with posttraumatic stress disorder: A meta-analysis. *Journal of Traumatic Stress*, *26*, 299–309.

Schwartzer, R. (1992). Self-efficacy in the adoption and maintenance of health behaviours: Theoretical approaches and a new model. In R. Schwartzer (Ed.), *Self-efficacy: Thought control of action* (pp. 217–243). Washington, DC: Hemisphere.

Spielberger, C. D. (1980). *Manual for the state–trait anxiety inventory*. Palo Alto, CA: Consulting Psychologists Press.

Stevens, A., & Price, J. (2016). *Evolutionary psychiatry: A new beginning*. London: Routledge.

Temoshok, L. (1987). Personality, coping style, emotion and cancer: Towards an integrative model. *Cancer Surveys*, *6*(3), 545–567.

Wickramasinghe, V. (2010). Work-related dimensions and job stress: The moderating effect of coping strategies. *Stress and Health*, *26*, 417–429.

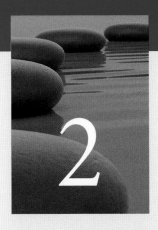

2 THE STATE OF RELAXATION

DR CAROLINE BELCHAMBER

CHAPTER CONTENTS

LEARNING OBJECTIVES

The aim of this chapter is to draw attention to the state of relaxation and its effect on the body both physically and mentally.

By the end of this chapter you will be able to:

1. Understand the meaning of relaxation
2. Appreciate the evidence that underpins relaxation techniques
3. Understand relaxation processes and mechanisms
4. Identify different relaxation techniques
5. Recognize various coping strategies
6. Discern the effect relaxation techniques have on the body and mind

This chapter will conclude with key points and time for reflection, providing learning opportunities through case studies.

INTRODUCTION TO RELAXATION

Relaxation suggests a state of ease which is characterized by limited body tension and freedom from unnecessary worries and fears. It is associated with feelings of warmth and tranquillity and a sense of being at peace with oneself. Thus the state of relaxation involves a complex interplay of psychological and physiological systems which include the nerves, muscles and major organs such as the heart, lungs, kidneys, liver and spleen.

INTRODUCTION TO EVIDENCE

Relaxation techniques described in this book are known as mind–body approaches and include techniques such as muscle relaxation, meditation and imagery. Measurement in this field has only developed in the last few decades, accounting for a relatively small research base, its development having possibly been delayed by the centuries-old dominance of the medical model. However, in recent years this research base has been growing and the evidence points to a variety of physical and psychological health benefits.

Reviewing the literature in 2003, Astin and colleagues found evidence to support the use of mind–body interventions. These included relaxation techniques in a variety of conditions such as cardiac rehabilitation, headache, insomnia, postsurgical pain, incontinence, chronic low back pain, cancer and the symptoms related to its treatment in the form of nausea and vomiting. For these conditions the evidence was considerable. Less robust evidence was found to support the use of mind–body techniques for hypertension and arthritis. The review excluded psychological disorders. On the basis of these results, Astin et al suggested that mind–body interventions be employed as adjuncts to conventional treatment.

A subsequent review in 2005 looked at the effects of relaxation techniques in a broader range of conditions that included psychological difficulties and disorders. It identified benefit in hypertension, cardiac arrhythmias, chronic pain, insomnia, anxiety, mild and moderate depression, premenstrual syndrome and infertility (Stefano & Esch 2005).

Evidence of the effect of relaxation techniques in reducing anxiety is shown in the systematic review of Manzoni et al (2008), in which relaxation techniques were found to be of consistent and significant benefit. State anxiety was shown to be more responsive to treatment than trait anxiety (see Chapter 1 for definitions of state and trait anxiety), but equal benefit was derived from both group and individual sessions. Anxiolytic effects were markedly greater in participants who practised relaxation techniques, and a gradient of benefit related to the intensity of training could be seen.

With regard to depression, relaxation techniques can be seen as a potentially effective treatment. This is the conclusion drawn in a Cochrane review of 15 trials where relaxation techniques were found to be more effective than no treatment or minimal treatment, although less effective than cognitive–behavioural therapy (CBT). However, this latter treatment is not always available, in which case relaxation techniques may be a useful first-line psychological treatment (Jorm et al 2008). Thus important research developments are

taking place and in 2018 a systematic review and meta-analysis was carried out on the effects of relaxation therapy on anxiety disorders. This study provides evidence of the effectiveness of relaxation techniques for people with anxiety disorders and concludes that relaxation techniques can be a useful intervention to reduce negative emotions in people with anxiety disorders (Kim & Kim 2018).

In many cases, relaxation techniques have been evaluated as a component of a larger scheme of stress management. Consequently it is not known what proportion of the success is due to the relaxation technique. Another problem concerns inconsistency in the research findings; it reflects limitations in the methodology such as inadequate allocation, concealment and non-blinded outcome assessment including self-report. Other factors relate to procedural variability – for example, different interpretations of the method. However, not all relaxation techniques have been through the systematic review process and this limits the drawing of conclusions in the field. At this moment, there is insufficient evidence to state that one relaxation technique is better than another.

THEORIES OF RELAXATION

Mechanisms thought to be responsible for bringing about the state of relaxation have been explored, giving rise to a number of theories. Some of these emphasize physiological aspects such as autonomic activity and muscle tension, whereas others focus on psychological elements such as self-perceptions and interpretation of life events. The major theories are briefly described next.

PHYSIOLOGICAL THEORIES

Body systems related to the states of stress and relaxation include both the autonomic and endocrine systems and the skeletal system. An integrated response of all these systems occurs in the presence of stress.

The Autonomic Nervous System and the Endocrine System

Physiological arousal is governed chiefly by the autonomic nervous system. This has two branches: the sympathetic, which increases arousal when the organism is

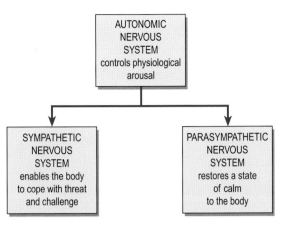

Fig. 2.1 ■ The autonomic nervous system.

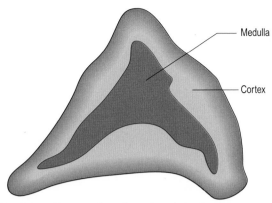

Fig. 2.3 ■ Cross-section of an adrenal gland.

under threat, and the parasympathetic, which restores the body to a resting state. Their actions are involuntary and designed to enable the organism to survive (Fig. 2.1). Organs involved in activating these changes include the adrenal glands, situated above the kidneys (Fig. 2.2). These glands consist of an inner part or medulla and an outer part or cortex (Fig. 2.3). Receiving directions from the hypothalamus via the spinal cord, they release hormones which modify the action of the internal organs in response to environmental stimuli.

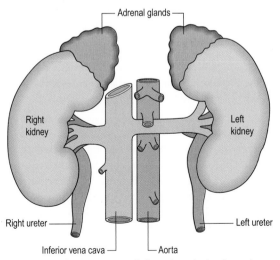

Fig. 2.2 ■ The positions of the adrenal glands and some of their associated structures. (From Wilson 1990 with permission.)

When a situation is perceived as threatening, the brain immediately responds via the spinal ganglia by stimulating the adrenal medulla to release catecholamines such as adrenaline and noradrenaline into the bloodstream. The function of these neurotransmitters is to prepare the organs for action in a manner which has been collectively known as the 'fight or flight' response. It is characterized by an increase in heart rate and a redistribution of the blood from the viscera to the voluntary muscles. Blood pressure and respiratory rate are also increased, alertness and sensory awareness are heightened, muscle tension is raised and there is a mechanism for losing body heat. These factors enable the person to make a physical response. The autonomic systems and their actions are shown in greater detail in Figs 2.4 and 2.5.

Some of the changes which occur as a result of sympathetic stimulation produce noticeable symptoms, for example, faster breathing, stomach cramps and sweating. States such as fear and anger illustrate this and underline the link between emotion and the internal organs. When the changes are pronounced and occur frequently, the organs concerned can become fatigued, and this has given rise to the concept of psychosomatic illness.

Closely associated with the autonomic system but acting in the longer term, the pituitary gland releases the adrenocorticotrophic hormone (ACTH). This stimulates the adrenal cortex to produce substances, the most important of which is cortisol, which helps maintain the fuel supply to the muscles.

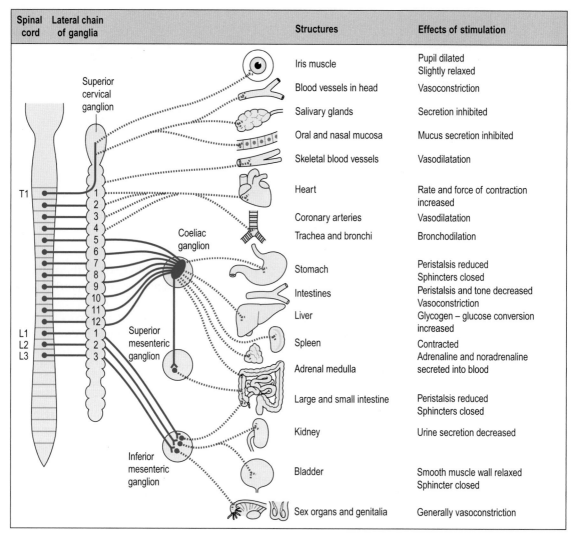

Spinal cord	Lateral chain of ganglia		Structures	Effects of stimulation
			Iris muscle	Pupil dilated Slightly relaxed
			Blood vessels in head	Vasoconstriction
			Salivary glands	Secretion inhibited
			Oral and nasal mucosa	Mucus secretion inhibited
			Skeletal blood vessels	Vasodilatation
			Heart	Rate and force of contraction increased
			Coronary arteries	Vasodilatation
			Trachea and bronchi	Bronchodilation
			Stomach	Peristalsis reduced Sphincters closed
			Intestines	Peristalsis and tone decreased Vasoconstriction
			Liver	Glycogen – glucose conversion increased
			Spleen	Contracted
			Adrenal medulla	Adrenaline and noradrenaline secreted into blood
			Large and small intestine	Peristalsis reduced Sphincters closed
			Kidney	Urine secretion decreased
			Bladder	Smooth muscle wall relaxed Sphincter closed
			Sex organs and genitalia	Generally vasoconstriction

Fig. 2.4 ■ The sympathetic outflow, the main structures supplied and the effects of stimulation. *Solid lines,* preganglionic fibres; *broken lines,* postganglionic fibres. (From Waugh & Grant 2006, Fig. 7.42, p171, with permission.)

In this way it supports the action of the catecholamines (Waugh & Grant 2014). There is also evidence suggesting that the stimulation of normal levels of cortisol enhances the immune system (Yoshiano et al 2015). High levels of cortisol such as those created by prolonged stress or by pharmacological doses are, however, associated with a suppressed immune system.

When faced with acute stress, all these hormones are released (Fig. 2.6).

When the situation of challenge passes and the stress response is no longer needed, neurotransmitters are released to restore balance to the autonomic system. The organs which were previously stimulated now weaken their hold and their actions subside as a state of equilibrium settles on the body metabolism. A shift occurs away from sympathetic dominance towards parasympathetic dominance. If the products of sympathetic activity are not burnt up in physical activity, they lie in the bloodstream, where they can irritate

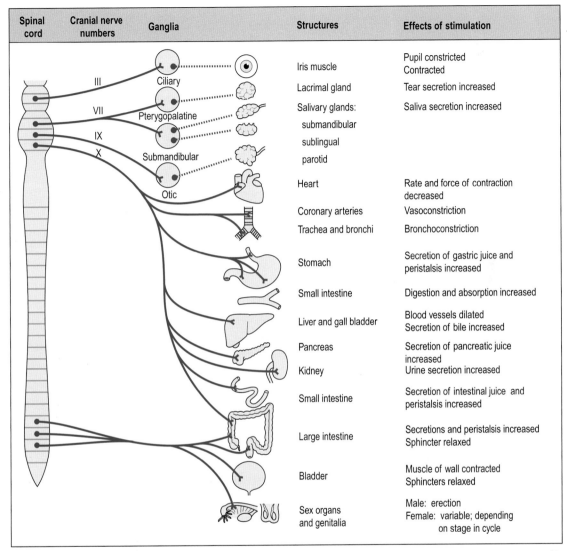

Fig. 2.5 ■ The parasympathetic outflow, the main structures supplied and the effects of stimulation. *Solid lines,* preganglionic fibres; *broken lines,* postganglionic fibres. (From Waugh & Grant 2006, Fig. 7.43, p172, with permission.)

other organs and promote the development of vascular deterioration (Gill 2008). It is important, therefore, to reduce their impact, and this can be done either by controlling the stressor or by introducing a method of relaxation. The relaxation response method of Benson aims to counteract the effects of sympathetic activity by promoting the action of the parasympathetic, thereby exploiting the reciprocal nature of the two parts of the autonomic nervous system (see Chapter 22).

Activity of the parasympathetic, however, is not always benign (Poppen 1998). Asthma is exacerbated by bronchial constriction and gastric ulcers by acid secretion. Both bronchial constriction and acid secretion are associated with parasympathetic dominance, yet the conditions of asthma and gastric ulcer are often relieved by relaxation and aggravated by stress. The theory is not consistent Chapter 18 and 19).

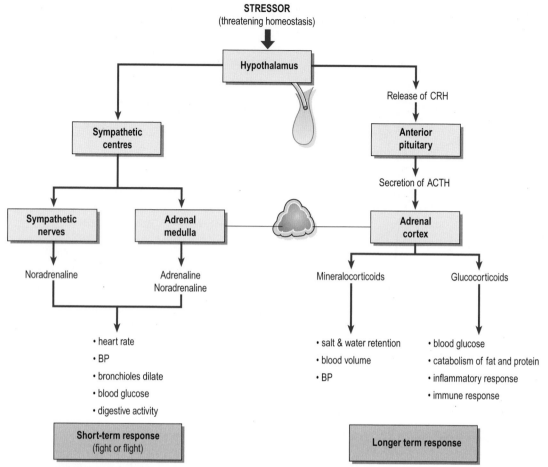

Fig. 2.6 ■ Responses to stressors that threaten homeostasis. *ACTH,* Adrenocorticotrophic hormone; *CRH,* corticotrophin-releasing hormone. (From Waugh & Grant 2006, Fig. 9.12, p224, with permission.)

PSYCHOLOGICAL THEORIES

Three types of psychological theory concerning relaxation are discussed in this section:

Cognitive
Behavioural
Cognitive–behavioural.

Cognitive Theories

'Our thoughts define our universe', writes Piero Ferrucci in *What We May Be* (2000). The way we perceive what happens to us determines how we feel about it. This idea epitomizes the cognitive approach which sees feeling as a function of thought. Interpretations, perceptions, assumptions and conclusions will all give rise to particular feelings, which in their turn govern our behaviour. This means that our experience of stress and anxiety is related to the way we interpret events in our lives: we may, for example, appraise situations in ways which make them appear unnecessarily threatening (Lazarus & Folkman 1984).

Ellis (1962, 1976), a psychotherapist, attributes much anxiety to the irrational responses made by individuals, and cites the following example:

If person X puts me off, it must mean they don't like me, and if they don't like me it's probably because I'm unlikeable.

In this example the person is basing his or her view of the self on one isolated event. Ellis also indicates that such a person tends to think in terms of absolutes; for example, 'I must be liked by everyone, otherwise I'll feel worthless'. Individuals locked into this pattern of thinking are doomed to disappointment and anxiety because of the impossible standards they have set for themselves. Therefore from Ellis's perspective good mental health is a result of rational thinking. From this foundation Ellis developed the ABC model to explain how irrational thoughts affect our behaviour and emotional state:

A – *Activating event,* such as poor exam results
B – *Beliefs,* such as believing you are a failure
C – *Consequences,* where the belief triggers depression or anxiety

Belief is the key to this model because it determines the consequences. Ellis states that where individuals have irrational beliefs they believe life is always meant to be fair. Ellis (1987) extended the ABC model to ABCDE, adding D – *Dispute,* and E – *Effect.*

Treatment consists of identifying the irrational beliefs, challenging them and considering more rational alternatives. These ideas form the basis of Ellis's rational emotive behaviour therapy (REBT). Where a person may say how unfair circumstances have been, the REBT therapist would challenge this irrational belief, with the intended effect to change the person's thinking. This may involve disputing whether there is evidence to support the belief or whether the negative thought logically follows the facts. There have been several updates to this original model, with a greater emphasis now placed on biological aspects of emotional disturbance (Dryden 1994).

Beck (1984), a contemporary psychiatrist, also sees anxiety (and depression) as stemming from negative thinking. To Beck, the distress is created by faulty information processing, which results in the individual having a distorted view of events. For example:

■ An individual blames himself or herself whenever something goes wrong although he or she is not responsible.
■ An individual feels unemployable after one job rejection.

■ An individual blows up a minor mistake into a catastrophe: accidentally scratching his or her car, the person sees it as irredeemably damaged.

Such people tend to magnify their weaknesses and to see their minor mistakes as disasters; they dwell on their failures and dismiss their achievements. Beck argued that these individuals developed a dysfunctional view of themselves which was caused by a negative triad:

1. A negative view of the world, seeing it as a cruel place and therefore having no hope
2. A negative view of the future, such as that his or her situation will never improve, where thoughts enhance depression and reduce hope
3. A negative view of self such as 'I am a failure' which enhances depression and confirms low self-esteem

The first step in therapy is to identify the automatic thoughts that make up the faulty thinking patterns. This is done by keeping a diary of anxiety-related events together with a description of the thoughts and fantasies and levels of emotion which accompany them. These thoughts are then tested against reality by asking what evidence there is to justify them. Are they plausible? Should they be challenged? Does it matter if what the person fears happens? If the automatic thoughts do not stand up to reality testing, the person will need to modify them. Another common error is that of overestimating danger and underestimating coping abilities. Recognizing when stress is caused by habitual thinking errors and not by a specific event immediately reduces the impact of the event or situation. Some thought patterns may need to become more positive and less negative, but the principal aim of therapy is to help these persons adopt a more realistic view of themselves, their world and their future (Beck 1976).

Recognition of the value of Beck's cognitive therapy is increasing. Over the last 30 years its effects on a variety of major mental health problems have been compared with those of pharmacological treatments, behaviour therapy and interpersonal psychotherapy and found to be either superior or of equal efficacy (Butler et al 2006, Elkin et al 1989, Gloaguen et al 1998, Hollon et al 2005).

Both Ellis and Beck see these people as having the ability to control their thoughts, and thus having the power to modify their feelings and their behaviour if they want to. Ellis and Beck's models are respectively concerned with challenging irrational thoughts and questioning faulty thinking patterns. Such approaches belong to the area of cognitive restructuring – that is, the combatting of 'self-defeating thought patterns by reordering the person's perceptions, values and attitudes' (Lichstein 1988). Although their theories are similar in many ways, their styles of therapy differ: Ellis adopts a confrontational approach while Beck is more collaborative (Neimeyer 1985).

Although cognitive theory is referred to several times in this book, the theories of Beck and Ellis are particularly relevant to the chapters on stress (Chapter 1), cognitive–behavioural therapy (Chapter 16) and goal-directed visualization (Chapter 19).

A further researcher whose work has been influential in the cognitive field is Seligman (1992). He focused on the degree of control people perceive themselves to have over their environment. People who lack this kind of control are subject to a state he termed 'learned helplessness', which predisposes them to depression. Seligman's work has been called 'positive psychology'. This work provides guidance on how to lead a meaningful and fulfilling life. Its principles are based on positive emotions, positive psychological traits and positive-minded institutions (Seligman & Csikszentmihalyi 2002). More recently Seligman has refined his work on 'positive psychology' and now describes five pillars, Engagement, Relationships, Meaning and Accomplishment (PERMA), which enable feelings of 'well-being' and ability to 'flourish' (Seligman 2012).

Cognitive methods may be seen to include most approaches involving the mind. Thus self-talk and mental diversion are cognitive, as are other techniques which aim to restructure the thoughts. Some of these, however, are less amenable to scientific investigation than the structured approach of Beck (1984).

Behaviour Theory

Behaviour theory, by contrast, is concerned with observable actions. Discounting what goes on in the mind, it sees behaviour as conditioned by external events. Such events are seen as leading the person to act in predictable ways. In the case of classical conditioning, behaviour is governed by associations; for example, Pavlov's dog learned to salivate at the sound of a bell because the sound of the bell was associated with the smell of food. This automatic association has helped to explain how fear responses can develop. Any stimulus that regularly occurs within a situation where fear is elicited will itself come to trigger a fear response.

In the case of operant conditioning, behaviour is governed by a system of reinforcement (Skinner 1938). *Positive reinforcement* refers to a response which is strengthened by adding something to the situation; for example, giving an employee a bonus every time he or she makes a profit for the firm. This results in the employee continuing to work hard. *Negative reinforcement* refers to the strengthening of a response by removing something from the situation; for example, when a headache is relieved by taking an aspirin, the likelihood of taking an aspirin to relieve the next headache is increased. Together, these two concepts can be used to shape behaviour.

Since these theories were first propounded, behaviour theory has developed in ways which take it away from its original reductionist models. However, it still retains its central principle, that observable behaviour is more worthy of investigation than behaviour which is only inferred (i.e., mental processes).

Behavioural approaches include muscular relaxation, distraction, graded exposure and social skills training. Muscular relaxation is described in the Chapters 6, 7, and 8 of this book; distraction consists of activity which diverts the attention; graded exposure offers a step-by-step approach towards mastery over a feared object or situation; and social skills training concerns interpersonal communication and covers verbal and non-verbal behaviour. Assertiveness techniques, developed in the 1970s by Alberti and Emmons, are a central component of social skills training and are a form of behaviour therapy designed to help people empower themselves. These writers define the concept as behaviour where people are acting in their best interests without experiencing undue anxiety and without denying the rights of others (Alberti & Emmons 2017). Topics included in assertiveness training are:

- Exercising personal rights
- Setting personal priorities
- Expressing views

- Making requests
- Refusing requests
- Countering manipulative behaviour in others
- Allowing oneself to make mistakes

Behaviour styles can range from aggressive to submissive, but the style of choice in most situations is the assertive one. Knowing when and how to use it is one of the social skills.

Initially it was considered by behavioural therapists that thoughts and emotions were unnecessary to the understanding of behaviour. However, over time it became evident that such matters could not be fully considered in isolation and that a certain overlap between cognitive and behavioural methods existed (Homme 1965). It can be seen from the previously listed items, for example, that assertiveness training contains a strong cognitive element. This has led some researchers to combine the two approaches.

Cognitive–Behaviour Theory

This theory brings together the ideas from both philosophies. The combined approach was referred to as cognitive–behavioural training. Both Beck and Ellis acknowledged the value of this new development and included behavioural exercises in their cognitive therapies (Davidson 2008). Research has shown it to be at least as effective as medication in a wide range of anxiety disorders (Blackburn & Twaddle 1996, Davis et al 2019). As a component of cognitive–behavioural interventions, relaxation techniques play a key part in the treatment of the physiological symptoms in anxiety and other clinical disorders (Donaghy 2008). However, although relaxation may be helpful in reducing stress, it is likely that in the management of anxiety disorders it will be used in conjunction with other interventions such as CBT or medication.

Stress can express itself in any of three modes: the somatic (physiological), the cognitive (psychological) and the behavioural (observable actions). It has been proposed that the pattern of changes produced by cognitive relaxation techniques will be different from those produced by physiological ones, and that benefit can be derived from matching the treatment to the problem. For example, tension headache may be more likely to respond to a somatic approach such as releasing muscle tension than to a cognitive one such as

correcting faulty thinking patterns (Lehrer 1996, Yung et al 2005). Current thinking in cognitive–behavioural theories favours a model in which interactions occur among somatic, cognitive and behavioural processes; for example, a painful joint is not simply a physical symptom, but one which also involves psychological factors such as worry and behaviours such as avoidance of certain activities which are associated with pain (Eccleston et al 2013, Gatchel & Rollings 2008, Vlaeyen & Morley 2005). Although different techniques may be used to influence the various aspects of anxiety, the aim of any therapeutic intervention is the seamless integration of its different elements (Ralston 2008, Sage et al. 2008). More recently this has included mindfulness-based cognitive therapy (MBCT), which combines mindfulness meditation with principles and strategies derived from CBT (Crane 2017).

Cognitive–behavioural principles are described in Chapter 16. They also underlie some of the coping strategies to relieve stress in Chapter 1, and feature in the goal-directed visualizations described in Chapter 19 and mindfulness-based meditation in Chapter 23.

COPING STRATEGIES

Coping has been defined as the way a person manages the demands of a situation when that situation is appraised as stressful. It refers to the thoughts an individual has about it, as well as any particular behaviour it evokes (Lazarus & Folkman 1984). People who cope well may be employing one or more strategies to reduce the stress. For example, it is often possible to change the environment: if the monitor screen is too low and gives you a backache, it could be raised. This is problem-focused coping. Another way of coping is for the person to change his or her response to the situation; instead of reacting angrily when things go wrong, the person could practise one of the strategies in anger management. This is emotion-focused coping (Lazarus & Folkman 1984).

Higgins and Endler (1995) add a further category which describes the avoidance practised by some people; that is to say, by avoiding situations which are likely to create stress, they feel they are coping adequately. Developing these theories, other researchers have suggested an approach which protects against future stress. This is the proactive coping style (Aspinwall &

Taylor 1997, Folkman & Moscovitz 2004). It searches out potential stressors and prepares a reserve of coping styles for handling them. For example, in situations of uncertainty it is useful to have built up a store of information together with strategies to help retain one's control of the situation, in case it should develop in a negative way (Kovacs 2007, Van den Brande et al 2016).

Coping strategies are a useful topic to offer a group of people in practice and for the purposes of this book, two of these topics, anxiety and coping, are considered.

PUTTING THEORY INTO PRACTICE

When offering relaxation techniques to a group of people, the health care professional may wish to include certain topics and a discussion. This has been found to enhance outcomes (Payne 1989). However, the type of education delivered must be considered carefully as implementation can vary (Alexander et al 2012). The topics must relate to those conditions which group members are experiencing – for example, anxiety, panic attack, depression and life changes.

Listed here are examples of coping strategies which could feature as topics for discussion in group meetings.

1. Getting as much control over the stressor as circumstances allow. While accepting the restrictions of the situation, there may be areas of freedom which a person can develop.
2. If control is not possible or expedient, a person can change the way he or she thinks about the stressor: for example, instead of being irritated by traffic queues, the person could see the time as an opportunity to listen to music.
3. Training oneself to predict stressful situations to weaken their impact.
4. Being task oriented and not letting emotions take over. Emotions fuddle the mind and interfere with problem solving. If the emotion is strong, it can first be acknowledged and then separated from the issue, which can then be judged dispassionately.
5. Avoidance of blaming; the latter tends to arouse anger. A more constructive attitude is to see mistakes as the result of a series of events which simply happened.
6. Dealing with anger. Some anger may serve a useful purpose; much anger, however, is purely destructive. The energy that goes into its arousal could often be more profitably spent in solving the problem. Ways in which anger can be controlled include the following:
   - Reinterpreting the stimulus in a more positive light; many situations contain ambiguities which allow reinterpretations to be made
   - Being realistic in one's expectations of other people
   - Modifying one's internal dialogue to include self-statements such as 'I am easygoing' or 'I keep my cool'
   - Focusing on the issue rather than the personality
7. Giving oneself permission to make a mistake. It is part of being human to make mistakes occasionally.
8. Distancing oneself. If circumstances seem to be overwhelming, one can try stepping back mentally to get a more objective view (Chapter 1). It is sometimes useful to visualize another person coping with the same problem.
9. Introducing humour at suitable moments. When a person smiles and laughs, the relaxation response takes over.
10. Managing time efficiently. Priorities need to be established and time allotted to tasks proportionately. If time is short, inessentials can be cut out and tasks delegated. It is sometimes possible to say 'no' to demands when time is restricted.
11. Having someone to confide in.
12. Rewarding oneself for a job well done.
13. Living in the present. This means savouring the moment, enjoying the journey as well as the arrival. It is useful to remember that the future is to a large extent determined by the way we handle the present. A lot of stress arises from dwelling on the past with its regrets or on the future with its uncertainties.
14. Establishing good relationships. The support derived both from intimate relationships and the wider social network acts as a buffer to protect the person from the full effects of stressful events (Ganster & Victor 1988, Zukauskiene 2017). However, relationships, whether at work or at home, demand time and attention.
15. Taking exercise (see Chapter 15).
16. Learning to become more assertive.

TABLE 2.1
Stress-evoking factors and related coping strategies

Stress-evoking factor	Coping strategy
Faulty belief system	Cognitive restructuring
Unclear goals	Goal setting
Unmade decisions	Decision making
Low self-esteem	Building positive self-image
Bottling up feelings	Confiding, assertiveness
Deadlines and time constraints	Restructuring time
Deteriorating relationships	Enhancing personal interaction

Table 2.1 sets out some stress-evoking factors alongside appropriate coping strategies.

Self-Efficacy

In the context of the relaxation class, where self-efficacy is an issue, it may be helpful initially to invite such persons as observers or provide them with a video to show the outcome of relaxation techniques, thereby allowing the person to experience vicariously the success of others. The more strongly they believe in the benefits of the exercise, the more confident they will feel practising it and the greater will be the likelihood of success in managing the stress in their own life.

Although relaxation may be helpful in reducing stress, it is likely that in the management of anxiety disorders, it will be used in conjunction with other interventions such as CBT or medication. In addition, therapeutic interventions should consider the role of our emotions within which interactions occur among somatic, cognitive and behavioural processes.

Relaxation and Emotion

The conditions of stress and relaxation have both cognitive and somatic aspects. In the case of relaxation, the cognitive aspect refers to the experience of mental calmness while the somatic aspect refers to such physiological matters as diminished nerve and muscle activity. Emotions are feelings of love, joy, anger and jealousy that each person experiences with associated changes occurring in the body; for example, the experience of fear is accompanied by a fast-beating heart.

Like the emotions, relaxation is linked on the one hand to thinking processes and on the other to physiological ones. Connecting them is the area of our feelings. These are relayed to the mind, which makes sense of them; it processes the material in a way which is based on the information it receives. This leads to physiological changes. However, thoughts can spontaneously arise in the mind, triggering our feelings, which themselves lead to physiological changes in the body. Thus our thoughts can trigger our emotions as our emotions can trigger our thoughts (Donaghy 2007, Moreno et al 2017).

Deeply involved in this process is the hypothalamus, a key organ within the limbic system where emotions are thought to originate. The hypothalamus carries impulses in both directions and initiates the chemical changes which accompany emotional activity. A biological system of feedback thus underlies the integrated actions of emotion, cognition and physiology.

Fig. 2.7 shows this two-way flow between the cortex and the limbic system and on to the physiological structures which produce the body's response. In the cerebral cortex there is a complex interplay among the many neuronal connections. The result is that links involving thought, emotion and neurophysiological responses run throughout the brain, allowing it to make constant refinements to our behaviour (Gill 2008).

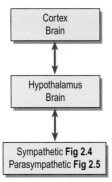

Fig. 2.7 ■ Two-way flow of impulses between the brain and the physiological organs.

EFFECTS OF RELAXATION TECHNIQUES

Some techniques, such as Benson's relaxation response, work by activating the parasympathetic division of the autonomic nervous system (Benson 1976, 1983). This is thought to decrease physiological arousal. Some techniques, such as progressive relaxation, reduce muscle tension. Others work by creating a distracting effect which draws attention away from the source of the stress, as in imagery, or by focusing attention on a specified emotionally neutral object, such as the breath in meditation. In all these the relaxation acts as a mediator, diminishing the impact of the stressor.

Most techniques, however, have several effects, the principal one tending to generalize across the entire organism because the mind cannot be separated from the body nor the body from the mind.

PRACTISING RELAXATION TECHNIQUES

All relaxation training involves the learning of new skills or the facilitation of already established ones. Practice is essential for the development of these skills and, for greatest benefit, should be undertaken daily. The length and quality of training and the dedication to home practice are vitally important to the outcome.

Borkovec and Matthews (1988) compared the anxiety levels of people trained in progressive relaxation with the levels of those untrained and found that the reduction in anxiety demonstrated in the trained group became considerably more pronounced as practice of the technique increased. A growing body of evidence confirms these findings (Ekkekakis 2013).

The learning process is aided by demonstration and feedback. People were also given information (printed as well as verbal), and this helped them to feel more in control of the procedure, provided the information was in a form which was meaningful to them. Feeling in control is thought to increase the person's motivation (Ekkekakis 2013, Pomeroy 2007, Wulf 2007). Motivation can also be stimulated by record keeping on the part of the person; for example, a diary could record times of practice and changes in anxiety levels.

For those who wish to teach the technique, some kind of training is necessary. However, where this is not available the principles which underlie some of the relaxation techniques can be woven into the skills already possessed by the health care professional. For example, attention to posture is a valuable and universal concept outside the domain of the Alexander technique, and images of warmth and heaviness can be induced without autogenic training.

The health care professional may sometimes feel inadequately equipped to deal with certain stress-induced conditions. Such a situation calls for consultation with a specialist in the area.

CHOOSING A RELAXATION TECHNIQUE

In selecting a technique for a particular disorder, the health care professional will be guided by the research. Chapter 30 contains research findings on a wide range of disorders for which relaxation training has been used, and Appendix 1 itemizes suggested applications for the different methods. It may be useful to consider the evidence alongside personal choice because a technique which gives the client a positive experience will probably have a relaxing effect.

Another guiding principle is the nature of the disorder and how it matches up with the technique. For example, a sports injury may respond best to a physical method such as progressive relaxation, whereas a cognitive disorder such as agoraphobia may benefit more from a psychological approach such as visualization. However, it is principally the evidence which should guide the practitioner in their choice of method to ensure that the best technique is selected for the particular situation.

Two examples will serve to illustrate how theory can inform practice. The first concerns a 55-year-old male office worker with tension headaches associated with pain in his neck and shoulders. The second relates to a 35-year-old housewife with agoraphobia. They would each benefit from a course of relaxation training, but whereas the first is a relatively straightforward problem, the second has more complex requirements.

KEY POINTS

1. Relaxation is a state of low physiological arousal accompanied by a calm state of mind.
2. It is possible to induce a state of relaxation in different ways, some focusing on the body and others on the mind. The state induced, however, will involve both mind and body.
3. Current evidence of effectiveness is presented, but the research base is too small to declare one relaxation technique superior to another.
4. Practicing the technique is essential. Greater practice leads to more effective results.

5. Relaxation can be used to ameliorate stress and feelings of anxiety. However, clinical anxiety may require additional interventions.
6. Coping skills can strengthen the person's perception of his or her ability to handle stressful situations. This helps turn a threat into a challenge.
7. An important coping skill is knowing how to relax.

Reflection

Describe how you relax.
What do you do to relax?
Why do you need to relax?
How do you feel?
What techniques/methods have you used for relaxation?

CASE STUDY LEARNING OPPORTUNITIES

The key points and reflection provide the background and knowledge required in relation to the case studies, Matthew (Case Study 1) and Angela (Case Study 2), to help deepen understanding of how relaxation techniques can help improve physical and mental well-being.

CASE STUDY 1

Tension Headache: *Relaxation Techniques for Matthew*

Matthew finds a therapist and arranges to meet at weekly intervals. His treatment begins with an investigation into his thoughts on the matter: what does he think causes the headaches? Does he have any thoughts which might help to find an explanation for his own particular headaches? It is explained to him that such a dialogue approach has been found to be an effective way of tackling the problem. He is asked to keep a diary to record headache occurrences, rating the severity of each one, the circumstances

in which it occurred and his feelings and thoughts about it.

In this way, the health care professional gently prepares the ground for Matthew to make his own contribution to the diagnosis. He begins to feel he has been expecting too much of himself; it doesn't work to be a perfectionist; it leads to unnecessary anguish when things go wrong. Instead, he learns to be more assertive.

CASE STUDY 2

Panic Disorder and Agoraphobia: Relaxation Techniques for Angela

One day Angela saw a class advertised for people suffering from agoraphobia. *This could be for me,* she hesitatingly thought. It was not easy getting there but she steeled herself to do so, arriving in a cold sweat with palpitations, hard breathing and butterflies in her stomach. It was a talking group whose members were all experiencing what she was going through. She began to relax. Talking was good. As well as being able to talk to people with the same problem, she learned what she could do about it. Change your thoughts, they said. But how? Why worry about a tomato stand? It's probably been knocked over before. The shop is used to it, we are sure nobody turned a hair. It's unlikely to happen to you again and, even if it does, it's not the end of the world. Get a diary, they say. Write down your fears as they occur and ask yourself what triggers them off. Are they justified? What is your way of dealing with them? We all have our particular solutions. This was magical talk to Angela. She felt soothed by this new way of thinking.

ACTIVITY

For each of the case studies:
1. List the relaxation technique that is helping with the condition.
2. Write down the impact relaxation is having from a physical perspective.
3. Write down the impact relaxation is having from a psychological perspective.
4. Write down the impact relaxation is having from an emotional perspective.
5. Consider the effects of the relaxation techniques on overall quality of life.

Chapter 3 will focus on preparing for relaxation to help put this learning into practice.

REFERENCES

Alberti, R., & Emmons, M. (2017). *Your perfect right: Assertiveness and equality in your life and relationships* (10th ed.). Oakland, CA: Impact Publishers.

Alexander, J., Bambury, E., Mendoza, A., & Reynolds, J. (2012). Health education strategies used by physical therapists to promote behaviour change in people with lifestyle-related conditions: A systematic review. *Hong Kong Physiotherapy Journal, 30*(2), 57–75.

Aspinwall, L. G., & Taylor, S. E. (1997). A stitch in time: Self-regulation and proactive coping. *Psychology Bulletin, 121,* 417–436.

Astin, J. A., Berman, B. M., Bausell, B., et al. (2003). The efficacy of mindfulness meditation plus qigong movement therapy in the treatment of fibromyalgia: A randomized controlled trial. *Journal of Rheumatology, 30*(10), 2257–2262.

Beck, A. T. (1976). *Cognitive Therapy and the emotional disorders.* New York: International Universities Press.

Beck, A. T. (1984). Cognitive approaches to stress management. In R. L. Woolfolk, & P. M. Lehrer (Eds.), *Principles and practice of stress management.* New York: Guilford Press.

Benson, H. (1976). *The relaxation response.* London: Collins.

Benson, H. (1983). The relaxation response: Its subjective and objective historical precedents and physiology. *Trends in Neurosciences, 6,* 281–284.

Blackburn, I. M., & Twaddle, V. (1996). *Cognitive therapy in action.* London: Souvenir Press.

Butler, A. C., Chapmen, J. E., Forman, E. M., et al. (2006). The empirical status of cognitive-behavioural therapy: A review of meta-analyses. *Clinical Psychology Review, 26,* 17–31.

Crane, R. (2017). *Mindfulness-based cognitive therapy* (2nd ed.). London: Routledge.

Davidson, K. (2008). Cognitive-behavioural therapy: Origins and developments. In M. Donaghy, M. Nicol, & K. Davidson (Eds.), *Cognitive-behavioural interventions in physiotherapy and occupational therapy* (pp. 3–18). Edinburgh: Butterworth-Heinemann.

Davis, M., Eshelman, R. E., & McKay, M. (2019). *The relaxation and stress reduction workbook* (7th ed.). Oakland, CA: New Harbinger.

Donaghy, M. E. (2007). Exercise can seriously improve your mental health: Fact or fiction? *Advances in Physiotherapy, 9*(2), 76–89.

Donaghy, M. E. (2008). Cognitive-behavioural approaches in the treatment of alcohol addiction. In M. Donaghy, M. Nicol, & K. Davidson (Eds.), *Cognitive-behavioural interventions in physiotherapy and occupational therapy* (pp. 105–120). Edinburgh: Butterworth-Heinemann Elsevier.

Dryden, W. (1994). Reason and emotion in psychotherapy: Thirty years on. *Journal of Rational-Emotive and Cognitive Behaviour Therapy, 12*(2), 83–99.

Eccleston, C., Morley, S. J., & Williams, A. C. (2013). Psychological approaches to chronic pain management: Evidence and challenges. *BJA: British Journal of Anaesthesia, 111*(1), 59–63.

Ekkekakis, P. (2013). *Routledge handbook of physical activity and mental health.* London: Routledge.

Ellis, A. (1962). *Reason and emotion in psychotherapy*. New York: Lyle Stuart.

Ellis, A. (1976). The biological basis of human irrationality. *Journal of Individual Psychology, 32*, 145–168.

Ellis, A., & Dryden, W. (1987). *The practice of rational-emotive therapy (RET)*. New York: Springer.

Elkin, I., Shea, M. T., Watkins, J. T., et al. (1989). General effectiveness of treatments. *Archives of General Psychiatry, 46*, 971–982.

Ferrucci, P. (2000). *What we may be*. London: Mandala.

Folkman, S., & Moscovitz, J. T. (2004). Coping: Pitfalls and promise. *Annual Review of Psychology, 55*, 745–774.

Ganster, D. C., & Victor, B. (1988). The impact of social support on mental and physical health. *The British Journal of Medical Psychology, 61*, 3–17.

Gatchel, R. J., & Rollings, K. H. (2008). Evidence informed management of chronic low back pain with cognitive behavioural therapy. *Spine Journal, 8*(1), 40–44.

Gill, J. S. (2008). Biomedical links between cognitions and behaviour. In M. Donaghy, M. Nicol, & K. Davidson (Eds.), *Cognitive behavioural interventions in physiotherapy and occupational therapy*. Edinburgh: Butterworth-Heinemann Elsevier.

Gloaguen, V., Cottraux, J., Cucherat, M., et al. (1998). A meta-analysis of the effects of cognitive therapy in depressed patients. *Journal of Affective Disorders, 49*, 59–72.

Higgins, J. E., & Endler, N. (1995). Coping, life stress and psychological and somatic distress. *European Journal of Personality, 9*, 253–270.

Hollon, S. D., de Rubeis, R. J., Shelton, R. C., et al. (2005). Prevention of relapse following cognitive therapy vs medications in moderate to severe depression. *Archives of General Psychiatry, 62*, 417–422.

Homme, L. E. (1965). Perspectives in psychology: XX1V control of coverants; the operants of the mind. *The Psychological Record, 15*, 501–511.

Jorm, A. F., Morgan, A. J., & Hetrick, S. E. (2008). Relaxation for depression. *Cochrane Database of Systematic Reviews, 4*, CD007142. doi:10.1002/14651858.CD007142.pub2.

Kim, H. S., & Kim, E. J. (2018). Effects of relaxation therapy on anxiety disorders: A systematic review and meta-analysis. *Archives of Psychiatric Nursing, 32*(2), 278–284.

Kovacs, M. (2007). Stress and coping in the workplace. *The Psychologist, 20*(9), 548–550.

Lazarus, R. S., & Folkman, S. (1984). *Stress, appraisal and coping*. New York: Springer.

Lehrer, P. M. (1996). Varieties of relaxation methods and their unique effects. *International Journal of Stress Management, 3*, 1–15.

Lichstein, K. L. (1988). *Clinical relaxation strategies*. New York: John Wiley.

Manzoni, G. M., Pagnini, F., Castelnuovo, G., & Molinari, E. (2008). Relaxation training for anxiety: A ten years' systematic review with meta-analysis. *BMC Psychiatry, 8*, 41.

Moreno, P. I., Wiley, J. F., & Stanton, A. L. (2017). Coping through emotional approach: The utility of processing and expressing emotions in response to stress. In C. R. Snyder, S. J. Lopez, L. M. Edwards, & S. C. Marques (Eds.), *The Oxford handbook of positive psychology* (3rd ed.). New York: Oxford University Press.

Neimeyer, R. A. (1985). Personal constructs in clinical practice. In P. C. Kendall (Ed.), *Advances in cognitive-behavioural research and therapy*. Orlando, FL: Academic Press.

Payne, R. A. (1989). Glad to be yourself: A course of practical relaxation and health education talks. *Physiotherapy, 75*, 8–9.

Pomeroy, V. M. (2007). Facilitating independence, motivation and motor learning. *Physiotherapy, 93*(2), 87.

Poppen, R. (1998). *Behavioural relaxation training and assessment* (2nd ed.). Thousand Oaks, CA: Sage.

Ralston, G. E. (2008). Cognitive behavioural therapy for anxiety. In M. Donaghy, M. Nicol, & K. Davidson (Eds.), *Cognitive behavioural interventions in physiotherapy and occupational therapy* (pp. 75–90). Edinburgh: Butterworth-Heinemann Elsevier.

Sage, N., Sowden, M., Chorlton, E., & Edeleanu, A. (2008). *CBT for chronic illness and palliative care: A workbook and tool kit*. Chichester, UK: John Wiley & Sons.

Skinner, B. F. (1938). *The behavior of organisms*. New York: Appleton-Century Crofts.

Seligman, M. E. P. (1992). *Helplessness: On depression, development and death*. San Francisco: Freeman.

Seligman, M. E. P. (2012). *Flourish: A visionary new understanding of happiness and well-being*. New York: Free Press.

Seligman, M. E. P., & Csikszentmihalyi, M. (2002). Positive psychology: An introduction. *American Psychologist, 55*(1), 5–14.

Stefano, G. B., & Esch, T. (2005). Integrative medical therapy: Examination of meditation's therapeutic and global medicinal outcomes via nitric oxide. *International Journal of Molecular Medicine, 16*(4), 621–630.

Van den Brande, W. V., Baillien, E., De Witte, H., Vande Elst, T., & Godderis, L. (2016). The role of work stressors, coping strategies and coping resources in the process of workplace bullying: A systematic review and development of a comprehensive model. *Aggression and Violent Behaviour, 29*, 61–71.

Vlaeyen, J. W. S., & Morley, S. (2005). Cognitive-behavioural treatments for chronic pain: What works for whom? *Clinical Journal of Pain, 21*, 1–8.

Waugh, A., & Grant, A. (2006). *Ross & Wilson anatomy and physiology in health and illness* (10th ed.). Edinburgh: Churchill Livingstone Elsevier.

Waugh, A., & Grant, A. (2014). *Ross & Wilson anatomy and physiology in health and illness* (12th ed.). Edinburgh: Churchill Livingstone Elsevier.

Wilson, K. J. W. (1990). *Ross and Wilson anatomy and physiology in health and illness* (7th ed.). Edinburgh: Churchill Livingstone.

Wulf, G. (2007). Self-controlled practice enhances motor learning: Implications for physiotherapy. *Physiotherapy, 93*(2), 96–101.

Yoshiano, K., Hironori, A., & Kazuyoshi, T. (2015). *Handbook of hormones. comparative endocrinology for basic and clinical research*. Edinburgh: Butterworth-Heinemann Elsevier.

Yung, P. M., Fung, M. Y., Chan, T. M. F., & Lau, B. W. K. (2005). Relaxation training methods for nurse managers in Hong Kong: A controlled study. *International Journal of Mental Health Nursing, 13*(4), 255–261.

Zukauskiene, R. (2017). *Interpersonal development*. London: Routledge.

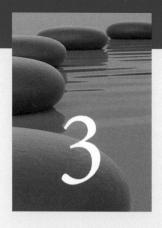

3

PREPARING FOR RELAXATION

DR CAROLINE BELCHAMBER

CHAPTER CONTENTS

LEARNING OBJECTIVES

The aim of this chapter is to provide a practical guide to generic aspects of relaxation training.

By the end of this chapter you will be able to:

1. Recognize key aspects of relaxation training procedures

2. Understand how to prepare and deliver relaxation training

3. Carry out a debrief session and know why it is important to do so

4. Identify the need for homework after a training session

5. Discern when it is appropriate to work with groups

This chapter will conclude with key points and time for reflection, providing learning opportunities through case studies.

INTRODUCTION TO RELAXATION TRAINING

The contents of this chapter may be helpful for preparing people for relaxation training, including students, self-help groups and health care professionals, whether the training is delivered in one-to-one sessions, in classes or through small group activity. The chapter starts with an introduction to the evidence of who is best qualified to teach relaxation techniques and the format in which to deliver the sessions. The importance of supervisory back-up for trainers is also discussed. After this, key aspects of relaxation training which apply to all relaxation techniques are presented, including setting, establishing confidentiality, position, introductory remarks, delivery, termination, debriefing, homework and number of sessions. Participant autonomy is then explored and different types of group work and potential pitfalls outlined.

INTRODUCTION TO EVIDENCE

Evidence around who is best qualified to teach relaxation techniques has been widely debated, psychologist Rachman (1965) and behavioural scientists Wolpe (1958) have used relaxation as part of their treatment for phobias and behavioural disorders. Occupational therapists working in the field of psychiatry have used group relaxation to manage various disorders such as anxiety and cardiovascular issues. The principles of relaxation have been used by physiotherapists for years in the management of conditions such as asthma and other respiratory, orthopaedic and neurological conditions (Elton et al 1978). Luthe (1970), referring to autogenic techniques, insists that only medically qualified practitioners are equipped to teach. Lichstein (1988) viewed this position as untenable, believing that health care professionals have much to offer, provided they use their judgement and recognize the limits of their training. He feels that the interests of society are best served by allowing and even encouraging such individuals to teach relaxation techniques. Lang and Stein (2001) list medical practitioners, physicians, psychotherapists, hypnotherapists, nurses, clinical psychologists and sports therapists as those who can employ relaxation techniques, whereas Varvogli and Darviri (2011) state that with proper training, health visitors, nurses, physicians and other health care professionals can safely and effectively use relaxation techniques for both the healthy population as well as those with a variety of conditions. The requirements for health care professionals who wish to teach relaxation methods include the following:

- Basic training as a health care professional
- Professional experience with the condition and type of group with whom they are working
- Arrangements for supervision on a regular basis
- Recognition that relaxation techniques are not a panacea, although they can be a powerful tool

Today there are validated courses on relaxation techniques which interested health care professionals are strongly advised to attend. Because relaxation training, in some form or other, has traditionally featured in the core training of many health care professionals, the health care professional environment is an appropriate setting for such work with individuals (Potter & Grove 1999).

Lichstein (1988) considered the delivery of relaxation techniques further and advocates the group format (discussed under Working with Groups later in this chapter) as an effective way of delivering relaxation. The group particularly lends itself to this function because an entire course can be worked out in advance. Relaxation training also occurs in facilitated and self-help groups; however, because the facilitators may not have had relevant training and experience, extra care should be taken in avoiding the pitfalls, described in the sections on Organization and Falling Asleep.

THEORIES BEHIND RELAXATION DELIVERY

Jacobson (1938) believed that all muscular tension was associated with all mental processes. Therefore relaxation was seen as a reduction of muscular tension through emotional and mental processes. Evidence for Jacobson's theory was demonstrated both clinically and experimentally. Wolpe (1958) supported Jacobson's views, demonstrating that relaxation was a key part of organized desensitization, and Hay and Madders' (1971) work reinforced this theory, demonstrating that a combination of relaxation and group discussion was successful in relieving migraine headaches. Jacobson's theory, however, did not focus on mental relaxation but saw it as an outcome of physical relaxation, and a number of studies (Davison 1966, Lader & Wing 1966, Rachman 1965) have since shown that 'suggestion' in the relaxation procedure is a vital element of the process.

Many techniques developed from theories can elicit relaxation. Therefore it is advisable for trainers to be familiar with a number of relaxation techniques and select those most appropriate for the person requiring relaxation and those they feel most comfortable delivering. In addition, supervisory back-up should be provided.

Supervisory Back-Up

The provision of supervisory back-up for the trainer is recommended for both individual and group relaxation sessions. The main purpose is to strengthen and maintain the skills of the trainer, which in turn ensure the value of the relaxation session received by participants. Supervision also helps protect trainers from emotional fatigue by providing an opportunity for them to release their own tensions, thereby guarding against the state of burn-out or exhausted empathy. In addition, supervision performs another function, namely, in helping trainers to handle their reactions if old wounds are re-opened during relaxation techniques, as they can be when past emotional experiences are stirred by listening to other people recounting theirs. Contact with a more experienced colleague is useful for resolving these and other problems which may arise in the course of work. Finding a supervisor is the responsibility of the trainer.

KEY ASPECTS OF THE PROCEDURE

Setting

Most authors advise a quiet, warm setting free from disturbance. However, others favour one that bears more resemblance to the normal environment, on the grounds that the relaxation skills learned will be more readily transferred to real life. Consequently, a background which includes faint external sounds may be deliberately sought because too heavy a silence can be artificial, even anxiety inducing.

Establishing Confidentiality

In the case of group work, confidentiality must be established at the outset and re-established each time a new participant joins. Confidentiality in this context means that nothing of a self-disclosing nature expressed by any group participant is referred to outside the session. Topics can be discussed outside but only in a general sense.

Position

For deep relaxation, lying is preferable to sitting because a totally supported body will more readily lose its tension. However, some people, for different reasons, do not like lying. Another drawback of the lying position is a tendency on the part of the trainee to fall asleep (Page 7). In addition, when lying on the floor, participants may find it comfortable to place a pillow under the knees as well as the head. Many groups meet in public buildings, such as schools or church halls, where the floors are wooden or tiled. These are hard,

but a length of foam or a beach or camping mattress provides a suitably softer surface and can be supplied at very little cost by the participants themselves. In defence of sitting, however, it can be argued that the skill of relaxing transfers to everyday situations more effectively if it is taught in a position in which stress is more likely to occur (i.e., sitting rather than lying). Thus it can be seen that both positions have value and may be used on different occasions during training. Whichever position is adopted, participants should be advised to wear suitable loose comfortable clothing, avoiding skirts, to gain the most from the exercises delivered during the relaxation session.

Various starting positions will be mentioned in later chapters. Mitchell (1990) lists three: lying supine, sitting and leaning forward with the arms and head supported on a high surface and sitting with the back and head supported. Jacobson (1938) mentions two: lying and sitting. Bernstein and Borkovec (1973) favour a reclining chair or an easy chair with a foot stool, as does Poppen (1998). Whichever relaxation position is chosen, relaxed postures have been validated and shown to reduce muscle activity (Poppen & Maurer 1984, Tatum et al 2006). Tatum and colleagues (2006) describe two categories, (1) how it feels to relax (behaviour) and (2) the relaxed position (operational definition): head, eyes, throat, shoulders, hands, body, feet, breathing, mouth and quiet. Breathing is an important element of relaxation training, and the trainer should incorporate the six key principles (see Chapter 4) into relaxation training. Whether the eyes are open or closed is determined by the nature of the approach and the preference of the participant. Introductory remarks can initiate the relaxation process.

Introductory Remarks

A short introduction will help to put the participants at ease.

Injury and illness can create stress, I think you'll agree. Stress is uncomfortable. It also interferes with the body's healing mechanisms because energy is diverted from the healing process in order to maintain a state of high alert. To reduce this state of high alert we need to promote a calm body and mind. Relaxation techniques can help to achieve this. There are different kinds of relaxation technique.

Some involve the muscles and breathing pattern while others involve the thoughts in the head. Often both are involved.

When presenting any particular relaxation technique it is believed that people want to know two things above all others: that the approach is well established and that it works (Lichstein 1988). A short rationale addressed to the participants is therefore appropriate. In addition, for the benefit of any participants who fear that they are going to be hypnotized, Hendler and Redd (1986) suggest adding a disclaimer to reassure the participants that such is not the purpose. A study by Taylor and Ingleton (2003) indicated that despite initial concerns around hypnotherapy, as described by Hendler and Redd (1986), participants were able to describe in detail how hypnotherapy had helped them, suggesting it is a valuable intervention. It can also reduce the possibility of unintentional trance induction.

A sample introduction might be:

This relaxation procedure is one that has been practiced for x [number of] years. It has been studied by researchers and found to be effective. You'll feel very relaxed and calm as a result. It is not the same as hypnosis and you will not lose consciousness at any point.

Because some relaxation techniques involve the musculature, the concept of muscle action could be described, as in the following paragraph.

Muscle Action

When a muscle contracts, its fibres shorten, making the muscle fat. On relaxing, the muscle returns to a resting state in which the fibres are by comparison long and thin. A contracting muscle feels hard to the touch. You can illustrate this by taking your thumb across the palm of your hand and, using the fingers of the other hand, feel the muscle below the thumb getting hard. Now, relax the thumb, and feel the muscle below it become soft.

This exercise demonstrates that the relaxation, as well as the contraction of skeletal muscles, is under the control of the will.

The introductory passages above need only be stated once; however, one of the two following passages may be used every time a session begins. These are used to help create the mood for relaxation by gently leading the participants into a calm frame of mind. The first approach is called 'sinking' and the second 'imaginary bubble'. It is not necessary to use both.

Sinking

Make yourself as comfortable as you can … become aware of the surface underneath you … let your body settle into it … notice how it supports you … notice the points of contact between you and the floor: your head … shoulders … spine … ribs … hips … heels … elbows … forearms and hands … feel your body sinking into the surface you are lying on … feel the tension leaving it … your body getting heavier as the tension ebbs away … feel at peace … Take one good breath and as you let it out, feel it carrying all your tensions away … then let your breathing settle into a gentle rhythm …

Imaginary Bubble

As you lie or sit, reflect on the idea that you are going to give the next half-hour to yourself. No telephone can ring for you; no doorbell can disturb you; no-one will call your name. You may hear sounds around you: voices, horns, sirens, bangs and revs … think of them as being outside your world. With these thoughts in mind, draw an imaginary circle around yourself, about 3 feet from the centre. Create an imaginary bubble … think of the interior as your space … your own private space. Feel how safe it is … safe to get in touch with yourself. Turn your thoughts inwards.

Delivery

Any relaxation procedure calls for a tone of voice that is quiet and calm. That does not imply that it should be hypnotic. Bernstein and Borkovec (1973) suggest that the tone should be conversational to begin with, but that the volume and pace of speech should be gradually reduced as the session wears on. They advise a tone which is 'smooth and quiet, perhaps even monotonous, but not purposely hypnotic'.

The pauses between instructions should always be long, to give the participants time to carry out the action or to evoke the image. Dots in the text indicate these pauses.

The 'live' voice is generally used for teaching. Tapes also have value; for example, the participants might learn initially from the live voice, then continue at home with a tape (preferably one containing the trainer's voice) until they know the technique. A disadvantage of tapes is that the participants may become dependent on them and unable to relax without them. Any advantage that tapes have in controlling the verbal aspect of the instruction is more relevant to research than to training.

Termination

All deep relaxation techniques should be brought to a gradual end, allowing the participants to make a slow return to the alert state. A variety of methods are described throughout this book. Some trainers use a counting process, others a simple sentence such as: 'When you feel ready, please open your eyes and sit up'. Some trainers recommend bending and stretching the limbs, whereas others advise sitting quietly for a few minutes. Most of the relaxation techniques mentioned in this book carry their own form of termination. The following is a sample procedure.

> I am going to bring this relaxation session to an end … I'd like you gradually to become aware of your surroundings … feel the floor/chair underneath you … in your own time open your eyes … give your limbs a few gentle stretches … make a few fists to stir up the circulation … have the feeling that you are alert and ready to carry on with your life …

Termination is sometimes referred to as 'arousal' or 'return to everyday activity'. In autogenic training, it is called a cancellation.

Debriefing

At the end of a relaxation session there is a de-briefing process, the object being twofold: to make the experience more satisfying for the participants and to provide the trainer with feedback. The trainer might open the discussion with questions such as: 'How did you find that experience?', 'Did it make you feel more relaxed?', 'Did you find the relaxation technique easy to follow?', 'Was anything about it confusing?' and 'Were you able to relate to the different parts of the body?'. Plenty of time should be allotted to the debriefing section to give participants the opportunity to express their reactions or confide their experiences, all of which helps the trainer to understand the participants better. Trainers should be prepared for feelings to be released during this period because thoughts related to past trauma can be unlocked by the relaxation experience.

Information gathered in this way is part of the ongoing assessment process and can help to increase the effectiveness of the following session.

Homework

Emphasis is placed on homework in every method of relaxation training because it leads to greater skill in using the relaxation technique. Skill is important because stress-related behaviour patterns tend to be resistant to change. Experienced use of the relaxation technique therefore increases its effectiveness.

Skill is built up by practice (see Chapter 2). Only by regular and frequent practice will behavioural change take place. The need to practice, therefore, is paramount, a point that needs bringing out because participants do not always appreciate its need. Investigating this topic in 1982, Hillenberg and Collins found significant levels of non-compliance in the home practice component of their study. However, a more recent study found that applying relaxation to real-world situations resulted in the participants being able to effectively use relaxation training as a coping response to daily life (Hayes-Skelton & Roemer 2013).

One way of increasing motivation is by introducing the record sheet or diary as a form of self-monitoring (see Chapter 2). Regular, time-recorded entries of homework sessions and their outcomes are made on the sheet by participants, and these provide feedback and encourage the participants to continue. As it is important that these practice sessions fit in with the participants' daily routine, convenient times can be discussed at the outset of the training session. Fig. 9.3 offers a useful model.

The frequency and duration of homework are conventionally set at two periods a day, each lasting 15 minutes (Bernstein & Borkovec 1973). Whether or not this should be carried out soon after meals has been debated, some researchers pointing to the benefits of postprandial low arousal. Others, however, favour avoidance of that time: Benson (1976) suggests that the process of digestion interferes with the physiological changes associated with meditation. Lichstein (1988), however, advises participants to experiment and find the times that best suit them. Breathing re-education as part of the homework should also be considered (see Chapter 4). It is advisable to carry out breathing exercises before eating to enable the diaphragm to move through its full range.

When the training session has come to an end, participants are urged to continue practicing, perhaps in some less frequent form, so that the benefits of training are not lost.

Number of Sessions

It is possible to learn most relaxation techniques in about six training sessions, assuming that attention is given to home practice. Transcendental meditation can be taught in six, and progressive relaxation in five to ten training sessions (Lichstein 1988). Many relaxation courses, however, cover several techniques and may do more than simply teach relaxation. They may include group discussion topics (see Page 7), mutual support and other concerns, thus extending the duration of the course beyond six sessions.

Participant Autonomy

Participant autonomy is a central feature of relaxation training, where the participant is seen as a self-determining being. Throughout all procedures, the person remains self-aware and free of control by outside forces. The state of relaxation the participants achieve is therefore of their own making. In so doing, they assume ownership of this state and responsibility for the progress they make. Relaxation training is firmly rooted in this principle.

Outcome Measures

Measurement of both physiological and psychological outcomes plays an important role in training delivery and is discussed in Chapter 28.

WORKING WITH GROUPS

The material in the succeeding chapters may be used with individuals or with groups of people. Because group work is a subject on its own, a short summary is relevant. Groups, in this context, may be of three kinds.

- *Led.* Here, a trainer offers a previously prepared programme. Although it is presented in a systematic way, the trainer displays flexibility when appropriate.
- *Facilitated.* Responsibility for the group is taken by a specific individual who, at the same time, imposes no strict format. The facilitator helps steer the group in the way the participants have decided it shall go but avoids telling them what to do. The facilitator's role is to suggest possibilities. If problems arise, however, the facilitator is responsible for dealing with them.
- *Self-help.* There is no designated trainer or facilitator. The style is informal, but the participants are usually highly committed, attending as they do for mutual help and support. Relevant information is collected for circulation among them, and their experiences are shared. A role of acting facilitator is often rotated.

Organization

Starting a group is one matter, but keeping it going can be more difficult. To build up and maintain group bonding, certain points need attention.

1. *Establishing and maintaining confidentiality.* The need for confidentiality was mentioned earlier. It is repeated here, as it cannot be overstated.
2. *Course programme.* A knowledge of what to expect enables participants to make plans. Dates should be supplied in advance together with, in the case of a formal course, a syllabus.
   Some classes offer relaxation alone; others begin each session with a topic related to the needs of the participants (Chapter 2), before moving into the area of relaxation itself.
3. *Participant choice.* The sense of belonging to the group is enhanced if participants are given some choice in the way it is run. How much choice depends on the nature of the group: in the formal

led group, less choice may be appropriate than in the informal self-help group. However, choice can still be introduced into the formal group by finding out from the participants at the outset why they joined and what they hope to get out of the meetings. This strategy helps the trainer to meet their needs and provides the participants with a more rewarding experience.

A system of paper slips can be used to collect the written answers. The alternative is to ask participants directly. However, many people find it threatening to have to voice their private thoughts in front of strangers; such an approach may also be non-productive if it draws false replies. In our experience, people prefer not to be asked such questions in front of a group but respond more favourably to the paper slip system (Payne 1989).

4. *Ice-breakers.* These are strategies for relaxing the atmosphere through their essential characteristic of physical participation. Some are designed for use in pairs, whereas others involve the whole group. An example of the first is seen when one participant of each pair tells the other about something pleasant that happened in the previous week; then they switch over. Another example of working in pairs is when person A talks to person B for 2 minutes, telling them who they are and what they do. Then B talks to A.

Whole-group activities are particularly useful for learning people's names. Remocker and Storch (1992) suggest a game in which each participant wears a name tag. The aim is to collect everyone's name in the shortest time.

5. *Discussion.* Exchanging information and sharing experiences are features of the group debriefing period and give the session an extra dimension. The trainer now occupies the role of facilitator, maintaining the focus of the group and seeing that all participants who wish to, get a chance to express their views. Participants tend to enjoy the discussion and normally display an eagerness to take part. There may, however, be a short period before participants have learned to trust each other, when a natural reticence holds them back from disclosing personal information. This can cause the discussion to dry up. It can

be revived by adopting the strategy of 'circular questions' (Powell & Enright 2015). This entails drawing one participant into conversation with another, for example: 'Peter, you've been in this situation. What would you say to Jenny, who is going through the same experience?'. In most circumstances, however, the discussion period helps hold the group together.

Although the discussion period has value, participants should not feel under any obligation to take part. The voluntary principle, which states that pressure should never be exerted on individuals, must be upheld (Heron 1998).

6. *Handouts.* Printed material setting out the points made in the session acts as an aide-memoire for participants. Handouts should relate to the topic currently being discussed: the information loses its relevance if it is produced a week later.

7. *Sharing the time.* Inevitably, some people talk more than others. Trainers are glad to have 'talkers' in the group: they liven it up. At the same time, it is part of the trainer's responsibility to see that the quiet ones have an opportunity to speak. Thus the trainer may feel that they sometimes have to intervene. A tactful way of doing this, is as follows: 'I don't want to dismiss what you are saying, but I wonder what X thinks about it?'.

8. *Friction-dispelling techniques.* Occasionally, friction arises; a participant may consistently disagree with the way the group is run. Calmly facing such a person and asking how they would like things changed, then putting it to the rest of the group, often resolves the matter.

Falling Asleep

There is a tendency in group work for some participants to fall asleep during the session. This is discouraged by most trainers. Bernstein and Borkovec (1973) take the view that it interferes with the learning of a skill and suggest strategies for preventing or dealing with it:

- Regularly asking for signals in the form of requests such as 'lift your index finger if you are beginning to feel relaxed'
- Directing the voice towards any sleeping participant
- Avoiding the early afternoon for teaching sessions

Keable (1997) suggests informing participants at the outset that they will be awakened with a light tap if they fall asleep. Others suggest that people who are inclined to fall asleep should sit in a chair rather than lie down because making people less comfortable reduces their tendency to fall asleep. Kokoszka (1992) refers to the effectiveness of focusing attention on a monotonous stimulus, such as counting breaths, for keeping people awake. Another study outlines the main components of wakefulness, which include specific postures (postures that do not encourage sleep), the position of the tongue and eyes, the use of mantra, breathing and the focus of attention accompanied by a belief system (AHRQ 2007).

Thus falling asleep tends to be seen in negative terms. Fanning (1994), however, takes the view that if people have come purely for respite from stress, they should be allowed to sleep.

KEY POINTS

1. Some training for the teacher is necessary.
2. The procedure described is suitable for both one-to-one sessions and groups.
3. A simple explanation at every stage can help to reassure the participant about the procedure.

4. Debriefing the participant after the session helps make it more effective for the participant.
5. Home practice is an important part of the learning process.

Reflection

Describe your experiences of delivering training.
How did you deliver the training sessions?
Why did you deliver the training sessions in that way?
What did you learn from delivering the training sessions?
What supervision / de-briefing did you put in place? Was it helpful?
What is your future action plan?

CASE STUDY LEARNING OPPORTUNITIES

The key points and reflection provide the background and knowledge required in relation to the case studies; Matthew (Case Study 1) and Angela (Case Study 2) to help deepen understanding of how preparing for relaxation can help improve the person's experience of relaxation.

CASE STUDY 1

Tension Headache: Relaxation Outcomes for Matthew

Matthew is introduced to posture exercises and stretchings to reverse the effects of the work posture. Perhaps his chair could be modified to make it more comfortable. Progressive relaxation is a further way of relaxing the tension, being a technique which has a direct effect on the muscles.

He responds favourably to all these procedures and is encouraged to integrate them into his work situation. He particularly likes the Jacobson technique, which he finds easy to learn, effective and something he can do without attracting the attention of other

people. Gradually, after a lot of daily practice, he begins to feel more at ease with himself and with his life. He stops worrying about the headaches, which grow less frequent and less intense, until after a few weeks, they stop altogether. He is delighted. Things start to improve at work, too. He seems to be getting on better with his colleagues; only yesterday he made a joke which made them all laugh. He feels happier; however, he realizes that the headaches could easily start again, so he decides to continue with daily exercise practice to ensure that he remains free of pain.

CASE STUDY 2

Panic Disorder And Agoraphobia: Relaxation Outcomes for Angela

The group facilitator taught a range of relaxation exercises: autogenics, passive muscular routines, imagery and visualizations. At first, Angela was afraid to surrender herself to the relaxation experience as she feared losing consciousness, but she was reassured that could not happen. The visualizations entailed picturing herself returning to the supermarket and successfully making purchases without the least trace of panic. Angela liked the visualizations; they showed her coming out on top. But it was made clear to her that to benefit from this teaching she would have to practise three times a day.

She went home after the first visit in a mood she did not recognize in herself and resolved to carry out the instructions.

Over the next couple of months, with weekly visits, Angela found things were beginning to improve. She practised hard and was delighted with her new skills. In time, she felt ready to start putting them to the test—gingerly at first, just walking up to the shop. Nothing terrible happened. Nobody took any notice of her. Gradually, over the next few days, she began to feel confident enough to enter the shop and still

nothing terrible happened. Her confidence grew over the next couple of weeks. She still had palpitations and butterflies, but she could control them, and as her confidence grew, her physical health improved.

She knew she had not fully thrown off the panic feelings, but now she had a way of dealing with them, and she was being invited to do some voluntary work, which made her feel herself again.

ACTIVITY

For each of the case studies:
1. List the key aspects used in the preparation for relaxation.
2. Write down the psychological outcomes experienced.
3. Write down the physical outcomes experienced.
4. Consider the outcomes on quality of life and overall well-being.

This chapter concludes Section I, setting the scene. Chapter 4 will begin Section 2, Somatic Approaches to Relaxation, which includes 12 different somatic approaches.

REFERENCES

Agency for Health Research and Quality (AHRQ). (2007). *Meditation practices for health: State of the research. Evidence Report / Technology Assessment Number 155*. Rockville, MD: AHRQ.

Benson, H. (1976). *The relaxation response*. London: Collins.

Bernstein, D. A., & Borkovec, T. D. (1973). *Progressive relaxation training: A manual for the helping professions*. Champaign, IL: Research Press.

Davison, G. (1966). Anxiety under total curaris. *Journal of Nervous & Mental Disorders, 443*.

Elton, D., Burrows, G. D., & Stanley, G. V. (1978). Relaxation theory and practice. *Australian Journal of Physiotherapy, 24*(3), 143–149.

Fanning, P. (1994). *Visualization for change* (2nd ed.). Oakland, CA: New Harbinger.

Hay, K. M., & Madders, J. (1971). Migraine treated by relaxation therapy. *Journal of the Royal College of General Practice, 24*, 1664.

Hayes-Skelton, S. A., & Roemer, L. (2013). A contemporary view of applied relaxation for generalized anxiety disorder. *Cognitive Behaviour Therapy, 42*(4), 1–12.

Hendler, C. S., & Redd, W. H. (1986). Fear of hypnosis: The role of labelling in patients' acceptance of behavioural interventions. *Behavior Therapy, 17*, 2–13.

Heron, J. (1998). *Catharsis in human development human potential research project* (revised ed.). Guildford: University of Surrey.

Hillenberg, J. B., & Collins, F. L. (1982). A procedural analysis and review of relaxation training research. *Behaviour Research Therapy, 20*, 251–260.

Jacobson, E. (1938). *Progressive relaxation* (2nd revised ed.). Chicago: University of Chicago Press.

Keable, D. (1997). *The management of anxiety: A guide for therapists* (2nd ed.). Edinburgh: Churchill Livingstone.

Kokoszka, A. (1992). Relaxation as an altered state of consciousness: A rationale for a general theory of relaxation. *International Journal of Psychosomatics, 39*, 4–9.

Lader, M. H., & Wing, L. (1966). *Physiological measurements, sedative drugs and morbid anxiety*. New York: Oxford University Press.

Lang, A. J., & Stein, M. B. (2001). Anxiety disorders. *Geriatrics, 56*(5), 24–30.

Lichstein, K. L. (1988). *Clinical relaxation strategies*. New York: John Wiley.

Luthe, W. (1970). Research and theory. In W. Luthe (Ed.), *Autogenic therapy* (4th ed.). New York: Grune and Stratton.

Mitchell, L. (1990). *Simple relaxation: The Mitchell method for easing tension* (revised ed.). London: John Murray.

Payne, R. A. (1989). Glad to be yourself: A course of practical relaxation and health education talks. *Physiotherapy, 75*, 8–9.

Poppen, R. (1998). *Behavioural relaxation training and assessment* (2nd ed.). Thousand Oaks, CA: Sage.

Poppen, R., & Maurer, J. (1984). Electromyographic analysis of relaxed postures. *Biofeedback and Self-Regulation, 7*, 491–498.

Potter, M., & Grove, J. R. (1999). Mental skills training during rehabilitation: Case studies of injured athletes. *New Zealand Journal of Physiotherapy, 27*(2), 24–31.

Powell, T. J., & Enright, S. J. (2015). *Anxiety and stress management*. London: Routledge, Taylor and Francis.

Rachman, S. (1965). Studies in desensitization, the separate effect of relaxation and desensitization. *Behaviour Research and Therapy, 3*, 245.

Remocker, A. J., & Storch, E. T. (1992). *Action speaks louder: A handbook of structured group techniques* (5th ed.). Edinburgh: Churchill Livingstone.

Tatum, T., Lundervold, T., & Ament, P. (2006). Abbreviated upright behavioral relaxation training for test anxiety among college students: Initial results. *International Journal of Behavioral Consultation and Therapy, 2*(4), 475–480.

Taylor, E., & Ingleton, C. (2003). Hypnotherapy and cognitive-behaviour therapy in cancer care: The patients' view. *European Journal of Cancer Care, 12*, 137–142.

Varvogli, L., & Darviri, C. (2011). Stress management techniques: Evidence-based procedures that reduce stress and promote health. *Health Science Journal, 5*(2), 74–89.

Wolpe, J. (1958). *Psychotherapy by reciprocal inhibition*. Stanford, CA: Stanford University Press.

Section 2

SOMATIC APPROACHES TO RELAXATION

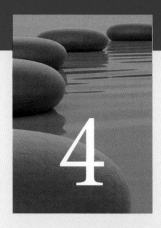

4 BREATHING

DR CAROLINE BELCHAMBER

LEARNING OBJECTIVES

The aim of this chapter is to provide an understanding of different breathing techniques used to induce a sense of relaxation.

By the end of this chapter you will be able to:

1. Understand the mechanism of breathing
2. Know why breathing increases during stressful situations
3. Recognize breathing exercises that induce a relaxed breathing pattern
4. Discern when to use different breathing techniques in relaxation training
5. Identify precautions to take when carry out breathing exercises

This chapter will conclude with key points and time for reflection, providing learning opportunities through case studies.

INTRODUCTION TO BREATHING

Breathing is an automatic process governed by centres in the brainstem (pons and medulla). These activate the diaphragm and costal muscles to open the rib cage, which expands in three directions: vertically (upwards), laterally (sideways) and anteroposteriorly (forwards and backwards). Negative pressure in the pleural cavity pulls the lungs out, causing air to be sucked in. Relaxation of the same muscles results in the recoil of the thoracic (rib) structures and the expulsion of air. The respiratory organs are illustrated in Fig. 4.1.

Oxygenated blood leaves the lungs bound for the heart, which pumps it around the body where its oxygen is exchanged for waste products, amongst them, carbon dioxide. These are carried back to the heart.

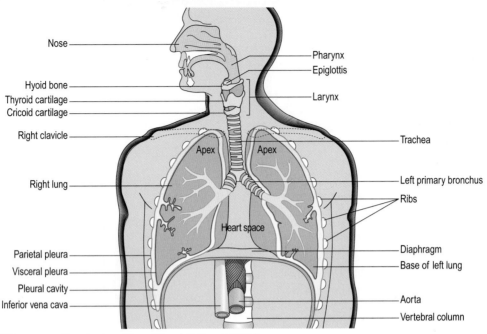

Fig. 4.1 ■ The organs of respiration. (From Waugh & Grant 2018.)

The spent blood is then returned to the lungs, where it gives up its carbon dioxide and collects a fresh supply of oxygen. The interchange of blood gases takes place in the alveoli (air sacs), which contain surfaces richly supplied with hairlike blood vessels through which the gases diffuse (pass through membranes). The direction in which the gases pass is determined by their concentration – that is, they move from a situation of high concentration to one of low concentration. Thus oxygen passes from the air in the bronchial tubes to the blood, and carbon dioxide passes from the blood to the air in the bronchial tubes. Each breath makes a contribution to the process. Fig. 4.2 shows the structure of a terminal bronchiole with its air sacs.

Chemoreceptors in the walls of the aorta and the carotid arteries help to control breathing and are sensitive to changes in the amount of carbon dioxide circulating in the blood (Waugh & Grant 2018). The levels of carbon dioxide influence physiological activity and are conventionally represented in terms of the partial pressure of carbon dioxide (PCO_2). The arterial PCO_2 ($PaCO_2$) may range from 4.7 to 6.0 kPa in the healthy individual (Hough 2001). Carbon dioxide

levels are measured using arterial blood gas samples or end-tidal airflow (air delivered at the end of exhalation and measured at the mouth or nostril); the results from either the blood or the airflow are very similar in normal lungs (Gardner 1996, Gardner & Bass 1989, Wilson 2018).

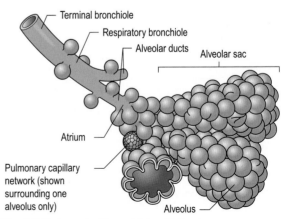

Fig. 4.2 ■ A terminal bronchiole with its air sacs.

Overbreathing and Underbreathing

Overbreathing (hyperventilation) leads to excessive loss of carbon dioxide and a lowered $PaCO_2$ (hypocapnia); underbreathing leads to a build-up of carbon dioxide and a raised $PaCO_2$ (hypercapnia). A small rise (mild hypercapnia) is associated with lethargy and symptoms resembling those of parasympathetic dominance, such as relaxation (Jardins 2012, Slonim & Hamilton 1987).

HYPERVENTILATION

In the state of hyperventilation, a person overbreathes: that is to say, the person processes a greater volume of air than is required by their body at that moment (Innocenti & Troup 2008). Thus a hyperventilating person is one who is breathing in excess of body needs: taking in too much oxygen and releasing too much carbon dioxide. This results in reduced levels of carbon dioxide in the arteries and body tissues. The $PaCO_2$, normally around 5.6 kPa, can fall to as low as 3.5 kPa (Innocenti 1983). Because carbon dioxide is acid, the pH value of the blood rises, creating alkalosis. This results in neuronal excitability, vasoconstriction and a widespread disturbance of the body chemistry, leading to the 'fight or flight' (see Chapter 1) response (Smith & Rowley 2011).

Hyperventilation is itself a symptom of stress; overbreathing thus creates symptoms on its own account, one of which is cerebral vasoconstriction (Gardner & Bass 1989). This is related to neurological symptoms (Duncan 2009, Smith & Rowley 2011) such as:

- Dizziness
- Agitation
- Confusion
- Fainting
- Hallucination
- Headache
- Visual disturbance

Other symptoms include the following (Hough 2001):

- Paraesthesia (tingling) caused by alkalosis
- Chest pain caused by coronary vasoconstriction
- Palpitations caused by paroxysmal dysrhythmia
- Anxiety and/or panic attack caused or aggravated by misattribution of physiological symptoms

Duncan (2009) also includes gastrointestinal symptoms and generalized muscle weakness with Smith and Rowley (2011), confirming that the musculoskeletal system is affected by the change in the physiological, psychological and neuronal states. In addition, the dysfunctional breathing pattern of a hyperventilating person displays irregularities which may involve any of the following (Birch 2015, Hough 2001):

- Rapid breathing, rising in some cases to 30 or more breaths per minute
- Sighing, yawning, excessive sniffing and throat clearing
- Halts in the breathing cycle
- Marked movement in the upper region of the chest
- Difficulty getting breath

These symptoms are collectively referred to as 'the hyperventilation syndrome' (HVS) or breathing pattern disorders (BPDs) (Smith & Rowley 2011). Many of them resemble the symptoms of sympathetic nervous system activity. The apprehension they create can itself release catecholamines, which reinforce the initial symptoms, setting up one vicious circle within another, as shown in Fig. 4.3.

Contrary to what might be supposed, overbreathing does not lead to a greater availability of oxygen because the hypocapnia causes vascular changes, which result

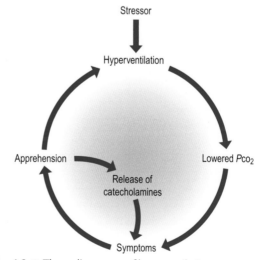

Fig. 4.3 ■ The cyclic pattern of hyperventilation.

in a decreased amount of oxygen being transferred to the tissues (Birch 2015, Lum 1981).

The condition may be acute or chronic. Acute hyperventilation, which occurs in some people during moments of extreme stress, can give rise to marked symptoms. In chronic hyperventilation, however, there are often few visible symptoms; a process of adaptation appears to take place where the respiratory control mechanism undergoes 'resetting' to a lower level of $PaCO_2$ (Gardner 1992). However, to maintain this level, the respiratory drive must be increased; that is, the individual must take deeper than normal breaths or suffer air hunger.

Although there is no conclusive way of testing for chronic hyperventilation, an indication of the state can be gained from simple tests. Four are described here:

Breathholding time: the individual is asked to hold his or her breath. This is best done on an empty chest rather than a full one (CSP Interactive 2008). Difficulty in holding it for less than 20 seconds suggests that the person may be hyperventilating. However, because people differ in the time they can hold their breath, the usefulness of the test lies in the repeated readings taken at regular intervals in the same person. As the breathing pattern becomes more stable, the breathholding time tends to increase (Innocenti & Troup 2008).

Provocation test: the person is asked to overbreathe rapidly for 3 minutes, after which the expired CO_2 is measured at the mouth. It is suggested that the end-tidal reading reflects the CO_2 level in the body (Bruton et al 2006). A fall in $PaCO_2$ of more than 1.33 kPa and a slow recovery after the test are factors which suggest that the person may be hyperventilating (Innocenti & Troup 2008). The test is often used as a diagnostic tool by medical practitioners, but it is not generally employed in therapy as people tend to get distressed by the symptoms it creates (CSP Interactive 2008, Meuret et al 2005). It is inadvisable where cardiac irregularities exist, and Innocenti and Troup (2008) draw attention to its low accuracy rate.

The Nijmegen questionnaire (Van Doorn et al 1982): this contains a list of 16 subjective symptoms (Fig. 4.4). Individuals mark the appropriate boxes, and the values are added up to give a final score. This is expressed as a fraction of 64, which is the maximum score. If they score greater than

	0 Never	1 Rarely	2 Sometimes	3 Often	4 Very often
Chest pain					
Feeling tense					
Blurred vision					
Dizzy spells					
Feeling confused					
Faster or deeper breathing					
Short of breath					
Tight feelings in chest					
Bloated feelings in stomach					
Tingling fingers					
Unable to breathe deeply					
Stiff fingers or arms					
Tight feelings around mouth					
Cold hands or feet					
Palpitations					
Feelings of anxiety					

Fig. 4.4 ■ The Nijmegen questionnaire (Van Doorn et al 1982). (From Hough 2001, with kind permission from Stanley Thornes.)

23, they are considered to be experiencing the hyperventilation syndrome. Validity has been reported but is not conclusive. However, the scale is a useful component of the screening process and is widely used, particularly at the beginning and end of a course of treatment.

Observing the respiratory rate and pattern over 1 minute: in health, the breathing pattern (chest movements) reflect the metabolic needs of the organism. Sickness, on the other hand, can be associated with a disordered (dysfunctional) breathing pattern. Correcting this disordered breathing pattern might help to promote recovery from sickness.

INTRODUCTION TO EVIDENCE

Dysfunctional breathing pattern (DBP) has been associated with asthma. The theory underpinning the claim suggests that asthma is exacerbated by over-breathing, with resulting hypocapnia and broncho-constriction (Kellett & Mullan 2002). Two approaches are based on this assumption: the Buteyko and the Papworth methods. The principal feature of the Buteyko method is breath control and breath holding to reduce ventilation and reset normal CO_2 levels. Thomas (2004) found the condition responded favourably to the approach while Bowler et al (1998) found the approach, resulted in a slightly decreased steroid use. Other researchers find the evidence lacking (Bruton & Lewith 2005), especially with regard to management of DBP, panic disorder or anxiety (Smith & Rowley 2011). However, a randomized controlled trial carried out in Canada comparing the Buteyko method with physiotherapeutic breathing exercises showed significant reductions in asthma symptoms in both groups, with no difference between them. Benefit was maintained at 6 months (Cowie et al 2008). The method bears some resemblance to the Papworth method, which employs diaphragmatic (abdominal) breathing, relaxation training and education to reduce hyperventilation. A randomized controlled trial of the Papworth method found that asthma symptoms were reduced by one-third in participants who practised the technique. The method appeared to ease respiratory symptoms and dysfunctional breathing. These benefits were maintained at follow-up 1 year later.

Accompanying depression and anxiety were also reduced (Holloway & West 2007), with Pinney and colleagues (1987) demonstrating that a programme of education, relaxation and abdominal breathing helped to relieve hyperventilation in 94% of participants. Breathing practice exercises have also been shown to reduce anxiety levels and re-establish normal breathing patterns (Tweeddale et al 1994).

Cowley (1987) demonstrated that 50% of those who experience DBP also suffered from panic attacks, whereas Kern and Rosh (2016) estimated that 25% of people with DBP also present with panic disorders. It is, however, often difficult to distinguish between hyperventilation in the acute form and panic attack. Similar symptoms occur in both conditions and have been linked to exhaustion syndrome (Ristiniemi et al 2014). This is a result either of overbreathing or of stimulation of the sympathetic nervous system. Some researchers discuss the likelihood of an interaction between the two conditions, a possibility which is supported by the tendency for panic attacks to decline after treatment that focuses on breathing control (Clark et al 1985). However, for this to be successful, the person needs to be self-motivated (Bott et al 2009). To cognitive researchers such as these, however, hyperventilation alone is not the cause of panic attacks. Cognitive factors predominate in their model in which it is suggested that resulting body sensations must be both perceived as unpleasant and interpreted in a catastrophic way for panic to develop. Fig. 4.5 illustrates this idea.

Matsumoto and Smith (2001) report that relatively little research has focused on breathing as a sole intervention. Breathing very often appears as a component of treatment but seldom on its own. Among the few published works on the topic is the comparison study of Bell and Saltikov (2000). These researchers compared the effectiveness of the Mitchell method inclusive of diaphragmatic (abdominal) breathing with diaphragmatic breathing alone in 45 healthy male participants. Using heart rate as an outcome measure, significant reductions were found in both intervention groups relative to the control condition of supine lying. However, no significant difference in effectiveness was found between the two groups themselves. In other words, diaphragmatic breathing appears to be an effective relaxation technique on its own and becomes

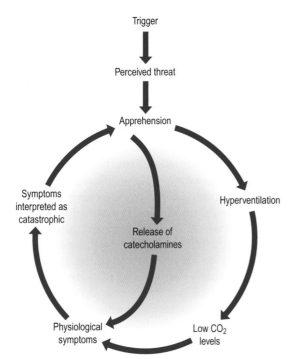

Fig. 4.5 ■ How hyperventilation might interact with cognitive factors to create a panic attack. (Adapted from Clark et al 1985.)

no more effective by being presented in conjunction with the Mitchell method. In their analysis, these researchers suggest that physiological benefits of the Mitchell method largely may be due to the component of diaphragmatic breathing, and that the technique of Mitchell may be only as effective as diaphragmatic breathing on its own (Bell & Saltikov 2000).

Gilbert (2003) reviewed evidence relating dysfunctional breathing patterns to cardiorespiratory conditions such as angina, hypertension and chronic obstructive pulmonary disease (COPD). Findings demonstrated that normalizing the breathing pattern through cardiac/pulmonary rehabilitation helped in some cases. An earlier study looked at the effects of focused breathing on recovery after cardiac surgery. Twenty-nine participants were trained preoperatively in breathing techniques. Investigating their reactions after surgery, Miller and Perry (1990) found significant decreases in both physiological responses and pain reports in the group who received the breathing techniques compared with those who did not receive it.

Some research has compared the effects of breathing re-education with those of drug therapy. The randomized trial of Kaushik et al (2005) compared biofeedback-assisted diaphragmatic (abdominal) breathing with propranolol in the long-term prophylaxis of migraine. Both approaches were found to be significantly effective, but the breathing group had a significantly greater long-term prophylactic effect than the propranolol.

Breathing re-education is important, as it has been shown to result in a slower breathing rate, a decrease in anxiety and a reduction in the frequency and intensity of panic attacks (Birch 2015, Han et al 1996). Lum (1981) proposed that slow breathing has a corrective effect on dysfunctional breathing patterns, whereas Garssen et al (1992) suggested that it may reduce stress for other reasons such as distraction. These are factors which make cognitive therapists reluctant to reject the benefits of breathing re-education (Meuret et al 2003) in breathing techniques.

THEORIES BEHIND BREATHING TECHNIQUES

For centuries in India and East Asia, breathing techniques have been considered important for physical, spiritual and mental wellbeing and a powerful antidote to stress and anxiety (Wilkinson et al 2002). In the Western world, a number of breathing techniques have emerged as a way of mitigating the effects of anxiety and stress. These breathing techniques have been proposed to induce relaxation and include slow breathing, deep breathing, breathing meditation and abdominal breathing. Using the natural breathing system as a means of gaining a relaxed state is clearly an accepted approach. Moreover, breathing techniques are easy to learn and can be carried out anywhere – a fact which makes them available in the stressful situation itself. Giving attention to the breathing is a feature of most relaxation techniques.

A number of relaxation techniques, such as imagery and muscle routines, influence the autonomic nervous system by indirect routes. However, breathing is different, as it is directly linked to the system which controls physiological arousal. This adds to its potential as a means of inducing physiological relaxation.

The kind of breathing which accompanies sympathetic arousal is quite different from the kind of breathing characteristic of parasympathetic arousal; the first tends to be fast and staccato, whereas the second tends to be slow and gentle. This connection between slow breathing and parasympathetic dominance has created a perception that slow breathing has stress-relieving properties and has led to its adoption as a relaxation technique (Sudsuang et al 1991, Wilkinson et al 2002). This breathing technique has been referred to as the 'slowing down respiration technique', an easy and effective way of controlling breathing to reduce tension, promote calmness and induce mental clarity (Wilkinson et al 2002). The approach is underpinned by physiological theory, but it also has cognitive elements in the form of the imagery which features in some of the breathing techniques. However, all of the breathing techniques have six key principles that are incorporated into relaxation training:

1. Breathing should occur at the natural pace of the individual.
2. It should be seen in terms of 'letting the air in' rather than 'taking a breath'.
3. A smooth transfer should take place between breathing in and breathing out, and between breathing out and breathing in, unless the breathing technique indicates otherwise.
4. Breathing through the nose is preferable to breathing through the mouth because the nasal passages both filter and warm the incoming air.
5. Although some breathing techniques may emphasize particular aspects of the breathing cycle, breathing should always remain gentle.
6. Artificially deep breaths should not be repeated in close succession because they can lead to hyperventilation.

When practising new breathing techniques, it is helpful to adopt an attitude of quiet self-awareness rather than one which is intent on scrutinizing the performance (Van Dixhoorn & Duivenvoorden 1989). This will involve a sense of breathing awareness.

Breathing Awareness

Breathing awareness is a phrase which refers to the focusing of attention on breathing patterns. It puts people in touch with their breathing and helps them to feel that they have some control over their breathing. As such, it forms a useful introduction to breathing techniques. Breathing awareness begins with an exploration of the movements of the chest and abdomen, which accompanies breathing in and out. To master this, the person needs to explore his or her breathing pattern.

Breathing Pattern Exploration

The exploration of breathing patterns should be carried out in a quiet environment, with plenty of time to allow the person to become aware of his or her breathing. When breathing in, the chest expands through all dimensions, and when breathing out, the chest returns to its original position. These breathing movements can be felt by adopting the following relaxation positions:

1. Lying or sitting

Place your hands on the lower edge of your ribs, fingertips a few centimetres apart. Feel your hands rise and separate as the air flows in and recoil as it flows out.

2. Sitting with head and arms resting on a table

With movement in the front of the chest now restricted, you can feel the chest expanding backwards.

3. Lying or sitting

Place your right hand over the solar plexus (the soft part between the ribs and the navel) and your left hand over the front of your chest below the clavicle (collar bone). Notice what happens under your hands when you breathe. As the air enters, feel the expansion growing, first under your right hand, then rising through the chest to reach the area under your left hand. Explore that idea for a minute or two.

After this exploration, the person should then consider his or her emotional state, as this can adversely affect the natural breathing pattern.

The Emotional State

Breathing is also subject to a person's emotional state.

Imagine for a few moments a situation that makes you feel uneasy … Next, imagine one in which you feel at ease … Did you notice any change in your breathing pattern from one to the other?

The natural pace of breathing in and out in a person resting (at ease) is slow, and because the oxygen requirement is low, breathing also tends to be rather shallow. The person may occasionally take a deep breath and find it profoundly relaxing, but the natural tendency is for such a breath to be followed by the original pattern of slow and fairly shallow breaths. Breathing in a relaxed state is associated with relaxed abdominal muscles and is characterized by visible movement of the upper part of the abdomen. Certainly, the breathing of a person who is not relaxed is itself often shallow, but the difference between tense and relaxed shallow breathing is that the former occurs at a fast rate and is accompanied by tight shoulder muscles that restrict the natural movements of the chest wall, whereas these factors are absent in a person who is relaxed.

Breathing in a stressed state is associated with a predominantly upper chest movement and often involves contraction of the muscles around the shoulders. In a relaxed state, the person's breathing tends to have a slow rate, whereas in a stressed state the person's breathing tends to be more rapid.

Relaxation is associated with a reduced rate of breathing; therefore slow breathing is one of many breathing techniques used to induce a state of relaxation.

BREATHING TECHNIQUES

Breathing techniques can be used to promote calmness and relaxation and help the person to gain a sense of control. This can be achieved using the following breathing techniques:

1. Abdominal breathing
2. Breathing pouch
3. 'Out tension, in peace'
4. Breathing meditation (1)
5. Breathing meditation (2)
6. Breathing with cue words (cue-controlled relaxation)
7. A yoga exercise
8. Breathing 'chi'
9. Sighing

One breathing technique is probably enough in one session. It can be repeated a few times, then dropped and taken up again later in the session. Allowing breaks between the exercises is a safeguard against overbreathing (hyperventilation), which may occur if the breathing techniques are carried out too enthusiastically.

Abdominal Breathing

Abdominal breathing refers to the kind of breathing which emphasizes the downward expansion of the chest cavity. It is useful at this point to inform or remind participants of the role of the diaphragm.

The diaphragm is a sheet of muscle whose edges are attached to the lower ribs, creating a floor to the chest. In the resting state, it is dome shaped. Contraction of the diaphragm flattens the dome, thereby lengthening the chest and drawing in air. Relaxation of the muscle causes it to reassume its dome shape, which helps push the air out. But the diaphragm also forms the roof of the abdomen, and as such, its movements affect the position of the internal organs: as the contracting diaphragm presses down on the organs, it causes the abdomen to swell slightly. Similarly, as the relaxing diaphragm releases its pressure on the organs, the abdomen sinks back again.

To carry out an abdominal breathing technique, participants should first make themselves as comfortable as possible and spend a few minutes quietly resting. The following instructions may then be given.

Spend a few moments running through a sequence of pleasant imagery … then, as your mind relaxes turn your attention to your breathing … lay one hand lightly over the solar plexus. Focus your attention on this area. Start the exercise with a breath out … a naturally occurring breath out. Notice a slight sinking of the area under your hand. Next, allow air to flow into the lungs, noticing the slight swelling which takes place under your hand. Then as the air is expelled, notice the area under the hand sinking back again. Allow the breathing to take place naturally.

Some trainers teach abdominal breathing by urging participants to 'think in and down' (Innocenti & Troup 2008). This helps create a natural abdominal movement.

Breathing Pouch

Breathing pouch, a variation of abdominal breathing, is a breathing technique that incorporates imagery. It is adapted from Everly and Rosenfeld (1981).

Concentrate on your breathing pattern without trying to change it. Become aware of your upper abdomen swelling as you breath in and sinking as you breath out. Picture an imaginary, hollow pouch lying inside your abdomen … as you breathe in, air travels down to fill the pouch, making the abdomen swell … breathing out empties the pouch, causing the abdomen to sink back … if you place your hand over your abdomen, you can feel gentle swelling and sinking taking place.

'Out Tension, in Peace'

This script follows the breathing listening technique, where participants focus on their breathing and emotions that they are currently feeling.

Listen to your breathing without altering its pattern … imagine your tensions being breathed out … imagine them being carried away, a little at a time with each breath out … and now, imagine that every time you breath in, you are breathing in peace, a little at a time with each breath … breathe out tension … breathe in peace … gently breathing … feeling peace flowing through your body … always keeping your breathing light …

Breathing Meditation (1)

This script focuses on relaxing the mind to improve inner awareness and make positive mental and/or physical changes.

Let your mind follow the path of the breath, taking care not to change its pace or pattern. Think of the air flowing in through your nostrils, along your nasal passages, down your windpipe and into your lungs … then, gently and smoothly turning, it is carried out along the same route … turning again as the air is drawn back in … notice the feel of the air … warm as it leaves, and cool as it enters … continue on your own with this idea for a few minutes.

Breathing Meditation (2)

This script illustrating 'breath mindfulness' is adapted from Lichstein (1988). It is particularly addressed to people with high blood pressure.

With your eyes closed, settle into your chair, couch or wherever you have chosen to be … let your body lose its tension and let your mind gradually become calm by using some pleasant imagery … allow your mind's eye to rest on the upper part of your abdomen … be aware of it swelling and sinking as you breathe … notice these breathing movements without trying to change them … just observe them in the knowledge that your body takes full care of your breathing … allow your breathing to continue on its own … flowing gently and smoothly … perhaps you can feel the rate getting slower … this is because your resting body doesn't need as much oxygen as when you are active … your heart rate also is lowered and your blood pressure falls, as a state of quiet settles on you … allow yourself to enjoy this feeling of tranquillity … let your mind continue to focus on your breathing for a few minutes longer.

Breathing With Cue Words

Breathing with cue words is described under the name of Cue-Controlled Relaxation in Chapter 9.

A Yoga Exercise

This script is quoted by Hough (2001).

Sit with your feet flat on the floor, and as you inhale, imagine the air being drawn in through the top of your head, travelling down through your body and passing out through your feet.

Breathing 'Chi'

This script follows the idea that 'chi' is an intelligent living energy that protects the body, balancing its functions.

> *Breathe in the energy force, 'chi', and let it flow into the solar plexus … then … on the breath out … let it flow to an area of your body that needs healing or soothing …*

Sighing

This script helps slow down the breathing rate and is one of the best preparations for relaxation.

> *Enjoy the feeling of being relaxed and notice your slowed breathing. As the air leaves your body on the next breath, let it go with a sigh … Aaaaah … and then resume normal breathing … two or three breaths later, repeat the sighing sound …*

Whenever a person is under stress, it is useful to employ breathing techniques that succeed in slowing the breathing rate to reduce ventilation as stress tends to increase ventilation. However, ventilation in a person in a stressed state can be increased to such an extent that it disturbs body systems and will require breathing re-education.

BREATHING RE-EDUCATION

In dysfunctional breathing, participants are first made aware of their existing breathing pattern, which is then gradually replaced by a new one through a process of gentle re-education. Treatment is aimed at raising the levels of dissolved carbon dioxide in the arterial blood and reprogramming the respiratory centre to trigger inspiration at these higher levels (Innocenti & Troup 2008). This can be achieved by modifying the breathing patterns in different ways.

- Altering the rate and depth, making the breaths slower and/or shallower
- Holding the breath for a few seconds
- Changing the composition of inhaled air by rebreathing exhaled air

Altering Rate and Depth

When people are asked to reduce their rate of breathing, they tend to take deeper breaths. This will not change the $PaCO_2$ level. If it is to be changed, the interaction of rate and depth needs to be considered. When reducing one, the other has to be held constant if the $PaCO_2$ is to be raised. The person can be reminded that slowing the rate means that the same volume of air is passing through, only travelling more slowly. A rate of 10 to 12 breaths a minute is a useful first target (Hough 2001). This can be reduced as the condition improves.

Breathing cycles which address rate and volume can be introduced (Innocenti & Troup 2008). For instance, a cycle for slowing the breath might consist of a gentle breath in, followed by a slow breath out. Counting strategies can be incorporated, such as counting 'in … two … three' on the breath in and 'out … two … three … four …' on the breath out.

A regularity of breathing pattern is aimed at throughout the treatment and an abdominal form of breathing encouraged (Innocenti & Troup 2008).

In the early stages of re-education, controlled breathing may create air hunger because the brain continues to maintain a high respiratory drive. Later, however, following daily practice, the respiratory centre will begin to make the necessary adaptation (Rowbottom 1992). Correcting the breathing pattern is also seen to diminish perceived breathlessness by reducing the effort of breathing in and consequently reducing anxiety (Smith & Rowley 2011).

Breath Holding

If, during re-education, this feeling of air hunger becomes too great, people may sometimes find themselves taking an excessively deep breath. This, of course, further lowers their $PaCO_2$ and temporarily worsens their condition. As a corrective measure, one breath hold is recommended lasting 5 or 6 counts (2 or 3 seconds), performed after the breath out. This compensates for the preceding unnaturally deep breath and helps normalize the breathing movement (Innocenti & Troup 2008). The same authors advocate the introduction of short gentle breath holds, performed at varying points in the breathing cycle, throughout the day (without altering the depth of the breathing).

Otherwise, breath holds do not feature in most current treatment programmes (CSP Interactive 2008).

Changing the Composition of Air

Air is made up of a variety of gases, of which, oxygen contributes 21% and carbon dioxide 0.04% (Waugh & Grant 2018). However, this applies only to the air which enters the lungs. The air which leaves the lungs contains a lower proportion of oxygen and a higher proportion of carbon dioxide (exhaled air contains about 4% carbon dioxide). If a person in a hyperventilated state (i.e., with a low $PaCO_2$) rebreathes their own exhaled air, the condition will be temporarily corrected. A convenient way of doing this is to breathe into cupped hands placed over the nose and mouth and without releasing the hands, continue to breathe into them four to five times, taking a rest, then repeating the process if necessary. Hough (2001) emphasizes that the rebreathing should be gentle.

Rebreathing exhaled air is useful in acute hyperventilation and particularly if symptoms rise to panic level. Where symptoms are chronic, however, rebreathing will do little more than temporarily relieve them (Gardner & Bass 1989). Treatment for chronic hyperventilation should focus on the re-education of normal breathing movements (as earlier).

People who habitually overbreathe need to understand that their symptoms are the result of a normal chemical reaction to stress. It occurs to some extent in everyone, particularly during crises. For certain people, however, it may become a habit, which they can be helped to overcome by correcting the breathing movement and learning to identify the precipitating factors.

PRECAUTIONS

1. Breathing exercises for inducing relaxation should not be seen as a substitute for medical treatment where a disorder exists. They may, however, be used as a complement if the doctor or physiotherapist agrees.
2. People should never feel as if they are straining or forcing the breaths; they must always feel comfortable.
3. Dizziness during the breathing exercises is probably a symptom of hyperventilation – that is, the breathing exercises are being performed too deeply or too quickly. It is advisable for the person to take a rest from the breathing exercise. It is useful if the trainer describes the condition of hyperventilation at the outset.
4. Because people vary in their breathing rates, routines imposed by the trainer are not recommended in a group situation. The instructions can be phrased in such a way that participants decide on a pace that suits them.
5. Although slow, abdominal breathing can be an effective way of inducing relaxation, it may not suit everyone. In particular, people who suffer from air hunger, for whatever reason, may not find it helpful to manipulate their breathing rate.
6. Although people who suffer from panic disorder have been shown to derive benefit from relaxation, a few people occasionally report the occurrence of panic attacks during periods of relaxation. Two possible explanations are offered here. One comes from Hough (2001), who points out that relaxation weakens the psychological defences and may allow disturbing feelings to rise to the surface. An alternative explanation is put forward by Ley (1988), who suggests that if a person who is currently hyperventilating begins to relax, they lower their metabolic rate. This reduces their production of carbon dioxide. If people do not make a corresponding reduction in ventilation, their hypocapnia will increase and their symptoms become more marked (Walton 2010).

HOME PRACTICE AND SELF-MANAGEMENT

For people who are chronically hyperventilating, training the respiratory centre to accept higher levels of PCO_2 takes time. Only practice can restore the correct breathing movements. This practice consists of slow, smooth, shallow, abdominal breathing performed for about 15 minutes three times a day (Hough 2001, Innocenti & Troup 2008, Walton, 2010). In addition to this programme, there are other strategies which can help to slow the breathing rate, such as humming and reading aloud (Hough 2001). People who hyperventilate may also need to examine environmental features which trigger or aggravate their condition and deal with them in an appropriate way.

RELAXATION

Because of the association between anxiety and dysfunctional breathing, relaxation has a part to play, both as a preliminary to breathing re-education and as a component of stress management.

Treatment incorporating breathing components for a range of conditions may be found in Chapter 30.

KEY POINTS

1. The respiratory system is strongly influenced by the emotional state.
2. Unlike other body systems, the respiratory system is directly linked to that which controls physiological arousal.
3. Breathing routines accompany most relaxation techniques.

4. Abdominal breathing plays an important role in the promotion of relaxation.
5. Hyperventilation can be corrected by breathing pattern re-education.

Reflection

Describe your breathing pattern in a relaxed state and in a stressed state.
How did you feel?
Why did your body respond in that way?
What did you learn from this experience?
What is your future action plan?

CASE STUDY LEARNING OPPORTUNITIES

The key points and reflection provide the background and knowledge required in relation to the case studies, Matthew (Case Study 1) and Angela (Case Study 2), to help deepen understanding of how breathing techniques can enhance relaxation techniques.

CASE STUDY 1

Tension Headache: *Breathing Techniques for Matthew*

The pain from Matthew's tension headaches often made him breath faster than normal, especially when the pain spread from his neck to his shoulders. Matthew's wife noticed that when Matthew worried, his breathing become more irregular, but the General Practitioner (GP) confirmed there was nothing organically wrong and concluded that the stress Matthew was under could also be contributing to his change in breathing rate.

As part of Matthew's relaxation training, the trainer explained the reasons for his change in breathing rate. The trainer also helped Matthew to explore his breathing pattern, and by becoming more aware of his breathing, he began to understand the effect stress was having on his breathing. Matthew was then introduced to breathing exercises

as part of the Jacobson's progressive relaxation technique. Starting with the breathing technique of gently breathing in, holding and then letting go enabled him to start to become aware of his body and the tension he was holding in his muscles. On breathing out, he could begin to feel his muscles relax, which prepared him for the rest of the progressive relaxation.

Matthew found that the breathing exercises helped him to become more aware of when he was becoming stressed at work. He also found that by applying the breathing techniques in his workplace, gradually with daily practice, he felt more relaxed, and that it was having a direct effect on his breathing pattern. Overall this made him feel much more in control of his situation.

CASE STUDY 2

Panic Disorder and Agoraphobia: Breathing Techniques for Angela

Whenever Angela allowed her thoughts to dwell on the supermarket incident, she could feel her mouth getting dry, her throat constricting and the butterflies returning. Sometimes her hand would shake. But most of all, she noticed a change in her breathing. It became halting, shallow and so high it was almost in her neck. She felt she might collapse. These panicky feelings accompanied every journey she made to the self-help class. The facilitator suggested she was hyperventilating – overbreathing, she said – and went on to explain how it caused loss of carbon dioxide and made her symptoms worse. She emphasized the need to breathe gently, slowly, smoothly and low down in her chest – so low in fact, that Angela could feel her stomach rising and sinking.

It certainly helped to calm her down. Angela decided to practise this breathing routine regularly. After a few days, she found she was able to calm herself down without help, and as the days went by, in an ever shorter time, as she became more skilled at the routine. The panic she felt as she made her way to the class was losing its intensity. What particularly pleased her was that, besides calming her physical symptoms, the breathing sequences also seemed to settle her fears. Her head became clearer, and she felt more able to choose her thoughts.

ACTIVITY

For each of the case studies:

1. List the factors that are contributing to breathlessness.
2. Write down the impact breathlessness is having from a physical perspective.
3. Write down the impact breathlessness is having from a psychological perspective.
4. Write down the impact breathlessness is having from an emotional perspective.
5. Consider how the above are affecting overall quality of life.

Chapter 5 will focus on progressive relaxation and the work of Edmund Jacobson.

REFERENCES

Bell, J. A., & Saltikov, J. B. (2000). Mitchell's relaxation technique: Is it effective? *Physiotherapy, 86*(9), 473–478.

Birch, M. (2015). Breathing retraining in anxiety and panic disorder. Clinical update. *Australian Nursing and Midwifery Journal, 23*(4), 31–33.

Bott, J., Blumental, S., Buxton, M., & Ellum, S. (2009). Guidelines for the physiotherapy management of the adult, medical, spontaneously breathing patient. *Thorax, 64*(suppl 1), i1–i51.

Bowler, S. D., Green, A., & Mitchell, C. A. (1998). Buteyko breathing techniques in asthma: A blinded randomized controlled trial. *Medical Journal of Australia, 169*, 575–578.

Bruton, A., Armstrong, M., Chadwick, C., Gibson, D., & Gahr, K. (2006). Preliminary investigations into the effects of end-tidal CO2 measures in patients with asthma and healthy volunteers during a single treatment session. *Physiotherapy, 93*(1), 30–36.

Bruton, A., & Lewith, G. T. (2005). The Buteyko breathing technique for asthma: A review. *Complementary Therapies in Medicine, 13*(1), 41–46.

Clark, D. M., Salkovskis, P. M., & Chalkley, A. J. (1985). Respiratory control as a treatment for panic attacks. *Journal of Behavior Therapy and Experimental Psychiatry, 16*, 23–30.

Cowie, R. L., Conley, D. P., Underwood, M. F., & Reader, P. G. (2008). A randomized controlled trial of the Buteyko method technique as an adjunct to conventional management of asthma. *Respiratory Medicine, 102*(5), 726–732.

Cowley, D. S. (1987). Hyperventilation and panic disorder. *American Journal of Medicine, 83*, 929–937.

CSP Interactive. (2008). *Respiratory care*. London: Chartered Society of Physiotherapy.

Duncan, D. (2009). Understanding hyperventilation syndrome. *Clinical Respiratory Independent Nurse, 28*–30.

Everly, G. S., & Rosenfeld, R. (1981). *The nature and treatment of the stress response*. New York: Plenum Press.

Gardner, W. N. (1992). Hyperventilation syndromes. *Respiratory Medicine, 86*, 273–275.

Gardner, W. N., & Bass, C. (1989). Hyperventilation in clinical practice. *British Journal of Hospital Medicine, 41*, 73–81.

Gardner, W. N. (1996). The pathophysiology of hyperventilation disorders. *Chest, 109*, 516–534.

Garssen, B., de Ruiter, C., & van Dyke, R. (1992). Breathing retraining: A rational placebo? *Clinical Psychology Review, 12*, 141–153.

Gilbert, C. (2003). Clinical application of breathing regulation: Beyond anxiety management. *Behavior Modification, 27*, 692–709.

Han, J. N., Stegen, E., de Valck, C., Clement, J., & van de Woestijne, K. P. (1996). The influence of breathing therapy on anxiety and breathing patterns in patients with hyperventilation syndrome and anxiety disorders. *Journal of Psychosomatic Research, 41*(5), 481–493.

Holloway, E. A., & West, R. J. (2007). Integrated breathing and relaxation training (the Papworth method) for adults with asthma in primary care: A randomized controlled trial. *Thorax, 62*, 1039–1042.

Hough, A. (2001). *Physiotherapy in respiratory care: An evidence-based approach to respiratory and cardiac management* (3rd ed.). Cheltenham, UK: Nelson Thornes.

Innocenti, D. M. (1983). Chronic hyperventilation syndrome. In P. A. Downie (Ed.), *Cash's textbook of chest, heart and vascular disorders for physiotherapists* (3rd ed.). London: Faber and Faber.

Innocenti, D. M., & Troup, F. (2008). Dysfunctional breathing. In J. Pryor, & A. Prasad (Eds.), *Physiotherapy for respiratory and cardiac problems* (4th ed., pp. 529–549). Edinburgh: Churchill Livingstone.

Jardins, T. D. (2012). *Cardiopulmonary anatomy and physiology: Essentials of respiratory care* (6th ed.). Chicago: Cengage Learning.

Kaushik, R., Kaushik, R. M., Mahajan, S. K., et al. (2005). Biofeedback-assisted diaphragmatic breathing and systematic relaxation versus propranolol in long-term prophylaxis of migraine. *Complementary Therapies in Medicine, 13*(3), 165–174.

Kellett, C., & Mullan, J. (2002). Breathing control techniques in the management of asthma. *Physiotherapy, 88*(12), 751–758.

Kern, B., Rosh, A. J. (2016). Hyperventilation syndrome. Available at: https://emedicine.medscape.com/article/807277-overview. Accessed February 2019.

Ley, R. (1988). Panic attacks during relaxation and relaxation-induced anxiety: A hyperventilation interpretation. *Journal of Behavior Therapy and Experimental Psychiatry, 19*, 253–259.

Lichstein, K. L. (1988). *Clinical relaxation strategies*. New York: John Wiley.

Lum, L. C. (1981). Hyperventilation and anxiety state. *Journal of the Royal Society of Medicine, 74*, 1–4.

Matsumoto, M., & Smith, J. C. (2001). Progressive muscle relaxation, breathing exercises and ABC relaxation theory. *Journal of Clinical Psychology, 57*(12), 1551–1557.

Meuret, A. E., Wilhelm, F. H., Ritz, T., et al. (2003). Breathing retraining for treating panic disorder: Useful intervention or impediment? *Behavior Modification, 27*(5), 731–754.

Meuret, A. E., Ritz, T., Wilhelm, F. H., et al. (2005). Voluntary hyperventilation in the treatment of panic disorder: Functions of hyperventilation, their implications for breathing training and recommendations for standardization. *Clinical Psychology Review, 25*(3), 285–306.

Miller, K. M., & Perry, P. A. (1990). Relaxation techniques and postoperative pain in patients undergoing cardiac surgery. *Heart Lung, 19*(2), 136–145.

Pinney, S., Freeman, L. J., & Nixon, P. G. F. (1987). Role of the nurse counsellor in managing patients with the hyperventilation syndrome. *Journal of the Royal Society of Medicine, 80*, 216–218.

Ristiniemi, H., Perski, A., Lyskov, E., & Emtner, M. (2014). Hyperventilation and exhaustion syndrome. *Scandinavian Journal of Caring Sciences, 28*, 657–664.

Rowbottom, I. (1992). The physiotherapy management of chronic hyperventilation. *Journal of the Association of Chartered Physiotherapists in Respiratory Conditions, 21*, 9–12.

Slonim, N. B., & Hamilton, L. H. (1987). *Respiratory physiology* (5th ed.). St Louis, MO: Mosby.

Smith, T. C., & Rowley, J. (2011). Breathing pattern disorders and physiotherapy: Inspiration for our profession. *Physical Therapy Reviews, 16*(1), 75–86.

Sudsuang, R., Chentanez, V., & Veluvan, K. (1991). Effect of Buddhist meditation on serum cortisol and total protein levels, blood pressure, pulse rate, lung volume and reaction time. *Physiology and Behavior, 50*, 543–548.

Thomas, S. (2004). Buteyko: A useful tool in the management of asthma? *International Journal of Therapy and Rehabilitation, 11*(10), 476–480.

Tweeddale, P. M., Rowbottom, I., & McHardy, G. J. R. (1994). Breathing retraining: Effect on anxiety and depression scores in behavioural breathlessness. *Journal of Psychosomatic Research, 38*(1), 11–21.

van Doorn, P., Colla, P., & Folgering, H. (1982). Control of end-tidal PCO_2 in the hyperventilation syndrome: Effects of biofeedback and breathing instructions compared. *Bulletin Européen de Physiopathologie Respiratoire, 18*, 829–836.

van Dixhoorn, J., & Duivenvoorden, J. A. (1989). Breathing awareness as a relaxation method in cardiac rehabilitation. In *Stress and tension control* (3rd ed., pp. 19–36). New York: Plenum.

Walton, T. (2010). Diversity of effective treatments of panic attacks: What do they have in common? *Depression and Anxiety, 27*, 5–11.

Waugh, A., & Grant, A. (2018). *Ross & Wilson anatomy and physiology in health and illness* (13th ed.). Edinburgh: Churchill Livingstone Elsevier.

Wilkinson, L., Buboltz, W. C., & Young, T. R. (2002). Breathing techniques to promote client relaxation and tension reduction. *Journal of Clinical Activities, Assignments & Handouts in Psychotherapy Practice, 2*(1), 1–14.

Wilson, C. (2018). Hyperventilation syndrome: Diagnosis and reassurance. *Journal of Paramedic Practice, 10*(9), 370–375.

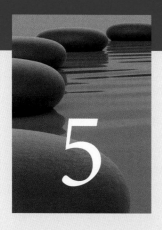

5 PROGRESSIVE RELAXATION

PROFESSOR TEENA CLOUSTON

CHAPTER CONTENTS

LEARNING OBJECTIVES

The aim of this chapter is to provide a practical guide to basic concepts of progressive relaxation.

By the end of this chapter you will be able to:

1. Understand the key principles and process of Jacobson's progressive relaxation

2. Discern the differences between the active and passive progressive relaxation approaches

3. Recognize the importance of the relationship between physiological muscle tension in the body and neurological responses

4. Identify the value of 'diminishing tension' in the body and how that helps you to learn to relax

5. Carry out a progressive relaxation session following Jacobson's original theory and method

This chapter will conclude with key points and time for reflection, providing learning opportunities through case studies.

INTRODUCTION TO PROGRESSIVE RELAXATION

To many people, relaxation training means learning techniques such as 'tense–release', that is, the tightening and letting go of specific muscle groups. In this approach, the tense–release action is an active process in the sense that individuals are actively and consciously working their muscles. Some muscle relaxation methods, however, are concerned only with the 'release' part of the sequence, and these could be described as passive muscular approaches.

This chapter introduces the work of Edmund Jacobson (1888–1938), a pioneer in this field of progressive relaxation. His work lays the foundation of both the tense–release and the passive approaches to relaxation which are generally used today. So important was Jacobson's work that, although the original process has been modified quite considerably over time, the technique of progressive relaxation is still synonymous with his name and is commonly known as Jacobsonian relaxation. This chapter describes Jacobson's original method of progressive muscular relaxation to (1 give you historical context and to set the scene for the more contemporary practical approaches that follow in Chapters 6 through 9; and 2) consider the specific application of Jacobson's techniques in present practice.

INTRODUCTION TO EVIDENCE

Jacobson's original ideas about progressive relaxation (PR) are based on what is known as a physiological approach because its procedures are concerned with physical organs (i.e., muscles and nerves). Although the act of focusing on muscular sensations gives it a cognitive slant, Jacobson proposed that it was a relaxed musculature that predominated in exerting a calming influence on the whole organism, including the mind. Essentially, Jacobson demonstrated that cognitive processes or thinking can be controlled through skeletal muscles, and that negative thoughts can dissipate in a state of deep physical relaxation (Jacobson 1938). He also maintained that people, can think more clearly when they are physically relaxed, and this, in turn, helps them to solve their emotional problems (Lehrer 1982).

What is important in Jacobson's work is that it promotes the value of the physical state of relaxation to address negative thinking or cognitive stress, and this physiological stance is notable. For Jacobson, PR was primarily used as a tool to address psychosomatic conditions – that is, stress-related conditions with physical manifestations. Lehrer (1982) maintains that Jacobson's original studies (Jacobson 1938) evidence excellent outcomes when used as an intervention tool to reduce physiological arousal. Thus this technique remains a therapeutically important approach in this context, suggesting that Jacobson's original approach still has merit and relevance today. This is an essential point to consider because his original method has become somewhat diluted and the underpinning theories forgotten in the context of the various modifications and applications of the PR technique today. Please be cognisant of this point as we look at the evidence base in more detail.

As previously noted, PR has changed over time, but in one form or another, it is widely used in the clinical field, and its effectiveness has been tested in many

conditions (Lehrer 1996). Although findings have been mixed, the general sense is that PR is an effective intervention in a variety of conditions.

In a comprehensive review of relaxation techniques, Kerr (2000) cites studies which have shown reductions in both physiological and psychological indicators of stress after a course of PR. Focusing on the treatment of pain in adults, Kwekkeboom and Gretarsdottir (2006) carried out a systematic review of randomized controlled trials to investigate the effectiveness of what they termed "progressive muscle relaxation" alongside that of a range of other mind–body methods. Eight of the fifteen trials reviewed contained evidence supporting their use. The intervention most often cited was PR, where arthritis pain was singled out as deriving particular benefit. Postoperative pain responded best to jaw relaxation and systematic relaxation. There was little evidence in favour of autogenic training and still less for rhythmic breathing or other techniques. Although these findings are positive, the authors note that inferences drawn are tentative, as the methodological quality of some of the studies warrant caution. They suggest that more research in the area of PR is needed.

Hui et al (2006) compared the effects of PR with qigong to determine their relative properties when applied to the quality of life among cardiac patients. A total of 65 patients with cardiac diseases ranging through myocardial infarct, valve replacement, post-coronary intervention and ischaemic heart disease took part in a study consisting of eight 20-minute sessions. Both interventions were effective in reducing blood pressure, but PR provided greater benefit. PR was also found to be more effective in somatic domains, whereas qigong seemed more effective in psychological ones.

More recent findings include a study by Vancampfort et al (2013), who carried out a systematic review to establish the effectiveness of progressive muscle relaxation on the psychological distress, anxiety symptoms and response/remission levels of people diagnosed with schizophrenia. Findings identified that PR could be a useful tool to reduce both anxiety and psychological distress and consequently improve subjective well-being.

A remarkably interesting study by Aiger et al (2016) compared the psychophysiological arousal levels of cancer patients while they were waiting for diagnostic screening, specifically, a positron emission tomography–computed tomography (PET-CT) scan. Half of the experimental group (n = 39) received Jacobson's PR techniques along with breathing exercises and visualization before the scan; the other half, the control group, did not. Results showed that the patients who performed the relaxation techniques were more attentive or present and calmer throughout the process (Aiger et al 2016).

Although these conclusions are positive in terms of PR, other studies have shown either equal outcomes when comparing PR with other stress-reducing approaches or no effects at all from a course of PR. In Salt and Kerr's (1997) study, for example, PR was compared with the Mitchell method of relaxation (see Chapter 13) in 24 normotensive participants. Findings evidenced significant reductions in heart rate, respiratory rate and blood pressure for both methods equally, without any significant difference in effectiveness between the two interventions. Similarly, Crist and Rickard (1993) found no difference in outcome between muscular and imaginal relaxation in 100 healthy students, but the pre- and posttrial effects were significant for both groups.

A systematic review by Conrad and Roth (2007) looked at the effects of what they term 'abbreviations' of the original Jacobsonian method on patients experiencing generalized anxiety disorder and panic disorder. Using a physiological approach that measured activation of the muscles and abnormal autonomic and respiratory responses, the authors were unable to find evidence to support the effectiveness of muscle relaxation in those conditions. Supporting the recommendations of Kwekkeboom and Gretarsdottir (2006), they further concluded that better designed studies were needed before firm conclusions could be drawn about the effectiveness of PR (Conrad & Roth 2007).

Overall, these studies would suggest that PR is an effective tool in reducing or diminishing muscle tension and inducing a sense of relaxation and calm. However, there is room for further high-quality research to take place and, because some of these studies may have used modified or abbreviated forms of the original Jacobsonian technique, aspects of the original theory may have been diluted.

THEORIES BEHIND PROGRESSIVE RELAXATION

Working as a physiologist-physician in the 1930s, Jacobson was investigating the startle reaction that follows a sudden loud noise. He noticed that people who were able to fully relax their muscles made no startled response. Thus he assumed from this that the state of the muscle influenced the magnitude of the reflex. To investigate his idea, he invented a technique for measuring the electrical activity in muscles and nerves which became known as electromyography (EMG); this allowed him to study hitherto unexplored aspects of physiology. Arising out of this new technology, he was able to demonstrate that thinking was related to muscle state, and that mental images, particularly those associated with movement, were accompanied by small but detectable levels of activity in the muscles concerned (Jacobson 1938).

This integrated activity between the mind and the muscles led him to view the brain centres and the voluntary muscles as working together 'in one effort circuit' (Jacobson 1970) – a neuromuscular circuit, because it was composed of both neural and muscular tissue. From this understanding, Jacobson proposed that just as a calm mind would be reflected in a tension-free body, so a relaxed musculature would be accompanied by the quietening of thoughts and the reduction of sympathetic activity, notions that would have relevance in the treatment of anxiety and associated conditions. The task facing Jacobson, therefore, was to find a way of inducing the skeletal muscles to lose their tension.

Muscle activity is accompanied by sensations so faint that we do not normally notice them. To promote awareness of tension, Jacobson emphasized the need to concentrate on those sensations, cultivating what he called 'learned awareness'. Once tension had been recognized, it would be easier to release it. If relaxation were then achieved, however, how deep would it be?

It is traditionally held that, in the waking state, healthy muscle, even during rest, is in a state of sustained, slight contraction. This is called muscle tone. Jacobson's EMG studies (1938) did not, however, support this notion. He found that voluntary muscle could achieve a state of complete relaxation during rest. He consequently formed the view that the aim of relaxation training should be to eliminate *all* tension, and relaxation could only be called complete if it proceeded 'to the zero point of tonus for the part or parts involved' (Jacobson 1938). Any tension that remained while resting a muscle was called 'residual', and it was this residual tension that Jacobson sought to eliminate in deep relaxation. 'Doing away with residual tension is … the essential feature of the present method' (Jacobson 1976, p 99).

Defining relaxation as the cessation of activity in the skeletal (voluntary) muscles, Jacobson devised a technique which he called progressive relaxation. It consisted of systematically working through the major skeletal muscle groups, creating and releasing tension. As a result, the trainee learned how to recognize muscle tension. Only one muscle action was carried out in each session, and it was repeated twice. The rest of the time was spent releasing tension. Jacobson (1938) insisted that his method be regarded as a skill to be learned. Unlike most other approaches, the use of suggestion was discouraged. Trainers were urged to avoid planting ideas of the kind: 'Your limbs are heavy/limp/relaxed' or even 'Notice how your limbs are feeling heavy/limp/relaxed'. This was because Jacobson wanted learners to make their own discoveries about their own unique neuromuscular body and mind circuit and, essentially, the influence of the motor act on the relaxed state (Munzert & Krüger 2018).

In addition to PR, Jacobson (1964) developed a method of instruction which he called 'self-operations control'. The principles of recognizing and eliminating tension are the same as those of PR. The emphasis, however, is placed on self-direction: the individual controlling muscle tension throughout the events of daily life, learning 'to go on and off … as different occasions may require' (Jacobson 1964). Through this process, the individual learns to monitor all sensations of tension, simultaneously and automatically, and to release those tensions which are not desired, in a continuing process (McGuigan 1984). The result is a decreased consumption of energy, which in effect extends to other body systems such as the autonomic nervous system, where sympathetic activity is reduced. Thought processes are also believed to benefit from the tension-decreasing effect (McGuigan 1981). This

method, however, takes as long to learn as Jacobson's original technique.

Jacobson (1938) also investigated the degree of tension necessary for carrying out a particular activity. He drew a distinction between those muscles actually performing the activity and those muscles not involved in it. The first group needed the minimum level of tension consistent with performing the task; the second group could be totally relaxed or as relaxed as possible. This differential in the degree of tension required was studied by Jacobson for the purpose of reducing both the excessive effort often used by the first group and the unnecessary effort often used by the second (Kyrios et al 2018). Differential relaxation is discussed in more detail in Chapter 11.

To summarize, Jacobson's fundamental theory was in fact quite complicated. His work was built over several years and focused on the physiological effects of mental motor imagery as well as progressive muscular relaxation (Munzert & Krüger 2018). He evidenced that progressive muscular relaxation could induce a relaxed state in both the mind and body. He did this by asking people to focus on a specific muscle to investigate the relationship between both physiological and mental processes. In this sense, he was a progenitor of psychophysiology, motor imagery and mental simulation theory as well as PR (Munzert & Krüger 2018).

KEY ASPECTS OF THE PROCEDURE

Ideal conditions for presenting PR include a quiet and private room where you will not be disturbed. If possible, the room should be big enough for trainees to lie down comfortably with plenty of room between them. This is important for personal comfort and a sense of safety. A large room with a carpeted floor is suitable for a group; however, equipment such as relaxation mats can be provided or trainees may be asked to bring a beach mattress or the equivalent to lie on, and a small pillow for the head. Lying is the position of choice; however, it is possible to learn PR in the sitting position, and comfortable but supportive chairs can be used. Before starting the training properly, the basis of the method must be introduced. With the trainees seated, the trainer describes the rationale of PR along the following lines.

Knowing how to rest the body enables body energy to be used more efficiently. It can also help to protect us from illness. This is a method of relaxing that involves the muscles. By creating and releasing tension, you will learn to tune into subtle feelings in the muscles, to recognize different levels of tension and to release that tension.

Muscle tension is believed to be closely associated with your state of mind: it is believed that muscles which are unnecessarily tense reflect their tension in the mind. If that muscle tension can be released, you will feel mentally calmer.

Your internal organs will also benefit in that pulse rate and blood pressure will be lowered while you are relaxing.

The method we are using is called progressive relaxation. It is not possible to learn it in one lesson. However, every bit as important as the lessons is the practice that you put in between them. Like any skill, the more you practise it, the more proficient you will become, and the more you will benefit from its effects, in this case relaxation.

The muscle action to be taught is then demonstrated, after which, trainees are asked to lie down, face upwards, with arms resting on either side of the body, legs uncrossed. The eyes are open to begin with, but after 3 or 4 minutes, trainees are asked to close them and to spend a few minutes quietly unwinding.

First Session: Wrist Bending Backwards

A first session would take the following form. The trainee is asked to extend the left wrist (bend it back) and to hold it in that position for 1 minute (Fig. 5.1).

The trainee then releases the tension, letting go all at once, and continues to relax the part for 3 minutes, during which, any residual tension is also released. This action is then repeated twice. The instruction might run as follows.

Would you please bend the left hand back at the wrist. Do this steadily without seesawing ... and avoid raising the forearm ... continue to hold the hand back for a full minute, noticing the different sensations you get from doing it.

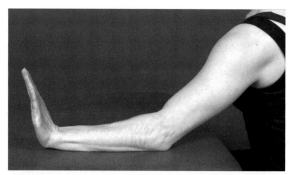

Fig. 5.1 ■ Wrist bending backwards.

Using Jacobson's technique, it is not suggested to the trainee what these sensations might be; the idea is that the trainee should discover them for themselves – that is, learned awareness is facilitated. However, in this case, sensations would include tension in the working muscles situated along the top of the forearm and across the back of the hand, together with some sensations of strain in the wrist joint and skin stretching in the palm. Of these, it is the muscle sensations that the trainee should learn to focus on.

As you continue to bend your wrist back, distinguish between the various feelings you are experiencing ... pick out particularly those related to the muscles ... concentrate on the sensation of tenseness ... keeping the action sustained until the minute is up ...

And now, discontinue the action ... allow the hand to fall by its own weight. Let it flop down. Avoid lowering it slowly or in any way controlling its descent.

Although you have let go as completely as you could, there may still be some tension there. Give it plenty of time to disappear ... give it at least 3 minutes as you focus on the sensation in the muscles ...

Now, bend the wrist back a second time ... feel the effort ... if you are finding difficulty in sorting out the feelings in the arm, allow the hand to fall down and try the following: with your right hand, pick up the left hand and gently press it back as if it didn't belong to you ... continue to press for about half a minute. Make sure the right hand does all the work. The feelings you're getting are coming from the wrist and from the palm. With your left hand still bent back, take away your right hand and as you do, transfer the power to your left arm. You are now using muscles in the left forearm to hold the left wrist back. Notice the new feelings you are getting … these are the feelings you are asked to concentrate on … continue to hold the wrist back for about a minute …

Now, cease the action and allow the hand to fall down, letting all the tension go … letting the muscle go negative … concentrating on the feelings you are getting from it … continue in that direction for the next 3 minutes …

The trainee is not asked to 'relax', which Jacobson felt might create tensions on its own account, but to 'discontinue', 'cease to bend' or 'go negative'. Relaxation occurs on its own as the learner releases tension.

One further repetition is carried out before the trainee adopts a state of continuous rest for the remainder of the hour when the session comes to an end.

Second Session: Wrist Bending Forwards

At the following session, a new action is introduced: wrist flexion (bending forwards). This action follows the same pattern as the previous one, except that the wrist is bent forwards instead of backwards (Fig. 5.2).

I'd like you to bend the left hand forward at the wrist … hold the position steadily … locate the feeling of tenseness (the underside of the forearm) … and (when the minute is up) … discontinue the action … let the hand fall back … continue

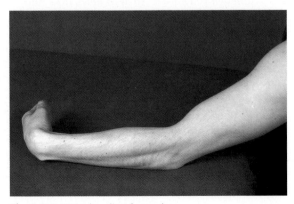

Fig. 5.2 ■ Wrist bending forwards.

letting go any remaining tension over the next few minutes … tuning in to the feelings in the muscle in the forearm …

Two repetitions are carried out, after which, the trainee rests. That marks the end of session number two.

Third and Subsequent Sessions

The third session does not contain any tensing component. Instead, the time is entirely devoted to releasing tension. Subsequent sessions are spent addressing other actions and may cover many weeks. The protocol is outlined below and laid out in full in Table 5.1.

- *Arms:* five items for each arm; tensing and releasing of arm and hand muscles.
- *Legs:* seven items for each leg; tensing and releasing of thigh, leg and foot muscles.
- *Trunk:* seven items; tensing and releasing of back, abdomen and shoulder muscles.
- *Neck:* four items; tensing and relaxing of muscles around the neck.
- *Eye area:* eight items; tensing and relaxing the muscles of the forehead and the eyes.
- *Visualization:* six items; imagining different objects, moving and stationary.
- *Speech area:* 15 items; tensing and relaxing muscles associated with speech; counting and reciting, first in a normal voice, then gradually getting fainter.
- Only one or two new actions are introduced at each period of tuition, and the whole programme takes about 50 sessions. In addition, an hour a day is devoted to home practice.

'Diminishing Tensions'

Jacobson avoided using the word *exercise* to describe the actions, since exercise, designed as it is to strengthen muscles, implies increasing effort. The wrist bending and other actions in PR are introduced simply to teach awareness of the different sensations that arise in activated muscle tissue. Learning to recognize these sensations requires differing levels of muscle tension. Of these, the lower levels are the most useful for picking up residual tension, as it is here that sensitivity to small fluctuations is greatest (Jacobson 1970,

TABLE 5.1	
Progressive relaxation: schedule of items (adapted from Jacobson 1964)	
Arms	Extend wrist (bend hand back)
	Flex wrist (bend hand forward)
	Relax only
	Flex (bend) elbow
	Extend elbow (straighten arm)
	Relax only
	Stiffen whole arm
Legs	Dorsiflex foot (bend foot up at ankle joint)
	Plantarflex foot (bend foot down at ankle joint)
	Relax only
	Extend (straighten) knee from a bent position
	Flex (bend) knee, dragging foot along floor
	Relax only
	Flex hip (raise bent knee towards chest)
	Extend hip (press thigh down into the supporting surface)
	Relax only
	Stiffen entire leg
Trunk	Contract (pull in) abdomen
	Extend spine (arch back slightly)
	Relax only
	Observe the action of breathing
	Brace shoulders back
	Relax only
	Flex shoulder joint (bring bent arm across chest)
	Repeat with the other arm
	Relax only
	Raise (hunch) shoulders
Neck	Press head back into pillow/headrest
	Raise head off pillow
	Relax only
	Bend head to right
	Bend head to left
	Relax only

(*Continued*)

TABLE 5.1 (CONT.)	
Progressive relaxation: schedule of items (adapted from Jacobson 1964)	
Upper face area	Raise eyebrows
	Frown
	Relax only
Eye area	Close eyes tightly
	Look left with eyes closed
	Relax only
	Look right with eyes closed
	Look up with eyes closed
	Relax only
	Look down with eyes closed
	Look forward with eyes closed
	Relax only
Visual imagination	Imagine a pen moving slowly, then fast
	Imagine a train passing, a person walking by
	Relax eyes
	Imagine a bird flying and stationary
	Imagine a ball rolling, the Houses of Parliament
	Relax eyes
	Imagine a horse grazing, a reel of cotton
	Imagine the Prime Minister
	Relax eyes
Jaw, voice and auditory imagination	Close jaws firmly Open jaws Relax only Bare teeth Pout Relax only Press tongue against teeth Pull tongue backwards Relax only Count aloud up to 10 Count half as loudly up to 10 Relax only Count softly up to 10 Count under your breath up to 10 Relax only Imagine you are counting Imagine you are reciting the alphabet Relax only Imagine saying: your name three times, your address three times, the Prime Minister's name three times

Lehrer et al 1988, Munzert & Krüger 2018). Thus the actions require an ever-*decreasing* intensity of contraction to fulfil their purpose.

To help the trainee become sensitized to low levels of tension, Jacobson devised a technique called 'diminishing tensions'. It is introduced as the learner becomes proficient in recognizing the sensation of tension. Returning to the action of wrist bending, the trainee would be instructed in the following way.

> *Bend your wrist back but this time using only half as much effort as you did the first time. Hold it back for about a minute, noticing the sensations you're getting from the muscle … and at the end of the minute … cease holding it back. Go negative … feel the tension leaving … allow plenty of time for the remaining tension to disappear … allow 3 minutes … then bend the wrist back again, this time tensing the muscle half as much as last time … hold it for about a minute, tuning in to the sensations … then release the tension … release it further … and further still … allow 3 minutes … now, raise the wrist the smallest amount possible … hold it there … for 1 minute … discontinue … allow 3 minutes … and finally, make the action just a thought … hold the thought for 1 minute … go negative … spend 3 minutes continuing to go negative…*

These progressively diminishing tensions train the individual to recognize differing levels, thus increasing individual control over the voluntary musculature.

Jacobson's assigning of every third session exclusively to passive relaxation is evidence of the high value he placed on the relaxation phase and the relatively low value he gave to the contraction phase, using it simply as a means of cultivating sensitivity to the tension sensation. Many of his successors have, by contrast, attached great importance to the contraction, claiming that it leads to a deepening of the subsequent relaxation. Jacobson argued that the reverse may be the case – namely, that tensions which build up during the contraction phase would continue to persist for some time, thus hindering relaxation. In untrained participants, he showed that muscle tension continues to remain elevated for up to several minutes after a contraction, even when the participant is co-operating

with appeals to 'go negative' (Jacobson 1934). Thus deliberate muscle tensing may, in the short term at least, actually obstruct the relaxation process.

The issue of tense–release versus a release-only approach has not been satisfactorily resolved. It has been common in clinical practice to favour tense–release. However, the results of a 1991 study (Lucic et al 1991) support the view that initial tensing is detrimental to relaxation, and this finding may have strengthened interest in passive approaches. Little formal research has been carried out on this topic since, but it is worth considering that both views may have some merit and can be used in practice.

Eye Movements

The procedures for the eye and forehead and for the area of the speech muscles differ somewhat from those of the trunk and limbs. Consequently, they are presented in more detail.

Although Jacobson (1938) indicated that only one or two actions should be carried out in each session, it is customary today to work through all the eye actions in a single session. Plenty of time should still be allowed for 'going negative'.

Jacobson's studies had demonstrated the effectiveness of PR in reducing muscle tension. He had also been able to show that a relaxed musculature had a calming effect on the mind (Jacobson 1938). Muscle relaxation could thus be seen as a mental relaxant. But Jacobson went further: he claimed that in deep relaxation, thought itself disappeared. In the totally relaxed body, the mind would be a blank.

The eye muscles were considered by him to be particularly closely related to thought, since thinking created mental images which were accompanied by a sense of tension around the eyes. Releasing tension from the eyes, Jacobson believed, had the effect of cancelling those images. The following sequences are adapted from Jacobson (1970). Time should be allowed between the items for the trainee to absorb the message.

> *With your eyes open, raise your eyebrows … feel the tension … and release it … frown … feel the tension … and discontinue … shut your eyes tightly … feel the tension … and let it go … with your eyes still closed, spend a few minutes releasing tension in this part of your face …*

Moving on to the eyes themselves (they are still closed) … without moving your head, turn your eyes upwards as if you were looking at the ceiling. As you do so, notice the sensation you get in the eye region … next, turn your eyes downwards as if you were looking at your feet, again taking note of the feelings around the eyes … repeat that several times, until you become familiar with the sensation in the eye muscles … then discontinue, going negative for a minute or so … still with your eyes closed, turn your eyes to the left for a few moments … now to the right … repeat this a few times to experience the transient sensations in the muscles … then, cease the action … do nothing for a few minutes …

Would you now, still with your eyes closed, imagine you are looking at the ceiling and the floor; do not actively look up and down, but simply think of looking up and down … notice the feelings (that is, the same sensations as when you deliberately turned your eyes up and down, although to a much lesser degree) … when you have identified the feeling, let your eye muscles go negative … notice what happens to the images … rest for a few minutes …

Now, imagine that you see the wall on your left … and the wall on your right … imagine seeing one after the other, noticing that slight tensions accompany the images … now, let your eyes go … and notice what happens to the images …

Similar effects can be created by imagining objects from everyday life: imagine a car passing … or a ball bouncing up and down … notice the sensation that accompanies the image … then let the eye muscles go negative and notice what happens to the images …

Multiply 16 by 80 in your head … when you have got the answer, notice how the eyes felt during the task … then, rest the eyes and notice what happens to the figures …

If the eyes are completely relaxed, the image disappears, and the thought dies (Jacobson 1964). The individual, however, has made no effort to stop the thought process. Rather, he or she is asked only to release tension, 'letting other effects come as they may' (Jacobson 1976). Whether thought does in fact disappear in a totally relaxed body has not been scientifically established. Jacobson (1938) was, however, able to produce clinical evidence of the success of ocular relaxation in overcoming insomnia.

Speech Movements

The speech muscles are also closely related to thought. Thinking with the use of words causes minute flickers of tension in the muscles of the tongue and jaw. Conversely, when these muscles are relaxed, thinking with the use of words is no longer possible (Jacobson 1970).

The following script begins with tensing of the speech muscles and ends with sequences of counting using 'diminishing tensions'. As with the eye actions, it is customary today to present the whole group in one session. As a rough guide, 5 to 10 seconds can be allowed for each action and 30 to 40 seconds for 'going negative'. Each action is repeated once.

Close the jaws firmly, noticing the sensations you get from the action … hold it … and … discontinue … let your jaw drop … feel the tension leaving you … and continuing to leave you … then repeat the sequence…

Next, bare your teeth … feel the tension in the cheeks … hold it for a few seconds … and cease the action …

Make a tight 'O' with your lips … hold it, while you register tension in the lips … and … go negative …

Press your tongue against your teeth … feel the pressure … and discontinue …

Now, pull the tongue back towards the throat. Feel the muscles drawing it back and note the sensations you get from this action … and … let it go negative …

Tune in to the presence of residual tension in any of the muscles associated with speech and let that tension recede … and go on receding …

(Allow several minutes for the last phase.)
A counting sequence follows, using diminishing tensions.

Count aloud slowly from one to ten, picking up the sensations you get from the muscles in the mouth, throat, face and chest. Repeat it a few times … then stop counting ... allow time for the full release of tension ...

Now, count again, half as loudly ... noticing the reduced amount of tension in the speech muscles ... discontinue ... next time, count softly ... notice the tension ... and let it go ... and now, under your breath ... still concentrating on the feelings you get in the mouth, jaw and throat ... rest a moment ... and now, simply imagine the counting ... here perhaps you can detect a flickering in the speech muscles ... finally, cease to count altogether ...

When the speech muscles ceased to be involved, Jacobson (1938, 1964, 1976) claimed that it was no longer possible to think in verbal terms. The notion that thought disappears in states of deep muscle relaxation is consistent with a theory which sees mental processes being influenced by the state of the skeletal musculature (Lehrer 1982).

PRECAUTIONS

The precautions described cover Chapters 5, 6, 7, 8 and 9. In general terms, it would seem that PR is appropriate in any circumstances where rest and relaxation are prescribed (McGuigan 1984). The method is unlikely to create negative effects, and Jacobson did not refer to any. Some points, however, need to be considered.

1. Training in relaxation should never be viewed as a substitute for medical treatment; wherever a disorder is present or suspected, medical help should be sought.
2. Variations in the blood pressure may occur in the course of relaxation training: it can rise when limbs are being tensed and fall during deep relaxation. The fall in blood pressure which accompanies deep relaxation is only that which occurs under any resting condition. After a session of relaxation, it is important to allow time for the individual to adjust before becoming active to avoid the risk of fainting.
3. The feet and legs should not be crossed during relaxation. This can lead to a temporary increase in blood pressure.
4. Driving or operating machinery should be avoided immediately after relaxation; time should be given to become fully present and self-aware first.
5. PR should not be practised when driving or during any other activity that requires the individual's full attention and concentration.
6. For people whose blood pressure is already high and for cardiac patients, a release-only method (see Chapter 8) is preferable to one which consists of tensing the muscles.
7. Active (i.e., tense and relax) progressive muscle relaxation may be contraindicated in antenatal or labouring mothers because of the possibility of interference with uterine contractions. Release-only forms (i.e., passive relaxation) would, however, be appropriate.
8. Tense–release procedures performed with excessive tightening may lead to cramp. To avoid this, trainees can be advised to shorten the tension period (Bernstein et al 2000). Recurrent cramp would indicate the unsuitability of the technique for that individual. Over tensing the spine and the neck should also be avoided because it can lead to spinal damage.
9. Some individuals find that focusing on the body intensifies their perception of pain (Snyder 1985), and for them, muscular approaches may be less useful than cognitive ones, such as imagery or meditation.
10. Trainees who, because of disability or disorder, are in doubt as to the suitability of any exercise should begin by performing it very gently. This applies, for example, to individuals with back or neck problems.
11. Some tense–release scripts make use of imagery. They will therefore, in addition, be subject to the precautions listed in Chapter 18.

APPLICATION

PR is widely used in the clinical field for reducing mental and physical tension. It has a particular use in helping trainees to understand the link between the physical and mental state. This is because it requires them to actively tense and relax muscle groups, or uses a passive relax-only approach, using mental imagery to focus on the muscles, and release them through the power of thought. It is an excellent method to begin to learn and understand what a relaxed state actually feels like physically and this, in turn, calms the mind. In its early form, however, it is seldom practised; its great length, accompanied by problems of time and money, constitute a major disadvantage. It has in many instances been replaced by modifications, one of which is described in the following chapter.

KEY POINTS

1. Jacobson formulated his progressive relaxation programme as a result of his experiments on the startle reaction.
2. The programme is based on the notion that a relaxed musculature exerts a calming influence on the mind.
3. The progressive relaxation programme itself consists of the alternative tensing and releasing of skeletal muscle groups, during which, the trainee is asked to take note of the sensations in the working muscle groups.
4. In particular, Jacobson asks the trainee to recognize and release residual tension.
5. As the trainee becomes more proficient, the tension component is dropped, and attention is focused exclusively on release.
6. Progressive relaxation is a skill, the mastery of which depends on daily practice.

Reflection

Describe your understanding of the technique of progressive muscular relaxation.

How did you feel when you completed your own progressive relaxation, and how do you think it could be applied in practice?

Why do you think Jacobson focused on 'learned awareness' as an important aspect of applying the method?

What did you learn about the 'neuromuscular circuit', and how this underpinned Jacobson's psychophysiological approach to relaxation?

What is the main learning point you will take away from this chapter?

What is your future action plan in terms of progressive relaxation?

CASE STUDY LEARNING OPPORTUNITIES

The key points and reflection provide the background and knowledge required in relation to the case studies; Bronwen (Case Study 1) and Morgan (Case Study 2) help to deepen understanding of how Jacobson's traditional approach to progressive muscular relaxation can be applied in practice.

CASE STUDY 1

Insomnia: *Progressive Relaxation Outcomes for Bronwen*

Bronwen has been suffering from insomnia for months. She is waking at around 3 a.m. every morning and cannot get back to sleep. Bronwen was introduced to and has been successfully practising a modified or abbreviated progressive relaxation approach based on the principles of Jacobson's technique and has developed a regular bedtime routine. She has learned to relax her muscles passively and can diminish tensions in her body. She has found that this is helping her to 'let go' and to fall to sleep; moreover, the quality of her sleep seems to have improved.

However, when she wakes in the early hours of the morning, she is still finding it difficult to get back to sleep because her mind is so active and is filled with negative thoughts. To address this ongoing issue, Bronwen is introduced to Jacobson's original method of ocular relaxation and, with use of a digital recording, learns to follow the exact script given in the 'eye movement' practice noted in this chapter (see also Table 5.1). Using her headphones to follow the recorded script at night, Bronwen has found that the method is assisting her to 'let go' of the images in her mind, and as they dissipate, so the associated thoughts are disappearing. Consequently, she is able to drop back off to sleep and thus finding this a positive intervention when she wakes in the early hours.

CASE STUDY 2

Headaches and Jaw Clenching: Progressive Relaxation Outcomes for Morgan

Morgan has a history of clenching his teeth and has been using progressive relaxation in a modified and abbreviated form of tensing and releasing muscles for some time. It has helped him to understand how muscle tension in his jaw, face and neck is related to his headaches. He can now release and diminish tension in his face and neck, and with daily practice, he feels he has reduced the frequency of his headaches. However, he has also found that once the headaches start, he cannot use his modified progressive relaxation techniques to break the cycle and thus prevent them getting worse. In other words, he cannot 'diminish tension' or 'let go' at this critical point, and the neuromuscular circuit spirals and increases the muscle tension he is experiencing. When this happens, the only intervention that works is medication and lying down in a darkened room.

On discussion with Morgan, his trainer suggests practising Jacobson's original script for focusing on the jaw, voice and auditory imagination (see speech movement script in text and Table 5.1). After just one practise session, Morgan notes some key points of residual tension in his jaw and tongue that he had not been aware of previously; he realizes this subliminal tension was possibly causal to the ongoing headaches and is related to his negative thoughts. Morgan has been using the script daily and is now finding that not only are the headaches diminishing in frequency, but that he can actually use the technique successfully to break the cycle when headaches do start, enabling him to manage this more proactively. He is continuing his practice in the hope that he will be able to reach a point where his speech muscles are so completely relaxed that he cannot think in verbal terms at all, and that, consequently, the negative thoughts will disappear completely.

ACTIVITY

For each of the case studies:

1. List key aspects used in the progressive relaxation approach.
2. Consider why this approach was taken.
3. Write down the impact progressive relaxation is having from a psychological perspective.
4. Write down the impact progressive relaxation is having from a physical perspective.
5. Write down the impact progressive relaxation is having from an emotional perspective.

Consider the outcomes on quality of life and overall well-being for both individuals.

Chapter 6 will focus on Bernstein and Borkovec's (1973) progressive relaxation training. This is an adapted form of Jacobson's traditional approach that promotes the value of tension to facilitate relaxation.

REFERENCES

Aiger, M., Palacín, M., Pifarré, P., Llopart, M., & Simo, M. (2016). Effectiveness of relaxation techniques before diagnostic screening of cancer patients. *Suma Psicológica, 23*(2), 133–140.

Bernstein, D. A., & Borkovec, T. D. (1973). *Progressive relaxation training: A manual for the helping professions.* Champaign, IL: Research Press.

Bernstein, D. A., Borkovec, T. D., & Hazlett-Stevens, H. (2000). *New directions in progressive relaxation training: A guide book for helping professionals.* Westport, CT: Praeger.

Conrad, A., & Roth, W. T. (2007). Muscle relaxation therapy for anxiety disorders: It works, but how? *Journal of Anxiety Disorders, 21*(3), 243–264.

Crist, D. A., & Rickard, H. C. (1993). A 'fair' comparison of progressive and imaginal relaxation. *Perceptual and Motor Skills, 76,* 691–700.

Hui, P. N., Wan, M., Chan, W. K., & Yung, P. M. (2006). An evaluation of two behavioral rehabilitation programs, qigong versus progressive relaxation, in improving the quality of life in cardiac patients. *Journal of Alternative and Complementary Medicine, 12*(4), 373–378.

Jacobson, E. (1934). Electrical measurements concerning muscular contraction (tonus) and the cultivation of relaxation in man: Relaxation times of individuals. *American Journal of Physiology, 108,* 573–580.

Jacobson, E. (1938). *Progressive relaxation* (2nd ed.). Chicago: University of Chicago Press.

Jacobson, E. (1964). *Anxiety and tension control.* Philadelphia: J B Lippincott.

Jacobson, E. (1970). *Modern treatment of tense patients including the neurotic and depressed, with case illustrations, follow-ups and emg measurements.* Springfield, IL: Charles C Thomas.

Jacobson, E. (1976). *You must relax.* London: Souvenir Press.

Kerr, K. M. (2000). Relaxation techniques: A critical review. *Critical Reviews in Physical and Rehabilitation Medicine*, *12*, 51–89.

Kyrios, M., Ahern, C., Fassnacht, D. B., Nedeljkovic, M., Moulding, R., & Meyer, D. (2018). Therapist assisted internet based cognitive behavioural therapy versus progressive relaxation in obsessive compulsive disorder: Randomised controlled trial. *Journal of Medical Internet Research*, *20*(8), e242.

Kwekkeboom, K. L., & Gretarsdottir, E. (2006). Systematic review of relaxation interventions for pain. *Journal of Nursing Scholarship*, *38*(3), 269–277.

Lehrer, P. M. (1982). How to relax and how not to relax: A re-evaluation of the work of Edmund Jacobson. *Behaviour Research and Therapy*, *20*, 417–428.

Lehrer, P. M. (1996). Varieties of relaxation methods and their unique effects. *International Journal of Stress Management*, *3*, 1–15.

Lehrer, P. M., Batey, D. M., Woolfolk, R. L., Remde, A., & Garlick, T. (1988). The effect of repeated tense-release sequences on EMG and self-report of muscle tension: An evaluation of Jacobsonian and post-Jacobsonian assumptions about progressive relaxation. *Psychophysiology*, *25*, 562–567.

Lucic, K. S., Steffen, J. J., Harrigan, J. A., & Stuebing, R. C. (1991). Progressive relaxation training: Muscle contractions before relaxation? *Behavior Therapy*, *22*, 249–256.

McGuigan, F. J. (1981). *Calm down: A guide for stress and tension control*. Englewood Cliffs, NJ: Prentice-Hall.

McGuigan, F. J. (1984). Progressive relaxation: Origins, principles and clinical applications. In R. L. Woolfolk, & P. M. Lehrer (Eds.), *Principles and practice of stress management*. New York: Guilford Press.

Munzert, J., & Krüger, B. (2018). Task-specificity of muscular responses during motor imagery: Peripheral physiological effects and the legacy of Edmund Jacobson. *Frontiers in Psychology*, *9*, 1–5.

Salt, V. L., & Kerr, K. M. (1997). Mitchell's simple physiological relaxation and Jacobson's progressive relaxation techniques: A comparison. *Physiotherapy*, *83*(4), 200–207.

Snyder, M. (1985). *Independent nursing interventions*. New York: John Wiley.

Vancampfort, D., Correll, C. U., Scheewe, T. W., et al. (2013). Progressive muscle relaxation in persons with schizophrenia: A systematic review of randomised controlled trials. *Clinical Rehabilitation*, *27*(4), 291–298.

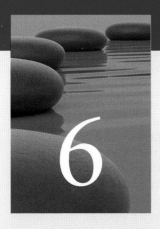

6

PROGRESSIVE RELAXATION TRAINING

PROFESSOR TEENA CLOUSTON

CHAPTER CONTENTS

LEARNING OBJECTIVES

The aim of this chapter is to provide a practical guide to basic concepts of progressive relaxation training.

By the end of this chapter you will be able to:

1. Recognize the differences between Jacobson's progressive relaxation and progressive relaxation training

2. Describe the aims of progressive relaxation training

3. Identify the underpinning argument for the use of muscle tensing and suggestion in progressive relaxation training

4. Understand the key differences between progressive relaxation training and hypnosis

5. Discuss when progressive relaxation training may be appropriate to use in practice

This chapter will conclude with key points and time for reflection, providing learning opportunities through case studies.

INTRODUCTION TO PROGRESSIVE RELAXATION TRAINING

Although Jacobson's method of relaxation (see Chapter 5) was found to reduce both pulse rate and blood pressure, it was time consuming and unlikely to have wide appeal as it stood; some form of abbreviation was needed. The first major attempt at shortening the format was made by Wolpe (1958), who reduced the training to six sessions and later reduced it further to one. Countless other modifications have followed, of which, Bernstein and Borkovec's (1973) modification is one of the best known.

Named 'progressive relaxation training (PRT)' by its authors, the approach is defined as learning to relax specific muscle groups while paying attention to the feelings associated with both the tensed and relaxed states. Its aims are to achieve a state of deep relaxation in increasingly shorter periods and to control excess tension in stress-inducing situations (Bernstein & Given 1984).

The trainee works through the sequential tensing and releasing of 16 muscle groups. These are reduced to seven in the next stage and to four in a subsequent stage. The tension component is then withdrawn, in what is called 'relaxation through recall', and the final stage consists of a mental summary of the previously learned techniques. Proficiency at each level depends on the skill obtained in the previous stage. The tense–release element of PRT is described in this chapter. Relaxation through recall is presented in Chapter 8. Two additional components are described in later chapters: 'cue-controlled' or 'conditioned relaxation' in Chapter 9 and 'differential relaxation' in Chapter 11.

DIFFERENCES BETWEEN PROGRESSIVE RELAXATION AND PROGRESSIVE RELAXATION TRAINING

Although PRT is founded on Jacobson's principles of recognizing and eliminating tension, there are important differences between the two approaches (Table 6.1). The most significant elements are as follows.

The Contraction Phase

One of the notable differences is the prominence given to the tensing component in the modified version. Bernstein and Borkovec (1973) describe an effect whereby the strength of the contraction determines the depth of the relaxation which follows it, in the manner of a pendulum which, when lifted high on one side, swings back to the same height on the other side. Thus the stronger the initial contraction, the deeper the subsequent relaxation. Jacobson (1938, 1970) does not share this view. He sees the contraction phase simply as a means of cultivating the individual's sensitivity to the presence of muscle tension. He never intended it as a means of 'producing' relaxation (Lehrer et al 1988).

The strength of the contraction is not specified by Jacobson, except in such terms as 'Do not stiffen your arm to the point of extreme effort, but only in moderation' (Jacobson 1964), and the command to 'tense', even at greatest magnitude, is taken to convey only a comfortable level, because the object is merely to enable the individual to identify the sensation of tension. To Jacobson, the lower the level of the contraction, the more useful it was. Bernstein and Borkovec (1973), in contrast, use phrases such as 'tight fist' and refer to 'trembling neck muscles', suggesting a high level of tension. Wolpe and Lazarus (1966), similarly, in their

TABLE 6.1		
Differences between Jacobson's progressive relaxation method and Bernstein & Borkovec's progressive relaxation training		
	Progressive relaxation	Progressive relaxation training
Position of relaxation	Lying or sitting	Reclining
Total number of muscle groups worked	401	16
Number of new muscle groups worked in one session	1 or 2	All groups
Emphasis of technique	Releasing tension	'Producing' relaxation through tense–release cycles
Perceived value of the contraction	To alert the individual to the tension sensation	To deepen each relaxation component by providing a 'running start'; a strong contraction leads to a deep relaxation
Part played by suggestion	None: the technique is purely a muscular skill	Indirect suggestion is used to enhance the effect
Use of tapes	Not used	Advised against
Number of sessions needed	501	8–12

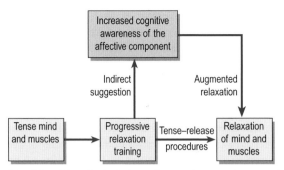

Fig. 6.1 ■ How the inclusion of suggestion may increase the effect of a muscular procedure.

version, urge trainees to clench their fists 'tighter and tighter'.

Use of Suggestion

Both Jacobson (1938) and Bernstein and Borkovec (1973) discuss suggestion in their approaches to relaxation, with the former discouraging it, and the latter supporting its use (Table 6.1; see Chapter 5). The argument in favour of using suggestion is that it increases cognitive awareness of the affective component, which is believed to enhance the overall effect and deepen the sense of relaxation (Fig. 6.1).

This is achieved through the use of indirect and subtle suggestions, such as 'Notice how your muscles are feeling more and more relaxed' and 'Let a feeling of relaxation flow through your limbs'. Voice modulations to reinforce the distinction between tension and relaxation are also encouraged: crisp tones during the tensing component and soothing tones during the relaxation component. While advocating the use of suggestion, Bernstein and Borkovec (1973) do point out that PRT uses a form of indirect suggestion, and that this differs from hypnotic techniques that use a more direct form of induction aiming to place people into a trance state. They suggest that in hypnosis, maximum use is made of direct suggestion, such as 'Now your arm is limp', and although this type of direct suggestion is crucial in hypnosis, it is not appropriate in relaxation. Interestingly, Paul (1969), in his early seminal studies, was able to show that relaxation training was more effective than hypnosis at reducing muscle tension. Moreover, several later studies have shown that PRT and hypnosis combined can be more

effective if used together than applied separately to address conditions such as anxious-depressive symptoms and insomnia (Borkovec & Fowles 1973, Holdevici 2014). This would suggest that these approaches are compatible in use for some individuals and conditions despite their different stance in terms of direct and indirect suggestion.

To Jacobson, however, even indirect suggestion is unacceptable in his relaxation theory. He sees progressive relaxation exclusively as a muscular skill, the mastery of which is impeded by any kind of suggestion. This is a critical difference in the two techniques.

INTRODUCTION TO EVIDENCE

PRT has produced favourable results in many conditions, such as anxiety (Dolbier & Rush 2012, Pan et al 2012, Rasid & Parish 1998), obsessive compulsive disorder (Kyrios et al 2018, Twohig et al 2010), depression (Safi 2015), cancer (Shahriari et al 2017), hypertension (Yung et al 2001), insomnia (Bootzin & Perlis 1992), asthma (Nickel et al 2006, Vázquez & Buceta 1993), epilepsy (Puskarich et al 1992), rheumatic pain (Stenstrom et al 1996) and dyspnoea and anxiety in chronic obstructive pulmonary disease (Gift et al 1992). Improvements in quality of life are commonly reported as notable outcomes across these studies (Cheung et al 2003, Dehdari et al 2009, Nickel et al 2006, Pan et al 2012, Shahriari et al 2017).

Looking particularly at people presenting with multiple 'somatoform disorders' (i.e., physical symptoms without an apparent organic cause), Schröder et al (2013) concluded that progressive muscle relaxation based on Bernstein and Borkovec's (1973) approach was an effective intervention for this condition. Exploring delivery through an online platform, Kyrios et al (2018) identified moderate improvements for people suffering from obsessive compulsive disorder (OCD) using PRT (n = 90) over a 12-week period. Dolbier and Rush (2012) focused their study on college students and found that a form of abbreviated progressive relaxation had significant short-term effects in lowering levels of anxiety and cortisol.

A randomized controlled trial specifically investigating the effectiveness of Bernstein and Borkovec's (1973) progressive relaxation on levels of depression in women with multiple sclerosis found that PRT was successful in reducing depression and increasing reported levels of quality of life (Safi 2015).

Pan et al (2012) explored the effects of PRT on levels of anxiety and health-related quality of life of women with ectopic pregnancy who were receiving methotrexate treatment. The results showed a marked improvement in both scores (i.e., anxiety and health) for women practising PRT over a short 3-day inpatient period; results also evidenced enhanced progress overall for the PRT trainees compared with the control group.

Using more long-term interventions structured over an 8-week period, Nickel et al (2006) found significant improvements in quality of life for pregnant women suffering from asthma, and Dehdari et al (2009) reported that a 6-week period of PRT improved the quality of life of cardiac patients suffering from anxiety. Similarly, a randomized controlled trial by Cheung et al (2003) to evaluate the effectiveness of PRT on anxiety and quality of life among patients with colorectal cancer following surgery showed a significant reduction in anxiety and an improved quality of life for patients practising the relaxation technique.

A more recent study by Shahriari et al (2017) found that PRT, used in tandem with diaphragmatic breathing and guided imagery, was a cost effective and convenient intervention for improving quality of life for older people with either prostrate or breast cancer. This suggests that PRT can work effectivity with other treatments, although the influence of PRT as a standalone intervention could not be identified.

An early comparative study by Stenstrom and colleagues (1996) considered the effects of dynamic muscle training with those of PRT in 54 patients with inflammatory rheumatic disease. Participants in both interventions trained for half an hour, 5 days a week, for 3 months. At the end of that time, the relaxation group exhibited marked improvements in muscle function, which were significantly greater than those recorded in the dynamic exercise group. Alternatively, a study by Crist and Rickard (1993) showed equal efficacy, where muscular relaxation was compared with imaginal relaxation in 100 healthy college students. Other studies offer a more tentative stance; for example, Carlson and Hoyle (1993) evaluated studies

featuring several forms of abbreviated progressive relaxation across a variety of conditions. Their findings indicated that PRT was most effective in treating tension headache, with other conditions, such as cancer and hypertension showing smaller effect sizes.

Finally, a study by Twohig et al (2010) compared the effectiveness of eight sessions of acceptance and commitment therapy (ACT) with eight sessions of PRT for adults with OCD. Findings showed that quality of life was reported as marginally better for those receiving ACT, signifying that it was more effective than PRT in outcome. This indicates that additional research comparing PRT with other traditional and more contemporary methods of intervention, such as ACT, would be valuable to investigate its efficacy further. Generally, however, findings in terms of the effectiveness of PRT as an intervention tool report either moderate or marked improvement in stress, anxiety and quality of life across a range of conditions, and thus the evidence for its use in practice is robust.

Shortened and standardized versions of progressive relaxation, such as Bernstein and Borkovec's (1973), are, in general, favoured by researchers and clinicians alike because of the length and complexity of the original approach. As noted in Chapter 5, Lehrer's (1982) re-evaluation of Jacobson's work argued for the superior benefit of the lengthy original, noting that abbreviated practice did not necessarily capture Jacobson's original theory and approach in its true form and thus missed the essential elements of its effectiveness. However, an early systematic review by Lichstein (1988) comparing the two approaches found the evidence inconclusive in terms of which was more effective. Because this study is now outdated, it could be argued that its relevance is negligible; indeed, Bernstein et al reviewed their approach to PRT in 2000 and published their revised directions for its application in a guidebook for the health care professional (Bernstein et al 2000). This would suggest that studies after this date are now more appropriate to consider in terms of evidence and effectiveness and perhaps a comparative study of Jacobson's original method with the abbreviated versions would now be worthy of investigation. That said, the present pressures in health care services would probably preclude the application of the full Jacobsonian method if explored in that setting.

THEORIES BEHIND PROGRESSIVE RELAXATION TRAINING

As noted previously, the main theory behind PRT is Jacobson's progressive muscle relaxation. However, whereas Jacobson's approach focused on recognizing and releasing tension in the muscles, PRT is more interested in the trainee experiencing the differences between a tense and relaxed state. This adaptation emerged through Wolpe's (1958, 1964) work around systematic desensitization. Based on behavioural approaches and classical conditioning, Wolpe taught his patients an adapted form of progressive relaxation to help them counteract a panic response to a phobia or traumatic stimulus. He began by teaching them how to relax using his method of PRT. This was marked by the use of the tension–release cycle; that is, he taught his patients to focus on different parts of the body, such as the hand or the shoulders, experience the tension and then release that tension to experience the ensuing state of relaxation; he also used deep breathing exercises to support his technique. Bernstein and Borkovec have both continued to develop their theories of PRT particularly in the field of anxiety. Borkovec carried PRT into the cognitive–behavioural field, where he has integrated it with other components of that approach (Borkovec et al 2002, Newman & Borkovec 2002).

Interestingly, the early debates about the value of the initial contraction phase have not been resolved over time. Although some authors, such as Bernstein and Borkovec, continue to see the contraction as a means of promoting relaxation, others support Jacobson's view and claim that it obstructs the process, pointing to increased muscle–nerve sympathetic activity resulting from the isometric contractions which feature in methods such as PRT (Farrell et al 1991). Ritz (2001) has suggested that tensing might provide benefit in the treatment of some respiratory conditions because the tension component is associated with sympathetic activity and thus dilation of the pulmonary air passages; the release component, on the other hand, is associated with parasympathetic activity and constriction of the air passages. Supported by Nickel et al (2006) and Vázquez and Buceta (1993), if this is so, then PRT has application in the treatment of asthma (see Chapter 30). This is an interesting point

and suggests, as noted in the previous section, that further studies comparing Jacobson's progressive relaxation with PRT could be useful.

KEY ASPECTS OF THE PROGRESSIVE RELAXATION PROCEDURE

The First Session

In Bernstein and Borkovec's (1973) approach, training is governed by a fixed procedure.

1. The rationale of the technique is presented to the trainee, and the items involving the 16 muscle groups are then described and demonstrated. (See introductory remarks section next.)
2. For the procedure itself, the trainee is seated in a reclining chair. If this is not available, the trainee can sit in a chair with a high, sloping back and arm rests.
3. The procedure starts with the trainee being asked to focus attention on a given muscle group. (See item one in the following section.)
4. A signal, such as the word 'Now', indicates that the muscle group is to be tensed.
5. The contraction is carried out all at once, not gradually.
6. Tension is maintained for 5 to 7 seconds, during which, the instructor asks the trainee to focus on the sensations of muscle contraction.
7. On a predetermined cue, such as the 'Release', 'Relax' or 'Let go', the muscle group is relaxed (again, all at once).
8. As the muscle group relaxes, the trainee is asked to notice the feelings that accompany the relaxation, while the trainer maintains a pattern which is indirectly suggestive of relaxation.
9. This continues for the duration of the relaxation period, which is 30 to 40 seconds.
10. All 16 muscle groups are worked in the first training session.

Introductory Remarks to Trainees

The method you are going to learn is called 'progressive relaxation training' and it consists of tensing and releasing muscle groups throughout the body. The object is to produce relaxation and this occurs after the tension is released. A firm contraction can lead to a deep relaxation, rather like a pendulum swinging high on both sides. You will be asked to concentrate on the feelings that accompany the tension and the relaxation; feelings that up to now, you may have taken for granted. There are 16 muscle groups to be tensed and released and it takes about 40 minutes to complete the whole schedule. First, I'll run through the items, demonstrating them and giving you a chance to try them out.

The trainer demonstrates the following items.

1. Making a fist with the dominant hand without involving the upper arm.
2. Pushing the elbow of the same arm down against the arm of the chair (activating the biceps), while keeping the hand relaxed.
3/4. The non-dominant arm is worked separately.
5. Raising the eyebrows.
6. Screwing up the eyes and wrinkling the nose.
7. Clenching the teeth and pulling back the corners of the mouth.
8. Pulling the chin in, and pressing the head back against a support, tensing the neck muscles.
9. Drawing the shoulders back.
10. Tightening the abdominal muscles (making the stomach hard).
11. Tensing the thigh of the dominant leg by attempting to contract the knee flexors and extensors together.
12. Pointing the dominant foot down (plantarflexion).
13. Pulling the dominant foot up towards the face (dorsiflexion).
14/15/16. The non-dominant leg is worked separately.

The trainer continues:

When we begin, I'll first describe each item but please do not tense the part until I give you the cue word 'Now'. Similarly, let it go only when I give you the cue word 'Relax'. Then let it go completely. Would you please close your eyes?

Item One

The first item involves the muscles of the right hand and forearm; the hand is drawn into a fist (Fig. 6.2).

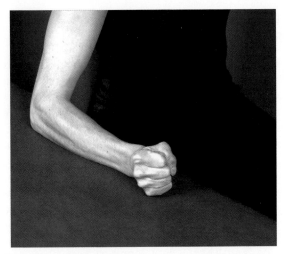

Fig. 6.2 ■ Making a fist.

We'll start with the right hand and forearm. I'm going to ask you to tense the muscles in the right hand and lower arm, by drawing up your hand into a tight fist … Now … clench the hand … keep it tight … feel the tension in the muscles as you pull hard … and … Relax … let go immediately and as the fingers uncurl, notice the feelings you now have in the muscles of the hand … focus on the sensations you are getting in the muscles of the forearm also, as they lose their tension … feel relaxation flowing into the area as the muscles get more and more deeply relaxed … completely relaxed … notice the way your muscles feel at this moment, compared to how they felt when tensed.

All items are performed a second time, after which there is an extended relaxation phase lasting a full minute. Trainees can be asked to raise the little finger of the right hand to indicate that they are fully relaxed before the next item is introduced.

Item Two and Subsequent Items

Item two involves the muscles of the right upper arm: the bent elbow is pressed down into the arm of the chair (Fig. 6.3). A wooden arm rest can be softened with a cushion.

Let the hand and forearm go on relaxing while you transfer your attention to the muscles in the right upper arm. I'd like you this time to press your elbow down against the arm of the chair. Do this without

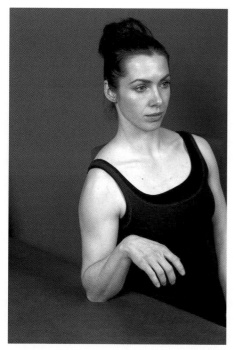

Fig. 6.3 ■ Pressing the elbow down onto the arm of a chair.

*involving the muscles of the hand and forearm …
Now… feel the tension in your upper arm as the elbow
presses down… and… Relax… let it go completely…
focus your attention on the relaxing muscles… feel
the tension flowing out … enjoy the pleasant feelings
of the muscles unwinding… experience the feeling of
deep relaxation and of comfort… then notice if the
upper arm feels as relaxed as the lower arm… if it
does, then signal with your little finger.*

The previous items give an idea of the nature of
PRT, and in the first session, the remaining 14 items
are also worked through. Bernstein et al (2000) have
introduced a slight change in procedure from the
original schedule. It requires the trainee to take a deep
breath and hold it before carrying out each of the
items which involve the trunk and legs. The breath is
released as the muscle group relaxes.

Ending the Session

At the end, the trainer terminates.

*I am going to bring the session to an end by counting
backwards from four to one. four… start to move*

*your legs and feet… three… bend and stretch your
arms and hands… two… move your head slowly…
and… one… open your eyes, noticing how peaceful
and relaxed you feel… as if you'd just woken from a
short sleep.*

Practice

Two daily practice sessions of 15 to 20 minutes each
are considered essential, the trainee picking moments
when he or she is not under any pressure.

Summarized Versions

When the trainee has learned the previous procedure,
it can be regrouped in a summarized form, enabling
the trainee to cover the process in a shorter time.

1. Right arm items combined.
2. Left arm items combined.
3. Face and head movements worked together.
4. Neck and shoulder region combined.
5. Torso items worked together.
6. Right leg items combined.
7. Left leg items combined.
8. A further summary cuts the process down to
   four items.
9. Both arms are worked together.
10. Face, head and neck items worked together.
11. Shoulder and torso movements combined.
12. Both legs are tensed together. (People who find
    this difficult should work the legs separately.)

Relaxation Through Recall

PRT continues with relaxation through recall. This is
described in Chapter 8.

PRECAUTIONS

The precautions of muscular approaches are listed in
Chapter 5.

APPLICATION

As with progressive relaxation, it is proposed that relaxing the musculature exerts a calming effect on the
whole organism, including the mind. The contraction phase in PRT, however, is given greater prominence because it is believed that initial tensing actually

produces relaxation (Bernstein et al 2000, Bernstein & Borkovec 1973). PRT is commonly used in the clinical field; indeed, it supersedes progressive relaxation and tends to dominate in its abbreviated and thus shortened forms.

KEY POINTS

1. PRT is one of the many modifications of progressive relaxation.
2. This particular modification places emphasis on the supposed value of the tensing component which precedes the release.
3. PRT also promotes the use of suggestion, which its authors believe augments the effect of the tense-release sequence.
4. The programme is also presented over a much shorter time than progressive relaxation – that is, 8 to 12 sessions instead of 50.
5. As a skill, PRT requires regular practice.

Reflection

Describe your understanding of the technique of progressive relaxation training.

How did you feel when you completed your own progressive relaxation training session?

Why do you think Bernstein and Borkovec focused more on contraction and suggestion than Jacobson?

What did you learn about the difference between hypnotic induction and suggestion in PRT?

What is the main learning point you will take away from this chapter?

What is your future action plan in terms of using and applying PRT in practice?

CASE STUDY LEARNING OPPORTUNITIES

The key points and reflection provide the background and knowledge required in relation to the case studies; Arwen (Case Study 1) and Tyrion (Case Study 2) help to deepen understanding of how PRT can be applied in practice.

CASE STUDY 1

Dissociative Seizures Non-Epileptic Seizures: PRT Outcomes for Arwen

Arwen has been suffering from non-epileptic dissociative seizures for some time. She has been trying cognitive–behavioural therapy (CBT); this has been helping in terms of addressing her negative thoughts and has reduced the frequency of her seizures. However, she has found that when she is in certain stressful situations her anxiety spirals and a seizure is the common outcome.

On discussion with Arwen, it becomes clear that she can actually feel the anxiety rising and begins to panic. Together, you discuss the option of learning progressive relaxation training techniques to see if this will help her to break the anxiety cycle at this critical point.

After the first session, she reports noting a sense of relaxation after tensing the muscles in her shoulders, neck and face. She loves the imagery of the pendulum and begins practising the tense–relax cycle on her own time. She realizes after a week that she is also holding tension in her abdomen and chest, and this is a surprise. As practice continues, she begins to realize that tension in her face, shoulders, neck, chest and abdomen are all precursors to the seizures that occur in stressful situations: this understanding offers her a sense of control over her seizures that she feels is a key to self-management, and is something she is continuing to develop. She is systematically reducing the process to instigate face, neck and head together, then shoulders and torso so she can use her learnt approach quickly whenever necessary.

Depression and Low Back Pain: *PRT Outcomes for Tyrion*

Tyrion's depression is getting worse. He is feeling very low and his feelings of helplessness and hopelessness are growing. He is also suffering from low back pain, which his GP thinks may be osteoarthritis; this is affecting his ability to walk his dog Jacob, as he finds he cannot manage uneven ground or long distances without discomfort. For Tyrion, this is yet another challenge, because his walks with his dog are his 'lifeline' and keep him calm and 'feeling positive'.

Tyrion wants some practical support and agrees to try PRT. Because his lower back is so tender, Tyrion is seated in a supportive, high-backed chair. After the first session he is surprised to realize that he has become aware of the level of tension he is holding in his body. He also recognizes that actually the relaxation process allows him to tense and relax his buttocks, thighs and lower back without pain, although he does find he needs to work on the legs separately, not together. He also learns that he is holding tension in his back and thighs and is 'protecting' his lower back to avoid pain, which is preventing free movement. Finally, Tyrion is finding that the 'letting go' phase really does induce a sense of release, relaxation and calm. This is making a real difference to his mood and general outlook on life; that practising

PRT is alleviating his depression is a revelation. The positive impact on both his physical and psychological health has motivated Tyrion to keep using PRT. He is now feeling more confident and has found he is able to walk Jacob over short distances if he uses some of the tense–relax strategies he has learned; he is aiming to build this up slowly.

ACTIVITY

For each of the case studies:

1. List key aspects used in the progressive relaxation training approach.
2. Consider why this approach was taken.
3. Write down the impact PRT is having from a psychological perspective.
4. Write down the impact PRT is having from a physical perspective.
5. Write down the impact PRT is having from an emotional perspective.
6. Consider the outcomes on quality of life and overall well-being for both individuals.

Chapter 7 focuses on a tense-release script that trainers can follow drawing on both the traditions of Jacobson's progressive relaxation and the adapted approaches of progressive relaxation training.

REFERENCES

Bernstein, D. A., & Borkovec, T. D. (1973). *Progressive relaxation training: A manual for the helping professions.* Champaign, IL: Research Press.

Bernstein, D. A., Borkovec, T. D., & Hazlett-Stevens, H. (2000). *New directions in progressive relaxation training: A guidebook for helping professionals.* Westport, CT: Praeger.

Bernstein, D. A., & Given, B. A. (1984). Progressive relaxation: Abbreviated methods. In R. L. Woolfolk, & P. M. Lehrer (Eds.), *Principles and practice of stress management.* New York: Guilford Press.

Borkovec, T. D., & Fowles, D. C. (1973). Controlled investigation of the effects of progressive and hypnotic relaxation. *Journal of Abnormal Psychology, 82*(1), 153–158.

Borkovec, T. D., Newman, M. G., Pincus, A. L., & Lytle, R. (2002). A component analysis of cognitive-behavioral therapy for generalized anxiety disorder and the role of interpersonal problems. *Journal of Consulting and Clinical Psychology, 70*(2), 288–298.

Bootzin, R. R., & Perlis, M. L. (1992). Non-pharmacological treatments of insomnia. *Journal of Clinical Psychiatry, 53*(suppl), 37–41.

Carlson, C. R., & Hoyle, R. H. (1993). Efficacy of abbreviated progressive muscle relaxation training: A quantitative review of behavioural medicine research. *Journal of Consulting and Clinical Psychology, 61*(6), 1059–1067.

Cheung, Y. L., Molassiotis, A., & Chang, A. M. (2003). The effect of progressive muscle relaxation training on anxiety and quality of life after stoma surgery in colorectal cancer patients. *Psycho-Oncology, 12*(3), 254–266.

Crist, D. A., & Rickard, H. C. (1993). A 'fair' comparison of progressive and imaginal relaxation. *Perceptual and Motor Skills, 76*, 691–700.

Dehdari, T., Heidarnia, A., Ramezankhani, A., Sadeghian, S., & Ghofranipour, F. (2009). Effects of progressive muscle relaxation training on quality of life in anxious patients after coronary artery bypass graft surgery. *Indian Journal of Medical Research, 129*, 603–608.

Dolbier, C. L., & Rush, T. E. (2012). Efficacy of abbreviated progressive muscle relaxation in a high stress college sample. *International Journal of Stress Management*, *19*(1), 48–68.

Farrell, P., Ebert, T., & Kampine, J. (1991). Naloxone augments muscle sympathetic nerve activity during isometric exercise in humans. *American Journal of Physiology*, *260*, E379–E388.

Gift, A. G., Moore, T., & Soeken, K. (1992). Relaxation to reduce dyspnoea and anxiety in chronic obstructive pulmonary disease. *Nursing Research*, *41*(4), 242–246.

Holdevici, I. (2014). Relaxation and hypnosis in reducing anxious-depressive symptoms an insomnia among adults. *Procedia Social and Behavioural Sciences*, *127*, 586–590.

Jacobson, E. (1938). *Progressive relaxation* (2nd ed). Chicago: University of Chicago Press.

Jacobson, E. (1964). *Anxiety and tension control*. Philadelphia: J. B. Lippincott.

Jacobson, E. (1970). *Modern treatment of tense patients including the neurotic and depressed, with case illustrations, follow-ups and EMG measurements*. Springfield, IL: Charles C Thomas.

Kyrios, M., Ahern, C., Fassnacht, D. B., Nedeljkovic, M., Moulding, R., & Meyer, D. (2018). Therapist assisted internet based cognitive behavioural therapy versus progressive relaxation in obsessive compulsive disorder: Randomised controlled trial. *Journal of Medical Internet Research*, *20*(8), e242.

Lichstein, K. L. (1988). *Clinical relaxation strategies*. New York: John Wiley.

Lehrer, P. M. (1982). How to relax and how not to relax: A re-evaluation of the work of Edmund Jacobson. *Behaviour Research and Therapy*, *20*, 417–428.

Lehrer, P. M., Batey, D. M., Woolfolk, R. L., et al. (1988). The effect of repeated tense-release sequences on EMG and self-report of muscle tension: An evaluation of Jacobsonian and post-Jacobsonian assumptions about progressive relaxation. *Psychophysiology*, *25*, 562–567.

Nickel, C., Lahmann, C., Muehlbacher, M., et al. (2006). Pregnant women with bronchial asthma benefit from progressive muscle relaxation: A randomized, prospective, controlled trial. *Psychotherapy and Psychosomatics*, *75*, 237–243.

Newman, M. G., & Borkovec, T. D. (2002). Cognitive behaviour therapy for worry and generalized anxiety disorder. In G. Simos (Ed.), *Cognitive behaviour therapy: A guide for the practising clinician* (pp. 150–172). East Sussex, UK: Brunner-Routledge.

Pan, L., Zhang, J., & Li, L. (2012). Effects of progressive muscle relaxation training on anxiety and quality of life of inpatients with ectopic pregnancy receiving methotrexate treatment. *Research in Nursing & Health*, *35*, 362–382.

Paul, G. L. (1969). Physiological effects of relaxation training and hypnotic suggestion. *Journal of Abnormal Psychology*, *74*, 425–437.

Puskarich, C. A., Whitman, S., Dell, J., Hughes, J. R., Rosen, A. J., & Hermann, B. P. (1992). Controlled examination of effects of progressive relaxation training on seizure reduction. *Epilepsia*, *33*(4), 675–680.

Rasid, Z. M., & Parish, T. S. (1998). The effects of two types of relaxation training on students' levels of anxiety. *Adolescence*, *33*(129), 99–101.

Ritz, T. (2001). Relaxation therapy in adult asthma: Is there new evidence for its effectiveness? *Behavior Modification*, *25*(4), 640–666.

Safi, S. Z. (2015). A fresh look at the potential mechanisms of progressive muscle relaxation therapy on depression in female patients with multiple sclerosis. *Iranian Journal of Psychiatry and Behavioral Sciences*, *9*(1), e340.

Schröder, A., Heider, J., Zaby, A., & Göllner, R. (2013). Cognitive behavioural therapy versus progressive muscle relaxation training for multiple somatoform symptoms: Results of a randomised control trial. *Cognitive Therapy and Research*, *37*, 296–306.

Shahriari, M., Dehghan, M., Pahlavanzadeh, S., & Hazini, A. (2017). Effects of progressive muscle relaxation, guided imagery and deep diaphragmatic breathing on quality of life in elderly with breast or prostate cancer. *Journal of Education and Health Promotion*, *6*, 1–6.

Stenstrom, C. H., Arge, B., & Sundbom, A. (1996). Dynamic training versus relaxation training as home exercise for patients with inflammatory rheumatic diseases: A randomized controlled study. *Scandinavian Journal of Rheumatology*, *25*, 28–33.

Twohig, M. P., Hayes, S. C., Plumb, J. C., Pruitt, L. D., Collins, A. B., & Hazlett-Stevens, H. (2010). A randomized clinical trial of acceptance and commitment therapy versus progressive relaxation training for obsessive-compulsive disorder. *Journal of Consulting and Clinical Psychology*, *78*(5), 705–716.

Vázquez, M. I., & Buceta, J. M. (1993). Psychological treatment of asthma: Effectiveness of a self-management program with and without relaxation training. *Journal of Asthma*, *30*(3), 171–183.

Wolpe, J. (1958). *Psychotherapy by reciprocal inhibition*. Stanford, CA: Stanford University Press.

Wolpe, J. (1964). Behavior therapy in complex neurotic states. *The British Journal of Psychiatry*, *110*(464), 28–34.

Wolpe, J., & Lazarus, A. A. (1966). *Behaviour therapy techniques*. New York: Pergamon Press.

Yung, P., French, P., & Leung, B. (2001). Relaxation training as complementary therapy for mild hypertension control and the implications of evidence-based medicine. *Complementary Therapies in Nursing and Midwifery*, *1*(2), 59–65.

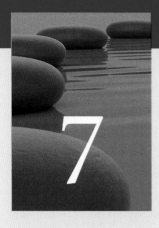

7

A TENSE–RELEASE SCRIPT

PROFESSOR TEENA CLOUSTON

CHAPTER CONTENTS

LEARNING OBJECTIVES

The aim of this chapter is to provide a tense–release script which can be followed and used as a template to deliver progressive relaxation training.

By the end of this chapter you will be able to:

1. Follow and deliver a progressive relaxation session.

2. Describe how the techniques of progressive relaxation and progressive relaxation training are interlinked.

3. Recognize the value of diminishing tension in the body to the practice of learning to relax.

4. Identify the need to become aware of tension in the mind and body to learn to relax.

5. Reflect on the effectiveness of an abbreviated and adapted progressive relaxation session following Jacobson's tradition of progressive relaxation.

This chapter will conclude with key points and time for reflection, providing learning opportunities through case studies.

INTRODUCTION TO A TENSE–RELEASE SCRIPT

The script set out here lies in the tradition of progressive relaxation. In procedure, however, it more closely resembles the abbreviated versions of progressive relaxation training, except that reduced effort is put into the repeats in the manner of Jacobson's diminishing tensions. The exercises themselves are drawn from a variety of sources. Trainees may be lying or sitting in a high-backed chair to perform them, although while the procedure is being introduced, a sitting position is more suitable.

INTRODUCTION TO EVIDENCE

Evidence supporting Jacobson's progressive relaxation (PR) can be found in Chapter 5 and its abbreviated or modified forms, such as progressive relaxation training

(PRT), in Chapter 6. These should be read in tandem with this section.

Tense–release scripts like this one are commonly used in practice and are considered a useful method for stress relief in a variety of conditions (Sundram et al 2016). Because a tense–release approach to relaxation has little or no evidence of any contraindications with medication, it can generally be used without concern of adverse reactions with pharmacological treatments.

As evidenced in Chapters 5 and 6, the tense–release approach has been used with success in anxiety reduction (e.g., Dolbier & Rush 2012), depression with a variety of underlying causes (e.g., Pan et al 2012, Safi 2015), obsessive compulsive disorder (e.g., Kyrios et al 2018) and schizophrenia (Vancampfort et al 2013) to name but a few effective studies; all share the common outcome of improving the quality of life and subjective well-being of the participants.

Dolbier and Rush (2012) suggest that when using a tense–release script, a state of relaxation can be achieved successfully in a single 20-minute session. They reported that a group of high-stress college students (n = 66) experienced significantly greater levels of mental and physical relaxation than the control group (n = 62), as well as significant short-term effects in relation to functioning and performance, after a single session of progressive muscle relaxation using a tense–release approach.

In other studies, Limsanon and Kalayasiri (2015) used a single tense–release session of 20 minutes duration with a group of smokers (n = 6). They found that compared with the control group (n = 6), cigarette cravings, withdrawal symptoms and blood pressure were significantly reduced for those who participated in the relaxation session.

Ikemata and Momose (2017) used a tense–release approach for people with dementia in care homes in Japan. Participants (n = 18) participated in a 15-minute session of progressive relaxation each day for a duration of 90 days. The control group (n = 19) continued with their normal daily routines, which did not include the relaxation sessions. Results showed a significant reduction in agitation, anxiety, apathy and irritability in participants who took part in the relaxation sessions. Further, there were notable improvements in volition, social relationships and daily living activities for this group.

These findings suggest that a tense–release script can be an effective tool to use with people who have variety of conditions and who live in different settings. It also evidences that the tense–release approach can be implemented effectively with measurable outcomes in sessions of 15 to 20 minutes duration.

THEORIES BEHIND A TENSE–RELEASE SCRIPT

As noted in the introduction to the chapter, this practical tense–release script lies in the tradition of progressive relaxation but in its procedure is more akin to progressive relaxation training. Thus the theories behind the practical approach and its application can be found in Chapter 5, which explores Jacobson's traditional approach to progressive relaxation and Chapter 6, which looks at the abbreviated and modified approaches under the heading of progressive relaxation training.

Please be cognisant of the fact that in this chapter the exercises themselves are drawn from a variety of sources and thus represent a customized form of a tense–release script that can be adapted further by the trainer/trainee or practitioner.

KEY ASPECTS OF THE PROCEDURE

To introduce the method the trainer should use the following script:

> I am going to lead you through some of the major muscle groups of the body, asking you to contract and relax them, one by one. Tensing and releasing muscles can help to induce a feeling of physical relaxation. You may also feel mentally relaxed. As you carry out the items, you'll experience sensations in the muscles. These sensations indicate tension which you will learn to identify and to release. This is a skill which enables you to relax yourself any time you want to and the more you practise it, the easier it will become.

The following exercises should then be demonstrated by the trainer to familiarize participants with the procedure. Participants are then invited to try them out. It is worth spending time on the demonstration so that group members or individual participants feel they know the exercises before the instruction begins.

THE EXERCISES

The exercises are as follows:

- Breathing (1)
- Arm: spider hand, rod-like arm
- Leg: plantar- and dorsiflexion (foot bending down and up), toe flexion (bending down) and extension (bending up)
- Breathing (2)
- Abdominal muscle tensing
- Shoulder bracing
- Shoulder hunching
- Head pressing back
- Upper face: brow raising, frowning, eye exercises
- Lower face: jaw, lips, tongue

Authors hold varying opinions as to the optimal duration of the tension and relaxation periods. Based on their collective judgements, we suggest 5 seconds for tensing and 30 to 40 seconds for relaxing.

It is explained to participants that each tension phase is carried out on the command 'Now'. The signal for the release of tension is the word 'Relax'. When calling the items, the tone of voice can be varied from slightly crisp during the tension phase to soothing during the relaxation phase.

Participants may have their eyes open or closed. When they have taken up their lying positions, the instructor begins.

Breathing (1)

The section on hyperventilation in Chapter 4 is relevant to this exercise.

Please make yourself as comfortable as you can. Let your breathing settle down and observe its natural rhythm. After a minute or two, follow a natural breath out, making it a little bit longer than usual ... then let the air in ... let it gently fill your lungs ... and ... breathe out slowly, releasing your tensions with the air ... and now let your breathing take care of itself ... do not immediately repeat this deep breath ...

You will recognize the exercises which follow. Please wait for the word 'Now' to perform the action.

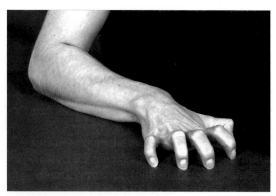

Fig. 7.1 ■ Spider hand.

Arm

Spider Hand

This is adapted from Wallace (1980) (Fig. 7.1).

I'd like you to focus attention on your right arm, whether it's lying alongside you or resting on the arm of your chair. With the hand placed palm downwards, slowly press the fingertips into the surface, drawing them towards your palm so that your hand gradually takes on the shape of a spider ... don't force the movement, just put a moderate amount of effort into it ... Now ... as you hold the position, notice the tensions in the hand and the underside of the forearm ... feel them build up ... then ... Relax ... let the tension go ... relax the muscles ... let the tension disappear and go on disappearing as you give the hand time to get more and more relaxed ... notice how it feels when it's fully relaxed ...

The 'spider' exercise is repeated once using less effort.

Rod-like Arm (Fig. 7.2)

If you are seated, start with your right arm in your lap. Lying participants will have their right arm alongside them. I want you slowly to tense up all the muscles so that the arm becomes rigid. Begin with a little tension in the fingertips ... let it grow until the fingers are drawn into the palm, making a fist shape. Then stretch out the arm, creating tension in the forearm and upper arm until the arm gets rigid

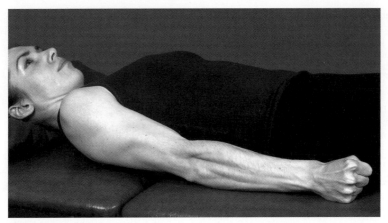

Fig. 7.2 ■ Rod-like arm.

like a rod ... Now ... feel the tension throughout the arm, but don't overdo it ... and ... Relax ... let it flop down ... feel the muscles going slack and the arm becoming limp ... notice the relief, the pleasant tingling and the sense of warmth ... let the arm go on relaxing ... and relaxing a bit more ... imagine the last remnant of tension flowing out through your fingertips ... notice how the arm muscles feel when they are fully relaxed.

The exercise is performed again, using less effort the second time.

'Spider' and 'rod' are then carried out with the left arm.

Leg

Next is a group of leg exercises. The first two are for those lying down and the second two are for those who are seated.

Feet Pointing Away from Face

In this exercise the supine participant is asked to point their feet away from the face (Fig. 7.3).

Turning your attention to your legs which are lying flat on the ground, I'd like you to point your feet down, as if you were using them to indicate something. Don't overdo it, especially if you are prone to develop cramp ... Now ... as you hold the position, study the tensions in your calves ... and

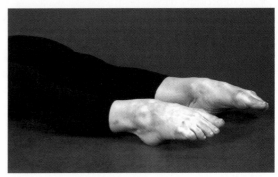

Fig. 7.3 ■ Feet pointing away from face.

then ... Relax ... let go ... let all the tension dissolve ... feel comfort returning to your lower legs ... notice the sensations you get from relaxing the muscles ... continue letting go until you feel they won't relax any further ...

Feet Pointing Towards Face

The feet are now pointed towards the face (Fig. 7.4).

This time, point your feet up towards your face, keeping the backs of your knees on the ground ... Now ... hold the position and notice the sensations you are getting in the working muscles around the shin bones ... and then ... Relax ... as you let go of your leg muscles, feel the tension leaving them ... feel it draining out as your legs and feet become more and more relaxed ...

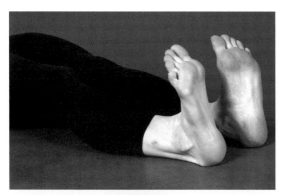

Fig. 7.4 ■ Feet pointing towards face.

These two exercises are repeated once with reduced tension.

The following two leg exercises are addressed to seated participants.

Heel Raising

Here seated participants are asked to raise their heels off the ground (Fig. 7.5).

Begin by making sure your feet are flat on the floor … then, keeping your toes firmly in contact with the floor, raise your heels up in the air … Now … feel the tension in your calf muscles … hold the

action … then … Relax … drop your heels to the ground … notice the relief … the comfort … the warm, tingling sensation in your calves … the enjoyable feeling of relaxing your feet … go on letting those feelings continue until your feet and calves are completely relaxed … then, a little bit further …

Toe Raising

In the toe-raising exercise, the front part of the foot is raised off the ground (Fig. 7.6).

This time, keep your heels on the ground, and raise the front part of your feet as if you were about to tap a rhythm … Now … keep your toes up in the air while you take notice of the tension sensation in the muscles around the shinbones … and … Relax … let the feet fall down … notice the relief in the shin area … feel the tension leaving you … draining out through your feet and toes … and continuing to drain out a bit longer …

These two exercises are repeated with diminished tension.

The next exercise is addressed to both lying and seated participants.

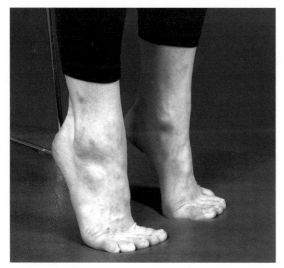

Fig. 7.5 ■ Heel raising.

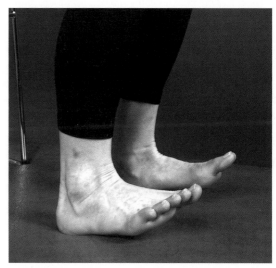

Fig. 7.6 ■ Toe raising.

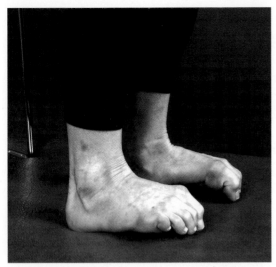

Fig. 7.7 ■ Toe flexion.

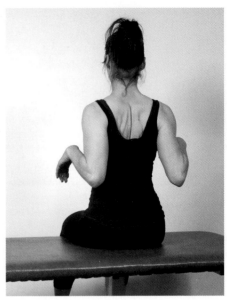

Fig. 7.8 ■ Shoulder bracing.

Toe Flexion and Extension

As in toe raising, in this exercise the front part of the foot is also raised off the ground (Fig. 7.7).

> *Let your attention focus on your toes. Whether you are lying or sitting, curl your toes down, restricting the action to the toes themselves. Some people can do it more easily than others, but just do what you can … Now … feel the tension in the sole of the foot and the calf of the leg … then … Relax … let it go … feel the muscles going slack … feel them going slacker as the tension disappears … notice how the muscles feel when they are relaxed.*

The exercise is repeated once using less tension.

It is followed by a similar exercise in which the toes are bent upwards. Here, muscle tension is felt along the top part of the foot and the shin.

Breathing (2)

At least a minute can be allotted to this item.

> *Turn your attention to your breathing again … notice its rhythm … place one hand over your upper abdomen and notice the gentle swell and recoil of the area underneath it … avoid any inclination to alter the rhythm … just let the breathing take care of itself …*

Abdominal Muscle Tensing

> *Focus next on the abdominal muscles … make the area over your internal organs go flat and hard as you pull the muscles in … Now … feel the tension under your ribs, over your organs and around the back of your pelvis … then … Relax … let go … allow your muscles to spread themselves … feel a sense of deep relaxation … and let that relaxation become deeper as the moments pass …*

One repeat is carried out using less tension.

Shoulder Bracing (Fig. 7.8)

> *Moving to the region of the back, bring your attention to the blade bones behind your shoulders. Draw them back so that they get nearer to each other (without putting too much effort into it) … Now … feel them being gently squeezed together … notice also how your chest is lifted away from the supporting surface … and then … Relax … release the tension … let the muscles soften … feel your back lying once again in contact with the supporting surface … notice the feeling of relaxation and let that feeling continue on and on …*

The exercise is repeated once with less tension.

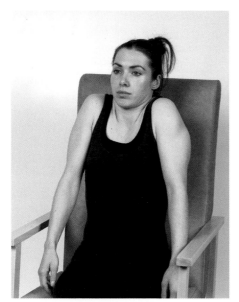

Fig. 7.9 ■ Shoulder hunching.

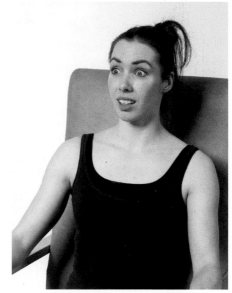

Fig. 7.10 ■ Eyebrow raising.

Shoulder Hunching (Fig. 7.9)

Moving to the neck region, I'd like you to lift your shoulders … hunch them up as if to touch your ears … Now … feel the tension in the lower neck … register the sensation … and … Relax … let the shoulders drop … and go on dropping … further and further as the tension ebbs away … feel your shoulders completely relaxed …

The exercise is performed once more using diminished tension.

Head Back

And the head: keeping your chin in, press your head back against the support (against the floor or back of the chair) … press it back, making double chins in the front … stop short of discomfort … Now … notice the feelings you get from the working muscles … tension in the back of the neck … and … Relax … let go … feel the area relax … notice the sense of ease that floods into the area … allow the relaxation to deepen until all the tension has left your neck …

One repeat is carried out using less tension.

Upper Face
Eyebrow Raising (Fig. 7.10)

Moving to the face, to the many muscles which control your facial expressions: would you now raise your eyebrows … raise them high, creating horizontal furrows … Now … feel the tension in the muscle that stretches across the brow … and … Relax … let the tension flow out … feel the furrows being smoothed … continue until there is no tension left in your brow … then a little bit further …

The repeat is carried out using less tension.

Frowning (Fig. 7.11)

Focus on your frowning muscle … bring the eyebrows closer together, buckling the skin between them into a deep frown … Now … hold it a few moments, taking note of the sensation you get from the action … then … Relax … release the tension … feel the eyebrows spread sideways … imagine the space between them getting wider and continuing to get wider … notice the comfortable feeling that accompanies this idea… continue until all the tension dies away …

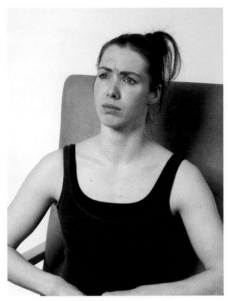

Fig. 7.11 ■ Frowning.

The exercise is repeated once using diminished tension.

Eyes

We come to the eyes. First, I'd like you to screw them up and notice the sensation you get from the action ... Now ... spend a moment registering it ... then ... Relax ... let go ... let the muscles loosen ... notice the feeling you get from loosening them ... feel the skin smoothing out ...

The exercise is performed once more using diminished tension.

For the following exercise, the trainee's eyes should be closed. The format is slightly different in that because there are so many eye movements, the relaxation is postponed until the end.

Next, without moving your head, turn your eyes upwards behind your closed lids ... Now ... hold your gaze up for a few moments ... notice the tension in the muscles ... and ... bring your eyes back to a central position ... and look down, as if towards your feet ... Now ... hold it a few moments ... then return to the centre ... look to the right ... Now ... keep a steady hold ... and return to the

front ... and, to the left ... Now ... hold it ... then bring your eyes back to the front ... and ... as they rest in a middle position, notice how they feel ... compare this with how they felt when they were working ... let them go on relaxing ... continue relaxing for a full minute ...

Finally, roll your eyes in a clockwise circle ... Now ... notice the sensations of tension ... pause ... roll them in an anticlockwise direction ... Now ... notice the feelings ... and ... Relax ... let them fully relax ... let them go on relaxing until all the tension has left them ...

One repeat may be carried out using less tension.

A further exercise consists of focusing at different distances behind closed lids: first on a faraway object, then on an object placed close to the eyes (adapted from Madders 1984).

With your eyes still closed, imagine you are looking at an object on the distant horizon. You can't see it clearly but you are trying to make it out ... Now ... notice how it feels as you strain to identify it ... then, releasing the tension, bring your eyes to focus on a piece of writing held very close ... Now ... notice the sensations as you make the effort to read the words ... and ... Relax ... let your eyes settle on the middle distance ... feel the relief as you let go of the tension in the muscles which control the focusing ... enjoy the feeling of releasing that tension ...

After a short rest, repeat the action with reduced tension.

Lower Face

Jaw

Bring your back teeth together ... do it firmly but without actually clenching them ... Now ... feel a sensation in your jaw as if you'd been chewing tough meat ... hold it ... and ... Relax ... release the jaw muscles ... feel the tension fading ... continuing to fade ... and then further still ...

The exercise is repeated with diminished tension.

Lips

Press your lips tightly together as if you were rejecting some unpleasant medicine … Now … hold your lips pursed … then … Relax … let them go … and as they relax, notice feelings such as the warmth of the blood flowing back into your lips … tune in to the feelings of relaxation …

One repeat is carried out using less tension.

Tongue

Finally, the tongue: press your tongue against the roof of your mouth and hold it there … Now … feel the tension in the tongue … and … Relax … notice how it feels when you relax it … and press it against the inside of your right cheek … Now … hold … and … Relax … and against your left cheek … Now … hold … and … Relax … and pull it back towards your throat (not too strongly) … Now … hold … and … Relax … and then let your tongue settle in the middle of your mouth, just touching the backs of your front teeth … feel it releasing tension … let it go on relaxing … enjoy the feeling of relaxation … let that feeling spread throughout your mouth and over your face, making them feel warm, glowing and relaxed … then, let it spread to cover your neck and shoulders … your arms … back … abdomen … and legs, so that your entire body experiences a feeling of complete relaxation … continue relaxing for several minutes …

Termination

And so, I'm going to bring this session to an end … gradually I'd like you to return to normal activity, but first I'll count from one to three to help you make the adjustment … when I get to three, I'd like you to open your eyes, feeling fresh and alert and ready to carry on with your day … one … two … three … before getting up, give a few gentle stretches to your arms and legs.

PRECAUTIONS

Precautions can be found at the end of Chapter 5.

APPLICATION

A tense–release script can be used individually or with groups. As noted previously, the method is suitable for use by people suffering from a wide range of conditions and in a variety of settings but can also be used as a general tool for maintaining or improving a state of well-being for all.

It is a very common method of relaxation and is extensively used in practice. Please see the case study examples given at the end of Chapters 5 and 6, as well as those at the end of this chapter for illustrations of its varied applications.

Tense–release scripts are readily and often freely available online and can be accessed from a wide range of apps. As a method, it can be used with people of all ages, children to older adults, and is an effective tool for stress relief and to create a sense of calm and well-being (Sundram et al 2016). Although the tense–release technique has few contraindications, guidance from a qualified practitioner is recommended before use and if any unusual reactions or discomfort are experienced practice should be stopped and advice sought.

KEY POINTS

1. This script is in the tradition of Jacobson's progressive relaxation and uses his technique of diminishing tensions; however, in practice it more closely resembles progressive relaxation training.
2. It is important for the trainer to demonstrate the process first.
3. The exercises are drawn from a variety of sources and so are an adapted form of both the Jacobson and Bernstein and Borkovec approaches.
4. Trainees can be sitting or lying down to do this procedure but sitting may be beneficial initially.
5. The script is suitable for use with individuals or in groups.
6. Learning to breathe deeply and release tension through the breath is an important part of the process.

Reflection

Describe your experiences of delivering the tense–release script training.

Why did you deliver the training sessions in the way that you did?

What did you learn from delivering the training sessions?

How do you think you might do this differently in future?

What is the main learning point you will take away from this chapter?

What is your future action plan?

CASE STUDY LEARNING OPPORTUNITIES

The key points and reflection provide the background and knowledge required in relation to the case studies; Arwen (Case Study 1) and Tyrion (Case Study 2), help to deepen understanding of how a tense–release script can be applied in practice.

CASE STUDY 1

Breathing: *Tense-Release Script Outcomes for Arwen*

Arwen (see Case Study 1 in Chapter 6) joins a relaxation class. The script found in this chapter is used in the sessions.

From the first session Arwen feels she is benefiting. She lies supine on a relaxation mat and feels focusing on her breath is very relaxing and calming; she also likes the 'diminishing tension' approach. Over time, she finds she can translate the breathing techniques she has learned to enhance the relaxation strategies she is using to calm her anxiety in stressful situations. She also feels that focusing on her breath actually helps prevent her hyperventilating, a response that she feels she has struggled to get under control previously. She intends to spend more time on becoming aware of her breathing and following its rhythm so she can adapt any shallow or fast breathing by slowing down her breath.

Spending time in a group was a big step for Arwen because she panics in social situations; however, she feels that this has, in fact, been beneficial for her. She is overcoming her fear of having a fit in front of others and this, in turn, is building her confidence in terms of her belief in her own ability to control and manage them.

CASE STUDY 2

Tense–Release Cycle: *Tense–Release Script Outcomes for Tyrion*

Tyrion (see Case Study 2 in Chapter 6) joins a relaxation class. The script found in this chapter is used in the sessions and he enjoys the class immensely. Because of his low back pain Tyrion sits in a high back chair. He is pleased to find that the group trainer requests that he modifies some of the exercises to support his back pain. First, he is told to sit rather than lie down. Then he is asked to ensure he is sitting with his back supported in the chair with his bottom at the back of the seat, his spine straight and his hips at 90 degrees at all times. He is also relieved that the trainer redraws his attention to this positioning before doing the abdominal and back tense-release cycle.

He finds that the abdominal breathing and muscle tension stage is helping to raise his awareness of even deeper levels of tension in his lower back; the release stage allows him to experience a deeper sense of 'letting go' of this tension. Although the tense-release cycle makes him aware that his lower back is very tense, he also notes that, alternatively, his abdominal muscles are not: they are slack.

On discussion with the trainer, he begins practising a tense–release cycle at home giving particular attention to his abdominal muscles. Following guidance, he makes sure his lower back is comfortable and gently pressed flat into the back of the chair when he pulls his abdominal muscles in. He is finding this exercise is very beneficial to his progress and he also realises that by holding his abdomen muscles in more when walking his dog, Jacob, his lower back is feeling stronger and his posture is improving. The tense–release practice is also improving his psychological state because it helps him think more positively; however, he also finds that the group support is helping lift his mood, and this is an added bonus he had not expected.

ACTIVITY

For each of the case studies:

1. List key aspects used in the tense–release cycle approaches.
2. Consider why this approach was taken.
3. Write down the impact that the tense–release script is having from a psychological perspective.
4. Write down the impact that the tense–release script is having from a physical perspective.
5. Write down the impact the tense–release script is having from an emotional perspective.
6. Consider the outcomes on quality of life and overall well-being for both participants.

Chapter 8 will focus on passive muscular relaxation, so called because the contraction or active phase is absent. The chapter will describe how the trainee is taught to focus on different parts of the body to spot any tension and then release it without contracting or tensing first.

REFERENCES

Dolbier, C. L., & Rush, T. E. (2012). Efficacy of abbreviated progressive muscle relaxation in a high-stress college sample. *International Journal of Stress Management, 19*(1), 48–68.

Ikemata, S., & Momose, Y. (2017). Effects of a progressive muscle relaxation intervention on dementia symptoms, activities of daily living, and immune function in group home residents with dementia in Japan. *Japan Journal of Nursing Science, 14*(2), 135–145.

Kyrios, M., Ahern, C., Fassnacht, D. B., et al. (2018). Therapist assisted internet based cognitive behavioural therapy versus progressive relaxation in obsessive compulsive disorder: Randomised controlled trial. *Journal of Medical Internet Research, 20*(8), e242.

Limsanon, T., & Kalayasiri, R. (2015). Preliminary effects of progressive muscle relaxation on cigarette craving and withdrawal symptoms in experienced smokers in acute cigarette abstinence: A randomized controlled trial. *Behavior Therapy, 46*(2), 166–176.

Madders, J. (1984). *Stress and relaxation: Self-help ways to cope with stress and relieve nervous tension, ulcers, insomnia, migraine and high blood pressure.* London: Martin Dunitz.

Pan, L., Zhang, J., & Li, L. (2012). Effects of progressive muscle relaxation training on anxiety and quality of life of inpatients with ectopic pregnancy receiving methotrexate treatment. *Research in Nursing & Health, 35*, 362–382.

Safi, S. Z. (2015). A fresh look at the potential mechanisms of progressive muscle relaxation therapy on depression in female patients with multiple sclerosis. *Iranian Journal of Psychiatry and Behavioral Sciences, 9*(1), e340.

Sundram, B. M., Dahlui, M., & Chinna, K. (2016). Effectiveness of progressive muscle relaxation therapy as a worksite health promotion program in the automobile assembly line. *Industrial Health, 54*(3), 204–214.

Vancampfort, D., Correll, C. U., Scheewe, T. W., et al. (2013). Progressive muscle relaxation in persons with schizophrenia: A systematic review of randomized controlled trials. *Clinical Rehabilitation, 27*(4), 291–298.

Wallace, J. M. (1980). Muscular relaxation. *Look after yourself.* London: Health Education Authority.

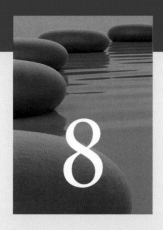

8

PASSIVE MUSCULAR RELAXATION

PROFESSOR TEENA CLOUSTON

LEARNING OBJECTIVES

The aim of this chapter is to provide a practical guide to basic concepts of passive muscular relaxation.

By the end of this chapter you will be able to:

1. Understand the key principles and process of passive muscular relaxation.

2. Describe the differences between the passive and active relaxation approaches.

3. Recognize why understanding the tense–release response before progressing to passive muscular relaxation is beneficial.

4. Identify the practical advantages of passive relaxation over the active approaches.

5. Carry out a passive relaxation session following the theories and methods in this chapter.

This chapter will conclude with key points and time for reflection, providing learning opportunities through case studies.

INTRODUCTION TO PASSIVE MUSCULAR RELAXATION

Muscular relaxation is a process by which contractile tension in voluntary muscles is reduced. The methods described in the previous three chapters are examples of the tense–release technique. Because of the contraction component, this is essentially an active procedure. When the contraction component is withdrawn, however, relaxation becomes a passive procedure. Jacobson's work covers both tense–release and passive relaxation.

Passive muscular relaxation consists of a systematic review of the skeletal muscle groups in the body. As attention is focused on each one in turn, the individual spots any tension and then releases it. Passive relaxation has certain practical advantages over 'active' methods in that:

- the sequences can be carried out without drawing attention to the individual performing them. They are thus potentially useful in the workplace or other public locations where stress arises.
- passive routines take less time to work through than tense–release ones.
- the method is available to those who find 'tensing' challenging or with physical disabilities, the nature of which might preclude some of the tension routines.

INTRODUCTION TO THE EVIDENCE

Evidence of the value of passive relaxation comes from Lucic et al (1991), whose work supports the view that muscles relax more fully when the process is not preceded by a strong contraction. In other words, the tensing of muscle groups before relaxation may actually hinder their capacity to relax. These findings are thus in line with the view of Jacobson (1938), whose work was essentially passive (though he did not use that word to describe it). Although his method has already been described in Chapter 5, reference must be made here to the position Jacobson holds as the preeminent exponent of the passive muscular approach. It is true that he used tensing procedures, but the emphasis of his work lay in the release of residual tension.

Interestingly, a study by Adler et al (2011) using passive and active relaxation techniques found that both methods improved the overall levels of anxiety for women in the third trimester of pregnancy equally well, with no preference for either method (n = 39). However, they also found that both methods of relaxation were more effective in women who had lower levels of anxiety and thus personality and high levels of anxiety could impact on the effectiveness.

Although little empirical research is available, Madders' methods (1980, 1984, 1989) are commonly used by occupational therapists and physiotherapists in the National Health Service. For example, occupational therapists in Guy's and St Thomas' NHS Foundation Trust use this approach to address stress and anxiety in cardiovascular patients (Guy's and St Thomas' NHS Trust 2019), and the Regional Department of Neurotology in Sheffield Teaching Hospital NHS Foundation Trust teaches Madders' 'emergency stop' technique to support patients to 'cope immediately with a stressful situation' (Sheffield Teaching Hospitals NHS Foundation Trust 2019, p2). In general, Madders' work purports that passive relaxation can reduce stress, nervous tension, ulcers, insomnia, migraine and high blood pressure (Madders 1980, 1984). She has also developed a technique to support children in expressing emotions and learning to relax (Madders 1989). Her method has been commended for use with migraine sufferers and in pregnancy (Lewis & The Migraine Action Association 1998).

McCallie et al's (2006) systematic review of progressive muscular relaxation identified that relaxation through recall and counting was added to Bernstein and Borkovec's (1973) method to promote deeper levels of relaxation for individuals in their personal home practice sessions. Lehrer et al (2007) support this notion but maintain that the effective use of this method requires the trainee to practice and be proficient in the tense–release cycle before using this modified approach.

A randomized controlled study by Hidderley and Holt (2004) using a type of autogenic passive relaxation identified that women with early stage breast cancer had strong statistical improvements in levels of anxiety and their immune responses compared with the control group, suggesting that either Everly and Rosenfeld (1981) or Kermani's (1990) scan method could be effective in this context.

THEORIES BEHIND PASSIVE MUSCULAR RELAXATION

Passive muscular relaxation, on the whole, requires previous knowledge of the tense–release approach. It is through tense–release that individuals learn to become aware of the sensations associated with muscle state, sensations that help them identify and release the tension. As noted previously Jacobson's (1938) philosophy is central to this approach as an underpinning principle. However, in terms of practice several theoretical approaches can be used.

The work of the following authors is described here:

- Bernstein and Borkovec (1973)
- Everly and Rosenfeld (1981)
- Madders (1984)
- Kermani (1990)

These authors have been included primarily because of the precise form of their presentations. Bernstein and Borkovec (1973) describe a release-only routine which they call 'relaxation through recall' in which muscle groups are relaxed by recalling the sensations associated with the release of tension.

Everly and Rosenfeld (1981) have developed a release-only approach which they call 'passive neuromuscular relaxation', defining it as a focusing of sensory awareness on particular muscle groups followed by their relaxation. These researchers see passive neuromuscular relaxation as a form of mental imagery which, together with its overtones of suggestion, departs from the strictly physical nature of Jacobson's progressive relaxation. On this account, the precautions for visualization (see Chapter 18) as well as those for muscular relaxation (see Chapter 5) should be read when adopting this approach.

The authors mentioned here are psychologists. Madders, a physiotherapist, includes passive relaxation in her book *Stress and Relaxation* (1984), whereas Kermani (1990), an autogenic training therapist, presents a scanning procedure.

KEY ASPECTS OF THE PROCEDURE

There are various techniques that can be used to practise passive relaxation. The four methods described here are relaxation through recall (Bernstein & Borkovec 1973), passive neuromuscular relaxation (Everly & Rosenfeld 1981), Madders' (1984) passive relaxation approach and Kermani's (1990) scanning method. Reference is also made to Öst's (1987) release only component in his applied relaxation approach, but this method is discussed in depth in Chapter 9.

RELAXATION THROUGH RECALL

While giving prominence to tense–release sequences in progressive relaxation training (see Chapter 6), Bernstein and Borkovec (1973) also offer a release-only

technique. 'Relaxation through recall' is the name given to this technique which is described here in an adapted form. It requires the trainee to have first learned the active form of progressive relaxation training because the passive form is based on the memory of those routines.

The muscle groups involved are the final summarized groupings of arms, head and neck, trunk and legs noted in Table 5.1 in Chapter 5. Two steps are involved:

1. Individuals focus on one of the groups, noticing any tension.
2. They then recall the sensation associated with releasing tension and spend 30 to 45 seconds relaxing any tension that they find.

Trainees are prepared by a short introduction.

Tensing and relaxing has made you highly sensitive to the feelings which accompany changes in the muscles, and now that you know the technique, I want to lead you to a more advanced version of it. I would like you to cast your mind back to the four-group tense–release procedure, but this time, to drop the tensing part. As we travel through these four groups, I'm going to ask you simply to look for any tension, and then, by recalling the sensations associated with its release, to let it go.

The trainee sits in a reclining chair or something that resembles it and the following script is presented.

Would you close your eyes please? I'd like you first to concentrate on the muscles of your hands and arms. See if you can identify any feeling of tension in them. If so, notice where it is notice how it feels … and relax it away, remembering previous feelings of releasing tension in these muscles … go on releasing tension as you recall those sensations … go on until the muscles become more and more deeply relaxed … until you feel relaxation flowing through all the muscles of your arms … until they are totally free of tension … signal with a lifted finger when the arms feel fully relaxed.

The trainer continues in this way for 30 to 45 seconds.

Next, bring your mind to focus on the muscles of your face and neck. Is there any tension there? If so, notice where it is and what it feels like … then, recalling the feeling of letting the tension go, relax it … feel the tension leaving the muscles … note the pleasant feeling of relaxation … allow the relaxation to deepen and go on deepening as you concentrate on the peaceful state of those muscles …

Next, concentrate on the muscles of the trunk. Pick up any sensation of tension you may find … notice where it is and what it feels like … remember what it felt like when you previously relaxed tension in those muscles … and relax them now … relax any tension you find … continue letting the tension go until your muscles feel quite loose. Go on relaxing them … feel them getting looser and looser.

Finally, give your attention to your legs … do you notice any tension there? … notice exactly where it is … notice how it feels … and release it … recalling the sensation of releasing it … remembering that feeling … letting all the tension dissolve … further … then further still … until the muscles feel entirely relaxed …

By practising relaxation through recall, the trainee will be able to reduce the time it takes to relax each muscle group from 45 to perhaps 15 seconds.

Relaxation Through Recall With Counting

When the trainee feels skilled at relaxing through recall, the procedure can be still further shortened by introducing counting. Here, recited numbers correspond to the groups in the recall procedure as follows.

I'm going to count slowly from one to ten. As I count, I'd like you to focus on the same muscle groups as in the recall procedure, relaxing them as you did then.

One … two, focusing on the arms and hands as they become more relaxed … three … four, relaxing the face and neck muscles … five … six, focusing on the muscles of the chest, back, shoulders and abdomen, feeling them becoming more and more relaxed … seven … eight, allowing relaxation to flow through the muscles of the legs and feet … nine … ten, relaxed all over …

It is suggested that the counting be done at a pace which corresponds with the trainee's respirations.

Once mastered, this technique can be used by the trainee when faced with challenging situations.

PASSIVE NEUROMUSCULAR RELAXATION

The technique described here is the work of Everly and Rosenfeld (1981). This method owes much to autogenic training (see Chapter 20) in its use of suggestion and its images of warmth and heaviness. It is, however, considered by its authors to be a muscular method and so belongs in this chapter.

Trainees are introduced to the approach with a short explanation on the following lines.

Tension in the muscles is associated with tension in the mind. If tension is eliminated from the muscles, then the subjective feeling of stress is reduced. In this method you will be asked to focus attention on one muscle group at a time, releasing any tension that exists. No activity is involved; the method is a passive one. It has been found that by concentrating on the muscles in this way, deep levels of relaxation can be achieved. Of course, the more you practise, the more effective it becomes.

The necessary conditions include a warm, quiet room where interruptions are unlikely to occur and a comfortable chair to sit in or flat surface to lie on. The following script is adapted from Everly and Rosenfeld (1981).

Settle into the chair you're in or the surface you are lying on, letting your body weight sink into it. Close your eyes. To start with, I'd like you to turn your attention to your breathing … follow the next breath out … then, let the air in … feel it gently filling your lungs … pause for a moment … and breathe out slowly … then allow your breathing to follow its natural rhythm: gentle and slow … getting gentler and slower …

Now bring your attention to the muscles of your head. Begin to feel a slow warm wave of relaxation gathering at the top of your head and beginning to descend towards your forehead … focusing on the muscles above your eyes … feel those muscles becoming heavy and relaxed ... concentrate on the heavy feeling you are getting from them ... now shift your attention to the muscles of your eyes and cheeks and feel them also becoming heavy and relaxed ... now, focus on the muscles of your mouth and jaw ... allow them to grow heavy and relaxed ...

Pause for 10 seconds.

As your head and face continue to relax, let the wave of relaxation slowly descend into your neck ... focus your attention on the neck muscles and feel them becoming slacker and more relaxed with every moment that passes ...

Pause for 10 seconds.

The wave of relaxation continues to roll down, this time spreading warmth over your shoulder muscles ... focus on this area ... allow it to become heavy and relaxed as you concentrate your attention on it.

Pause for 10 seconds.

The head, neck and shoulders remain relaxed while you focus on your arms ... letting the wave of relaxation bring heaviness and warmth to them ... concentrate on the feelings in the arms ...

Pause for 10 seconds.

Now feel the wave of relaxation descending into your hands as you focus on them ... feel the muscles of your palms and fingers relaxing ... feel warmth flowing into them as they become more relaxed ...

Pause for 10 seconds.

Now, as the upper part of your body remains in deep relaxation, switch your attention to your abdomen and the wall of muscle covering your internal organs ... let those muscles loosen and spread ... then feel the wave of relaxation beginning to descend into your thigh muscles ... and as you concentrate on them, feel your thighs becoming heavy ... heavy as lead ...

Pause for 10 seconds.

The wave of relaxation continues to descend into your lower legs ... focus on your calf muscles ... feel the sense of heaviness and relaxation in your calves ...

Pause for 10 seconds.

Now, as the rest of your body remains relaxed, turn your attention to your feet ... feel the warm wave of relaxation descending into your foot muscles ... feel them becoming warm, heavy and relaxed ...

Pause for 10 seconds.

Then, as you feel all your muscles to be in a state of relaxation, start to recite the phrase, 'I am relaxed'; repeat it every time you breathe out.

After a 5-minute pause:

I'd like you now to bring your attention back to the room in which you are lying. I am going to count from one to five, and as I count, begin to feel more and more awake, more and more refreshed, with a clear head. When I reach five, I'd like you to open your eyes. One, begin to feel alert ... two ... three, more alert still ... four ... five ... open your eyes and gently stretch your arms and legs ...

The Relaxation 'Ripple'

Closely related to the previous method is the relaxation 'ripple'. Adapted from Priest and Schott (1991), the technique consists of one continuous wave of relaxation which begins at the crown of the head and progresses down through the body to the toes. As the wave descends, individuals briefly scan the muscle groups, releasing tension. If they are lying down, all tension can be released; if they are standing, excess tension can be released. The effectiveness of the exercise is increased if it is timed to coincide with the outbreath. However, participants should be discouraged from extending the outbreath for too long.

The exercise can be better understood if the first relaxation ripple is preceded by a tensing of the whole body (Schott & Priest 2002). Thereafter, it can be performed in a passive manner.

A PASSIVE RELAXATION APPROACH

The script presented here is adapted from Madders (1984). It is addressed to trainees who are lying down. A supplementary section enables the instructor to adapt it for the seated participant.

Introductory Remarks to Trainees

This is a method which helps to relax your muscles and your thoughts. It consists of focusing on different parts of the body in turn and releasing any tension you find. There are no physical actions involved; relaxation occurs by virtue of a thought process. In spite of its length, the method is one which you can easily use to induce relaxation on your own.

Procedure for Participants Who Are Lying Down

A firm support with a soft surface is needed, such as a length of foam spread out on the floor. The script could begin with the passage called 'Sinking' in Chapter 3 and continue as follows:

With your eyes closed, notice how slow and regular your breathing is becoming … easy, calm and even … leaving you more relaxed than you were before …

I'm going to ask you to take a trip round the body, checking that all the muscle groups are as relaxed as possible and letting go of any tension that might still remain. If outside thoughts creep in, hold them in a bubble and let them float away. I'll begin with the feet.

Bring your attention to your toes … are they lying still? If they are curled or stretched out or in some way not entirely comfortable, waggle them gently. As they come to rest, feel the tension ebbing away … feel the tension leaving them as they lie motionless …

Let your feet roll out at the ankles. This is the most relaxed position for them. Let all the tension flow out of them … enjoy the sensation of just letting them go.

Moving on to the lower legs: feel the tension leaving the calf muscles and the shins. As the tension

goes, so they feel heavier … so they feel warm and pleasantly tingling.

The thighs next: to be fully relaxed they need to be slightly rolling outwards … feel the relaxing effect of this position … make sure you have released all tension, and feel your thighs resting heavily on the floor.

Focus for a moment on the sensation of sagging heaviness throughout your legs … let the muscles shed their last remaining hint of tension and settle into a deep relaxation.

And now, think of your hips. Let them settle into the surface you are lying on … recognize any tension that lingers in the muscles … then relax it away … let it go on relaxing a bit further than you thought possible.

Settle your spine into the rug or mattress … become aware of how it is resting on the floor. Let it sink down, making contact wherever it wants to … all tension draining out of it.

Let your abdominal muscles lose their tension. Let them go soft and loose. Feel them spreading as they give up their last vestige of tension … notice how your relaxed abdomen rises and falls with your breathing … rises as the air is drawn in and falls as the air is expelled … abdominal breathing is relaxed breathing.

Moving up to your shoulders, to muscles which are prone to carry tension … feel them letting go … feel them spreading … feel them easing into the floor, limp and heavy … feel them dropping down towards your feet … imagine them shedding their burdens … and as the space between your shoulders and your neck opens out, imagine your neck a bit longer than it was before.

Now, direct your thoughts to the muscles of your left arm. Check that it lies limply on the ground. Notice the feeling of relaxation and allow this feeling to sweep down to your wrist and hand. Think of the fingers, are they curved and still? … neither drawn up nor stretched out … in a hand that is neither open nor closed, but gently resting … totally relaxed. As you breathe out, let the arm relax a little bit more … let it lie heavy and loose … so heavy and loose that if someone were to pick it up, then let go, it would flop down again like the arm of a rag doll.

Repeat the previous steps with the muscles of the right arm.

Your neck muscles have no need to work with your head supported, so let them go … enjoy the feeling of 'letting go' in muscles which work so hard the rest of the time to keep your head upright. If you find any tension in the neck, release it and let this process of releasing continue, even below the surface … feel how pleasant it is when you let go of the tension in these muscles.

Bring your attention now to your face, to the many small muscles whose job it is to manage your expressions. At the moment there's no need to have any expression at all on your face, so allow your muscles to feel relaxed … imagine how your face is when you are asleep … calm and motionless …

Now, think about the jaw … and as you do, allow it to drop slightly so that your teeth are separated … feel it relaxing with your lips gently touching. Check that your tongue is still, and lying in the middle of your mouth, soft and shapeless. Relax your throat so that all tension leaves it and the muscles feel smooth and resting.

With no expression on your face, your cheeks are relaxed and soft. If you think of your nose, let it be just to register the passage of cool air travelling up your nostrils while warmer air passes down … breathe tension out with the warm air … breathe stillness in with the cool air.

Check that your forehead is smooth … not furrowed in any direction … and as you release its remaining tension, imagine it being a little higher and a little wider that it was before … let this feeling of relaxation extend through your scalp muscles, over the crown of your head and down behind your ears … feel a sense of calm as you do this.

Let your attention focus on your eyes as they lie behind gently closed lids. Think of them resting in their sockets, floating rather than fixed … and as they come to rest, so do your thoughts also.

Spend a few minutes continuing to relax, deepening the effect of the above sequences …

You have now relaxed all the major muscle groups in your body. Think about them now as a whole … a totally relaxed whole … and soothed by your gentle breathing rhythm, feel the peacefulness of this idea …

Images may drift in and out of your mind … see them as thoughts passing through. Feel yourself letting go of them. Say to yourself: 'I am feeling calm, I am feeling peaceful'. Let your mind conjure up a scene of contentment.

Trainees can relax quietly for a few minutes before the session is brought to an end.

Termination

I am going to ask you to bring yourself slowly back to the room you are lying in. Gradually become aware of it. Gently move your arms and legs … wriggle your spine, and in your own time, allow your eyes to open. Slowly sit up and take in your surroundings. Give your body plenty of time to adjust from the relaxed to the alert state.

Before the meeting breaks up, the value of practice should be emphasized. If carried out on a daily basis, the technique will help the trainee to relax more effectively.

Adapted Procedure for Seated Trainees

The trainee picks the chair they find most comfortable, although in a public building the choice may be limited. For deep relaxation the body needs to be well supported. The procedure begins in the following way.

Settle into your chair, sitting well back into the seat, your feet flat on the floor and your hands in your lap. Close your eyes. Become aware of the parts of your body that touch the chair and the floor. Feel the weight of your body passing through those points: hips, thighs, feet, back and arms, some of them carrying more weight than others. If the back of the chair is high enough, use it to support your head. If not, your head may be dropping forwards which is all right if you find it comfortable, but it tends to put a strain on the neck muscles if held for a long time. Try raising your head and seeing it as a weight supported by a pole. If you can balance it in this way, on your spine, you will be giving your neck muscles a rest.

The same script as for the lying position may be used, substituting the words 'sitting' for 'lying' and 'chair' for 'floor'. The paragraph about the neck muscles can be deleted, and also the one referring to the feet.

KERMANI'S SCANNING TECHNIQUE

Akin to Everly and Rosenfeld's (1981) passive neuro-muscular relaxation, Kermani's work has also emerged from autogenic approaches (see Chapter 20). To 'scan', in this sense, is to run the attention over all the voluntary muscles.

Scanning may be used for at least two purposes: as a means of checking to see if tension exists, and as a device to enable the individual to feel in touch with their body as a whole. Both purposes are relevant in the context of relaxation, and the method forms a quick and simple version of the passive relaxation approach.

Here is an example adapted from Kermani (1990).

I'll ask you to spend a moment getting in touch with the different parts of your body, acknowledging them as part of you and checking that they feel relaxed and comfortable. Begin by bringing your attention to your feet. First the toes … working up through the ankles … to the calves and shins … over the knees … along the thighs … the abdomen … then the chest. Think now of your shoulders … of travelling down to the elbows … through the forearms … and into the wrists … hands and fingers. Become aware even of your fingertips.

Next, move across to the lower spine and the pelvis. Give your attention to the lumbar region … rising to the back of the chest and the shoulder blade bones … continuing up into the neck and scalp … to the crown of the head … then slowly begin to descend to the forehead … ending with the jaw … feel that every part of your body is relaxed …

You might like to think of a giant paint brush sweeping over your body, following the same route.

ANOTHER PASSIVE METHOD

A release-only method is described in Chapter 9 as one component of Öst's (1987) applied relaxation.

PRECAUTIONS

Passive relaxation is subject to the precautions of other muscular approaches (see Chapter 5). Because passive methods often include imagery and suggestion, the precautions relating to visualizations should also be taken into account (see Chapter 18).

APPLICATION

Passive muscle relaxation is widely used in practice for reducing mental and physical tension in a broad range of conditions. Although theoretically predicated on an understanding of the tense–release approach, it can be used with people who have difficulty with the tensing stage or active contraction of muscle groups. The use of mental imagery enables trainees to use the power of thought to release tension in the muscles and engender positive thinking to relax the mind and body.

KEY POINTS

1. Different authors have proposed variations of passive relaxation. Four are included in this chapter: Bernstein and Borkovec, Everly and Rosenfeld, Madders and Kermani.
2. Passive muscular relaxation is derived from Jacobson's progressive relaxation but differs from it in its absence of the 'tensing' component.
3. Summarized versions of these methods constitute scanning procedures.
4. Passive forms of relaxation are useful for people who cannot tolerate tensing actions.
5. Passive relaxation is a skill and as such requires regular practice.

Reflection

Describe your understanding of the technique of passive relaxation.

What did you learn about the differences between the four methods of passive relaxation in this chapter? How do you think these could be applied in practice?

How did you feel when you completed your own passive relaxation session?

What is the main learning point you will take away from this chapter?

What is your future action plan in terms of passive relaxation?

CASE STUDY LEARNING OPPORTUNITIES

The key points and reflection provide the background and knowledge required in relation to the case studies;

Mali (Case Study 1) and Lewis (Case Study 2) help to deepen understanding of how passive relaxation can be applied in practice.

CASE STUDY 1

Early Stage Breast Cancer and Anxiety: PMR Outcome for Mali

Mali has been diagnosed with early stage breast cancer. She has received a lumpectomy and adjuvant radiotherapy. Her prognosis is good, but she is suffering from anxiety and depression and tells you that she just cannot "shake of the dark clouds" she feels are hanging over her. She also feels like she has a band strapped around her chest; this is constricting her and affecting her breathing, which is shallow.

You suggest she join an 8-week relaxation course based around Everly and Rosenfeld's (1981) passive neuromuscular approach. You explain to her that this is quite an advanced relaxation technique because the trainee has to 'visualize' relaxing muscle groups and remember what it feels like to actually be relaxed. The technique also uses imagery and imagination to facilitate the relaxation.

Initially Mali is unsure, but you explain that she has the skills to do this as she completed a course of progressive relaxation training and is an experienced yogi who has practised 'shavasana' (relaxation at the end of a yoga session) and 'yoga nidra' (guided yoga meditation) for years. Following your recommendation Mali joins the course. She benefits in mood immediately and starts practising deeper abdominal breathing in between classes as well as doing a daily PMR session on her own at home. By the end of the 8-week programme not only has the feeling of constriction in her breast reduced but she is experiencing lower levels of anxiety and depression, and her sleep and immune responses have also improved. She has been envisaging the wave of relaxation flowing down her body and is finding this extremely beneficial. Mali is so pleased with the result that she intends to keep on practising passive muscular relaxation daily.

PMR, Passive muscular relaxation.

CASE STUDY 2

Cardiac Rehabilitation: PMR Outcomes for Lewis

Lewis is recovering from a myocardial infarct (heart attack). He has been discharged and is living at home but is still feeling very anxious. He is particularly concerned about returning to work. He has joined the 6-week cardiac rehabilitation course at the hospital in the hope that the stress management component will alleviate his worries.

On arrival at his first session, Lewis explains to the group leader that he has never practised any form of relaxation before and is, in fact, quite worried about that. His fears are allayed by the trainer explaining that the first group relaxation session will help him to identify the difference between a tense and relaxed

state by offering the opportunity to practise Bernstein and Borkovec's (1973) tense–release cycle.

In the relaxation room Lewis just follows the leader's instructions and to his surprise he can feel the tension in his body and does experience some sense of relief at the relaxing stage. With the help of a CD, he practises this method at home during the week.

At the second session, the group members are introduced to Madders' (1984) method of relaxation. Lewis enjoys the script and finds he can in fact 'let go' of tension by focusing on the parts of the body with his mind. He takes a CD of this method home and practises it daily, usually before going to bed.

Although his anxiety is improving, he is still concerned about returning to work and wants to use his relaxation to help him manage stressful situations in the workplace. The group leader suggests learning a couple of shortened versions of passive relaxation and offers training in relaxation through recall and counting to help Lewis with this. He finds he can use this technique in a more 'on the spot' way to help him relax, and this in itself is helping him feel more able to manage his anxieties about returning to work.

*CD, *; PMR,* Passive muscular relaxation.

ACTIVITY

For each of the case studies:

1. List key aspects used in the passive relaxation approaches.
2. Consider why this approach was taken.
3. Write down the impact that passive muscular relaxation is having from a psychological perspective.
4. Write down the impact that passive muscular relaxation is having from a physical perspective.
5. Write down the impact that passive muscular relaxation is having from an emotional perspective.
6. Consider the outcomes on quality of life and overall wellbeing for both individuals.

Chapter 9 will focus on Öst's (1987) method of applied relaxation. Using progressive relaxation as its core technique this method teaches the individual to relax in successively shorter periods and to then transfer this technique to everyday situations.

REFERENCES

Adler, J., Urech, C., Fink, N., Bitzer, J., & Hoesli, I. (2011). Response to induced relaxation during pregnancy: Comparison of women with high versus low levels of anxiety. *Journal of Clinical Psychology in Medical Settings, 18*(1), 21–31.

Bernstein, D. A., & Borkovec, T. D. (1973). *Progressive relaxation training: A manual for the helping professions.* Champaign, IL: Research Press.

Everly, G. S., & Rosenfeld, R. (1981). *The nature and treatment of the stress response.* New York: Plenum Press.

Guy's and St Thomas' NHS Foundation Trust. (2019). *The Jane Madders Relaxation Technique.* London: Guy's and St Thomas' NHS Foundation Trust.

Hidderley, M., & Holt, M. (2004). A pilot randomised trial assessing the effects of autogenic training in early stage cancer patients in relation to psychological status and immune system responses. *European Journal of Oncology Nursing, 8*(1), 61–65.

Jacobson, E. (1938). *Progressive relaxation* (2nd ed.). Chicago: University of Chicago Press.

Kermani, K. S. (1990). *Autogenic training.* London: Souvenir Press.

Lehrer, P. M., Woolfolk, R. L., & Sime, W. E. (2007). *Principles and practice of stress management* (3rd ed.). New York: The Guilford Press.

Lewis, J., & The Migraine Action Association (1998). *The migraine handbook: The definitive guide to the causes symptoms and treatments.* London: Vermilion.

Lucic, K. S., Steffen, J. J., Harrigan, J. A., & Stuebing, R. C. (1991). Progressive relaxation training: Muscle contractions before relaxation? *Behavior Therapy, 22*(2), 249–256.

Madders, J. (1980). Group relaxation in the treatment of migraine a multifactorial approach. In F. J. McGuigan, W. E. Sime, & J. M. Wallace (Eds.), *Stress and tension control* (pp. 141–145). Boston: Springer.

Madders, J. (1984). Stress and relaxation: Self-help ways to cope with stress and relieve nervous tension, ulcers, insomnia. *migraine and high blood pressure.* London: Martin Dunitz.

Madders, J. (1989). Introducing relaxation methods to young children. In F. J. McGuigan, W. E. Sime, & J. Macdonald Wallace (Eds.), *Stress and relaxation in education* (pp. 201–208). New York: Plenum Press.

McCallie, M. S., Blum, C. M., & Hood, C. J. (2006). Progressive muscular relaxation. *Journal of Human Behavior in the Social Environment, 13*(3), 51–66.

Öst, L. G. (1987). Applied relaxation: Description of a coping technique and review of controlled studies. *Behaviour Research and Therapy, 25*(5), 397–409.

Priest, J., & Schott, J. (1991). *Leading antenatal classes: A practical guide.* Oxford: Butterworth-Heinemann.

Schott, J., & Priest, J. (2002). *Leading antenatal classes: A practical guide* (2nd ed.). Oxford: Books for Midwives, Butterworth-Heinemann.

Sheffield Teaching Hospitals NHS Foundation Trust. (2019). *A Guide to Short Relaxation Exercises.* Sheffield, UK: Sheffield Teaching Hospitals NHS Foundation Trust.

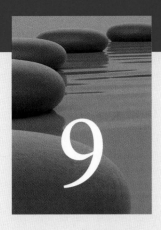

9 APPLIED RELAXATION

PROFESSOR TEENA CLOUSTON

CHAPTER CONTENTS

LEARNING OBJECTIVES

The aim of this chapter is to provide a practical guide to the basic concepts of applied relaxation.

By the end of this chapter you will be able to:

1. Understand the key principles and process of applied relaxation.

2. Identify the key elements necessary to utilize applied relaxation when required in the everyday life situation.

3. Recognize the importance of the physiological, cognitive, psychological and behavioural components of anxiety and how applied relaxation techniques can mitigate these.

4. Describe how applied relaxation has developed from Jacobson's and Wolpe's original methods.

5. Follow the principles of applied relaxation and evaluate its effectiveness.

This chapter will conclude with key points and time for reflection, providing learning opportunities through case studies.

INTRODUCTION TO APPLIED RELAXATION

The methods described in previous chapters have, on the whole, been concerned with the induction of deep relaxation. Their purpose is to equip the individual with routines to be performed in the privacy of their own home. As such, these methods are useful for unwinding after a stressful day but may not provide strategies for coping with stress as it occurs. For this, some kind of shortened version that can be linked into life activities is required.

Jacobson's (1938) differential relaxation (Chapter 11) and Wolpe's (1958) systematic desensitization represent early attempts at applied formats. However, it was Goldfried (1971) who, recognizing the extent of the gulf between relaxation in the therapeutic environment and relaxation in the stressful situation, focused expressly on the issue of the application of the skills.

He emphasized the need for a portable and shortened form of progressive relaxation; a form which could be used to defuse anxiety as it occurred, and one which the individual could use as a general coping skill in everyday life. In so doing, he gave individuals a new role, defining them as an active agent in their own treatment rather than passive clients. The approach was called 'training in self-control' because it implied active mastery of anxiety by the individual who practised it.

Öst's (1987) applied relaxation method is a more recent version of Goldfried's approach. Using progressive relaxation as a core technique, the method teaches the individual to relax in successively shorter periods and to transfer these relaxation effects to everyday situations. In Öst's (1987, p397) own words 'the purpose of this treatment method is to teach the patient coping skills which will enable him/her to relax rapidly, to counteract, and eventually abort the anxiety reactions altogether.' Thus, through learning to recognize the early stages of anxiety symptoms and learning to respond to this through the application of applied relaxation techniques, so the individual is equipped with a strategy to control reactions to stressful events as they occur.

The method consists of six components, in each of which a particular aspect of relaxation is taught:

- Tense–release technique
- Release-only technique
- Cue-controlled (conditioned) relaxation
- Differential relaxation
- Rapid relaxation
- Application training

It is estimated that by using the tense–release method taught here (Wolpe & Lazarus 1966), the trained individual can achieve a relaxed state in 15 to 20 minutes; by using the release-only technique it can be achieved in 5 to 7 minutes; using the cue-controlled, in 2 to 3 minutes; the differential technique, in 60 to 90 seconds; and using rapid relaxation, in 20 to 30 seconds. The final goal is to be able to apply relaxation skills to the experience of every day stressful events.

The components must be taught in a precise order since progression to each depends largely on mastery of the preceding one. A total of 8 to 12 sessions of tuition is required, backed up by home practice which should be carried out twice a day, and is itself an important part of the programme.

INTRODUCTION TO THE EVIDENCE

Developed in the 1970s, Lars-Göran Öst's method of applied relaxation addresses four modes of anxiety with the applied relaxation approach: the physiological, the cognitive, the psychological and the behavioural (Hayes-Skelton et al 2012, 2013a). The physiological aspect is addressed through muscle relaxation, the cognitive through the cue word, and the psychological and behavioural through differential relaxation and exposure to the stressor. A multivariate approach such as this has advantages in a condition like anxiety where changes occur in different modes.

As a method, applied relaxation has been tested in a wide variety of complaints, including phobia, panic disorder, headache, epilepsy and tinnitus. In all these it has been found significantly more effective than no treatment or placebo conditions. Follow-up at varying times from 5 to 19 months showed that effects were maintained and, in some cases, augmented (Öst 1987, 1988). In particular Öst's approach has been deemed an effective intervention with generalized anxiety disorder.

Studies comparing applied relaxation with psychological methods have often reported very little difference in effectiveness; for example, in a study comparing the method with cognitive therapy on a population of 33 people experiencing generalized anxiety disorder, it was not possible to declare one method superior to the other. Both, however, were found to be effective (Öst & Breitholtz 2000). Using the same comparators, later studies by Arntz (2003) and Siev and Chambless (2007) supported these findings. Similarly, studies comparing applied relaxation with cognitive–behavioural therapy (Donegan & Dugas 2012, Dugas et al 2010), acceptance-based therapy (Hayes-Skelton et al 2013b) and worry exposure (Hoyer et al 2009) all had similar results. Although this is still positive in terms of the evidence base for applied relaxation, Hayes-Skelton et al (2012) and Hayes-Skelton et al (2013a) have cogently argued that in many cases the process of training in terms of applied relaxation is often unclear in these studies and thus the validity and, consequently, efficacy of the applied relaxation method cannot be effectively measured. They argue this may mean that the technique could, in fact, be far more effective than studies to date suggest.

An early study that addressed this shortfall by Spence and colleagues (1995) tested the effect of applied relaxation on chronic upper extremity pain caused by cumulative trauma. Forty-eight patients were randomly allocated to four groups: applied relaxation, electromyographic feedback, a combination of both and a waiting list control. After treatment twice weekly for 4 weeks, significant reductions in pain, depression, distress and anxiety were found in all the relaxation groups while minimal change occurred in the waiting list control. However, the greatest benefit, in the short term at least, was reported in the group who received applied relaxation. This study therefore supports the contention that the method could in fact be far more effective than the majority of existing research evidenced.

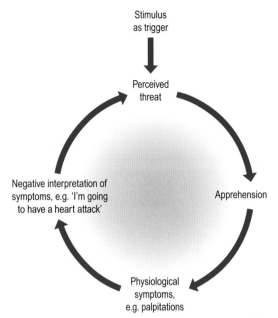

Fig. 9.1 ■ A cognitive model of panic attacks. (Adapted from Clark 1986.)

THEORIES BEHIND APPLIED RELAXATION

As with all versions of progressive relaxation, applied relaxation is said to calm the thoughts as a result of relaxing the musculature. Thus it can be used for coping with day-to-day stress. Öst's method, however, was designed principally for use with people who suffer from panic and other kinds of anxiety. In this context, an understanding of anxiety as a state is crucial to the success of the training and an explanation should be given to the participant at the outset.

Anxiety may be seen as having four aspects: the physiological, the cognitive, the psychological and the behavioural. The physiological aspect is represented by such phenomena as raised heart rate and blood pressure, sweating and increased muscle tension; the cognitive aspect by negative thoughts such as 'This is too much for me to cope with' or 'I'm going to have a heart attack', the psychological aspect by overwhelming feelings like panic or stress and the behavioural aspect by tense posture and different kinds of unrelaxed activity. These effects can escalate with one inflaming the other. In particular, the physiological,

psychological and cognitive aspects can create a vicious circle with negative thoughts leading to sympathetic changes which are themselves interpreted in an unhelpful way (Clouston 2015[*]). The result can be a spiralling of anxiety (Clark 1986, Clouston 2015) (Fig. 9.1).

One way of breaking the circle would be to reinterpret the body changes in a more positive light; that is, instead of thinking they are about to collapse with a heart attack, individuals could try adopting reassuring thoughts like 'everyone gets palpitations sometimes'. This constitutes a cognitive and affective or psychological approach, facilitating individuals to address the negative or distorted pattern manifest in their thinking and feelings. Clouston (2015, p114) suggests a five-step approach to address this as follows:

Step 1: recognize the negative thoughts as errors or distortions in judgement and accept that they do not reflect the reality of the situation.

Step 2: begin to rationalize this incongruence and revise the pattern of thinking and the usual response to the situation.

---

[*]This book provides an in-depth overview of why we get stressed in modern life and the physiology of the human stress response, as well as a variety of practical mindfulness and relaxation techniques.

Date	Situation	Reaction, i.e. anxiety signals	Intensity (0–10)	Action taken

Fig. 9.2 ■ Form for recording self-observed early anxiety signals. (Adapted from Öst 1987.)

Step 3: identify a more accurate and evidence-based appraisal of the situation and begin to apply this more realistic version to the situation.

Step 4: put that accurate and more positive response into action.

Step 5: review the situation in terms of feelings, behaviours, thoughts and physiological responses; revise if necessary and repeat the process. Practising the new approach is the key to its success.

Another way of breaking the circle would be to neutralize the anxiety with the use of a relaxation technique such as progressive relaxation. This draws on physiological theory. A third way would be to introduce graded exposure to the feared item, which represents a behavioural approach. All three are incorporated in Öst's applied relaxation, which can thus be seen as a cognitive–behavioural method (Heimberg 2002).

Because anxiety is easier to relieve when it is mild, it should be addressed before it reaches a peak. Early signals or signs of rising anxiety levels such as a pounding heart, sweating, fast breathing or tense muscles can be used as cues to employ the technique. Experiences of anxiety-provoking events can be recorded by means of 'self-monitoring', where the individual notes on a printed form the situations, the intensity of their anxiety and the remedial action taken by them to address this (Fig. 9.2). This form, over time, builds to reflect the successful strategies adopted and thus the progress in coping with such events.

KEY ASPECTS OF THE PROCEDURE

Conditions for Training Sessions

It is suggested that participants sit for the exercises because daily stress often occurs in this posture rather than in a lying one. The chair should be comfortable and have arm rests. The procedures are first demonstrated by the trainer and carried out by the trainee to ensure that they have been understood. Trainees then closes their eyes while the instructor runs through the programme. At the end, trainees rate the degree of relaxation gained on a 0 to 100 scale.

Each component requires 1 to 2 weeks of practice for trainees to become proficient in it.

Introductory Remarks to Participants

Before beginning the programme of relaxation, the rationale of the treatment is presented to participants.

As its name suggests, this method will show you how to apply relaxation skills in everyday life. This means the techniques have to be quick-acting and unobtrusive. The aim is to be able to relax in 20 to 30 seconds and to transfer this skill to situations of stress.

When people experience anxiety they tend to react in four different ways: a physiological way in which their blood pressure rises and they become breathless with a pounding heart and a cold sweat; a cognitive and psychological way in which distressing thoughts and feelings go through their head; and a behavioural way whereby they find themselves trying to escape.

If the physiological symptoms are viewed as threatening, the body will respond by intensifying those symptoms, which in turn will make the thoughts and feelings more negative. This is the way a panic attack develops.

However, this vicious circle can be broken and one way of doing this is by learning not to react so strongly. This will reduce your feeling of distress and your symptoms will tend to subside.

I am going to lead you through a well-tested method which will help you to achieve this. You'll be learning a skill so it's important to practise it, but once you've mastered it, you'll find it useful in nearly all situations.

The approach starts by introducing you to progressive relaxation which consists of tensing and releasing the muscles throughout the body. When that is learned and practised daily, the tensing part of the exercise is dropped.

Next, you'll be asked to repeat the word 'relax' to yourself when you are in a state of relaxation. Attaching the word to the state has the effect of turning the word into a cue; a cue to invoke a state of relaxation. This only happens, of course, after repeated associations.

Learning how to use reduced amounts of muscle tension when carrying out specific tasks is the next procedure, followed by a rapid-acting technique for maintaining low levels of stress throughout the day. Finally, these skills are applied to particular situations of stress.

These exercises enable you to achieve relaxation in progressively shorter periods of time. Success depends on practice.

Tense–Release

Two sessions of tuition are devoted to learning this version of progressive relaxation.

First Session

The first session is spent working on the hands, arms, face, neck and shoulders. Each muscle group is taken through one tense–release cycle in which 5 seconds are allotted for the tension and 10 to 15 seconds for the release, as follows:

Begin by clenching the right hand … make a fist … make it tight … notice the sensation of tension in the hand and forearm while you hold it for 5 seconds … then let it go … feel the hand and forearm becoming relaxed and comfortable … warm and relaxed … relaxed and heavy …

The release is continued for 10 seconds.

The other actions featuring in session one are as follows:

- Clenching the left hand
- Bending the right elbow
- Straightening the right elbow by pressing the wrist down on the arm of the chair
- Bending the left elbow
- Straightening the left elbow
- Raising the eyebrows and wrinkling the forehead
- Bringing the eyebrows together and frowning
- Screwing the eyes up tight
- Biting the teeth together
- Pressing the tongue against the roof of the mouth
- Pressing the lips together
- Pressing the head against the back of the chair
- Pressing the chin down on to the collarbone
- Hunching the shoulders up to the ears
- Bracing the shoulders back to bring the blades together.

Termination. When the previous exercises have been worked through, the session is brought to an end.

The relaxation session is over now, and to help you return to activity, I'm going to count from one to five, and when I get to five, I want you to open your eyes, feeling calm and relaxed … one, feeling calm … two, feeling relaxed … three, very calm … four, very relaxed … five … open your eyes, feeling ready to carry on with your everyday life.

A debriefing period follows (Chapter 3). Participants are instructed to practise for 15 minutes twice daily. They are asked to record the level of relaxation achieved, using a 0 to 100 scale where 0 equals total relaxation, 100 equals maximum tension, and 50 represents normal. They are also asked to keep a note of the length of practice time taken to reach the level achieved. The form shown in Fig. 9.3 serves to motivate the individual to practise as well as to record the details of the homework session.

Second Session

Session two starts with a review of the work done in the first session followed by tense–release exercises for

0 = totally relaxed
100 = maximum tension

| Date | Time | Component | Degree of relaxation (0–100) | | Time taken to achieve it |
			Before	After	

Fig. 9.3 ■ Form for recording relaxation training homework. (Adapted from Öst 1987.)

the chest, stomach, back, legs and feet. These are as follows:

- Tensing the muscles which pull the stomach in
- Arching the back so that the spine leaves the back of the chair
- Tensing the buttock muscles by pressing the feet down into the floor
- Raising the heels with the toes remaining on the ground
- Raising the front part of the foot, keeping the heels on the ground.

The second session is terminated in the same way as the first and trainees are reminded to practise.

Release-Only

In the release-only phase of instruction, the 'tension' part of the sequence is eliminated, leaving just the 'release' part. As a result, the relaxed state can be achieved in less time than when working with the full sequence; 5 to 7 minutes are suggested instead of the 15 of the tense–release session.

The training session begins with breathing instructions, followed by a scanning of all the voluntary muscles starting with the head and working down to the toes. The following instructions are adapted from Öst (1987).

In a moment I'm going to ask you to focus your attention on your breathing and, in particular, on the movement of your upper abdomen … notice how it swells slightly as you breathe in, and sinks back as you breathe out … do not change it in any way … just tune in to its rhythmic pattern … feel yourself relaxing more with each breath … feel your muscles letting go from the top of your head … your forehead … eyebrows … eyelids … cheeks … temples … jaws … throat … tongue … lips … feel your entire face relaxed … now … your neck … shoulders … arms … and down to the tips of your fingers … and while you are doing this, let your breathing continue at its own pace, expanding the stomach region in particular … Now, relax your back … now, the lower part of your body … hips … thighs … knees … calves … shins …. feet … toes … still breathing gently and noticing the relaxing effect of each breath … feel yourself relaxing more and more …

The sequence is terminated in the same way as for the first component.

Again, the homework assignment is a twice-daily practice, the trainee being asked to record afterwards the level of relaxation achieved and how long it took to reach it.

Cue-Controlled or Conditioned Relaxation

This component of the training focuses on the breathing. It begins by asking the trainee to relax by employing the release-only method of progressive relaxation. Once relaxed, the trainee is asked to begin silently to recite the word 'relax'; this should be recited once each time they breathe out. After many repetitions, an association is built up between the word and the relaxed state whereby the word alone becomes capable of inducing a measure of relaxation. The word has thus become a cue. The stronger the association, the greater the power of the cue word. Expressed in other terms, a conditioning process has been set up, as a result of which the trainee feels relaxed whenever he or she thinks of the word 'relax'.

The trainer introduces the exercise in the following manner.

Spend a few moments with your eyes closed … relax yourself by running through the release-only routine … signal to me by raising your right index finger when you feel fully relaxed … if you are ready, turn your attention now to your breathing … tune in to its rhythm … let it adopt its own pace … do not be tempted to alter it … and just before you breathe in, think the word 'inhale' … just before you breathe out, think the word 'relax' …

Leading with the instructions of 'inhale' and 'relax' for five breaths, the trainer then asks participants to continue on their own for a further five breaths. After a few minutes' rest, the full sequence is repeated.

If there is more than one participant, the trainer will not attempt to synchronize their respirations but will let them conduct their own exercise. As proficiency increases, the command 'inhale' can be dropped, and the word 'relax' used on its own.

Homework consists of 20 pairings a day of the word 'relax' with the state of relaxation. Participants should be warned against overbreathing – that is, allowing the breathing to become deeper or more rapid (see Chapter 4). The trainee keeps a record of the level of relaxation achieved and the time taken to reach it.

Once learned, it takes only 2 to 3 minutes to become fully relaxed by this method.

Differential Relaxation

So far, the sessions have been concerned with teaching basic techniques. The application of those skills now begins. Differential relaxation focuses on controlling the levels of muscle tension while the individual is engaged in some activity. Although some tension is needed to carry out the task, the level is often greater than is necessary and may need to be reduced. Also, there may be unnecessary tension in the muscles not directly engaged in the task. Different levels of tension (or relaxation) are required for each.

Because an ability to recognize muscle tension at its varying levels is essential for developing this skill, differential relaxation is presented after the individual has been trained in progressive relaxation.

Two sessions of tuition are indicated, one dealing with sitting and the other with standing activities. Both sessions begin with a revision of cue-controlled relaxation.

The First Session: Sitting

In the first session, the trainee, seated in an armchair, is instructed to make certain movements while maintaining a relaxed state in the rest of the body.

Please make yourself as comfortable as possible. Settle into the chair with your feet flat on the floor. With your eyes closed, relax yourself using your cue word with breathing … when you are ready, would you raise your right index finger … I'd like you now to open your eyes and look around the room without moving your head … notice the tension in the eye muscles but keep the body relaxed …

Next, look around the room allowing your head to move in order to increase your range of vision. Keep a minimum of tension in the neck muscles while you do this, and check that the rest of your body is free from tension …

Would you now lift one arm, and as you do, remember to keep the other parts of your body relaxed … and lower the arm. Continue to scan your body for signs of unnecessary tension.

Now, lift one leg off the ground, keeping the rest of your body as relaxed as possible … and let it down.

If you had any difficulty with this exercise, perhaps we could discuss it before moving on.

The routine is then carried out on the other arm and leg, after which trainees are moved from the armchair to an upright chair. Trainees relax in this new sitting position before being led through the same procedure of eye, head and limb movements. Next, trainees are seated at a table and asked to write something short such as their name and address, using the minimum of muscle tension needed to accomplish the task. As an alternative, in practice sessions, they could make a short telephone call, adopting the same relaxed state.

The Second Session: Standing

In the second session of differential relaxation, trainees stand. The position should be near a wall or some form of support, in case they feel unsteady, but they should not be leaning on it. The session begins with cue-controlled relaxation, after which the same schedule of head, arm and leg movements is worked through.

Lastly, trainees are asked to practise relaxation while walking. Emphasis is placed on finding an easy way of moving and on relaxing the muscles not used, such as those of the face and hands. Any initial awkwardness will disappear as individuals discover more relaxed ways of holding their body.

With the skills they have learned and practised, individuals will be able to achieve a state of relaxation consistent with effective task performance within 60 to 90 seconds. Differential relaxation is expanded in Chapter 11.

Rapid Relaxation

As its name implies, the rapid relaxation component is designed to reduce still further the time it takes to become relaxed; it also gives the trainee the opportunity to practise in everyday situations. First, the trainee's environment is arranged so that a regularly used appliance acts as a cue to relax; for example, the wristwatch or the telephone are marked with a coloured dot which reminds individuals relax whenever they see it. Every

time they look at their watch or makes a telephone call, they are reminded to release tension. This means that stress is, in general, held at low levels in the everyday setting. Rapid relaxation consists of the following routine performed each time the individual sees the coloured dot.

Take a slow breath … think 'relax' … then exhale. Repeat this twice … scan the body for unnecessary tensions … and release them.

Regular practice of this short sequence (15 to 20 times a day) makes the technique more effective and results in the trainee being able to relax in a still shorter space of time. It has been found that after 1 or 2 weeks' practice, the trainee can relax by this method in as little as 20 to 30 seconds.

Application Training

Applying relaxation skills to situations of potential stress is the subject of the application phase. With the use of a system of graded exposure (see Chapter 2), the trainee is encouraged to face the situation of stress. Anxiety-provoking situations should, however, be presented at a level of challenge which the trainee can cope with, neither too high nor too low.

Take yourself to a situation that you know is likely to provoke stress for you. Relax yourself before entering the scene. Observe your reactions. If you feel anxiety levels beginning to rise, bring out your cue word 'relax'. Continue to apply it until you feel your anxiety levels falling.

It may not work the first time because, like any skill, practice is necessary to achieve success, but gradually you will find you are gaining more control over your anxiety levels.

As a preliminary, individuals could visualize themselves successfully coping in the stress-provoking situation before being exposed to the same event in real life (see Chapter 19).

Maintenance Programme

However successful the treatment, Öst suggests keeping up the habit of scanning the body for unnecessary tension and using rapid relaxation to release it.

PRECAUTIONS

Because applied relaxation is based on progressive relaxation, it is subject to the same precautions. Because visualization is also used, these too need to be considered. These can be found in Chapter 5 and Chapter 18, respectively.

APPLICATION

Applied relaxation is a multivariate method and as such is particularly useful for treating conditions, such as anxiety, which present with a complex range of physiological, cognitive, psychological and behavioural symptoms. Although effective therapies for anxiety exist, many individuals refrain from seeking treatment because of the embarrassment associated with seeking help. Internet-based self-help programmes supplemented by weekly telephone calls can be an alternative. Exploring the benefits of this approach, Carlbring et al (2003) randomly divided 22 participants experiencing panic disorder into two self-help groups. One was trained in cognitive–behavioural therapy, the other in applied relaxation. Therapist contact was minimal. Both trainings were found to be effective, achieving significant medium to large effects, providing support for the use of Internet-administered self-help.

A further study by Carlbring et al in 2007 compared Internet-directed cognitive–behavioural therapy with a waiting list control in people experiencing social phobia. Results of this randomized controlled trial showed greater reductions in anxiety in the treatment group than in the control group. Moreover, there was 93% adherence to the Internet programme with benefit maintained 1 year later. These results strengthen support for the use of Internet self-help programmes and suggest that it could be an effective method for delivering training in applied relaxation.

KEY POINTS

1. Öst was one of many researchers who sought to apply the work of Jacobson to everyday life.
2. The method uses a multivariate approach which addresses the physiological aspect through muscle relaxation, the cognitive and the psychological through the cue word and behavioural through exposure to the stressor.
3. Öst's approach was designed to be learned in 8 to 12 sessions compared with the 50 of Jacobson's.
4. Applied relaxation is a skill which has to be learned and therefore home practice is essential.
5. As the trainee becomes more proficient, the state of relaxation can be achieved in ever shorter periods.

Reflection

Describe your understanding of the technique of applied relaxation.

How do you think the multivariate approach of applied relaxation could be used in practice?

Why do you think this is an appropriate use of the method?

What did you learn about the use of the 'cue word' and how this can be used in everyday situations?

What is the main learning point you will take away from this chapter?

What is your future action plan in terms of applied relaxation?

CASE STUDY LEARNING OPPORTUNITIES

The key points and reflection provide the background and knowledge required in relation to the case studies: Vala (Case Study 1) and Huw (Case Study 2) help to deepen understanding of how applied relaxation can be applied in practice.

CASE STUDY 1

Performance Anxiety: *Applied Relaxation Outcomes for Vala*

Vala is an actor and has just been offered the opportunity to play Miranda in *The Tempest* by the Royal Shakespeare Company. She is over the moon but has been suffering from what she describes as 'stage fright' or performance anxiety over the last few months and she fears this is getting worse.

When asked to describe her thoughts, feelings and behaviour, Vala tells you that since the death of her mother 6 months ago she has been suffering from anxiety and insecurity at work. When rehearsing she feels reasonably ok, although she has noticed that her confidence has been very low since her mother's death. However, when she has to perform in front of an audience, she has been becoming more and more anxious. She has experienced palpitations, sweating, sickness and diarrhoea and more recently mild panic attacks. She has managed them so far, but they are getting worse and she has had to ring in sick on three occasions feigning ill health. As she does not have a big part in this play, she feels it has not had a huge impact on the show ... but Miranda is a different situation entirely; if this continues, she will be missed and her understudy may take over the show.

She has not spoken to any of her family, colleagues or friends about it because she is embarrassed and fears ridicule; she is also concerned about her reputation and career: 'How can an actor fear going on stage and acting?' she asks. She has a 3-month break between her present job finishing and rehearsals for *The Tempest* starting. She is keen to address the problem if possible.

Vala is offered an online package of applied relaxation which she can practise in her own time and without fear of being 'found out' by her family, friends or colleagues. It comprises 12 weekly sessions which must be worked through chronologically;

the procedure follows the sessions described in this chapter. She is also offered a follow-up appointment or phone call with a therapist/trainer. After sessions 1 and 2 (tense–release), she begins to see how her physiological responses in terms of tension in her muscles are linked to her negative thoughts and the behavioural reaction (i.e., a flight and/or freeze response). After practising the release-only cycle (sessions 3 and 4) and the cue control (sessions 5 and 6) she begins to feel some sense of autonomy and uses the cue word 'relax' daily. She finds the differential relaxation practise (sessions 7 and 8) quite astounding because she realises how much tension she is holding her body – she is rigid and stiff on stage both sitting and standing. In the rapid relaxation training (sessions 9 and 10), Vala begins to use her thumb ring as the cue to help scan her body, check for tension and release this. Finally, at the application stage (sessions 11 and 12), Vala imagines herself on stage; she works on this twice daily and continues to do so when she begins rehearsals.

Although the anxiety is still present, Vala is feeling that she can and will get on the stage on the opening night of *The Tempest*. She has also read that several famous actors suffer from the same condition and use various techniques to manage it; for some it appears to have wider implications and be related to social anxiety disorder. This has made her feel more normal, and she is positive about her progress: 'If they can do it, so can I' has become her mantra.

CASE STUDY 2

Agoraphobia: Applied Relaxation Outcomes for Huw

Huw's general practitioner has referred him for a 12-week course of applied relaxation training. Huw tells you he has never suffered from anxiety previously, but recently he has been experiencing pain in his chest, palpitations, sweating and breathing difficulties. The first time it happened he was in Tesco with his wife. He thought he was having a heart attack and was going to die. An ambulance was called, but when he got to Accident and Emergency, they said it was a panic attack. Since then, things have got worse and he panics just at the thought of going out 'in

case I have an attack'. Because Huw cannot leave the house, he is visited at home by the trainer.

In the first session they work through the human stress response; this helped Huw to understand what was going on in his body and he now feels he can appreciate the physical, cognitive, psychological and behavioural components of anxiety a little more. He also practised the tense–release cycle and he feels this has really helped him to recognize tension in his body; he had no idea before that he had this tension there.

As he progresses through the sessions, he feels a greater sense of control and begins to apply his learned techniques to visualizing leaving the house: first just standing at the door, then stepping over the front door, to progressing down the path to the gate, to walking to the local shop for his paper. He is still working on the latter in visualization, but he has managed to actually walk down the path to his front gate, first with the trainer and then with his wife. He is now practising going to the gate every day with his wife using his cue word 'relax' and using his breathing.

The trainer has told Huw that next week he is actually going to open the gate and step through it. Although anxious, Huw keeps visualizing this in his twice-daily practice and uses his breathing and cue word when he begins to feel panic. He is also rationalizing his thinking by telling himself, 'What's the worst that can happen? Nothing. If I feel any panic, I can step right back into the garden again and shut the gate'.

ACTIVITY

For each of the case studies:
1. List key aspects used in the applied relaxation approach.
2. Consider why the methods were chosen.
3. Write down the impact that applied relaxation is having from a psychological perspective.
4. Write down the impact that applied relaxation is having from a physical perspective.
5. Write down the impact that applied relaxation is having from an emotional perspective.
6. Consider the outcomes on quality of life and overall well-being for both individuals.

Chapter 10 will focus on behavioural relaxation training. Based on the work of Schilling and Poppen (1983), this type of relaxation is based on the principle that a relaxed body displays a different posture from a stressed body. Because it requires a lot of feedback from the trainer for the trainer to learn to adjust body positioning and gain self-awareness it is classed as a behavioural approach.

REFERENCES

Arntz, A. (2003). Cognitive therapy versus applied relaxation as treatment of generalized anxiety disorder. *Behaviour Research and Therapy*, 41(6), 633–646.

Carlbring, P., Ekselius, L., & Andersson, G. (2003). Treatment of panic disorder via the internet: A randomized controlled trial of cognitive behavioural therapy versus applied relaxation. *Journal of Behavioral Therapy and Experimental Psychiatry*, 34(2), 129–140.

Carlbring, P., Gunnarsdóttir, M., Hedensjö, L., Andersson, G., Ekselius, L., & Furmark, T. (2007). Treatment of social phobia: Randomised trial of internet-delivered cognitive-behavioural therapy with telephone support. *British Journal of Psychiatry*, 190, 123–128.

Clouston, T. J. (2015). *Challenging stress, burnout and rust-out: Finding balance in busy lives.* London: Jessica Kingsley.

Clark, D. M. (1986). A cognitive approach to panic. *Behaviour Research and Therapy*, 24(4), 461–470.

Donegan, E., & Dugas, M. J. (2012). Generalized anxiety disorder: A comparison of symptom change in adults receiving cognitive behavioral therapy or applied relaxation. *Journal of Consulting and Clinical Psychology*, 80(3), 490–496.

Dugas, M. J., Brillon, P., Savard, P., et al. (2010). A randomized clinical trial of cognitive-behavioral therapy and applied relaxation for adults with generalized anxiety disorder. *Behavior Therapy*, 41(1), 46–58.

Goldfried, M. R. (1971). Systematic desensitization as training in self-control. *Journal of Consulting and Clinical Psychology*, 37(2), 228–234.

Hayes-Skelton, S. A., Usmani, A., Lee, J. K., Roemer, L., & Orsillo, S. M. (2012). A fresh look at potential mechanisms of change in Applied Relaxation for generalized anxiety disorder: A case series. *Cognitive and Behavioral Practice*, 19(3), 451–462.

Hayes-Skelton, S. A., Roemer, L., Orsillo, S. M., & Borkovec, T. D. (2013a). A contemporary view of applied relaxation for generalized anxiety disorder. *Cognitive Behavioural Therapy*, 42(4), 292–302.

Hayes-Skelton, S. A., Roemer, L., & Orsillo, S. M. (2013b). A randomized clinical trial comparing an acceptance-based behavior therapy to applied relaxation for generalized anxiety disorder. *Journal of Consulting and Clinical Psychology*, 81(5), 761–773.

Heimberg, R. G. (2002). Cognitive-behavioural therapy for social anxiety disorder: Current status and future directions. *Biological Psychiatry*, 51(1), 101–108.

Hoyer, J., Beesdo, K., Gloster, A. T., Runge, J., Höfler, M., & Becker, E. S. (2009). Worry exposure versus applied relaxation in the treatment of generalized anxiety disorder. *Psychotherapy and Psychosomatics*, 78(2), 106–115.

Jacobson, E. (1938). *Progressive relaxation* (2nd ed.). Chicago: University of Chicago Press.

Öst, L. G. (1987). Applied relaxation: description of a coping technique and review of controlled studies. *Behaviour Research and Therapy*, 25(5), 397–409.

Öst, L. G. (1988). Applied relaxation versus progressive relaxation in the treatment of panic disorder. *Behaviour Research and Therapy*, 26(1), 13–22.

Öst, L. G., & Breitholtz, E. (2000). Applied relaxation versus cognitive therapy in the treatment of generalized anxiety disorder. *Behaviour Research and Therapy*, 38(8), 777–790.

Schilling, D. J., & Poppen, R. (1983). Behavioural relaxation training and assessment. *J. Behav. Ther. Exp. Psychiatry*, *14*, 99–107.

Siev, J., & Chambless, D. L. (2007). Specificity of treatment effects: Cognitive therapy and relaxation for generalized anxiety and panic disorders. *Journal of Consulting and Clinical Psychology*, *75*(4), 513–522.

Spence, S. H., Sharpe, L., Newton-John, T., & Champion, D. (1995). Effect of electromyographic biofeedback compared to applied relaxation training with chronic, upper extremity cumulative trauma disorders. *Pain*, *63*(2), 199–206.

Wolpe, J. (1958). *Psychotherapy by reciprocal inhibition*. Palo Alto, CA: Stanford University Press.

Wolpe, J., & Lazarus, A. A. (1966). *Behaviour therapy techniques*. New York: Pergamon Press.

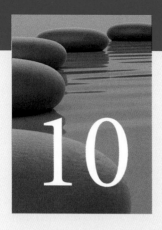

10

BEHAVIOURAL RELAXATION TRAINING

PROFESSOR TEENA CLOUSTON

CHAPTER CONTENTS

LEARNING OBJECTIVES

The aim of this chapter is to provide a practical guide to basic concepts of behavioural relaxation training.

By the end of this chapter you will be able to:

1. Understand the key principles and process of behavioural relaxation training.

2. Identify why adopting a relaxed posture can induce a state of feeling relaxed.

3. Recognize why feedback from the trainer is important in behavioural relaxation training.

4. Describe why behavioural relaxation training can be appropriate when working with people with learning disabilities.

5. Carry out a behavioural relaxation training session following Schilling and Poppen's 1983 method.

This chapter will conclude with key points and time for reflection, providing learning opportunities through case studies.

INTRODUCTION TO BEHAVIOURAL RELAXATION TRAINING

A person who is tense adopts a characteristic pattern of muscular activity in the form of frowning, clenching and general body tenseness. The muscles of a relaxed person, by contrast, are free from excessive muscle tension. As a result, people who are tense look different from people who are relaxed. Their feelings are associated with a different posture in each case. Don Schilling, a psychologist working in the early 1980s, found the converse also occurred; that is, people adopting a relaxed posture reported feeling more relaxed.

Schilling, who was teaching progressive relaxation to adolescent boys, noticed they were better at tensing than relaxing; in fact, they found it difficult to respond to the request to relax. He suggested to his pupils that instead of trying to become relaxed, they should adopt the more concrete objective of trying to look relaxed: to take up postures they would expect to see in people who *were* relaxed. The result was that the pupils not only succeeded in looking relaxed but reported actually feeling more relaxed. Thus, by adopting postures characteristic of relaxation, they had induced a subjective feeling of relaxation.

The idea is reminiscent of the facial and postural feedback hypotheses, which state that feedback from facial expression and posture induces feelings that match those expressions and postures. In other words, people feel the emotions that correspond with their poses.

Based on these ideas, Schilling and Poppen (1983) set up a method of relaxation which they called behavioural relaxation training (BRT). Liberal feedback from the trainer provided reinforcement or corrective adjustment. The method is thus underpinned by behaviourist principles.

INTRODUCTION TO EVIDENCE

Behavioural relaxation training has been found to be effective in a variety of conditions ranging from learning disabilities (Lindsay et al 1997, Lindsay & Morrison 1996), autism and behavioural problems (Paclawskyi 2002) to acquired brain injury (Guercio et al 2001) and hyperactivity in children (Raymer & Poppen 1985).

Raymer and Poppen's (1985) study was small, using only three children. However, the method was rigorous and findings were positive in terms of improvements for all the children measured from multiple perspectives; this included the Hyperactivity Index of the Conners Parents Rating Scale, objective observation of the relaxed state and reduction in frontalis muscle tension (Donney & Poppen 1989). The study also identified that support from the parents was essential in terms of homework and that parents could be trained effectively in BRT to enable them to then teach their own hyperactive children to relax. Further, Donney and Poppen (1989) purported that practice could be generalized to other settings, including school and everyday life situations, and that beanbags offered a more supportive and effective sitting position for children when learning the postures.

Lindsay and colleagues carried out a series of studies charting the effect of BRT on cognitive performance. Lindsay and Morrison's (1996) analysis showed that where the disability was severe, short-term memory and learning significantly improved after 12 sessions of BRT compared with quiet reading, where no significant differences were reported. In a later study, Lindsay et al (1997) tested concentration and responsiveness in eight participants, this time with profound learning disabilities. Four stress-relieving procedures were compared: snoezelen, aromatherapy massage, BRT and active therapy. After each therapy participants were set simple concentration tasks. The treatments which led to the most successful outcomes were snoezelen and BRT, in which significant effects were recorded. There was no improvement in the aromatherapy group, and the active group even showed a deterioration.

Studies by Paclawskyj (2002) investigated the use of BRT for children with autism spectrum disorder, developmental disabilities and severe behavioural problems. Findings identified that teaching the 10 stages of BRT in a structured sequence, moving from large muscle groups to small, was more effective than when a random order was used. Moreover, when using this structured method, behavioural difficulties such as compulsive skin picking, tantrums in response to noise, self-injury and aggression in tandem with agitation and screaming were markedly improved.

Brain injury is another area where the approach has been applied. Guercio et al (2001) taught BRT skills to one adult with an ataxic tremor resulting from an acquired brain injury (ABI). Having learned the skills, the participant was then connected to a biofeedback facility. Results demonstrated a significant reduction in the severity of the tremor. Denmark and Gemeinhardt (2002) reviewed the causes of anger in ABI and maintained that anger and relaxation could not co-exist in one person at the same time. Thus they suggested that relaxation can in fact be taught to manage anger in people with ABI.

Finally, evidence suggests that the benefits of behavioural relaxation training can be seen after very little teaching: Schilling and Poppen (1983) observed benefit within as few as two training sessions. They also reported that effects were retained at follow-up 4 to 6 weeks later. Paclawskyj's work (2002) maintained that a shortened structured method could be learned in a little as 2 hours.

THEORIES BEHIND BEHAVIOURAL RELAXATION TRAINING

Behavioural relaxation training teaches trainees to adopt 10 overt postures and behaviours through the use of modelling, prompting and performance feedback (Poppen 1998, Raymer & Poppen 1983, Schilling & Poppen 1995). Token reinforcement, prompting and praise are all useful methods to improve effectiveness and learning for the trainee (Donney & Poppen 1989). Consequently, it is based on the behavioural approach and owes much to Jacobson's original theory of progressive relaxation – that is, that by relaxing muscles, a state of not only physical but also psychological and cognitive relaxation can be induced.

Behavioural relaxation training offers both therapy and a means of assessment. As a therapy, it provides a form of body scanning in which relaxed postures are adopted and feelings of relaxation experienced. As an assessment tool, it provides a numerical measure of the level of relaxation present in the musculature.

The approach does not ask participants to recognize subtle degrees of arousal or to be conscious of different levels of relaxation; the method is easily learned and readily applied. These attributes make it a convenient technique for reducing anxiety in people with learning disabilities (Michulka et al 1988).

KEY ASPECTS OF THE PROCEDURE

Setting

The ideal setting is a warm, quiet room with dimmed lighting. A padded recliner is the chair of choice but, because this may not be available, any flat surface will serve. Pillows may be used under the knees, forearms and head, as required. Wearing comfortable trousers is beneficial because trainees can then adopt the positions required with ease.

Introduction of Method to Participants

Participants are introduced to the method in the following way.

We can all recognize signs of tension: tightly drawn face muscles, clenching of teeth and fingers. These are typical postures that people adopt when under stress. When people are relaxed, muscle tensions are released and a new posture results. The central idea of behavioural relaxation training is that by adopting the posture of a relaxed person, we can make ourselves feel more relaxed.

In this method you will be asked to make different parts of your body look as relaxed as possible and then to notice the effect the new position has on you; to notice how the new position feels. I'll describe and demonstrate each item before we begin. Please try out the items on yourself.

The postures, as described in Table 10.1, are then demonstrated and the trainee asked to copy them. The unrelaxed postures are also demonstrated to emphasize the point. Feedback is provided by the trainer in the form of praise or corrective instructions. The trainee is asked particularly to take note of the proprioceptive events – that is, the joint and muscle feelings which convey the sense of body position as each new posture is adopted.

After the demonstration, the trainee rests quietly with their eyes closed. After a few minutes, the instructor may make an initial assessment (see the section on the Behavioural Relaxation Scale, See Page 6).

Training Procedure

The training procedure is then presented in its entirety. Following is a slightly paraphrased version of the protocol laid out in Poppen (1998), where it is suggested that each relaxed posture be held for 30 to 60 seconds. Trainees are asked to close their eyes.

Feet

Starting with the feet: these are relaxed when you feel they are flopping, with the toes slightly pointing away from each other. No effort is involved; it is the posture of rest. If you are putting any effort into it, then your muscles will be working and your feet will be tensed. Notice how your feet feel in the relaxed position.

Body

The next item is called 'body'. Your body is relaxed when your hips and shoulders are in line with each other and resting on the supporting surface. If you are lying in a crooked fashion, your body is not relaxed. If there is any movement, you are not

	TABLE 10.1	
	Relaxed and unrelaxed behaviours (adapted from Poppen 1998, with permission from the author)	
Item	**Relaxed**	**Unrelaxed**
Breathing	Breaths regular and fewer in number than recorded on the baseline	Breaths irregular and greater in number than recorded on the baseline
Quiet	No audible sounds such as sighs, words or movements	Talking, whispering, sighing, coughing, snoring or other audible sounds
Body	Symmetrical and fully resting on supporting surface	Holding any part tense or twisted
Head	Motionless and supported with nose in midline	Head turning or other movements; head unsupported or tilted; nose outside midline
Eyes	Lids lightly closed with eyes still	Eyes open or, if closed, darting about under tense and fluttering lids
Mouth	Lips parted at centre of mouth with teeth separated	Lips firmly closed with teeth held together or mouth uncomfortably open
Throat	No activity	Swallowing, twitching or preparing to speak
Shoulders	Dropped and level with each other; resting against support	Both hunched or one higher than the other; not resting on support
Hands	Both resting at sides, on armrests or on lap; palms down, fingers gently curled	Clasped, clenched tight or gripping the armrest
Feet	Comfortably rolled out so that the toes point away from each other	Pointing vertically, crossed or excessively rolled out

relaxed. Make a note of the sensation of having a relaxed body.

Hands

This posture is called 'hands'. Your hands are relaxed when they are resting on a surface with the fingers gently curled, that is to say, neither clenched nor stretched out. Notice the sensations in your hands as you relax them.

Shoulders

And now the shoulders: these are relaxed when they are level and dropped. If you feel one is twisted or higher than the other, then they are not relaxed. Register the feeling of having relaxed shoulders.

Head

The next posture is called 'head'. Make sure your head is resting on its cushion and facing forwards. Feel it being supported. Any attempt to turn or twist it will cause your neck muscles to work. Notice the feelings you get as you relax your neck muscles.

Mouth

The next posture is called 'mouth'. Your mouth will be relaxed if your teeth are parted and your lips gently touching. If you are smiling, grimacing, licking your lips or pressing them together, your mouth is not relaxed. Take note of the feelings you get as you relax your mouth.

Throat

Now the area called 'throat': this is relaxed when you can feel no movement there. If you are swallowing or if your tongue is twitching, then your throat is not relaxed. However, if you need to swallow, do so, then return to your relaxed state. Notice the sensations in your throat as you relax it.

Breathing

The next item is called 'breathing'. Relaxed breathing is slow and gentle. Unrelaxed breathing is rapid, jerky and may be interrupted by coughing, sighing and yawning. Register the effect of your relaxed breathing.

Quiet

And now we come to an item called 'quiet'. This means that you are not making any sounds such as sniffing, umm-ing or talking. If you feel you have to clear your throat, that's all right, but return to your state of quiet afterwards, noticing the sensation of stillness.

Eyes

The last relaxed area is called 'eyes'. These are relaxed when the lids rest over them in a lightly closed position and when the eye movements are brought to rest. Eyes are unrelaxed when they dart about and when the lids are twitching. Notice the feelings you are getting from your eyes as you relax them.

The order is not important, but it is suggested that the eyes are left until the end because the trainee needs to use them to mentally observe the other behaviours (Poppen 1998).

A training session will last about 15 to 20 minutes, after which the trainee is instructed to continue relaxing as they silently review the items for a further 10 to 15 minutes. At the end of this period, the trainer may carry out a posttreatment assessment (see Page 6).

Arousal

Arousal takes place in the following manner.

Very slowly, I would like you to prepare to end the session. To help you transfer from your deeply relaxed state, I am going to count slowly from one to five: one … two … three, open your eyes … four … five … begin to move your limbs … and in your own time, sit up.

Variations of the Protocol

Variations of the previous protocol exist for different situations: first, where the only available chair is an upright chair, and second, where the need for relaxation occurs in the middle of a task (termed 'mini-relaxation' by Poppen (1998)).

Script for Trainee Sitting in an Upright Chair

When the trainee is seated in an upright chair, the following four areas of legs, back, arms and head should be substituted for feet, body, hands and head in the protocol given earlier.

Legs

This area is called 'legs', and these are relaxed when you have both feet flat on the floor with a right angle at the knees. Allow the knees to fall outwards into a comfortable position. The legs are unrelaxed when crossed, extended or tucked under the chair. Notice the sensations in your legs when they are in the relaxed position.

Back

The next area called 'back'. It is relaxed when your shoulder blades and hips touch the chair symmetrically. It is unrelaxed when you are bending forwards, arching backwards or leaning to one side. Register the feelings you get from the relaxed posture.

Arms

Next is the area called 'arms'. These are relaxed when the wrists are resting on the thighs; they are unrelaxed when hanging down, when crossed or when being leant on. Notice the sensations as you relax your arms.

Head

Now we come to the area called 'head', and this is relaxed when it is held upright and looking forwards. The head is unrelaxed when it is tilted or turned in any direction. Notice the feelings you get from holding your head in the relaxed position.

'Mini-Relaxation'

Tension can arise in the course of any task or situation. For example, while talking, the individual might develop tension in the hands; while typing, in the shoulders, and while focusing on a difficult job, in the mouth and throat. Breaking off to release these tensions is what Poppen means by mini-relaxation. He suggests that a person, when engaged in any task, should take mini-relaxation breaks periodically. Thus mini-relaxation can be seen as a form of differential relaxation (see Chapter 11).

Mini-relaxation can be practised throughout the day, and reminders to do so provided by placing reminders in your mobile phone or smart speaker or using coloured dots on the telephone, watch, steering wheel, typewriter, kettle handle or any other frequently used appliance.

THE BEHAVIOURAL RELAXATION SCALE

There are no universally accepted procedures of assessment in relaxation; a reliable and valid measuring device has yet to be found. Schilling and Poppen's (1983) Behavioural Relaxation Scale (BRS) is an attempt to fill one aspect of this gap. It was designed as an easy method for measuring the motor element of relaxation (i.e., that relating to the voluntary muscles). Although it specifically measures the behaviours taught in BRT, it may be used to assess the motor aspect of any relaxation procedure.

The scale is based on the assumption that a person who feels relaxed also looks relaxed. As a result, some kind of judgement of the degree to which a person is relaxed can be made by an onlooker. Using the same items that feature in BRT, the scale allows an objective assessment to be made, without the need for expensive equipment such as electromyographic instruments. Each posture is checked for its degree of relaxation with reference to the table of relaxed and unrelaxed postures (see Table 10.1). The order of the items in Table 10.1 is suggested by Poppen (1998) as being the most convenient for assessment purposes.

Using the Behavioural Relaxation Scale

Establishing the Baseline Breathing Rate

The first measure concerns the breathing rate. This is counted over a 30-second interval (each count representing a complete cycle of inhalation and exhalation). The process is repeated 15 times and the total sum of the respirations divided by 15 to give the mean or average number of respirations in 30 seconds. The mean is then entered in the box marked 'breathing baseline' on the score sheet (Fig. 10.1). A diaphragmatic form of breathing is recommended (see Chapter 4).

General Assessment

A general assessment covers five 1-minute periods in which the individual is observed for outward signs of relaxation. Each minute begins with a further count of the breathing rate lasting 30 seconds; it is entered in the empty box in the column marked '1' in Fig. 10.1. If the answer is less than the baseline rate, then the adjacent plus sign is ringed; if it is more, the minus sign is ringed. The following 15 seconds are spent scanning the trainee's key postures, picking out any unrelaxed ones and repeating the appropriate word label – for example, 'shoulders' for a hunched arm. The succeeding 15 seconds are spent ringing the items: plus for

Name .... Date .... Time .... Session no. ....

Breathing baseline ☐

+ relaxed
− unrelaxed

INTERVALS

	1			2			3			4			5		Total
Breathing	−	☐	+	−	☐	+	−	☐	+	−	☐	+	−	☐	+	
Quiet	−	+		−	+		−	+		−	+		−	+		
Body	−	+		−	+		−	+		−	+		−	+		
Head	−	+		−	+		−	+		−	+		−	+		
Eyes	−	+		−	+		−	+		−	+		−	+		
Mouth	−	+		−	+		−	+		−	+		−	+		
Throat	−	+		−	+		−	+		−	+		−	+		
Shoulders	−	+		−	+		−	+		−	+		−	+		
Hands	−	+		−	+		−	+		−	+		−	+		
Feet	−	+		−	+		−	+		−	+		−	+		

Self-ratings 1 2 3 4 5 6 7   Score ☐

Fig. 10.1 ■ Behavioural relaxation scale score sheet. (Adapted from Poppen 1998 with permission from the author.)

relaxed postures, minus for any that continue to be unrelaxed.

After the first minute, the procedure is repeated and the answers recorded under the figure '2', and so on until five columns have been completed. The ringed plus signs are added up and entered under 'total'.

Working Out the Score

Scoring is expressed as a percentage arrived at in the following way: the total number of ringed 'plus' signs is counted and the sum divided by the total number of observations (i.e., the 10 behaviours multiplied by the five testings). The resulting figure is then multiplied by 100. For example, if there were a total of 40 ringed plus signs, they would be divided by the 50 observations. After multiplying the resulting fraction by 100, a figure of 80% would be obtained.

The Pretreatment Baseline

At the beginning of the course one pretreatment assessment is carried out. It acts as a baseline against which to measure progress, but should itself be carried out after a short period of rest to avoid confusing the effects of training with those which occur naturally whenever a person enters a restful environment (Lichstein et al 1981). Thereafter, assessment follows each training session to monitor progress.

Reliability and Validity of the Behavioural Relaxation Scale

The reliability of the scale (i.e., its ability to produce the same scores when used on different occasions) has been tested. It was found that higher levels of reliability were obtained with trained observers than with untrained ones. Thus the training of observers is important.

Two forms of validity have been demonstrated: one procedural, where participants receiving other accepted forms of relaxation training showed statistically significant changes in relaxation scores on the Behavioural Relaxation Scale, whereas controls did not (Schilling & Poppen 1983); and the other concurrent. Here, significant correlations were found between electromyographic measures of frontalis muscle and BRS scores; that is, low electromyography (EMG) readings were associated with scores which reflect relaxed postures as described in the BRS, whereas high readings were associated with scores which reflect unrelaxed postures (Poppen & Maurer 1982). Further work has tended to strengthen confidence in these results (Norton et al 1997), but more research is needed.

OTHER METHODS OF ASSESSMENT OF BEHAVIOURAL RELAXATION TRAINING

Because relaxation involves responses in subjective, physiological and behavioural spheres, a full assessment would take account of all three modalities. Poppen indicates the need to view behavioural assessment as part of a broader system of measurement. One of its components is self-report.

Self-Report

Because relaxation and anxiety are subjective states, it is appropriate and customary to include a self-rating measure when assessing trainees' personal perspectives on their levels. Self-report can take the form of free description, but because this is difficult to quantify, preset descriptive phrases with associated numbered ratings are often used. The individual rings the number corresponding with the phrase that most accurately reflects their perceived state.

A behavioural relaxation self-rating scale, adapted from Poppen (1998), is shown here:

1. Feeling extremely tense and upset throughout my body.
2. Feeling generally tense throughout my body.
3. Feeling some tension in some parts of my body.
4. Feeling relaxed as in my normal resting state.
5. Feeling more relaxed than usual.
6. Feeling completely relaxed throughout my entire body.
7. Feeling more deeply and completely relaxed than I ever have.

Discrepancy Between Self-Report and Objective Testing

There are often wide discrepancies between self-reports and objective measurements. One of the reasons is that self-report may be coloured by factors of social desirability – for instance, where trainees give the answer they think is expected of them. These matters are discussed further in Chapter 28.

PRECAUTIONS

As with any relaxation approach, precautions should be considered before taking it up. Chapter 5 contains a discussion of potential hazards relating to muscular approaches.

APPLICATION

Behavioural relaxation training is a method in which tense postures are replaced by relaxed ones. The trainee is required to take up specified relaxed postures based on the way people look when they are relaxed. This enables them to then register the feeling engendered by the posture itself. Because behavioural relaxation training is a skill, practice is necessary. Trainees are urged to spend 20 minutes a day practising. Poppen (1998) suggests that benefit can be derived from combining BRT with cognitive relaxation methods such as autogenics or meditation. In this way, the one can augment the effects of the other.

KEY POINTS

Behavioural relaxation training rests on the principle that a relaxed body displays a different posture from a stressed body. The trainee is asked to look as relaxed as possible.

1. The training procedure focuses on each muscle group in turn, checking it for relaxed appearance.
2. Trainees are asked to register the 'feel' of the relaxed postures.

3. As a therapy it provides a form of body scanning in which relaxed postures are adopted and feelings of relaxation experienced.
4. As an assessment tool it provides a numerical measure of the level of relaxation present in the musculature.
5. The approach can be used by anyone. However, on account of its simplicity it has particular application for people with learning disabilities.

Reflection

Describe your understanding of the technique of behavioural relaxation training.

How do you think behavioural relaxation training could be applied in practice?

Why do you think this is an appropriate use of the method?

What did you learn about the application of behavioural relaxation training?

What is the main learning point you will take away from this chapter?

What is your future action plan in terms of behavioural relaxation training?

CASE STUDY LEARNING OPPORTUNITIES

The key points and reflection provide the background and knowledge required in relation to the case studies; Dylan (Case Study 1) and the Learning Disabilities Group (Case Study 2) help to deepen understanding of how behavioural relaxation training can be applied in practice.

CASE STUDY 1

Acquired (Traumatic) Brain Injury: Behavioural Relaxation Training Outcomes for Dylan

Dylan was an avid biker, loving father and husband before his road traffic accident. He was a self-employed painter and decorator and enjoyed his job. He does not remember much about the accident, but he knows he was on his motorbike going over the Brecon Beacons when a car pulled out in front of him. He was in hospital for several weeks and, after rehabilitation with occupational therapists and physiotherapists, is walking and independent in daily living. His memory and concentration, however, are still poor; he also struggles with problem solving and managing his emotions. As a result, he cannot return to work and is feeling very angry and depressed. He is short tempered at home and this is affecting his relationships with his wife and children.

On discussion with the therapist, Dylan tries behavioural relaxation training. He works through the table of postures (see Table 10.1) with the therapist and begins to realize that he is holding a lot of tension in his body and is unrelaxed most if not all of the time; he becomes very upset and starts to cry.

By supporting Dylan and talking this through with him it becomes clear that he is very angry about his accident and what has happened to him. He knows his personality has changed and that he is less tolerant with his family. He agrees to practise 'relaxed' postures daily and also sets up a reminder on his mobile phone and smart speaker to do mini-relaxations throughout the day.

Dylan also agrees to use the self-report scale on a daily basis and to discuss the outcomes of this with his wife. This helps Dylan to reflect on his subjective description of his tension and to recognize how his wife perceives the situation. He has struggled with empathy in terms of how his wife might be feeling about the accident and Dylan's state of health and well-being, so this is giving them a shared space to talk more frankly about their feelings.

Dylan is keen to reclaim his premorbid calm 'self' and become a more relaxed person at home. Since beginning BRT, Dylan has noted that his memory and concentration are improving; this is helping him feel better in himself, and his mood and general demeanour are improving.

CASE STUDY 2

The Group Sessions: Behavioural Relaxation Training Outcomes for Students With Learning Disabilities

Mr Davies' students in Green Acres special school are struggling to concentrate on their work, and disruptive behaviours are becoming more common. Each of the students has a personal plan which includes concentrating in class and working well to complete achievable and agreed goals, but recently high spirits and hyperactivity have been preventing accomplishing these successfully. Mr Davies has tried introducing music sessions, exercise and relaxation classes, and although these do help, the impact is short lived.

Mr Davies explains the students are between 15 and 16 years old and are 'an active and excitable group'. It is a small class of 12 students, 5 females and 7 males, with a range of learning disabilities and needs. On the whole they like each other and work well together, accommodating differences and unique characteristics; but lately they have become less tolerant of each other and more reactive to each other's behaviours, resulting in the present problems. As a therapist in the school, you suggest a more pragmatic approach to relaxation and propose BRT.

To begin, you ensure that you can book the relaxation room for a regular slot of 1 session per week over a 6-week period and ensure there are sufficient beanbags in the room for student use. You then discuss the plan with the students and explain that you are going to explore with them what it 'looks like' to be relaxed.

In the first session you follow the protocol and go through the postures in Table 10.1. You encourage the students to feed back on their own experiences and share ideas with others. After a short break you go through the relaxation process in its entirety and ask them to discuss what they learned. You then set a goal for them to practise during the week. To do this, you ask them to start noticing their own and others, relaxed postures in the classroom and to help each other look more relaxed by giving feedback on how they are looking throughout the week. You ask Mr Davies to use this exercise as a cue to help students focus when they are becoming high spirited.

In the second session, you ask for feedback on how they have been using the idea of 'looking' relaxed and helping each other; you then go through the relaxation procedure again. By week 4 Mr Davies tells you that he has noticed quite a marked difference in the students' ability to concentrate and that they are more focused and respectful to each other after he reminds them to scan themselves, observe others and adopt relaxed postures.

The students tell you they are enjoying the relaxation and are trying to see who can have the most relaxed postures in class. You discuss with them the difference between relaxation practice and being relaxed during activities so they can differentiate between the two. You introduce the idea of mini-relaxation to help with this and thus change the game of observing each other in class to focus on being relaxed during tasks. You hope to build on this so that students can use relaxed postures to engage in activities more meaningfully.

ACTIVITY

For each of the case studies:
1. List key aspects used in the behavioural relaxation training.
2. Consider why this approach was taken.
3. Write down the impact behavioural relaxation training is having from a psychological perspective.
4. Write down the impact behavioural relaxation training is having from a physical perspective.
5. Write down the impact behavioural relaxation is having from an emotional perspective.
6. Consider the outcomes on quality of life and overall well-being for Dylan and the group participants.

Chapter 11 will focus on differential relaxation to gain a deeper understanding of minimising tension within the muscles.

REFERENCES

Denmark, J., & Gemeinhardt, M. (2002). Anger and its management for survivors of acquired brain injury. *Brain Injury, 16*(2), 91–108.

Donney, V. K., & Poppen, R. (1989). Teaching parents to conduct behavioral relaxation training with their hyperactive children. *Journal of Behavioral Therapy & Experimental Psychiatry, 20*(4), 319–325.

Guercio, J. M., Ferguson, K. E., & McMorrow, M. J. (2001). Increasing functional communication through relaxation training and neuromuscular feedback. *Brain Injury, 15*(12), 1073–1082.

Lichstein, K. L., Sallis, J. F., Hill, D., & Young, M. C. (1981). Psychophysiological adaptation: an investigation of multiple parameters. *Journal of Behavioral Assessment, 3*, 111–121.

Lindsay, W. R., & Morrison, F. M. (1996). The effects of behavioral relaxation on cognitive performance in adults with severe intellectual disabilities. *Journal of Intellectual Disability Research, 40*(4), 285–290.

Lindsay, W. R., Pitcaithly, D., Geelen, N., Buntin, L., Broxholme, S., & Ashby, M. (1997). A comparison of the effects of four therapy procedures on concentration and responsiveness in people with profound learning disabilities. *Journal of Intellectual Disability Research, 41*(3), 201–207.

Michulka, D. M., Poppen, R. L., & Blanchard, E. B. (1988). Relaxation training as a treatment for chronic headaches in an individual having severe developmental disabilities. *Biofeedback and Self-Regulation, 13*, 257–266.

Norton, M., Holm, J. E., & McSherry, W. C. (1997). Behavioral assessment of relaxation: The validity of a behavioral rating scale. *Journal of Behavioral Therapy & Experimental Psychiatry, 28*(2), 129–137.

Paclawskyj, T. R. (2002). Behavioral Relaxation Training (BRT) with children with dual diagnoses. *The NADD Bulletin, 5*, 81–82.

Poppen, R. (1998). *Behavioural relaxation training and assessment* (2nd ed.). Thousand Oaks, CA: Sage.

Poppen, R., & Maurer, J. (1982). Electromyographic analysis of relaxed postures. *Biofeedback and Self-Regulation, 7*(4), 491–498.

Raymer, R., & Poppen, R. (1985). Behavioral relaxation training with hyperactive children. *Journal of Behavioral Therapy & Experimental Psychiatry, 16*(4), 309–316.

Schilling, D. J., & Poppen, R. (1983). Behavioural relaxation training and assessment. *Journal of Behavioral Therapy & Experimental Psychiatry, 14*(2), 99–107.

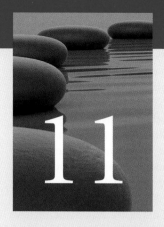

11

DIFFERENTIAL RELAXATION

PROFESSOR TEENA CLOUSTON

CHAPTER CONTENTS

LEARNING OBJECTIVES

The aim of this chapter is to provide a practical guide to basic concepts of differential relaxation

By the end of this chapter you will be able to:

1. Describe the key principles and process of differential relaxation.

2. Understand why task or activity analysis is important in applying differential relaxation in practice.

3. Recognize the importance of understanding what muscles need to be engaged or active for the primary activity and which can be relaxed in everyday action.

4. Identify the value of using muscle groups appropriately in everyday activities and how that helps you to learn to relax.

5. Carry out a differential relaxation session.

This chapter will conclude with key points and time for reflection, providing learning opportunities through case studies.

INTRODUCTION TO DIFFERENTIAL RELAXATION

Differential relaxation, a phrase introduced by Jacobson (1938), means, in his own words, 'the minimum of tensions in the muscles, requisite for an act, along with the relaxation of other muscles' (Jacobson 1976, p131). This is to say that the muscles engaged in performing any activity, such as typing, should exhibit a minimum level of tension consistent with task efficiency, whereas those not directly engaged in the task are relaxed. This leaves the body as relaxed as it can be while achieving the objective (i.e., typing the page). Thus differential relaxation is progressive relaxation applied to everyday tasks.

We need muscle tension to live our lives. It is essential for carrying out purposeful activity of the type that Jacobson (1976, p136) calls 'primary'. Purposeful activity, however, may be accompanied by tension in muscles whose action does nothing to promote the outcome, such as grimacing while writing. This is referred to by Jacobson (1976, p136) as 'secondary activity'. Differential relaxation calls for the recognition and elimination of all secondary activity, and of any excessive tension in the muscles performing or helping to perform the primary activity.

INTRODUCTION TO EVIDENCE

Differential relaxation is based on the premise that trainees can learn to avoid unwanted tension in the body during activity by learning to release unnecessary tension in muscles during activity. In particular, the method is reported to be effective in addressing inappropriate body positioning and tension in everyday situations (Gilman & Yaruss 2000). The technique can be particularly relevant where these may be habituated and thus 'normalized' by the individual. Essentially, the trainees learn to recognize how to exert just the right amount of muscle tension in the relevant muscle group required to perform a particular movement, and to release tension or activation in muscles that are not necessary for the task at hand. This means that energy is used efficiently and effectively, and thus poor positioning and the use of inappropriate muscle tension is addressed. Many elite athletes use this technique to their advantage in terms of both performance and reducing levels of anxiety in their sport (Kent 2006).

The Alexander technique, with its concept of 'balanced use' (see Chapter 12), is grounded in the principle of differential relaxation. Here, the crucial elements are the relationships of head, neck and spine, which, when correct, allow the body to adopt balanced and relaxed postures while engaged in activity. Alexander's procedures for the actions of sitting down and rising are essentially techniques of differential relaxation. Alexander suffered from functional dysphonia, a voice disorder without an apparent physical cause (Behlau et al 2015). He developed his techniques through addressing the effects of his own condition and found that by positioning himself appropriately and relieving unnecessary muscle tension, he could improve his overall presentation in both physical and vocal terms;

associated levels of anxiety were also reduced. He later translated his work to successfully treat people who stuttered (Schulte & Walach 2006).

More recent studies have evidenced the effectiveness of the Alexander technique in treating chronic back pain (Beattie et al 2010, Hollinghurst et al 2008, Yardley et al 2010) by improving postural tone (Cacciatore et al 2011) and sustaining an increase in activity levels for people suffering with Parkinson's disease (Stallibrass et al 2002, 2005). Woodman and Moore (2012), in a comprehensive systematic review, also suggested that the Alexander technique can lead to improvements in balance skills for the elderly, general chronic pain, posture, respiratory function and stuttering, but they do note that the evidence is limited (see Chapter 12 for detailed explanations of the Alexander technique).

Mitchell (1987) is advocating differential relaxation when she urges the partial use of her schedule during task performance; for example, practising 'joint changes' for the shoulders and the jaw while driving or typing. Her 'key changes' can also be seen as a differential technique, in that they are directed at switching off unnecessary global tension while allowing specific movements to take place (see Chapter 13).

Poppen's mini-relaxation (1998) is another differential form. Here, relaxed-looking postures are adopted in the muscle groups not engaged in the task; for example, the legs can be relaxed while writing a letter (see Chapter 10).

THEORIES BEHIND DIFFERENTIAL RELAXATION

The approach is underpinned by the same theoretical principles as progressive relaxation (see Chapter 5). A thorough knowledge of progressive relaxation provides the skills to carry out differential relaxation.

Differential relaxation is concerned with minimum tension levels during activity and task performance. Consequently, there are two prerequisites: knowing which muscle groups are needed for each activity and which are not; and possessing the skill of muscle relaxation. Jacobson's (1938), Bernstein and Borkovec's (1973) and Öst's (1987) methods all provide a theoretical framework for differential relaxation.

Jacobson's Method

Jacobson has described a method in which he isolates the task, reduces muscle tension to less than the level at which the task can be performed, and then, gradually, reintroduces tension to the minimum level where the task can be carried out efficiently. He gives an example (Jacobson 1976, p135).

You are now to read, while relaxing the lower limbs; the back, so far as sitting posture permits; the chest, so far as can be done while inner speech continues; and the arms, so far as is possible while they hold the book or magazine. With the forehead and eyes extremely relaxed, you will of course not read. But you should relax these parts while holding the reading matter in order to become familiar with an extreme form of differential relaxation. A little more tension is then introduced; the words are to be read, but the eyes and other parts are to be kept as far relaxed as possible at the same time. Perhaps you find that you now follow the words but fail to get the meaning. This still represents too great a degree of relaxation. Accordingly, you are to read again, this time engaging in just enough contractions to get the meaning clearly but not more.

A similar routine can be applied to writing. For example, try the following:

Take up a pen with the intention of writing your name but using too little energy to make a mark on the paper. Repeat the action, this time putting a little more force into it. Continue putting slightly more force into it until you reach a point where you are able to write in a way which you recognize as your style. Keep it relaxed. You are now combining effective outcome with economy of effort.

A good time to test for the presence of secondary tensions is when opening the morning post or accessing your email. The anticipation and apprehension of what it might reveal can raise tension levels far beyond what is necessary for the simple task of opening envelopes or clicking on the email icon.

Bernstein and Borkovec's Method

In their manual on progressive relaxation training, Bernstein and Borkovec (1973) develop the idea of differential relaxation. They single out three aspects of complexity: position of the body, level of activity and the situation in which the activity takes place. Variations of each are worked into an eight-step schedule, starting with 'sitting, doing nothing in a quiet room' and ending with 'standing, performing some activity in a busy environment'. Four of the items occur in the sitting position while the level of activity and the situation are varied; the other four occur in the standing position. During the performance of these exercises, trainees are asked to monitor tension levels, using 'recall' (see Chapter 8) to enable them to relax.

Öst's Method

Öst's (1987) approach to differential relaxation is described in Chapter 9.

KEY ASPECTS OF THE PROCEDURE

As noted previously, differential relaxation is a form of progressive relaxation that can be applied in everyday situations to facilitate a minimum level of muscle tension consistent with task efficiency. The following offer typical examples where the technique can be used.

Seated at a Desk Typing

Using just enough power in the hands to control the keys, type a few sentences. Then break off to check your body for tension. If you find any, relax it away using 'recall' (Chapter 8) or cue-controlled breathing (Chapter 9). Resume typing, checking again for tension. Make a telephone call, maintaining a relaxed posture, using only enough tension to hold the receiver.

Driving to the Supermarket

As you settle yourself into the driving seat, spend a minute checking all your muscle groups for tension. Identify the muscles you need for driving. If you notice excess tension in any of these muscles, relax it. Check that the muscles you don't need, such as the face muscles, are relaxed. Maintain relaxation while steering and changing gear until you arrive at the store. Park the car and walk towards the entrance, relaxing any tension in your face and shoulders. Pick a trolley and as you push it around, continue to check your body, relaxing those muscles you do not need and putting the minimum of tension into the ones you need for the task. Pause regularly to scan your body for unnecessary tension.

Digging the Garden

As you pick up the spade, feel the weight of it in your hand, fleetingly judging the degree of muscle work required to use it. Remind yourself that you can put too much effort into tasks of this nature. Relax your face muscles while you carry out the digging.

Stressful Situations

Differential relaxation is relatively easy to achieve in activities which do not pose any threat, but is more difficult in situations of stress, such as delivering a speech. In such cases additional strategies may need to be employed, such as mental rehearsal of the event and positive self-talk, to help reduce excessive tension (see Chapter 19).

Standing and Walking

The principles of differential relaxation can also be applied to the postures of standing and walking, where certain muscle groups, such as those of the back and the legs, hold the body vertical and propel it along while uninvolved groups, such as those of the face, can be relaxed. The following two examples illustrate these ideas.

Standing

Have your eyes open. Stand with shoes off, feet parallel and 5 or 6 cm apart. Release excess tension with cue-controlled breathing. Unlock your knees, slightly bending and stretching them a few times to feel the weight falling evenly down through them to your feet. Rock forwards and backwards over them until you find a comfortable position for your hips. Feel your spine rising above your hips … feel it supporting your head, and let your head reach up as high as it wants to go. Nod it gently to find its best position. Relax your face muscles. Let your arms hang down by your sides with your shoulders dropped. Feel your body relaxed and resilient. Enjoy being inside it. There should be no effort involved.

When the posture feels as comfortable as possible, notice what makes it feel like that.

Walking

One way of finding your own energy-economical way of walking is to experiment with different kinds of walking. Marching, sailor's roll and tiptoeing are, of course, artificial ways of walking, but by exploring different styles, you may find it easier to distinguish between unnatural and natural forms, and thus be helped to find your own natural way of walking. This will be the one that gives you most comfort and ease. Practise it, enjoy it. Feel your whole body relaxing into the rhythm of your step. Feel that the muscles responsible for carrying you along are no more tense than they need to be … and that your face and shoulder muscles are relaxed.

PRECAUTIONS

As the effective implementation of differential relaxation is predicated on knowledge and practice of progressive relaxation or its modified approaches, precautions are as in progressive relaxation (see Chapter 5).

APPLICATION

In the context of differential relaxation, it is worth noting that knowledge of the muscle groups required in daily activities is necessary to apply the principles in practice. A task or activity analysis may need to be carried out or research undertaken around the active and passive muscles groups used in relevant activities.

Prerequisites therefore include knowledge of the muscles and the action required in the specified activities; knowledge of and ability to carry out a task or analysis of the activity; and application of this learning to the situation at hand in line with implementing any precautions necessary.

Trainees also need to have some experience of relaxation practice before applying differential relaxation techniques in practice. This is because they need to understand the difference between the tense and relaxed state to identify and relax any unnecessary muscle activity. If this has not been completed previously, then training in these techniques will need to be undertaken before practising differential relaxation.

KEY POINTS

1. Differential relaxation is a form of applied relaxation in which actions are performed with the minimum energy.
2. The muscles employed in carrying out the task are working with just enough effort to accomplish the task, whereas the muscles not directly employed are as relaxed as possible.
3. The approach can be illustrated in all activities. Examples given here are typing, driving and garden digging.
4. Practice is essential in order for the action to become automatic.

Reflection

Describe your understanding of the techniques of differential relaxation.

How do you feel about applying this technique in practice?

Why do you think it is important to understand what muscles are used in everyday tasks to apply differential relaxation appropriately?

What did you learn about using task or activity analysis and/or understanding the different muscle groups and their action in everyday activity?

What is the main learning point you will take away from this chapter?

What is your future action plan in terms of differential relaxation?

CASE STUDY LEARNING OPPORTUNITIES

The key points and reflection provide the background and knowledge required in relation to the case studies; Seren (Case Study 1) and Tom (Case Study 2) help to deepen understanding of how differential relaxation can be applied in practice.

CASE STUDY 1

Driving the Car: *Differential Relaxation Outcomes for Seren*

Seren is presenting with headaches and muscle tension in her neck and shoulders. The symptoms are worse after driving. On taking a detailed history it becomes clear that Seren's condition seems to be related to a car accident 6 months ago; she fears she may have jolted her back or neck at that time and is questioning whiplash.

After further investigation, these prove inclusive, and you investigate her sitting position in the car and observe her driving. She has been using a tense–release relaxation method and is quite proficient, but on investigation it becomes clear that she is tensing her shoulders, upper back, neck and facial muscles when seated in and driving the car; she is also clenching her teeth.

You ask Seren to sit in the car and follow Jacobson's notion of diminishing tension whilst sitting in the driving seat; then, after breathing and relaxing, you ask her to hold the wheel and adjust her position until she feels she is ready to drive. When accommodated in the position, you then question Seren about how her body feels and where the tension is. She describes feeling tightness in the lower back, shoulders, neck, face and jaw. At this point you ask her to breathe and relax, letting go of that tension and recalling the relaxed state.

When she is able to sit in a relaxed state in the car but has sufficient tension to drive – that is, to hold the wheel in a relaxed and comfortable way, and to activate the feet to accelerate, brake and change gear – you begin taking short drives.

Seren works on this for a few weeks, as well as translating what she is learning about which muscles need to be active and which do not into her daily driving. She reports she is beginning to realize she is holding a lot of tension in her jaw, face, neck, shoulders and back, including her lower back. By breathing, using her cue word 'relax' and checking (scanning) and adjusting her position, Seren is slowly adopting a more relaxed position in her driving, using only the muscles she needs to and relaxing the others; as a consequence of this practice she is reporting that her headaches are occurring far less frequently.

CASE STUDY 2

Working in the Allotment: Differential Relaxation Outcomes for Tom

Tom is 76 years old and suffers from palindromic rheumatism and osteoarthritis. He is finding his gardening is becoming harder and he is suffering from low back pain most of the time. He loves his allotment, grows his own veg and feels his life would be empty if he can't keep it going. He has been using passive relaxation techniques for some time. He finds this works best for him because when he uses the tense–release cycle it causes his fingers and feet to cramp or spasm. He is also quite good at pacing himself; he has learned the hard way that if he pushes it, his rheumatism flares up and his lower back, hips and knees ache a lot too; he says he knows that's his osteoarthritis playing up.

You wonder whether a review of the way Tom is gardening might help and explain to him that he might not be using his muscles in the most efficient way. Tom says he'll give anything a go if it keeps him active in the garden. You observe Tom hoeing, weeding and picking veg and can see that he is quite stiff, bends from the hips and stands with his legs apart. You also observe that he is holding tension in his hands, arms, shoulders, back and legs; far more than is necessary to complete the task at hand.

You complete a full activity analysis of the motor function necessary for gardening and share your findings with Tom. Armed with this knowledge, you teach Tom to scan and identify where he is holding tension in his body when he gardens, to relax this and activate only the muscles he needs to do the job. You also look at his standing posture, the most efficient way to bend to weed and to use the garden tools effectively. He finds he has really been overusing some of his muscles and overworking his body.

Tom reports that so far the adjustments he is making to his activities are definitely helping in keeping him going in the garden. He is also having more tea breaks in his shed and spending more time chatting to his mates in the allotments. This is a more psychological gain that is really benefiting Tom's overall mood and sense of well-being.

ACTIVITY

For each of the case studies:

1. List key aspects used in the differential relaxation approaches.
2. Consider why this approach was taken.
3. Write down the impact differential relaxation is having from a psychological perspective.
4. Write down the impact differential relaxation is having from a physical perspective.
5. Write down the impact differential relaxation is having from an emotional perspective.
6. Consider the outcomes on quality of life and overall well-being for both individuals.

Chapter 12 will focus on the Alexander Technique to gain a deeper understanding of how the principles of differential relaxation are applied.

REFERENCES

Beattie, A., Shaw, A., Yardley, L., Little, P., & Sharp, D. (2010). Participating in and delivering the ATEAM trial (Alexander technique lessons, exercise and massage) interventions for chronic back pain: A qualitative study of professional perspectives. *Complementary Therapies in Medicine, 18*(3–4), 119–127.

Behlau, M., Madazio, G., & Oliveria, G. (2015). Functional dysphonia: Strategies to improve patient outcomes. *Patient Related Outcome Measures, 6*(24), 243–253.

Bernstein, D. A., & Borkovec, T. D. (1973). *Progressive relaxation training: A manual for the helping professions.* Champaign, IL: Research Press.

Cacciatore, T. W., Gurfinkel, V. S., Horak, F. B., Cordo, P. J., & Ames, K. E. (2011). Increased dynamic regulation of postural tone through Alexander Technique Training. *Human Movement Science, 30*(1), 74–89.

Gilman, M., & Yaruss, J. S. (2000). Stuttering and relaxation: Applications for somatic education in stuttering treatment. *Journal of Fluency Disorders, 25*(1), 59–76.

Hollinghurst, S., Sharp, D., Ballard, K., et al. (2008). Randomised controlled trial of Alexander technique lessons, exercise, and massage (ATEAM) for chronic and recurrent back pain: Economic evaluation. *BMJ: British Medical Journal, 337*, a2656.

Jacobson, E. (1938). *Progressive relaxation* (2nd ed.). Chicago: University of Chicago Press.

Jacobson, E. (1976). *You must relax.* London: Souvenir Press.

Kent, M. (2006). *Oxford dictionary of sports science and medicine* (3rd ed.). Oxford, UK: Oxford University Press.

Mitchell, L. (1987). *Simple relaxation: The Mitchell method for easing tension* (2nd ed.). London: John Murray.

Öst, L. G. (1987). Applied relaxation: description of a coping technique and review of controlled studies. *Behaviour Research and Therapy*, 25(5), 397–407.

Poppen, R. (1998). *Behavioural relaxation training and assessment* (2nd ed.). Thousand Oaks, CA: Sage.

Schulte, D., & Walach, H. (2006). F.M. Alexander technique in the treatment of stuttering – a randomised single-case intervention study with ambulatory monitoring. *Psychotherapy and Psychosomatics*, 75(3), 190–191.

Stallibrass, C., Frank, C., & Wentworth, K. (2005). Retention of skills learnt in Alexander Technique lessons: 28 people with idiopathic Parkinson's disease. *Journal of Bodywork and Movement Therapies*, 9(2), 150–157.

Stallibrass, C., Sissons, P., & Chalmers, C. (2002). Randomized controlled trial of the Alexander technique for idiopathic Parkinson's disease. *Clinical Rehabilitation*, 16(7), 695–708.

Woodman, J. P., & Moore, N. R. (2012). Evidence for the effectiveness of Alexander technique lessons in medical and health related conditions: A systematic review. *International Journal of Clinical Practice*, 66(1), 98–112.

Yardley, L., Dennison, L., Coker, R., et al. (2010). Patients' views of receiving lessons in the Alexander technique and an exercise prescription for managing back pain in the ATEAM trial. *Family Practice*, 27(2), 198–204.

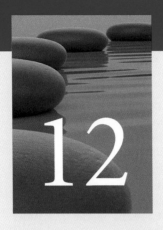

12

THE ALEXANDER TECHNIQUE

DR CAROLINE BELCHAMBER

CHAPTER CONTENTS

LEARNING OBJECTIVES

The aim of this chapter is to provide a practical guide to the Alexander technique.

By the end of this chapter you will be able to:

1. Understand the theory behind the Alexander technique.

2. Recognize the evidence that underpins the Alexander technique.

3. Describe what is meant by primary control and list the three components.

4. Identify faulty sensory perceptions and their relation to body movement.

5. Grasp the principles of the Alexander technique and application to practice.

The chapter will conclude with key points and time for reflection, providing learning opportunities through a case study.

INTRODUCTION TO THE ALEXANDER TECHNIQUE

'Posture' refers to the way people habitually hold themselves against the forces of gravity and is one of their recognizable features. A look round at our acquaintances tells us that they all have characteristic ways of holding themselves; each person stands differently, walks differently and sits differently. Although a person's posture may be largely of genetic origin and thus beyond their control, we are inclined to think that it is also governed by the way they look at and react to life.

Alexander technique trainers point to the way young children use their bodies, describing the effect as 'poise'. They also indicate how this natural poise can become distorted by emotional and physical influences as the child grows towards maturity, resulting in the development of tension habits which interfere with healthy functioning.

This notion captured the attention of Matthias Alexander, at a time when he was experiencing a problem with his voice. An actor by profession, he noticed that he was developing hoarseness and a painful throat whenever he began to perform. Intuitively, he felt that posture lay at the root of it. Mirrors revealed that he was pulling his head back and tightening his neck muscles to the extent that he could not breathe properly. By freeing his neck and lengthening his spine he discovered he could regain control of his voice, and the manner in which he accomplished this forms the basis of the Alexander technique (Alexander 1932).

The Alexander technique is among the few relaxation techniques to focus systematically on relaxation of the body while it is in motion (Woolfolk & Lehrer 1984). This is achieved by the trainer providing integrated spoken and hands-on guidance to enable both cognitive and experiential learning to improve mind and body function (Eldred et al 2015). As such, it is a form of kinaesthetic re-education. The technique is based on the assumption that the way we use our bodies affects our general functioning. However, there is no ideal; it is for each person to explore their possibilities and find better ways of using their body. For this and other reasons, the technique does not readily lend itself to systematic investigation and has not, until recently, begun to receive scientifically rigorous assessment.

INTRODUCTION TO EVIDENCE

The work of the anatomist Adams (Adams et al 1994, Adams & Hutton 1985) is relevant with regards to some of the postural claims made by Alexander. Adams studied the effect of actions which impose physical stress on the lumbar spine. He found that a moderate degree of flexion (i.e., flattening of the lumbar curve) is mechanically advantageous, which supports Alexander's views about the action of sitting down and the value of the monkey stance (Fig. 12.1), described under 'keeping length'. However, the research base at the time was small and not all studies met the requirements of being methodologically sound and clinically relevant. More research, both psychological and physiological, was recommended to help clarify the position. Until that has been carried out and conclusions drawn, the technique must, in Barlow's words, continue to be regarded as a hypothesis (Barlow 1975).

In 2000 Kerr carried out a critical review of relaxation techniques, which concluded that the Alexander technique may offer benefit in states of stress; it may also have a positive effect on conditions such as anxiety and depression. Positive changes in depression scores have since been demonstrated in Stallibrass et al's (2002) study. They tested the Alexander technique's efficacy in people experiencing symptoms of Parkinson's disease. Ninety-three participants were randomly divided into three groups: one received 24 lessons in the Alexander technique, one received 24 sessions of massage and there was a control which received no treatment. Results showed that, from pre- to postintervention, motor symptoms in the Alexander technique group improved significantly compared with the no treatment group, and this improvement was maintained at 6-month follow-up. These benefits were not demonstrated in the massage group. Both intervention groups, however, recorded positive changes on the Beck Depression Inventory (Beck 1988), whereas the control group registered no such changes.

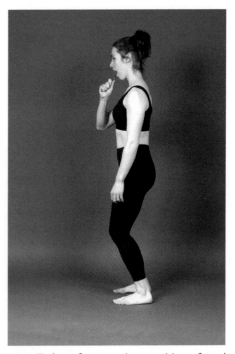

Fig. 12.1 ■ Task performance in a position of mechanical advantage (the monkey stance).

A systematic review of controlled clinical trials concluded that the evidence in favour of the Alexander technique is 'encouraging' rather than 'convincing' (Ernst & Canter 2003). Further research since this systematic review has been more conclusive, with Little et al (2008) suggesting that one-to-one lessons in the Alexander technique are effective for people with chronic back pain. In their randomized controlled trial of 579 patients, these researchers found that 24 lessons provided significant benefit in 3 months. At 12 months, the benefit was even greater. Little et al's (2008) study also demonstrated that it was possible to achieve a similar effect with fewer lessons: the researchers found that six lessons, followed by prescribed exercise, was almost as effective. Woodman and Moore's (2012) systematic review on health-related conditions corroborates Little et al's (2008) findings, and Macpherson et al's (2015) randomized controlled trial found that the Alexander technique led to long-term benefits for people with chronic neck pain, with pain and disability significantly reduced at 12 months. Wenham et al (2018) analyzed participants' perspectives from Macpherson et al's (2015) trial to gain an in-depth understanding of the impact of the Alexander technique. They concluded that the Alexander technique enabled behavioural change to improve self-care, leading to a sense of embodiment and, consequently, self-efficacy associated long-term reduction in pain. There is therefore a growing body of evidence to support the long-term benefits of the Alexander technique.

THEORIES BEHIND THE ALEXANDER TECHNIQUE

The Alexander technique is not underpinned by any established theory, but it is based on principles of body positioning:

- Primary control
- Use and misuse
- Faulty sensory perception
- Inhibition
- 'End-gaining' and the 'means whereby'
- Integration of mind and body

Primary Control

Alexander believed that the primary control of human posture lay in the relationships of the head to the neck and of the neck to the rest of the spine. So convinced was he of their crucial nature that an almost magical significance was attached to these relationships in his day. This status has, however, been modified over the years, and the Alexander technique trainer today sees primary control less as an inviolable principle than as a useful starting point.

Primary control has three components:

- A neck that is free and whose muscles contain only enough tension to keep the head upright
- A head moving forward and up (Fig. 12.2), not back and down to crumple the spine (Fig. 12.3)
- A spine that feels lengthened, thus counteracting any tendency towards sagging

Use and Misuse

'Use' refers to the characteristic way a person holds their body. It is a neutral term. When there is harmony between the tension necessary to support the body and

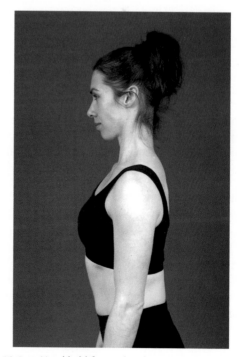

Fig. 12.2 ■ Head held forward and up.

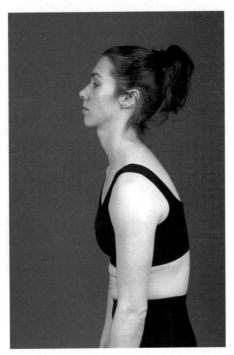

Fig. 12.3 ■ Head held back and down.

the relaxation necessary to allow it to move, the use is said to be 'balanced'. When, however, this is upset by too much or too little tension, a state of misuse is said to prevail (Barlow 1975). Examples of misuse are hunching of the shoulders, head sinking into the spine, and chin thrusting out.

The regaining of 'balanced use' means the recovery of natural movement patterns, which can only occur if people review the messages they are getting about the position of their body in space.

Faulty Sensory Perceptions

All movement in the healthy organism is accompanied by sensory feedback in the form of proprioceptive impulses from the moving part. This gives the person information about the position of body parts in space. In the young child, these messages lead to responses which are natural, economic (in terms of energy consumption) and uncontaminated by emotional factors, whereas those in the adult may be distorted by trauma (mental or physical).

Responses carried out repeatedly turn into habits, which are then interpreted by the higher centres as

normal; that is, the way people habitually use their bodies will feel normal to them simply because they are used to it. Alexander's experience with the mirror showed him he was still pulling his head back even after he felt he had corrected it. This could only be because his body had got used to the 'bad' posture and had internalized it as normal, so that even the smallest degree of correction was interpreted by his conscious mind as overcorrection.

The phrase 'faulty sensory perception' refers to the way messages are interpreted in a misused body.

Inhibition

Many of the body's movements are automatic. If they show patterns of misuse which require correction, it will be necessary to intercept them – that is, to examine them before they are automatically executed. A pause is necessary. This act of pausing constitutes what Alexander called 'inhibition'. It allows the person to question the validity of their response. It gives them the chance to reconsider their action and to redirect their movement.

Inhibition, not to be confused with the Freudian meaning, is what happens when people cease to react automatically to stimuli, thereby leaving them free to respond appropriately, to do nothing for a moment while the maladaptive, automatic response pattern is broken. 'When you stop doing the wrong thing, the right thing does itself' (Alexander 1932).

'End-Gaining' and the 'Means Whereby'

Inhibition provides the opportunity to focus on the means whereby the person achieves a certain end. It draws attention away from 'end-gaining,' where action is performed too quickly and too energetically for the person to give any thought as to the manner in which the end is gained. Alexander would say that if you pay attention to the means, the end will take care of itself (Maisel 2000).

Integration of Mind and Body

Central to the teachings of Alexander is a belief that the mind and the body are interdependent. Not only does the body posture reflect people's thoughts, but their mind responds to the way they use their body. Such notions introduce a new dimension to the concept of body movement, and can be said to lie at the heart of the statement that 'we *are* our posture' (Barlow 1975).

THE ALEXANDER TECHNIQUE

The Alexander technique itself re-educates the body to perform in a balanced and energy-economical way (Gray 1998). Habits of misuse are identified and replaced by more appropriate ways of using the body. Assessment and correction are carried out in positions of lying, sitting, standing and walking. Gently using a hands-on approach, the trainer guides the participant's body both in motion and at rest while the pupil mentally focuses on the message he or she is getting from the trainer's hands. For example, a person lying down might be told to think of the words 'shoulder release and widen', as the trainer is repositioning one of the shoulders. Thus, without actively performing the movement, the participant directs the body to co-operate.

Some of the principal instructions are listed here, beginning with the three elements of primary control:

1. 'Neck free'
2. 'Head forward and up'
3. 'Back lengthen'

Other instructions include the following:

4. 'Keeping length'
5. 'Back widen'
6. 'Shoulder release and widen'

The Three Elements of Primary Control

1. 'Neck Free'

'Neck free' means that the head is carried in such a way that no undue strain is put on the neck muscles. The image of the nodding dog in the back of the car may help to convey the feeling of a free neck.

2. 'Head Forward and Up'

'Head forward and up' is the phrase for those who are sitting or standing. It means that the head is held with the chin pointing to the toes, not poking out. It also means that the head is lifted up and out of the vertebral column. The result is that the person feels taller or longer, having 'grown' from a point at the back of the head. It is the opposite of a head which sinks into the shoulders with the chin thrust out. At the same time, no excessive effort should be made to extend the body. The effect described can often be achieved simply by

'thinking up'. Figs 12.2 and 12.3 illustrate the correct and incorrect ways of carrying the head.

3. 'Back Lengthen'

An erect spine anteroposteriorly (front to back) displays a succession of natural curves: concavities in the cervical and lumbar regions, convexity in the dorsal region. In urging 'back lengthen', it is not implied that efforts should be made to obliterate these natural curves, but rather that the curves should not be allowed to become overemphasized because that would result in crumpling or shortening of the spine. Actions which particularly shorten the spine are:

- overextension of the cervical vertebrae (thrusting out the chin).
- overextension of the lumbar vertebrae (exaggerated lumbar concavity) (Fig. 12.4).

Similarly, slumping is to be avoided. Slumping occurs when the whole spine is rounded into a long C-shaped curve, with the neck hyperextended to allow

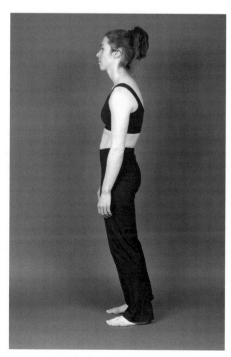

Fig. 12.4 ■ Standing with exaggerated cervical and lumbar curves.

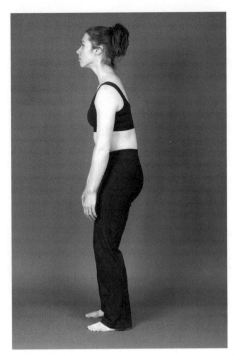

Fig. 12.5 ■ Standing with spine slumped into a long C-shaped curve.

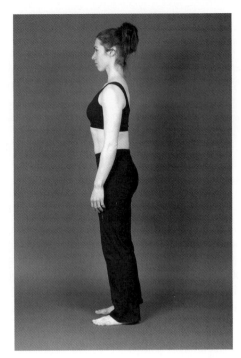

Fig. 12.6 ■ Balanced standing posture.

the eyes to look forwards. Slumping also creates shortening of the spine (Fig. 12.5).

'Back lengthen' indicates that the spine should be allowed to reach its full length (or height), as opposed to being either crumpled (where spinal curves are exaggerated) or slumped (where the back is too rounded). An image that evokes the idea of lengthening the back is that of a jet of water springing up in the spine and lifting it gently. The head should feel lightly balanced on top.

Alexander's view of a balanced standing posture is one in which the body weight passes through the front of the heel, the knees are unbraced and the pelvis is in midposition, with the 'tail' neither thrown out nor forcibly tucked under. The direction to 'think up' helps convey the idea of standing straight, but without making any forced effort to do so. Some trainers introduce the image of a helium-filled balloon lifting the head (Gray 1998). Fig. 12.6 illustrates the correct standing position.

'Neck free', 'head forward and up' and 'back lengthen' are fundamental to the technique.

Other Instructions

4. 'Keeping Length'

The instruction 'keeping length' is related to 'back lengthen'. Alexander applies it to the action of sitting down where he sees particular benefit to be gained from the avoidance of crumpling. His technique of lowering the body is illustrated in the following passage (Leibowitz & Connington 1999).

Place your feet slightly apart and positioned so that the backs of your legs are lightly in contact with the chair seat. Let your arms hang loosely by your sides. Before lowering yourself, let your mind focus on the idea of 'keeping length', that is, not crumpling the spine. Keep the head and neck in the same relation as they were in the standing position and as you lower yourself, flatten the lumbar curve. Although you are looking at the floor as you go down, make a point of thinking 'UP' to prevent any tendency of the spine to crumple.

Fig. 12.7 demonstrates the correct way of lowering the body into a chair.

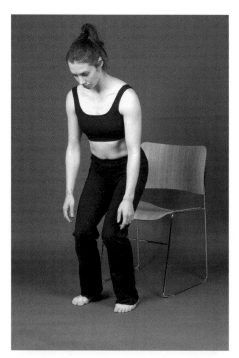

Fig. 12.7 ■ Sitting down with the spine 'keeping length'.

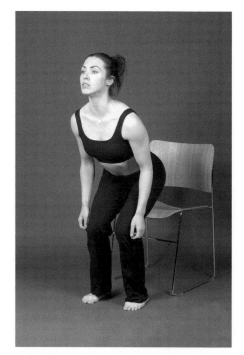

Fig. 12.8 ■ Sitting down with a 'crumpled' spine.

The wrong way of sitting down, according to Alexander, is to overextend both the neck and lumbar regions – that is, to thrust the chin out and exaggerate the lumbar concavity. Their combined effect crumples and shortens the spine (Gray 1998). Fig. 12.8 shows an incorrect way of lowering the body into a chair.

On rising from the chair, the head should start the movement and lead the body forwards. From that point the motions of sitting down are put into reverse.

What Alexander is saying is that the lumbar spine should be slightly flexed and the cervical spine prevented from extending itself in the actions of sitting down and rising. He urges applying the same ideas to other activities which carry the centre of gravity forwards, such as leaning over a basin to clean the teeth.

Alexander compared the action of tooth brushing in humans to the peeling of fruit by erect primates in the wild. Both actions take place anterior to the body itself. On noticing that primates adopted a particular stance to carry out their task, he concluded that mechanical advantage was being gained from it. The stance itself is characterized by bent knees and slightly flexed (flattened)

lumbar and cervical spines, a posture which is referred to as the 'monkey stance' (see Fig. 12.1).

The effect of the monkey stance is to keep the centre of gravity as close to the spine as possible, thereby relieving the strain on the lumbosacral junction. Where the monkey stance is not adopted for comparable tasks, a position of mechanical disadvantage is created. Fig. 12.9 illustrates this idea: the arms and head reach forwards, pulling the centre of gravity with them, while the cervical and lumbar spines retain their concavities.

Common to both the monkey stance and the act of sitting (as recommended by Alexander) is a slight flexion of the lumbar spine. Alexander's insistence on the value of this posture has been supported by research (Adams et al 1994, Adams & Hutton 1985, Dolan & Adams 2001).

5. 'Back Widen'

The phrase 'back widen' applies to the posterior part of the thorax, which should be allowed to feel wide to permit full expansion of the ribs. To convey the idea of 'back widen', Gray (1998) promotes the image of the rib cage filling out into the back as the air enters the lungs.

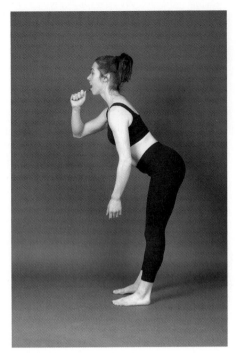

Fig. 12.9 ■ Task performance in a position of mechanical disadvantage.

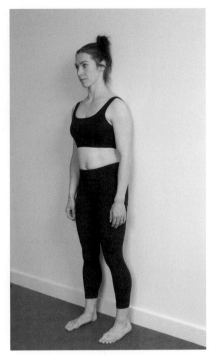

Fig. 12.10 ■ Testing for body alignment 1: leaning against wall.

6. 'Shoulder Release and Widen'

'Shoulder release and widen' is aimed at relaxing the muscles of the shoulder girdle, which are often held more tensely than they need to be.

Recognizing and Correcting Misuse

Test for Body Alignment

As mentioned in the section on faulty sensory perception, a habitual posture, whether balanced or not, will feel 'right' to its owner. This makes it difficult for people to recognize misuse in themselves. A procedure to solve this matter has been worked out by Barlow (1975).

Stand with your heels 5 centimetres (2 inches) from a wall, with your feet 46 centimetres (18 inches) apart. Let your body sway back until it touches the wall.

Fig. 12.10 shows this position.

If your shoulders and hips touch simultaneously with each side level, your alignment is correct. However, you may find that one side touches the wall before

the other, or that your shoulders touch before your hips. Do what you can to realign yourself. Next, bend your knees slightly and notice that this action will tend to bring the lumbar vertebrae into contact with the wall (lumbar curve flattened).

Fig. 12.11 demonstrates this effect.

If you can hold this position with relative comfort, then your body is not in a misused state. If you find it unduly tiring, then practice will make it easier and help to restore alignment.

Changing Posture

Alexander sees misuse as resulting, largely, from stress and the demands of contemporary life; in its turn, misuse can be the cause of physical stress, leading to muscle and joint problems.

People wishing to change their posture need to consider three points. They should:

■ be aware of the particular habit-governed movement that they want to correct.

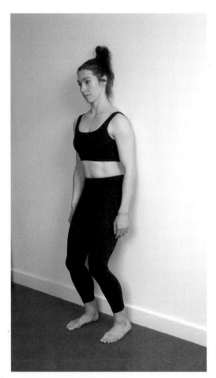

Fig. 12.11 ■ Testing for body alignment 2: flattening the lumbar concavity as the body is lowered.

- refuse to react automatically. This implies pausing to reassess the 'means whereby' – that is, being ready to say 'no' to the old response.
- redirect their muscles by a thought process. In the early stages of re-education this signifies *thinking* about the corrected movement rather than driving the muscles to perform it. Such an approach

allows the neuromuscular system to restructure its response. 'The mind gives the instruction, and little by little, the body absorbs the message' (Fontana 1994) until the corrected form of the movement becomes automatic.

Regularly practising new responses will result in a gradual weakening of the old ones and turn a pattern of misuse into one of more balanced use. There are no defined stages of progress nor specified goals of perfection. Individual problems call for individual remedies. Common to all remedies, however, is the cultivation of a sensitive approach to the movement of the person's own body (Barlow 1975).

Relaxation Effects

Although proponents speak of 'balanced use' rather than relaxation, the Alexander technique can nonetheless be seen as a method for promoting relaxation. Balanced use is associated with the elimination of excess muscular activity and is concerned with establishing minimum levels of muscle tension. These are concepts that are found in Jacobson's differential relaxation (see Chapter 11). For Alexander, however, they form the basis of his technique, whereas for Jacobson they are subsidiary to his main concern, which is the release of residual tension.

Alexander suggests a daily 15-minute session of rest, to be carried out in a crook lying position (knees bent up, feet flat on the ground) with a book under the head (where the height of the book is determined by the shape of the spine). The object is to allow the body to regain its natural symmetry; the procedure is also, however, a relaxing one (Fig. 12.12).

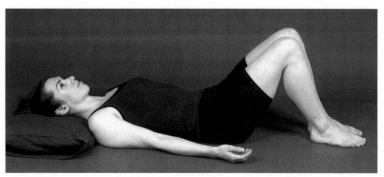

Fig. 12.12 ■ Promoting body symmetry in a relaxed position.

Teaching the Alexander Technique

The purpose of writing this chapter is to give a general idea of the principles underlying the Alexander technique, rather than to show how to teach it; such training involves a 3-year course. The principles, however, may be woven into other relaxation techniques, particularly where posture is a key item.

Alexander technique trainers often work in the field of performing arts in the belief that the approach can identify unwanted movement patterns which can interfere with performance (Batson 1996). However, the technique has universal relevance for a number of conditions (Woodman & Moore 2012).

KEY POINTS

1. The Alexander technique is a process of psychophysical re-education.
2. The re-education includes the unlearning of disadvantageous postural habits and the learning of alternative ones so that the muscles work in a more energy-economical way.
3. Posture plays a central role in this technique. Phrases such as 'spine lengthening' and 'head held forward and up' illustrate the basic principles of the Alexander technique.
4. Alexander's message is, *If the posture is right, the body will be relaxed and the mind also.*

5. By its emphasis on balance, the technique helps defuse body stress, and this has application in the area of the performing arts.
6. There is some evidence that the technique can help to reduce disability in Parkinson's disease. Different forms of paralysis, such as stroke and multiple sclerosis, may also respond favourably to the approach.

Reflection

Describe your posture in sitting, standing and lying.
How did you perceive your posture?
Why did your body respond in that way?
What changes did you make when you repeated these positions in front of a mirror?
What did you learn?
What is your future action plan?

CASE STUDY LEARNING OPPORTUNITY

The key points and reflection provide the background and knowledge required in relation to the case study, Low Back Pain: Alexander Technique Outcomes for Harry, to help deepen understanding of how the Alexander technique can be applied to practice.

CASE STUDY

Low Back Pain: *Alexander Technique Outcomes for Harry*

Harry is a 47-year-old man with a 20-year history of lower back pain. His lower back causes him pain on a daily basis. Harry works in a local factory and his job entails sitting at a computer or standing to give talks to his team. Standing for more than 20 minutes exacerbates Harry's lower back pain. Harry is not keen to have any surgery to relieve his pain and doesn't like to take medication if he can avoid it. However, the pain is sometimes so great he resorts to taking paracetamol.

Harry has found that walking helps relieve his low back pain; however, there are times when the pain is so severe that all Harry can do is curl up in a ball on

his side to try to relieve the pain. Harry's general practitioner (GP) therefore suggested seeing a physiotherapist trained in the Alexander technique, who would be able to assess Harry's low back pain and provide ways of managing his pain. However, he would need to commit to attending the lessons and have the time available to do so. Harry decided it was worth a try if it enabled him to manage his pain without surgery.

At the first appointment the physiotherapist explored Harry's current situation and pain levels, empowering Harry to lead his own care. Harry's goals were to be able to carry out activities of daily living pain free, such as working at the computer and standing, and to reduce his overall pain level. After this discussion, the physiotherapist then observed Harry's posture and noted that Harry's pelvis was tilted and rotated. There was also an increase in the curvature (kyphosis) of Harry's thoracic (chest) spine. In addition to this Harry's knees were hyperextended. After this observation the physiotherapist measured Harry's range of motion. There was asymmetry in Harry's lower back when he was asked to stand tall and then slide his hand down the side of his leg, first to the right and then to the left. When Harry bent forward his movement was restricted, with him only able to reach his knees. When he was asked to lean back, movement was limited to the lower part of his lumbar spine (L4 and L5), with no extension above this level. Muscle strength was also measured, and it was noted that Harry's abdominal muscles were weaker than his trunk extensor muscles.

Harry had weekly lessons lasting approximately 45 minutes each, with a total of 20 lessons over a 6-month period. Harry was taught the principles of the Alexander Technique in sitting, standing and lying postures. The trainer emphasized anatomical relationships when explaining the directions required, with the help of mirrors to manage self-perception of body position to correct the alignment. Towards the end of the sessions the trainer worked with Harry during daily activities, such as computer work. He was not given any exercises to perform outside the sessions, but was told instead to apply the principles learned in the sessions to his daily activities.

After the sessions Harry's postural co-ordination had improved and he reported that his pain had reduced to 1 to 2 days a month. In addition to this, he was now able to stand for several hours without pain and no longer had severe pain where he had to lie down to gain relief.

ACTIVITY

For the case study:
1. List key aspects of the Alexander technique in managing Harry's pain.
2. Write down the psychological outcomes experienced.
3. Write down the physical outcomes experienced.
4. Consider the outcomes on quality of life and overall well-being.

Chapter 13 will focus on the Mitchell (1987) method of relaxation. Mitchell's method is based on the physiological principle of reciprocal inhibition; that is, when one muscle group is acting on a joint, the opposing muscle group is obliged to relax.

REFERENCES

Adams, M. A., & Hutton, W. C. (1985). The effect of posture on the lumbar spine. *Journal of Bone and Joint Surgery, 67B*, 625–629.

Adams, M. A., McNally, D. S., Chinn, H., & Dolan, P. (1994). Posture and the compressive strength of the lumbar spine. *Clinical Biomechanics, 9*, 5–14.

Alexander, F. N. (1932). *The use of the self*. New York: Dutton.

Barlow, W. (1975). *The Alexander principle*. London: Arrow.

Batson, G. (1996). Conscious use of the human body in movement: the peripheral neuro-anatomic basis of the Alexander technique. *Medical Problems of Performing Artists, 11*(1), 3–11.

Beck, A. T. (1988). *The Beck depression inventory*. Sidcup, UK: Psychological Corporation.

Dolan, P., & Adams, M. A. (2001). Recent advances in lumbar spinal mechanics and their significance for modelling. *Clinical Biomechanics, 16*(1), S8–S16.

Eldred, J., Hopton, A., Donnison, E., Woodman, J., & MacPherson, H. (2015). Teachers of the Alexander Technique in the UK and the people who take their lessons: A national cross-sectional survey. *Complementary Therapy Medicine, 23*(3), 451e461.

Ernst, E., & Canter, P. H. (2003). The Alexander technique: A systematic review of controlled clinical trials. *Forsch Komplementarmed Klass Naturheilkd, 10*(6), 325–329.

Fontana, D. (1994). *The meditator's handbook: A comprehensive guide to eastern and western meditation techniques*. Shaftesbury, UK: Element.

Gray, J. (1998). *Your guide to the Alexander technique* (3rd revised ed.). London: Weidenfeld & Nicolson–Orion Publishing.

Kerr, K. M. (2000). Relaxation techniques: A critical review. *Critical Reviews in Physical and Rehabilitation Medicine, 12*, 51–89.

Leibowitz, J., & Connington, B. (1999). *The Alexander technique*. London: Souvenir Press.

Little, P., Lewith, G., Webley, F., et al. (2008). Randomized controlled trial of Alexander technique lessons, exercise and massage for chronic and recurrent back pain. *BMJ: British Medical Journal, 337*, 438.

MacPherson, H., Tilbrook, H., Richmond, S., et al. (2015). Alexander technique lessons or acupuncture sessions for persons with chronic neck pain: a randomised trial. *Annals of Internal Medicine, 163*(9), 653–662.

Maisel, E. (2000). *The Alexander technique: The essential writings of F. Matthias Alexander*. New York: Carol Publishing Group.

Stallibrass, C., Sissons, P., & Chalmers, C. (2002). Randomized controlled trial of the Alexander technique for idiopathic Parkinson's disease. *Clinical Rehabilitation, 16*, 705–718.

Wenham, A., Atkin, K., Woodman, J., Ballard, K., & MacPherson, H. (2018). Self-efficacy and embodiment associated with Alexander technique lessons or with acupuncture sessions: a longitudinal qualitative sub-study within the ATLAS Trial. *Complementary Therapies in Clinical Practice, 31*, 308–314.

Woodman, J. P., & Moore, N. R. (2012). Evidence for the effectiveness of Alexander technique lessons in medical and health-related conditions: A systematic review. *International Journal of Clinical Practice, 66*(1), 98–112.

Woolfolk, R. L., & Lehrer, P. M. (Eds.). (1984). *Principles and practice of stress management*. New York: Guilford Press.

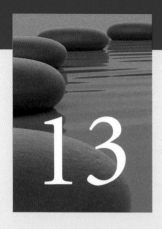

13

THE MITCHELL METHOD

DR CAROLINE BELCHAMBER

LEARNING OBJECTIVES

The aim of this chapter is to provide a practical guide to the Mitchell method of relaxation.

By the end of this chapter you will be able to:

1. Understand the rationale behind the Mitchell method.

2. Recognize the 'punching position'.

3. Describe the theory behind the Mitchell method.

4. Follow the procedure for delivering the Mitchell method.

5. Apply the relaxation technique to practice.

The chapter will conclude with key points and time for reflection, providing learning opportunities through a case study.

INTRODUCTION TO THE MITCHELL METHOD

In 1963 a new relaxation technique was introduced. Its originator was Laura Mitchell, a physiotherapist with a wide experience of teaching and practice in the field of obstetrics. She argued that it was useless to ask a person to notice tension in their muscles because there are no nerve endings in muscle tissue capable of conveying such information to the conscious brain. The sensory apparatus in the muscle connects only with the lower brain and spinal cord. Consequently, exhortations to become aware of the presence or absence of muscle tension are inappropriate. However, proprioceptive structures in the joints, and skin pressure receptors do have links with the conscious brain. The first tell us where our limbs are in space and the second tell us where the skin is being stretched or compressed. It is only, she claims, by moving the joints and stretching the skin that information about muscle state is relayed to the higher centres. Thus the joints and the skin are the organs on which we need to focus attention.

Both Jacobson (see Chapter 5) and Mitchell see their relaxation techniques as skills to be learned. Neither favours the use of tone of voice to influence the message. Instead, the participant is required simply to respond to the basic instruction. Again, like Jacobson, Mitchell avoids using the instruction 'Relax'. Her reason is that she finds it 'vague, generalized and ambiguous'. Jacobson avoided using it because he felt it provoked the participant into making an effort which was superfluous, when 'going negative' was the effect he wanted. On other points they are, of course, fundamentally opposed, Mitchell placing the highest value on joint and skin sensations and rejecting the idea of information coming from the muscles, whereas Jacobson is only interested in muscle feelings, dismissing any value that joint sensations might have.

Greater resemblance may be found between the Mitchell method and the Alexander technique (see Chapter 12) in the value placed on proprioceptive stimuli and awareness of posture. There is little difference between the 'three-point pull' of the Mitchell method (see Practice) and the 'neck lengthen' instruction of the Alexander technique (see Alexander Technique in Chapter 12).

The Mitchell method (Mitchell 1990) is composed of 13 actions, referred to as joint changes (although they do not all involve joint activity). These changes reverse different aspects of the 'punching position' described here:

- Shoulders hunched
- Arms held close to sides
- Fingers curled into the palms
- Legs crossed
- Feet dorsiflexed (drawn up towards face)
- Torso bent forwards
- Head held forwards
- Breathing rapid with noticeable movement in the upper chest
- Jaw clenched
- Lips pursed
- Tongue pressed into upper palate
- Brow furrowed into a frown

Mitchell does not suggest that the 'punching position' is actually adopted under stress; rather, that the muscles responsible for it are contracting to a slight extent.

The Mitchell method actions address tension in the whole body; however, many people have characteristic ways of displaying tension. This means that they are likely to benefit more from some joint changes than from others. The joint change that an individual finds most effective in reducing tension is referred to by Mitchell as the 'key change' because it is instrumental in releasing tension in other parts of the body. The key change can be identified by asking people how they tend to react when experiencing anger, pain, anxiety or conflict. If they tend to make fists, their key change will be finger lengthening; if they tend to clench their teeth, it will be jaw dropping. Key changes, by their generalizing effects, can promote a sense of ease throughout the whole body.

Mitchell applies the relaxation technique to everyday activities, using the concept of 'triggers of tension'– that is, events which tend to provoke feelings of stress, such as waiting at traffic lights or being interrupted by bells and alarms. She suggests sticking coloured tabs on potentially stressful appliances such as the steering wheel and the telephone as reminders to adopt the key change. Thus, to become more relaxed in daily life, there is first a need to recognize the triggers and second, a need to diminish their impact by using the key change to move the body into the ease position.

Benefit can also be gained from a partial use of the relaxation technique. Mitchell suggests that selected joint changes be used during specific activities; for example, the face actions can be carried out while driving or the leg actions while reading. The idea is not far removed from differential relaxation (see Chapter 11).

The Mitchell method promotes awareness of relaxed postures. The method is simple and quick and many of the 'changes' can be carried out unobtrusively. It is widely practised as a stress-relieving strategy and clinical findings testify to its effectiveness. Scientific evaluation of the Mitchell method, however, is limited.

INTRODUCTION TO THE EVIDENCE

Jackson (1991) studied four people with rheumatoid arthritis trained in the Mitchell method, comparing them with controls who simply rested. Using electromyography to measure activity in the frontalis muscle (a sensitive indicator of general muscle state), she found a marked reduction of tension in the study group and very little change in the control group. No statistical analysis was reported.

An interesting comparison between the Mitchell method and Jacobson's progressive relaxation technique was made by Salt and Kerr (1997). With a sample of 14 men and 10 women, these authors measured the effects of both approaches on the cardiovascular and respiratory systems. The study was designed with a control condition of supine lying. Participants were randomly assigned to three groups: the Mitchell method, the Jacobson's technique and the control condition, presented in different sequences to avoid order effects. Heart rate, systolic blood pressure, diastolic blood pressure and respiratory rate were recorded before and after every treatment. Results showed significant reductions after treatment on all measures for both relaxation techniques, with no significant differences between them. The control condition itself showed significant reductions in heart rate and respiratory rate; however, compared with the control, both relaxation techniques were found to be significantly superior on measures of systolic blood pressure. On a subjective level, there was some evidence of participants finding the Mitchell method easier to follow and less demanding in concentration than Jacobson's progressive relaxation. Thus, although each relaxation technique demonstrated greater effectiveness than supine lying on certain counts, the study has been unable to demonstrate a substantial difference in the separate capacities of the two relaxation techniques to induce physiological relaxation. This is the first study to investigate the Mitchell method using statistically analyzed data. A later study compared the Mitchell method with diaphragmatic breathing (Bell & Saltikov 2000) and also found a lack of significant difference between the two. However, a more recent study by Amirova and colleagues (2017) demonstrated that the Mitchell method is statistically effective in reducing pain, sleep problems and fatigue in people with fibromyalgia. In this study the relative high rates of reduction in both pain and fatigue suggest clinical significance. Walter and Shepard (2001) report that the Mitchell method is applied extensively in both women's health and mental health in the holistic management of anxiety, which has been verified by another study on postpartum eclampsia, stress and stress-induced convulsions (Paras 2013). This nationwide survey demonstrated that breathing re-education was an effective part of the management of anxiety. Therefore Mitchell's insistence that breathing should be slow and easy, and never include breath holding, is another reason for the method being favoured by those working in the obstetric field (Mantle et al 2004). For the same reasons the method is often adopted by those who work in the field of respiratory medicine (Hough 2001). Thus the Mitchell method lends itself to a range of conditions including insomnia, psychiatric disorders, dyspnoea, osteoarthritis and cardiac rehabilitation, as well as everyday stress. It is widely used in the field of obstetrics where its advantage lies in its avoidance of tensing procedures. The required relaxation is achieved by simply moving the body part as described later in this chapter.

THEORIES BEHIND THE MITCHELL METHOD

The Mitchell method is based on the theory of physiological principle of reciprocal inhibition; that is, when one group of muscles acting on a joint is working, the opposing group is obliged to relax. As the fibres of one group contract, the fibres of the opposing group become slack. It is a built-in mechanism to allow the smooth performance of movement.

Mitchell exploits this principle and makes it the nub of her approach. Stress-related posture, or what she calls 'the punching position' is studied, the working muscle groups are identified, and then relaxed by activating the opposing groups. The resulting changes of joint position and the accompanying skin sensations are then mentally registered as the part settles into the posture of ease. Thus her approach consists of moving the body out of the posture of defence or stress and training the mind to recognize the posture of ease or relaxation.

The aim of the procedure described here is to reduce stress and relax the mind. Mitchell proposes that the relaxation induced by this method spreads throughout the organism to include the mind.

PROCEDURE

Introductory Remarks

Participants are introduced to the relaxation technique by a short description of the Mitchell method rationale and procedure.

I just want to say something about the Mitchell method before we begin. When people are under stress, there is a position which they tend to adopt. We could call this 'the punching position'. Although people don't actually present themselves in a punching posture, the muscles which create it are tensing to a minute degree. This happens instinctively and helps to promote a feeling of being ready for anything.

If we move the body into the opposite of 'the punching position', we will be taking it into a position of ease or relaxation.

You might ask, 'How do we get the punching muscles to relax?' This is where the physiological principle comes in: when one group of muscles acting on a joint is tensed, the opposing group automatically relaxes.

The trainer demonstrates.

When I bend my wrist forwards, the bending-back muscles relax, and vice versa. It's a reciprocal mechanism without which smooth action could not take place.

The method itself consists of a succession of changes of position. Each change moves a body part out of its position of defence and into its position of ease. As the part settles into the position of ease, you'll be asked to notice how it feels. The aim is to learn to recognize the relaxed position so that you can reproduce it more easily. I'll first demonstrate the starting positions and actions.

Starting Positions

Three starting positions are described.

1. Supine lying with a pillow under the head (Fig. 13.1). A pillow under the thighs is optional.
2. Forward-lean sitting – that is, leaning forwards with head and arms resting on a table (Fig. 13.2).
3. Sitting in a high-backed chair with arm rests on which the hands are supported, palms downwards (Fig. 13.3).

Varying the starting position is useful to extend the range of application of the Mitchell method. The eyes may be open or closed.

Instructions

The trainer begins by giving an order to direct a part of the body away from its posture of tension. The order is followed by the word 'Stop'. This means that the part is no longer being actively moved; it also means that the muscles responsible for the movement are no longer contracting. The part then falls naturally into the position of ease. This position is then mentally registered. Following is a list of the items to be worked.

Actions

1. Pull your shoulders towards your feet.
2. Slide your elbows away from your body.
3. Stretch your fingers and thumbs.
4. Turn your hips outwards.
5. Move your knees until they are comfortable.
6. Push your feet away from your face.
7. Breathing.
8. Push your body into the support.
9. Push your head into the support.
10. Drag your jaw downwards.
11. Press your tongue downwards in your mouth.

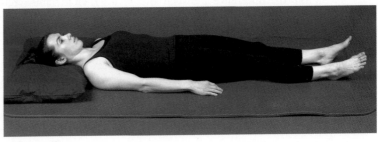

Fig. 13.1 ■ Starting position: supine.

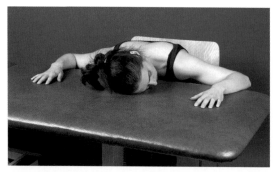

Fig. 13.2 ■ Starting position: forward-lean sitting.

12. Close your eyes.
13. Think of a smoothing action which begins above your eyebrows, rises into your hairline, continues over the top of your head and down into the back of your neck.

Each action is modelled by the trainer who asks the participant to copy it.

Process

The relaxation technique is then worked through in its entirety. It is presented here with the instructions expressed in inverted commas.

1. Shoulders

'Pull your shoulders towards your feet'. Do this gently, but go on until you can't pull them down anymore. Feel the space between your shoulders and your ears getting greater. 'Stop pulling'. Notice the feel of the new position. Take plenty of time to register the sensations you are getting from it.

2. Elbows

'Elbows out and open'. For participants lying supine or sitting in a high-backed chair: slide your elbows sideways, carrying your arms away from your body until you reach a comfortable point (Figs 13.4 and 13.5). For participants in forward-lean sitting: slide your arms away from your body, opening your arms at the elbow joint (Fig. 13.6). 'Stop moving'. Check that your arms are resting on the supporting surface and notice how it feels to have a space between your arms and your body. Feel this position.

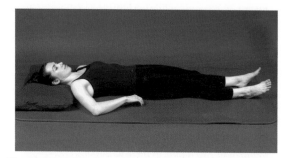

Fig. 13.4 ■ 'Elbows out and open' in supine position.

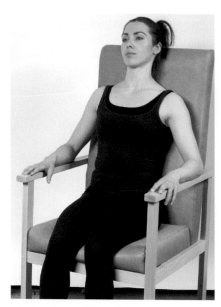

Fig. 13.3 ■ Starting position: sitting.

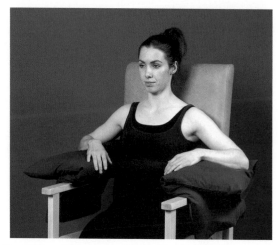

Fig. 13.5 ■ 'Elbows out and open' in sitting position.

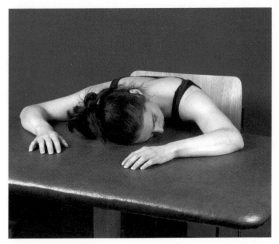

Fig. 13.6 ■ 'Elbows out and open' in forward-lean sitting position.

3. Hands

'Fingers and thumbs long'. Stretch and separate your fingers and thumbs while the heels of both hands remain in contact with the floor, the table or the arm of the chair. While the fingers and thumbs spread (Fig. 13.7), feel the palms getting taut. 'Stop'. As you stop, the fingers recoil and fall on to the supporting surface where they lie with the hand gently open, fingertips touching the surface underneath (Fig. 13.8). Notice how the hand feels; notice also, without disturbing your fingers, the texture of the surface under your fingertips. Spend a moment or two taking in these sensations.

Extra time should be spent on the hand because of its disproportionately large sensory area in the brain.

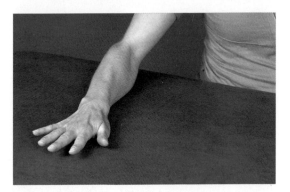

Fig. 13.7 ■ 'Fingers and thumbs long'.

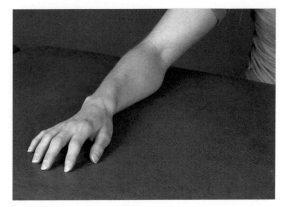

Fig. 13.8 ■ Fingers recoiling.

4. Hips

'Turn your hips outwards'. If you are lying, this means rolling your thighs outwards (Fig. 13.9). If you are sitting, it means swinging your knees apart. 'Stop'. Let your legs settle comfortably, noting how they feel in this position.

5. Knees

'Move your knees until they are comfortable'. This simply means adjusting their position in whatever way enhances their comfort. 'Stop' and register that sense of ease.

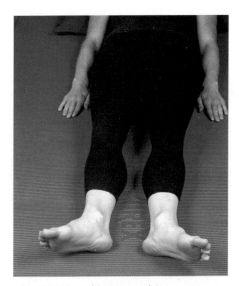

Fig. 13.9 ■ 'Turn your hips outwards'.

6. Feet and Ankles

'Push your feet away from your face'. If you are lying, point your feet and toes down (Fig. 13.10), being careful not to induce cramp. If you are sitting with your feet on the floor, keep your toes in contact with it and raise your heels (Fig. 13.11). You are working the calf muscles and reciprocally relaxing the muscles around the shin. 'Stop'. As you stop, your calf muscles stop working too. (If you are sitting, your heels drop down.) Take note of the feelings you are now getting from your feet and ankles. Spend a few minutes enjoying the sensation of ease in your legs.

7. Breathing

There are no orders for this item because people have their own breathing rates. I'll describe the action first, and then you can perform it in your own time.

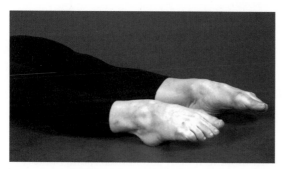

Fig. 13.10 ▪ 'Push your feet away from your face' in supine position.

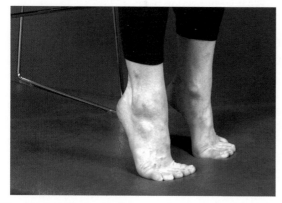

Fig. 13.11 ▪ 'Push your feet away from your face' in sitting position.

I'd like you to think of the soft triangle between the front edge of your ribs and your waist. As you breathe in you can feel it swelling slightly; at the same time you can feel your ribs spreading outwards. As you breathe out, that soft area sinks back and your ribs recoil.

Allow your breathing to take place slowly and comfortably, without putting any effort into it and without attempting to alter its rhythm.

8. Torso

'Push your body into the support'. Press against the support, whether it is underneath you or behind you. 'Stop'. Feel your body slumped into the floor, table or chair. Feel its weight being supported. Notice the points where your body touches the support.

9. Head

'Push your head into the support'. This will be the floor for those lying down, the table for those leaning forwards and the back of the chair for those seated. 'Stop'. As you stop pushing, notice that the support still carries the weight of your head. Feel your head being supported.

10. Jaw

'Drag your jaw downwards'. Let your teeth come apart and your jaw hang down inside your mouth. 'Stop'. Feel the new position. Notice also the contact between your gently touching lips.

Spend a bit longer on this action because the lips, in common with the fingertips, are richly supplied with sensory nerve endings.

11. Tongue

'Press your tongue downwards in your mouth'. Draw it away from the upper palate. 'Stop'. Feel your tongue lying loosely behind your teeth. Notice also your throat slackening.

12. Eyes

'Close your eyes' (if they are not already closed). Simply lower your eyelids and gently keep them down. Let your eyes be as still as they can be. Feel the peace of the darkness.

13. Forehead and scalp

'*Think of a smoothing action which begins above your eyebrows, rises up into your hairline, continues over the crown of your head, and down to the back of your neck*'. Savour the effect.

The previous 13 actions may be repeated.

Mind

Mitchell ends with a sequence for the thoughts.

Let your mind focus on a topic you find pleasant. Pick one that flows like a poem or a walk in the country and let it hold your attention as it develops. Continue for a few minutes.

Termination

When you are ready, I'd like you to begin to make a gradual return to normal activity. Give your arms and legs a good stretch. Sit up slowly, giving your body plenty of time to adjust to an active state.

PRACTICE

The Mitchell method of physiological relaxation is a skill which can be learned; the more it is practised, the greater will be the benefit gained from it. It is through practice that the person can cultivate their awareness of the relaxed posture, thus enabling them to reproduce it at will.

The 'three-point pull' is another action that is useful for stretching the joints in the neck and may be practised in public situations without attracting attention. This is a variation of the shoulder action where, in addition to pulling the shoulders down, the head gently reaches upwards. (It should be done without tilting the head backwards.)

PRECAUTIONS

The precautions are similar to those of other muscular relaxation techniques (see Chapter 5).

KEY POINTS

1. The Mitchell method is built around the physiological principle of reciprocal inhibition; that is, when one group of muscles acting on a joint is working, the opposing group is obliged to relax. Thus, for example, to relax a flexor group of muscles, the participant is asked to activate the extensor group.
2. Each session takes the participant through all the major voluntary muscle groups in the body.
3. Practice is essential to obtain maximum benefit.
4. 'Key changes' play an important role in the Mitchell method. These are particular actions in the relaxation technique that the participant finds most effective, such as jaw dropping, finger lengthening or shoulders dropped down. In their effectiveness, they act as a key to the whole body system.
5. Triggers are another important concept. These are stress-provoking events such as traffic lights, bells and alarms. Mitchell urges the participant to adopt stress-diffusing tactics in advance.

Reflection

Describe the key aspects of the Mitchell method.
How did you feel when you practiced the different exercises?
How did your body and mind respond to the relaxation technique?
Did you need to make any adjustments?
What did you learn?
What is your action plan?

CASE STUDY LEARNING OPPORTUNITIES

The key points and reflection provide the background and knowledge required in relation to the case study to help deepen understanding of how the Mitchell method can help improve the person's experience of relaxation.

CASE STUDY

Postpartum Depression: Mitchell Method Outcomes for Jane

Jane was referred to the physiotherapy department after the delivery of her baby girl. She was complaining of being restless and had had some seizures since labour. During Jane's prenatal check-up at 30 weeks of gestation, she was found to have high blood pressure and swelling of her hands and ankles. The blood pressures was recorded and monitored and the consultant gynaecologist prescribed 5 mg of nifedipine to be taken on a daily basis. Jane's blood pressure was normal during delivery, which was a vaginal birth with no complications. However, after the birth Jane experienced a convulsion of 8 minutes duration of which she was fully conscious but disorientated in place and time. Her blood pressure was high, and therefore Jane was hospitalized and given further medication. Jane's blood pressure was monitored regularly after discharge and found to be normal, so 6 days later Jane stopped all medication with the consultant's advice. Two days after stopping medication, Jane experienced further convulsions with resultant high blood pressure. Jane was given further medication for her high blood pressure and anticonvulsants to manage these symptoms. She was also referred for a magnetic resonance imaging scan and an electroencephalogram, both of which were normal. Because of Jane's high anxiety levels and depression she was referred for relaxation as part of her treatment plan.

The physiotherapist chose the Mitchell method as the preferred relaxation technique for Jane because it is an effective way to manage postpartum stress, depression and anxiety as well as postpartum eclampsia. After a number of sessions and regular practice at home, Jane was able to be slowly weaned off her medication and had no further convulsions. It was thought that Jane's convulsions were triggered by stress and altered posture after pregnancy, which can induce mental stress and pain. The posture correction exercises taught in the Mitchell method helped to reduce these symptoms and had an overall positive outcome for Jane.

ACTIVITY

For the case study:

1. List the key indicators for the Mitchell method.
2. Consider why this approach was taken.
3. Write down the impact the Mitchell method is having from a psychological perspective.
4. Write down the impact the Mitchell method is having from a physical perspective.
5. Write down the impact the Mitchell method is having from an emotional perspective.
6. Consider the outcomes on quality of life and overall well-being.

Chapter 14 will focus on stretching techniques for relaxation to gain a deeper understanding of the mechanism involved in stretching to induce relaxation of the muscle groups.

REFERENCES

Amirova, A., Cropley, M., & Theadom, A. (2017). The effectiveness of the Mitchell Method relaxation technique for the treatment of fibromyalgia symptoms: A three-arm randomised control trial. *International Journal of Stress Management, 24*(1), 86–106.

Bell, J. A., & Saltikov, J. B. (2000). Mitchell's relaxation technique: Is it effective? *Physiotherapy, 86*(9), 473–478.

Hough, A. (2001). *Physiotherapy in respiratory care: An evidence-based approach to respiratory and cardiac management* (3rd ed.). Cheltenham, UK: Nelson Thornes.

Jackson, T. (1991). An evaluation of the Mitchell method of simple physiological relaxation for women with rheumatoid arthritis. *British Journal of Occupational Therapy, 54*, 105–107.

Mantle, J., Haslam, J., & Polden, M. (2004). *Physiotherapy in obstetrics and gynaecology* (2nd ed.). Oxford, UK: Butterworth-Heinemann.

Mitchell, L. (1990). *Simple relaxation: The Mitchell method for easing tension* (2nd ed.). London: John Murray.

Paras, J. (2013). Effect of Mitchell relaxation technique and general mobility exercises on post partum eclampsia, stress and stress induced convulsions – A case study. *IOSR Journal of Dental and Medical Sciences, 10*(2), 23–27.

Salt, V. L., & Kerr, K. M. (1997). Mitchell's simple physiological relaxation and Jacobson's progressive relaxation techniques: A comparison. *Physiotherapy, 83*(4), 200–207.

Walter, J., & Shepherd, W. (2001). Anxiety disorders: A nation-wide survey of treatment approaches used by physiotherapists. *Physiotherapy, 87*(10), 536–548.

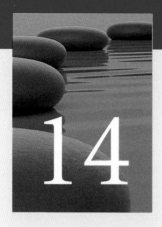

14

STRETCHING

DR CAROLINE BELCHAMBER

CHAPTER CONTENTS

LEARNING OBJECTIVES

The aim of this chapter is to provide knowledge of stretching as a relaxation technique.

By the end of this chapter you will be able to:

1. Understand the importance of stretching to maintain flexibility and joint mobility.

2. Appreciate the evidence that underpins stretching.

3. Understand the theory of stretching processes and mechanisms.

4. Recognize the process of stretching and its link with physiological principles.

5. Identify different stretches for activities of daily living.

6. Discern the effects of stretching.

This chapter will conclude with key points and time for reflection, providing learning opportunities through a case study.

INTRODUCTION TO STRETCHING

Flexibility is one of the properties of muscle tissue which mild stretching helps maintain. Gentle stretchings also help to promote the mobility of the joints and stimulate the flow of synovial fluid. This fluid lubricates the joint and creates a smooth action.

In the case of the spinal joints, stretchings help the discs to recover after activity which changes their shape. The intervertebral discs are soft structures whose shape is altered when the spine is moved. Bending in any direction transforms the discs into wedge-shaped bodies with their fluid content squeezed towards the thick end of the wedge. When a body position such as leaning over a desk, for example, is held for long periods and under load, even the load of the body's own weight, this effect becomes more pronounced (McGill 2007, Neumann 2010, Ryan et al 2012, Twomey 1993). This is known as 'creep' and is defined as the progressive deformation of a structure under constant load by forces which are not large enough to cause permanent damage (Kazarian 1975, Neumann 2010, Ryan et al 2012).

The condition rights itself as the body resumes its normal position, but it takes time. Stretchings in the opposite direction can aid the recovery and may help to reduce the risk of injury, since the spine is vulnerable during the interval.

For this reason, motorists who have driven long distances, creating conditions in which creep occurs, should avoid lifting heavy loads immediately afterwards and should perform stretchings, not only at the end of the journey but at regular intervals throughout its course (Twomey & Taylor 1987). Stretchings will not guarantee protection from injury but they may make it less likely to occur. (See the sections on Back Arching and Crouching/Squatting.)

Many jobs and everyday activities require postures which put strain on body structures and in particular increase mechanical stress in the low back through repetitive bending (Min-Hyeok et al 2013). Stretches help to relieve this strain. The stretch exercise is designed to carry the body or body part in the opposite direction from the posture determined by the work; for example, a seated worker could stand and stretch upwards, whereas a standing operator might arch himself backwards or crouch down on his haunches. Activities which involve precision movements with flexed arms and fingers would call for wide arm stretches.

Stretching is something we do unconsciously after being in one position for a long time. The body seems to ask for it. We stretch after sleeping, after working at a desk, after bending down to weed a flower bed. All three trigger the need or the desire to stretch the body. Subjectively, stretches result in a feeling of comfort, pleasure and relief.

INTRODUCTION TO EVIDENCE

It has long been held that stretching a muscle before use confers benefit; conventional wisdom has suggested it provides protection against muscle soreness, but this claim has often been challenged. Herbert and Gabriel (2002) in their systematic review, found no evidence to support the claim. These same researchers drew similar conclusions in a subsequent systematic review (Herbert & de Noronha 2007), adding, however, that stretching may have other advantages such as reducing injury and enhancing performance. The latter benefits suggest that stretching should be an established part of a warm-up session. In addition, relaxation training can take the form of stretch–release. This approach was adopted in a study to explore stress and relaxation in Hong Kong hospitals. Sixty-five nurse managers were randomly assigned to three groups: stretch–release, cognitive and test control. Mental health status was assessed using the Chinese versions of the State-Trait Anxiety Inventory and the General Hospital Questionnaire at three time points: pretreatment, after four sessions and at 1-month follow-up. In the results, both intervention groups were shown to derive benefit but no statistical analysis was reported (Yung et al 2004).

The muscle-tendon unit in the human skeleton exhibits properties of viscoelasticity and shows time-dependent properties when held at a constant force or torque (creep) and length (stress relaxation). The decrease in passive torque (stress relaxation) is often examined in research under constant-angle stretching (Magnusson et al 1998), whereas creep is investigated during constant-torque stretching protocols (Ryan 2010). In Ryan et al's studies (2008, 2009) constant-torque stretching was deemed to increase work on the muscle tendon unit, resulting in greater viscoelastic creep, which then translated into greater reduction in stiffness during repetitive stretching. Further research carried out by Ryan et al in 2010 examined the consistency of viscoelastic creep during a 30-second stretch and confirmed the response to be consistent. A 2013 study investigated whether acute viscoelastic responses (stress relaxation and creep) were influenced by differences in maximum range of motion and passive stiffness. The findings showed that viscoelastic responses during four consecutive 30-second stretches were influenced by passive stiffness but were not unaffected by differences in maximum range of motion. Thus people with stiff joints may exhibit less creep as they exhibit greater elastic resistance to stretch across the repeated stretches. These differences in creep response in people with high and low levels of passive stiffness may result from differences in tissue compliance or tissue quality (Sobolewski et al 2013). Passive stiffness increases with age (Ochala et al 2004), and it is therefore possible that acute viscoelastic stretch responses are altered (Sobolewski et al 2013). Understanding the effect of stretching and the theories that lies behind this relaxation technique is therefore important.

THEORIES OF STRETCHING

A number of theories have been proposed to explain increases in the extensibility of muscles after intermittent stretching. The majority of these theories describe the mechanical increase in length of the muscle being stretched (Weppler & Magnusson 2010), indicating that stretching is essentially a physical action. The process of stretching therefore links in with physiological principles in that the stretched group is responding in a reciprocal way to the action of the prime mover. Mechanical theories for increasing muscle extensibility include the following:

Viscoelastic deformation – Skeletal muscles are seen as viscous in their behaviour when they are stretched to a significant magnitude, duration or frequency (Magnusson 1998). They are also seen to demonstrate elastic properties as they resume their original length once a tensile force has been removed (Weppler & Magnusson 2010).

Viscoelastic stress relaxation – Occurs when there is a decline in resistance to a muscle which is being held in a stretched position for a time (De Deyne 2001, Enoka 2002).

Creep – Occurs in response to a constant stretching force, which causes mechanical length of the muscle to gradually increase (Enoka 2002, Taylor et al 1990).

Plastic deformation – An increase in muscle extensibility after stretching is due to plastic (Chan et al 2001, Feland et al 2001) or permanent (Draper et al 2004) deformation of the connective tissue (Taylor 1995).

Increased sarcomeres in series – Muscles adapt to a new functional length by changing the number and length of sarcomeres in series, so that it can optimize force production at the new functional length (Williams & Goldspink 1978). Short-term (3 to 8 weeks) stretching regimens can increase sarcomeres in series with a concurrent increase in length of the muscles being stretched (Folpp et al 2006, Gajdosik 2001).

Neuromuscular relaxation – Slowly applied static stretch associated with proprioceptive neuromuscular facilitation stimulates the neuromuscular reflexes that induce relaxation of the muscles undergoing the stretch (Nelson & Bandy 2004, Winters et al 2004). It is thought that this repeated stretch over time enhances the muscles' ability to relax and therefore increases its extensibility (Weppler & Magnusson 2010). However, a sensory theory has now been proposed suggesting that increases in muscle extensibility are due to a modification of sensation (Weppler & Magnusson 2010).

Charles Carlson, a psychologist at the University of Kentucky, looked at the effects of stretching and suggested mechanisms by which it might help to promote relaxation (Carlson et al 1990):

1. It has been found that a stronger contrast can be obtained between stretching and releasing than between tensing and releasing because more length-sensitive receptors in the muscle are activated during stretching than during tensing (Anderson 1983). This more pronounced contrast effect might make it easier for individuals to release body tensions.
2. Stretch-based exercises have been found to lower the excitability of the motor neuron pool (Scholz & Campbell 1980), a finding which suggests a resulting decrease in levels of muscle tension, pain and ischaemia.

Carlson and colleagues devised a procedure consisting of muscle stretchings on the lines of progressive relaxation training; that is to say, the tensing routines in the abbreviated version of Bernstein et al's (2000) protocol are replaced by stretch-based actions. Each stretch lasts 10 seconds and is followed by a relaxation period of 60 seconds (Carlson et al 1990). The purpose is to induce an overall sense of relaxation.

Stretchings presented here consist of a range of large body movements and are similar to those in Carlson's schedule. Each stretch is carried out slowly, held for 5 to 10 seconds, then released quickly. An interval of approximately 30 seconds can be allowed between each stretch (Heptinstall 1995). Participants are asked to notice the feelings in the relevant body part and to compare the sensations during and after the action.

INTRODUCTORY TALK TO PARTICIPANTS

The relaxation technique you are about to learn consists of a series of stretches. It is believed that stretching a muscle helps relax it and there is evidence to support this idea. The exercises are arranged so that each stretch lasts about 5 seconds after which there is a rest period of 30 seconds. Please don't overdo the actions – they should be comfortable, even pleasant. Let the stretch build up slowly and take note of the sensations that accompany it. Then, when you release it, register the feelings of relaxation and notice how they contrast with the feelings of the stretch. Settle into a comfortable position before starting the procedure.

PROCEDURE

The exercises are arranged according to their starting positions.

Lying

The floor or ground provides the best surface, softened by a mat or a carpet. Grass or firm sand also give the degree of hardness required. A bed is too soft.

Body Rotations (Fig. 14.1)

Lie flat on your back. Bend both knees and place the feet flat on the ground. Now roll your bent knees to one side; roll them as far as they will easily go. At the same time, carry both your arms and your head to the other side. You are now twisting your body and stretching one set of oblique trunk muscles.

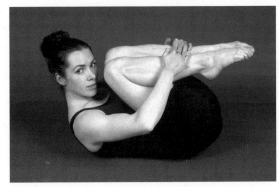

Fig. 14.2 ■ Curling into a ball.

Make it a comfortable stretch. Hold the position for a few seconds. Then bring your knees back to midline, resting your feet on the ground and your arms by your sides. Repeat the exercise in the other direction.

Curling into a Ball (Fig. 14.2)

Lie flat on your back. Draw your knees up. Gather them in your hands and gently pull them towards your face. Still holding your knees, release the pull. Repeat the pull a few times.

Here the soft structures on the posterior aspect of the spine are being stretched. Some lower back conditions respond favourably to this exercise and the previous one, Body Rotations.

Hip Joint Stretches (Fig. 14.3)

Sit on the ground (cushion optional) and draw your legs into a bent position with your knees pointing

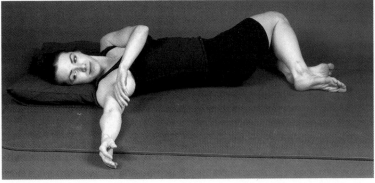

Fig. 14.1 ■ Body rotations.

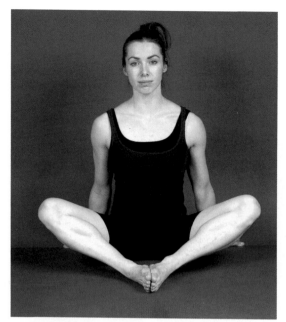

Fig. 14.3 ■ Hip joint stretches.

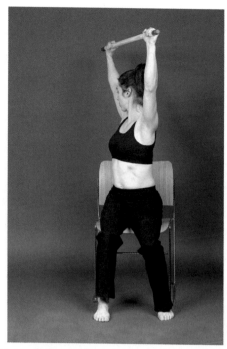

Fig. 14.4 ■ Body turning.

sideways. Have the soles of your feet facing each other and in contact. Place your hands around your ankles and rest your elbows on your thighs. Apply pressure to your thighs, gently and slowly. You should feel a comfortable stretching in the hip area. However, the range of movement in hip joints varies greatly, so do not compare yourself with other people. Perform the exercise just to the point where you feel it is giving you a comfortable stretching sensation and no further. Then take a rest. Reapply the pressure.

Sitting

An upright chair or stool is used for this group of stretchings. For the first item, a long stick such as a broom handle is needed, in an exercise which stretches the trunk and shoulder muscles. Other exercises in this group stretch the shoulder area in different ways.

Body Turning (Fig. 14.4)

Sit with your feet flat on the ground. Grasp the broom handle with your hands 90 cm (3 feet) apart and raise your arms so that the stick just clears your head (your elbows are bent). Turn the upper part of your body to the right. This moves the stick through

about 90 degrees. Just go as far as you need to in order to get a comfortable stretch. Do not overstretch or bounce. Then return to the starting position. Repeat in the other direction.

Shoulder Circling (Figs 14.5 and 14.6)

Bend your elbows and place your fingertips on your shoulders. With your elbows, slowly draw circles in the air. After two or three circles, break off and repeat in the opposite direction.

Arms Stretching Above Head (Fig. 14.7)

Bend your elbows and lift your arms above your head. Feel yourself pushing the air above you with your open hands. When your elbows are straight, spread your arms sideways and lower them to your sides. Let them rest limply. Repeat once or twice.

Head Pressing Backwards (Fig. 14.8)

Clasp your hands behind your head and, resting your head in them, arch backwards. Take care not to lean back too far if you are in a lightweight chair. Return your body to a vertical position.

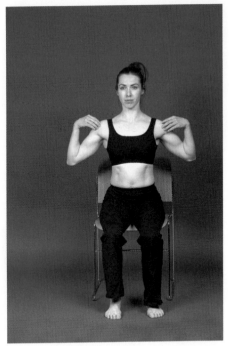

Fig. 14.5 ■ Shoulder circling: 1.

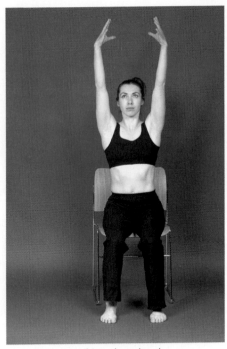

Fig. 14.7 ■ Arms stretching above head.

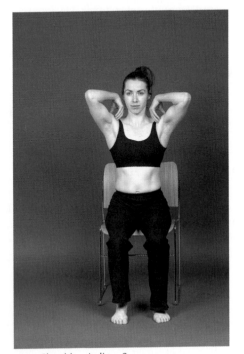

Fig. 14.6 ■ Shoulder circling: 2.

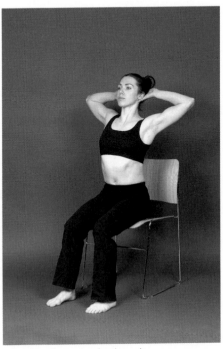

Fig. 14.8 ■ Head pressing backwards.

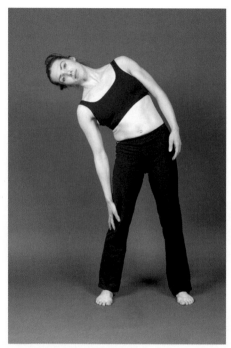

Fig. 14.9 ■ Trunk bending sideways.

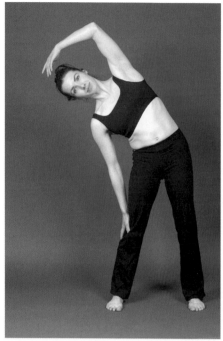

Fig. 14.10 ■ Arm and trunk bending sideways.

Standing

Trunk Bending Sideways (Fig. 14.9)

Stand with your feet apart and your hands by your sides. Bend your body sideways, giving it a good stretch. Return to the upright position and repeat on the other side.

Arm and Trunk Bending Sideways (Fig. 14.10)

This exercise resembles the previous one except that the sideways bend is performed with one hand over your head. Maintain an easy stretch in each direction.

Arms Stretching Back (Fig. 14.11)

Clasp both hands behind your back and straighten your elbows, drawing your shoulders back at the same time. Feel a stretch in the shoulder area, but do not overdo it. Then relax your arms and repeat the exercise.

Arms Reaching Upwards (Fig. 14.12)

Stand with your feet slightly apart. Clasp your hands, then raise your arms above your head, turning the palms towards the ceiling as you

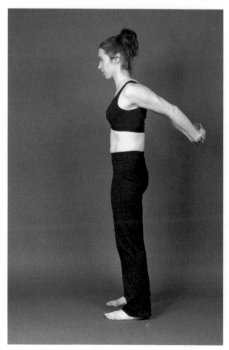

Fig. 14.11 ■ Arms stretching back.

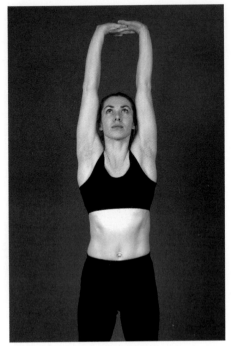

Fig. 14.12 ■ Arms reaching upwards.

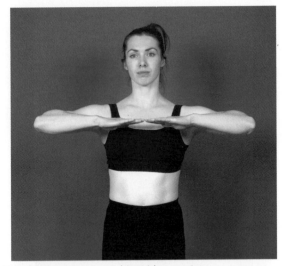

Fig. 14.13 ■ Arms stretching sideways: 1.

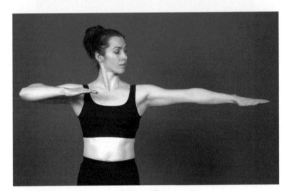

Fig. 14.14 ■ Arms stretching sideways: 2.

straighten your elbows. Hold them there a few seconds, then lower them.

Arms Stretching Sideways (Figs 14.13 and 14.14)

Stand with your feet apart, and your arms bent at the elbow and raised to shoulder level. Gently swing one arm sideways and as you do so, allow your elbow to straighten. Return your arm to the bent position. Repeat with the other arm.

The previous five exercises are particularly useful for people who are leaning over a desk or a workbench. The last two can also be performed in a sitting position.

Trunk Twisting (Fig. 14.15)

Stand with your hands on your hips. Slightly bend your knees and twist the upper part of your body to the left. Feel a comfortable stretch, then return to the starting position. Repeat on the other side.

Back Arching (Fig. 14.16)

Place the palms of your hands over the bones that run sideways from your lumbar spine. Using that

point as a fulcrum, bend over backwards. Go as far as is comfortable. No further! Then return to an upright position. Repeat. If the exercise makes you feel dizzy, keep your head and eyes looking forwards as you perform it.

Benefit can be gained from this exercise when driving long distances, brushing paths, vacuuming carpets or leaning over a table to sort papers.

Crouching/Squatting (Fig. 14.17)

Get into a crouching or squatting position. Hold the position for 10 to 20 seconds. If you can, lay your feet flat on the ground; otherwise, perch on your toes. That is all that most people can do.

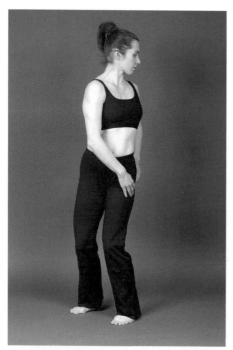

Fig. 14.15 ■ Trunk twisting

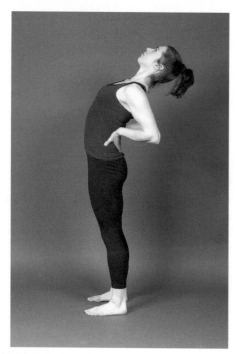

Fig. 14.16 ■ Back arching.

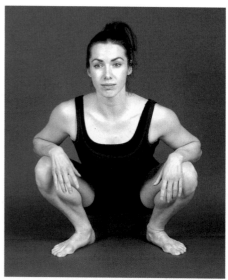

Fig. 14.17 ■ Crouching.

This is another exercise which may be found to ease the lumbar spine during long-distance drives. Its somewhat bizarre appearance will escape attention if the driver pretends to be examining the tyres of his vehicle. The squat position seems to be beneficial for back health in general because it has been found that in populations where it is habitually adopted, lumbar disc degeneration is rare (Fahrni & Trueman 1965). For people with painful knees, however, it may not be advisable.

Calf Stretching (Fig. 14.18)

Take your shoes off and stand facing a wall with your toes about 30 cm (12 inches) away from it. Have your feet parallel and 10 cm (4 inches) apart. Raise your arms and lean your forearms vertically on the wall. Rest your body weight on your forearms. With your heels on the ground and your knees straight, let your hips sink forwards.

You will feel a stretching in the calf muscles. Let it be a comfortable stretch, not a punishment. If you do not feel any stretching, take your feet further back until you do. As you stretch the calf muscles, hold the position for 5 seconds, then release it. Repeat a few times.

Inner Thigh Stretching (Adductor Stretching) (Fig. 14.19)

Stand with your feet about 50 cm (20 inches) apart, hands on your hips. Swing your weight over the left

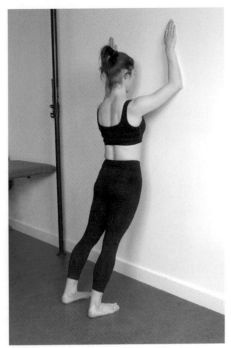

Fig. 14.18 ■ Calf stretching.

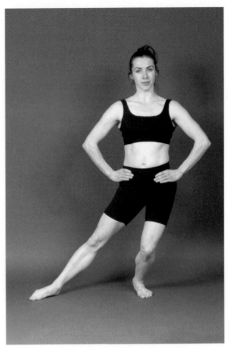

Fig. 14.19 ■ Inner thigh stretching.

knee, bending it as you do so. This puts a stretch on the inside of the right thigh. Hold the position for about 5 seconds, then release the stretch. Repeat. Then swing your weight over the other leg.

PRECAUTIONS

1. A participant may be undergoing medical treatment which contraindicates a particular stretching exercise. Priority should always be given to any medical instructions the participant has received.
2. The stretching must be done slowly to avoid causing microscopic tearing of the connective tissue (Anderson 1983). It should also be done without straining. At no time should any exercise feel uncomfortable. If it does, it should be stopped. Reasons for possible discomfort are that the participant:
   a. is overdoing it.
   b. has an innate restriction of joint movement.
   c. has an incipient disorder.
3. The number of repetitions carried out is a matter for the participants to decide. Only they know if they are still benefiting from the exercise.

4. When working with a group of people there is often a temptation to do better than, or at least as well as, the others. Minor injuries can occur when participants feel challenged by neighbours (perhaps older than they) who outshine them. People often feel they have a duty to prove themselves. This of course is mistaken thinking. The only 'duty' imposed on the person in this context is to make his or her body feel as comfortable as possible.

KEY POINTS

1. Gentle stretchings can make the body feel more comfortable. The increased comfort can promote relaxation.
2. A full programme of body stretches should include all the major groups of voluntary muscles.
3. Reductions in muscle tension have been noted in some studies after a course of stretchings.
4. It is suggested that stretch-based procedures be viewed as effective alternatives to tense–release.

Reflection

Describe how you stretch.

What do you do to stretch?

Why do you need to stretch?

How do you feel after stretching?

What techniques or methods have you used for stretching?

What is your future action plan?

CASE STUDY LEARNING OPPORTUNITY

The key points and reflection provide the background and knowledge required in relation to the case study to help deepen understanding of how stretching techniques can help improve physical and mental well-being.

CASE STUDY

Low Back Pain: *Stretching Outcomes for Duncan*

Duncan, a 57-year-old long-distance lorry driver with a history of low back pain (LBP), was referred for treatment. On assessment it was ascertained that Duncan's LBP had been ongoing for 11 months and during that time he had not received any specific treatment. He scored an 8 on the visual analogue scale (VAS) for pain. Further clinical examination, assessing stresses in flexion and rotation, confirmed a diagnosis of lumbar flexion-rotation syndrome. Trunk range of movement was measured with the following results: lumbar flexion angle of 50 degrees; extension angle 32 degrees; right rotation angle 50 degrees; left rotation angle 52 degrees. As well as the reduced range of movement. Duncan was anxious about his job because the pain meant he couldn't sit for long periods, which his job involved. It was also affecting his time management because he had to make frequent stops to relieve his LBP. This increased his stress levels and consequently the tension in his back, which was also affecting his pain levels.

Duncan's goals were to increase his range of movement, reduce his LBP and relieve his anxiety so that he could continue in his current job and improve his overall well-being. Treatment included two thoracic stretching exercises. The first stretching exercise involved back arching in standing followed by repeating this stretch on his knees and elbows, adding in neck flexion, and then on his hands and knees, ensuring lumbar movement

was limited when carrying out the stretches. Duncan was asked to 'hunch' his back on inspiration and 'arch' his back on full expiration. The thoracic region was stretched, making sure that Duncan did not overextend his neck. Duncan was asked to perform the two thoracic stretching exercises for a month, completing 10 sets of 10 repetitions a day.

After a month of thoracic stretching exercises Duncan's trunk range of movement had increased by 12% at lumbar flexion and extension, with an increase of 8% for right and left rotation. His VAS score for LBP had decreased to 5 and he was able to sit for longer periods, which relieved his anxiety because he was able to complete his journeys within the correct time frame.

ACTIVITY

For the case study:

1. List the stretching technique that is helping with the condition.
2. Write down the impact stretching is having from a physical perspective.
3. Write down the impact stretching is having from a psychological perspective.
4. Write down the impact stretching is having from an emotional perspective.
5. Consider the effects of the stretching techniques on overall quality of life.

Chapter 15 will focus on physical activity, helping to put this learning into practice.

REFERENCES

Anderson, B. (1983). Stretching and sports. In O. Appenzeller, & R. Atkinson (Eds.), *Sports medicine* (2nd ed.). Baltimore: Urban and Schwarzenberg.

Bernstein, D. A., Borkovec, T. D., & Hazlett-Stevens, H. (2000). *new directions in progressive relaxation training: A guide book for helping professionals.* Westport, CT: Praeger.

Carlson, C. R., Collins, F. L., Nitz, A. J., Sturgis, E. T., & Rogers, J. L. (1990). Muscle stretching as an alternative relaxation training procedure. *Journal of Behavior Therapy and Experimental Psychiatry, 21*(1), 29–38.

Chan, S. P., Hong, Y., & Robinson, P. D. (2001). Flexibility and passive resistance of the hamstrings of young adults using two different static stretching protocols. *Scandinavian Journal of Medicine & Science in Sports, 11*, 81–86.

De Deyne, P. G. (2001). Application of passive stretch and its implications for muscle fibers. *Physical Therapy, 81*, 819–827.

Draper, D. O., Castro, J. L., Feland, B., Schulthies, S., & Eggett, D. (2004). Shortwave diathermy and prolonged stretching increase hamstring flexibility more than prolonged stretching alone. *Journal of Orthopaedic & Sports Physical Therapy, 34*, 13–20.

Enoka, R. M. (2002). *Neuromechanics of human movement* (3rd ed.). Champaign. IL: Human Kinetics Publishers.

Fahrni, W. H., Trueman, G. E. (1965). Comparative radiological study of the spines of a primitive population with North Americans and Northern Europeans. *J. Bone. Joint. Surg., 47B*, 552–555.

Feland, J. B., Myrer, J. W., Schulthies, S. S., Fellingham, G. W., & Measom, G. W. (2001). The effect of duration of stretching of the hamstring muscle group for increasing range of motion in people aged 65 years or older. *Physical Therapy, 81*, 1107–1110.

Folpp, H., Deall, S., Harvey, L. A., & Gwinn, T. (2006). Can apparent increases in muscle extensibility with regular stretch be explained by changes in tolerance to stretch? *Australian Journal of Physiotherapy, 52*, 45–50.

Gajdosik, R. L. (2001). Passive extensibility of skeletal muscle: Review of the literature with clinical implications. *Clinical Biomechanics, 16*, 87–101.

Heptinstall, S. T. (1995). Relaxation training. In T. Everett, M. Dennis, & E. Ricketts (Eds.), *Physiotherapy in mental health* (pp. 188–208). Oxford, UK: Butterworth-Heinemann.

Herbert, R. D., & Gabriel, M. (2002). Effects of stretching before and after exercising on muscle soreness and risk of injury: Systematic review. *British Medical Journal, 325*, 468–470.

Herbert, R. D., & de Noronha, M. (2007). Stretching to prevent or reduce muscle soreness after exercise. *Cochrane Database of Systematic Reviews, 4*, CD004577.

Kazarian, L. (1975). Creep characteristics of the human spinal column. *Orthopedic Clinics of North America, 6*(1), 3–15.

McGill, S. M. (2007). *Low back disorders: Evidence-based prevention and rehabilitation* (2nd ed.). Champaign, IL: Human Kinetics.

Magnusson, S. P. (1998). Passive properties of human skeletal muscle during stretch manoevers: a review. *Scandinavian Journal of Medicine & Science in Sports, 8*, 65–77.

Magnusson, S. P., Aagard, P., Simonsen, E., & Bojsen-Moller, F. (1998). A biomechanical evaluation of cyclic and static stretch in human skeletal muscle. *International Journal of Sports Medicine, 19*, 310–316.

Min-Hyeok, K., Doh-Heon, J., Duk-Hyun, A., Won-Gyu, Y., & Jae-Seop, O. (2013). Acute effects of hamstring-stretching exercises on the kinematics of the lumbar spine and hip during stoop lifting. *Journal of Back and Musculoskeletal Rehabilitation, 26*, 329–336.

Nelson, R. T., & Bandy, W. D. (2004). Eccentric training and static stretching improve hamstring flexibility of high school males. *Journal of Athletic Training, 39*, 254–258.

Neumann, D. A. (2010). *Kinesiology of the musculoskeletal system: Foundations for rehabilitation* (2nd ed.). St. Louis: Mosby.

Ochala, J., Lambertz, D., Pousson, M., Goubel, F., & Van Hoecke, J. (2004). Changes in mechanical properties of human plantar flexor muscles in ageing. *Experimental Gerontology, 39*, 349–358.

Ryan, E. D., Beck, T. W., Herda, T. J., et al. (2008). The time course of musculotendinous stiffness responses following different durations of passive stretching. *Journal of Orthopaedic & Sports Physical Therapy, 38*, 632–639.

Ryan, E. D., Herda, T. J., Costa, P. B., et al. (2009). Determining the minimum number of passive stretches necessary to alter musculotendinous stiffness. *Journal of Sports Science, 27*, 957–961.

Ryan, E. D., Herda, T. J., Costa, P. B., et al. (2010). Viscoelastic creep in the human skeletal muscle-tendon unit. *European Journal of Applied Physiology, 108*, 207–211.

Ryan, E. D., Herda, T. J., Costa, P. B., Walter, A. A., & Cramer, J. T. (2012). Dynamics of viscoelastic creep during repeated stretches. *Scandinavian Journal of Medicine & Science in Sports, 22*, 179–184.

Twomey, L. T. (1993). Lumbar biomechanics and physical therapy. *Journal of the Organisation of Chartered Physiothearpists in Private Practice, 70*, 14–19.

Scholz, J., & Campbell, S. (1980). Muscle spindles and the regulation of movement. *Physical Therapy, 60*, 1416.

Sobolewski, E. J., Ryan, E. D., Thompson, B. J. (2013). Influence of Maximum range of motion and stiffness on the viscoelastic stretch response. *Muscle and Nerve*, 571–577.

Taylor, D. C., Dalton, J. D., Seaber, A. V., & Garrett, E. E. (1990). Viscoelastic properties of muscle-tendon units: the biomechanical effects of stretching. *American Journal of Sports Medicine, 18*, 300–309.

Taylor, B. F., Waring, C. A., & Brashear, T. A. (1995). The effects of therapeutic application of heat or cold followed by static stretch on hamstring muscle length. *Journal of Orthopaedic & Sports Physical Therapy, 21*, 283–286.

Twomey, L. T., & Taylor, J. R. (1987). *Physical therapy of the low back.* New York: Churchill Livingstone *Journal of the Organisation of Chartered Physiothearpists in Private Practice.*

Weppler, C. H., & Magnusson, S. P. (2010). Increasing muscle extensibility: a matter of increasing length or modifying sensation? *Physical Therapy, 90*(3), 438–449.

Williams, P. E., & Goldspink, G. (1978). Changes in sarcomere length and physiological properties in immobilized muscle. *Journal of Anatomy, 3*, 459–468.

Winters, M. V., Blake, C. G., Trost, J. S., et al. (2004). Passive versus active stretching of hip flexor muscles in subjects with limited hip extension: A randomized clinical trial. *Physical Therapy, 84*, 800–807.

Yung, P., Fung, M. Y., Chan, T. M. F., & Lau, B. W. (2004). Relaxation training methods for nurse managers in Hong Kong: A controlled study. *International Journal of Mental Health Nursing, 13*(4), 255–261.

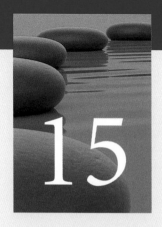

15

PHYSICAL ACTIVITY

DR CAROLINE BELCHAMBER

CHAPTER CONTENTS

LEARNING OBJECTIVES

The aim of this chapter is to provide an understanding of physical activity as a relaxation technique.

By the end of this chapter you will be able to:

1. Understand the importance of physical activity.

2. Appreciate the evidence that underpins physical activity.

3. Understand physical activity processes and mechanisms.

4. Recognize the transtheoretical model.

5. Identify the steps in a typical physical activity consultation session.

6. Discern the effects of physical activity.

This chapter will conclude with key points and time for reflection, providing learning opportunities through a case study.

INTRODUCTION TO PHYSICAL ACTIVITY

Any movement of the body which involves the expenditure of energy constitutes physical activity. It includes routines of daily living, domestic chores, gardening and walking. Exercise is a subset of physical activity and may be practised for health reasons or for leisure where it covers such activities as swimming, jogging, brisk walking, physical workouts and sport. The topic has been included to provide the reader with the evidence in favour of physical activity as a means of promoting mental and physical health. Throughout this chapter, the words 'physical activity' will be used synonymously with 'exercise'.

Physical activity is an effective way of relieving stress, whether the activity is practised on its own or as part of a stress management programme (Mikkelsen et al 2017, Tsatsoulis & Fountoulakis 2006). The effect of exercise on body systems resembles the effect of a stressful event or situation in that the same autonomic, musculoskeletal and endocrine systems are involved. The smooth integrated functioning of these systems, which takes place during exercise, can help resolve the stress-related effects of adverse events or situations. Thus exercise enhances the body's ability to deal with stress.

A lifestyle which incorporates exercise has the potential to promote physical and psychological well-being, limiting the risk of life-threatening disease and common mental health disorders (see also Chapter 30). Initially, research focused on vigorous exercise, such as running (Blair 1995); however, with further research the emphasis has shifted to moderate-intensity physical activity (such as brisk walking) because this has been linked to a reduction in the incidence of coronary heart disease, colon cancer, obesity and diabetes (Department of Health 2004, 2020; O'Donovan et al 2010; Pedersen & Fischer 2007; Warburton et al 2006). Such a programme is not only intuitively appealing, it is now supported by strong evidence.

Physically active lifestyles are beneficial to health and well-being (Khalil et al 2012, WHO 2004). Physical inactivity, on the other hand, is a major public health concern because it is now known that people who lead sedentary lives are at much higher risk of developing life-threatening conditions such as heart disease and cancer. In acknowledging these public health risks, the chief medical officer (CMO) in the UK published a position paper about physical activity titled *At Least Five a Week* which emphasizes the strength of the evidence for the relationship between physical activity and health (Department of Health 2004). The Physical Activity Guidelines (Department of Health 2020) have developed these recommendations further and are summarized in Box 15.1.

Alongside the prevention of life-threatening diseases, regular physical activity provides some protection

---

BOX 15.1
RECOMMENDED PHYSICAL ACTIVITY GUIDELINES FOR ADULTS IN THE UK (DOH, 2020)

Please note that the physical activity guidelines for adults are written for generally healthy adults and therefore should be tailored for individuals based upon their needs and abilities, particularly where there are disabilities and any specific health-related issues. The guidelines recommend the following:

Adults should aim to minimize the amount of time spent being sedentary and, when physically possible, should break up long periods of inactivity with at least light physical activity.

Engage in moderate-intensity aerobic physical activity for at least 150 minutes per week; this physical activity should be spread across the week; for example, engaging in at least 30 minutes on 5 or more days each week. Physical activity can be accumulated across multiple sessions throughout the week. Individuals should aim for sessions of at least 10 minutes of moderate intensity activity at a time.

Vigorous-intensity activity can also provide health benefits for adults, and 75 minutes of vigorous-intensity activity (also spread across the week) provides comparable health benefits to 150 minutes of moderate-intensity activity. In addition, combinations of moderate- and vigorous-intensity activities can provide health benefits, and this represents another way of achieving the recommended target volume of activity.

Undertaking muscle-strengthening activities involving the major muscle groups of the body on two or more days per week is recommended. Time spent carrying out muscle-strengthening activities should be in addition to the primary recommendation of 150 minutes. Stretching and flexibility training may also be beneficial.

Physical activity has an important role in healthy weight management and body composition. Overweight and obese adults achieving the recommended weekly volume of activity (5 × 30–150 minutes/week) will gain multiple health benefits even in the absence of reductions in body weight.

Physical activity aids prevention of mental illness (such as depression and dementia) and improving mental well-being (such as mood, self-perception and sleep). Those who are least active are most at risk of poor health and increasing physical activity (even if it does not meet the public health target of 150 minutes of moderate-intensity activity per week) will have health benefits. Higher volumes of activity (>150 minutes) are associated with even greater health benefits. The risks of ill health from inactivity are very high and outweigh the very low risk of injury from engaging in health-promoting physical activity.

For the older adult a gradual increase of physical activity levels should be achieved over time. This is particularly important for an inactive older adult with low fitness levels, where building up to the 10-minute session of physical activity is recommended. Older adults, at risk of falls should include balance training on 2 or more days per week.

DOH, Department of Health.

from depression. The evidence for this has been made available over the last 30 years from longitudinal studies undertaken with men and women in different countries: in the United States, examples include Paffenbarger et al (1994) and Motl et al (2004); in the Netherlands, van Gool et al (2003) and Bernaards et al (2006); in Germany, Weyerer (1992); in Finland, Lampinen et al (2006); in Australia, Mikkelsen et al (2017); in Taiwan, Chang et al (2017); and in the UK, Khalil et al (2012) and Rebar and Taylor (2017).

The evidence for the psychological benefits of exercise suggests that it is an effective treatment for common mental health problems such as anxiety and depression either as a treatment in its own right or as an adjunct to cognitive–behavioural therapy or medication (Biddle & Mutrie 2008, Donaghy 2007, Mikkelsen et al 2017). The psychological benefits of exercise include distraction from worries, release of frustrations, sense of achievement, a feeling of improved physical appearance, self-confidence, and enjoyment in the company of other individuals in the pleasant surroundings of the exercise activity. Where physical activity has been carried out in a natural environment a greater reduction in the risk of poor mental health has been noted and different types of environment may promote a variety of positive psychological responses (Calogiuri et al 2014, Mitchell 2012). In addition to these benefits, exercise is inexpensive, noninvasive and has few side effects.

INTRODUCTION TO EVIDENCE

There is a growing body of evidence which recognizes that physical activity has a positive effect on mood states, such as stress, anxiety and depression (Anderson & Shivakumar 2013, DeBoer et al 2012, Donaghy 2007, Mikkelsen et al 2017). Psychological outcomes from research suggest that a sense of well-being is derived from regular physical activity, with participants reporting less tension, fatigue, aggression, depression and insomnia (Biddle & Mutrie 2008, Mikkelsen et al 2017).

In a review of four meta-analyses on exercise and anxiety, Biddle and Mutrie (2008) conclude that exercise has a small-to-moderate positive effect on non-clinical levels of anxiety. There is also some evidence to suggest that people with high levels of aerobic fitness

have reduced levels of physiological arousal in reaction to psychological stressors (Biddle & Mutrie 2008), indicating the possibility of a protective factor for those who regularly participate in aerobic exercise. A recent review article of exercise and mental health research from 2007 to 2017 identified positive effects of exercise for anxiety, stress and depression through physiological and biochemical mechanisms. In addition, psychological mechanisms were shown to influence the effects of exercise on mood states. Inflammation was also shown to decrease through a variety of processes, which can contribute to improved health outcomes in individuals with mood disorders (Mikkelsen et al 2017). Therefore regular physical activity decreases depression and stress; it also improves cognitive function in fit older adults and has positive effects on mood, physical self-perceptions and body image (Biddle et al 2000, Mikkelsen et al 2017). Explanations from psychology suggest links between exercise and physical self-perceptions such as body image, physical self-worth and self-esteem (Mutrie & Faulkner 2003). The findings from a survey undertaken by the charity MIND support this explanation, with 50% of the participants stating that exercise boosted their self-esteem (MIND Survey 2001), and Mikkelsen et al's (2017) review article confirms these findings.

It is perhaps easier to accept that exercise (a high-arousal activity) could relieve depression (a low-arousal state) than that it could relieve anxiety, itself a high-arousal state. Nevertheless, exercise has been fairly consistently associated with decreased levels of state anxiety (see Chapter 2). Experimental studies support an anxiety-reducing effect for exercise, with benefits resulting from moderate exercise during activity and from moderate- and high-intensity exercise after activity (Biddle & Mutrie 2008, Mikkelsen et al 2017, Scully et al 1998). The most persuasive results have been found in the field of generalized anxiety, where a marked treatment response often occurs. Martinsen (1990) found that little benefit was gained in the field of panic disorder or agoraphobia. However, this conclusion has subsequently been challenged by the findings of Broocks et al (1998) in their study of 46 outpatients with moderate-to-severe degrees of panic disorder, where symptoms were reduced by a programme of exercise. Although exercise (aerobic) was found to be less effective than medication (clomipramine), its effect after 10 weeks was significant. However, persistent and untreated anxiety can lead to generalized anxiety disorder, which can itself be associated with panic and phobia. These and other forms of anxiety are discussed in Chapter 1). With regard to the effects of exercise in specific anxiety disorders, such as panic, Mikkelsen et al's (2017) review article confirms that panic disorders are improved with physical activity.

Evidence for the benefit of exercise in general has, in recent years, accumulated to the point where guidelines endorse its use as a treatment in its own right or as an adjunctive treatment for mild-to-moderate depression (Department of Health 2020, NICE 2003, SIGN 2009). The evidence associating exercise with relief from symptoms of depression has been gathering strength over the last two decades. This association has been demonstrated in randomized controlled studies looking at the efficacy of exercise in the treatment of adults with mild-to-moderate levels of clinical depression (Blumenthal et al 2007, Mead et al 2008). The consistency of the evidence makes a persuasive argument in the case of mild-to-moderate depression (Biddle & Mutrie 2008, Donaghy 2007, Wegner et al 2014). More recently a randomized controlled trial was carried out by Haller and colleagues (2018), who investigated individualized web-based exercise for the treatment of depression. Results indicated significant clinical improvements in depressive symptoms of people with moderate-to-severe depression. These results compare well with those of psychotherapy and cognitive–behavioural therapy (Fremont & Craighead 1987, Greist et al 1979, Klein et al 1985, Wegner et al 2014). Furthermore, when drug intervention is added to exercise and compared with exercise alone, no difference is shown (Babyak et al 2000, Blumenthal et al 1999). Patients themselves have also reported favourably on exercise, many of them adding that they would choose it as an intervention for clinical depression. The survey by the charity MIND found that 83% of people with mental health problems looked to exercise to lift their mood or reduce their stress, whereas two-thirds of them indicated that it helped to relieve their depressive symptoms (MIND Survey 2001). A commissioned report in the UK also came out strongly in favour of exercise as a first-line treatment for depression. This led to a raising of awareness through the publication of leaflets and posters distributed to general practitioner surgeries in England (Mental Health Foundation, 2019). Non-clinical populations have also been studied, showing that symptoms of depression in this population group can also be reduced by physical activity. The evidence comes from randomized controlled trials as well as cross-sectional and large-scale epidemiological studies (Biddle & Mutrie 2008).

Because exercise has been shown to confer substantial benefit as a treatment for depression, it has been hypothesized that it might also have some protective value in psychologically healthy members of the community. In a review of 11 prospective longitudinal studies, Donaghy (2007) found a positive association between physical activity and the reduced risk of depression. These studies included measures of exercise and depression at two or more time points. Research carried out in the United States, Netherlands and Finland (which includes populations of community dwellers, workers, adults, adolescents and older people) has produced similar results. These show that people who are physically active and exercise regularly are less likely to be diagnosed with depression in the period between baseline and follow-up.

One of the earliest prospective studies (Farmer et al 1988) produced findings which suggest that women who had engaged in little or no recreational activity were twice as likely to develop depression as women who had engaged in moderate or high levels of activity. The Harvard Alumni (Paffenbarger et al 1994), one of the largest longitudinal studies of its kind, confirms the protective effects of physical activity and the lowered risk of developing depression for men. Thus exercise has been found to be a protective factor for both men and women. Evidence for the protective action of exercise has also been demonstrated in studies of older people. Adults older than 65 who took part in a daily walking programme were followed for 3 years, providing evidence that exercise in this form reduced their risk of depression (Mobily et al 1996). Another US study with middle-aged and older adults confirmed these findings (Strawbridge et al 2002). Protective factors have also been found in studies undertaken in Europe: van Gool and colleagues in the Netherlands (2003) found that study participants who became depressed between baseline and follow-up had changed from an active to a sedentary lifestyle, and research undertaken in Finland (Lampinen et al 2006) found that mental well-being in later life is associated with mobility and physical activity. This research raises the question of whether these benefits are only available to people with a long-standing active lifestyle. Motl et al (2005) looked at vulnerability to depression when physical activity was introduced to formerly sedentary, older adults. Study participants were randomly assigned to 6-month conditions of either walking or low-intensity resistance and/or flexibility training. Findings showed that depressive symptom scores decreased after the 6-month intervention; this was followed by a sustained reduction over 1 to 5 years. The effect for both types of physical activity was found to be similar (Motl et al 2005). The authors concluded that there may be gains for previously sedentary populations. A study in the Netherlands looking at how much exercise was needed to offer protection found that those with sedentary jobs only needed to engage in strenuous physical activity once or twice a week to reduce their risk of depression and emotional exhaustion (Bernaards et al 2006). Interestingly, higher levels of activity, three or more times a week, did not offer this protection.

Adolescents also benefit from the protective effects of physical activity (Motl et al 2004). Findings indicate that a decrease in the frequency of leisure-time physical activity is related to an increase in depressive symptoms. Studies have been undertaken in a variety of community settings and workplaces and provide support for the transferability of findings across different populations. Some studies have followed up formerly clinically depressed populations to see if maintaining physical activity offers protection from recurring incidents. Harris et al (2006) investigated a clinical sample of 424 previously depressed patients (with a 1-, 4- and 10-year follow-up). They found that more physical activity was associated with less concurrent depression; physical activity appeared to be countering the effects of negative life events. However, not all studies concur with these results. Cooper-Patrick et al (1997) carried out a prospective study on 973 middle-aged physicians to explore the preventive capacity of exercise, but results did not indicate that exercise reduced the risk of developing depression. However, more recent research indicates that being physically active reduces depression and anxiety (Cooney et al 2013) as regular exercise increases resilience to both physical and emotional

stress, enabling people to adapt to difficult situations (Otto & Smits 2011).

Thus there is strong evidence that regular physical activity at the recommended level offers protection from life-threatening physical diseases and prolongs life expectancy (Department of Health 2004). It is therefore in everyone's interest to promote these key targets and messages. The evidence for protection against depression is less strong but there exist a number of randomized controlled trials that suggest that exercise is a useful intervention to reduce symptoms of depression. Exercise may also offer some protection against anxiety. Getting started and maintaining programmes of physical activity depend on motivational factors and social support; it is therefore recommended that people seek advice from a relevant health care professional or exercise consultant.

THEORIES BEHIND PHYSICAL ACTIVITY

As a therapy, physical activity is not underpinned by any particular theory. However, rather than being conceptualized as a theoretical approach, Mutrie and Faulkner (2003) suggest it should be viewed as a process through which therapeutic goals can be reached.

Many explanations, both physiological and psychological, are put forward in an attempt to explain the mechanism underlying the association between physical activity and mental wellbeing. For example, the increased blood flow to the brain stimulates the release of naturally occurring mood-enhancing chemicals which are similar to morphine and have been linked to the 'runner's high'. Their presence in blood samples of people following a bout of exercise has been demonstrated (Mutrie & Faulkner 2003). Studies on animals have also shown that chemicals associated with mood elevation are released into the bloodstream during exercise (Chaouloff 1997). Antidepressant medication such as Prozac works by boosting these chemicals. The finding may also partly explain why exercise offers protection against depression and is effective as a treatment intervention. A further benefit is an increase in levels of the brain-derived neurotrophic factor (BDNF). This is a substance associated with the enhancement of mood and the longer survival of brain cells and may be linked to improved cognitive function (Clow & Edmunds 2014, Donaghy 2007, Otto & Smits 2011). It has also been suggested that increased levels of phenylethylamine, a known stimulant in the brain produced during exercise, is linked to the release of dopamine and endorphins, which act as natural antidepressants (Clow & Edmunds 2014, Donaghy 2007).

This creates a persuasive picture but leaves many questions unanswered. For example, does the sense of physical well-being transfer to the psychological sphere, making the thoughts more positive? Does the active coping strategy engender a feeling of mastery? Mutrie and Faulkner (2003) refer to the association of regular exercise with raised self-esteem, but it is not known whether this is brought about by virtue of weight reduction, improved physical health or sense of achievement.

Then again, is there some connection with people's expectations? Do people feel positive mood changes after a bout of exercise because they expect to? Does distraction play a part?

La Forge (1995) has reviewed all the possible mechanisms. He sees them as integrated rather than separate. His model shows the mechanisms as overlapping, sharing the same neural pathways. In this light, an approach which addresses them as linked processes would seem more appropriate than one which studies them in isolation.

Transtheoretical Model

Many people find difficulty in starting an exercise programme. They may be vague about the choice of activity or lack the confidence to begin. Motivation to get started in an exercise programme, maintaining exercise over time and overcoming barriers to exercise have been extensively studied (Biddle & Mutrie 2008). This has led to the development of different theoretical models that provide plausible explanations for the choices people make. To provide the reader with some knowledge of the factors that influence decision making with regard to exercise participation, we have selected the transtheoretical model which also provides a framework for intervention strategies.

The transtheoretical model (DiClemente et al 1985) contains three key ideas. First, behaviour change in the individual is seen as a dynamic process that occurs in the following *stages*: 'precontemplation' (the individual is not considering exercising), 'contemplation' (the individual is considering exercise and is seeking information from the doctor, physiotherapist or others), 'preparation' (the individual makes efforts to start exercising by joining a class or planning a personal routine of physical activity), 'action' (the individual attends the exercise class/starts the programme of physical activity) and 'maintenance' (the individual maintains attendance at the class or keeps up the programme of physical activity). These stages represent different levels of behaviour change.

The second key idea is that progress through these stages is driven by a series of 10 *processes* specific to particular stages, including 'consciousness raising' (receiving information on how exercise may help or how exercise classes can be accessed), 'counter-conditioning' (using the positive aspects of exercise to counter fears and anxieties about future health) and 'stimulus control' (controlling situations that may trigger dropping out from the exercise class).

A third key idea refers to individuals' experience of accompanying problems such as their symptoms, the situational constraints, maladaptive cognitions, interpersonal conflicts and family problems. These may occur during any of the stages specified earlier. The advantage of this model is that it indicates the individual's readiness for change.

The knowledge given here can be applied by health care professionals and exercise instructors to enhance the likelihood of participants' continued attendance in an exercise programme. It is an approach which has been well received by health care professionals. However, although it is one of the most researched models, some misclassification of stages may occur as a result of the way those stages are operationally defined (Bulley et al 2007).

Central to the exercise and its planning is the setting and achieving of goals, the development of skills and the resulting increase in self-confidence; exercise may also provide a mechanism for social support if the exercise includes other people. In addition, the anxiety-reducing effects of exercise have been linked to improved cardiovascular fitness because they reduce the reactivity to psychosocial stressors and help to promote recovery from them (Biddle et al 2000).

The typical content of a physical activity consultation session has been outlined in step form by Biddle and Mutrie (2008).

Steps in a Typical Physical Activity Consultation Session

Step 1: Determine physical activity history: what the person previously enjoyed doing, why he or she wants to increase physical activity and the kind of activities he or she may now wish to engage in.

Step 2: Discuss what the person sees as being the 'pros' and 'cons' of increasing physical activity. Discuss how the 'cons' may be managed.

Step 3: Ask what kind of support the person will need and who can provide it, both for getting started and for continuing with the exercise.

Step 4: Help the person identify appropriate goals for gradually increasing physical activity. Write out action-related goals, such as 'In 4 weeks' time I would like to be walking for 30 minutes at moderate level of intensity (slightly out of breath) on at least 5 days of the week'.

Step 5: It is helpful also to discuss relapse strategies, such as what to do if the person misses sessions or if his or her motivation to continue wanes.

Step 6: Provide local information about leisure centres, sporting activities, walking paths and swimming pools. This makes a useful supplement to the discussion.

PRESCRIBING EXERCISE

Before prescribing exercise or participating in increased levels of physical activity, it is important to undertake an assessment on readiness to exercise. This should consider the individual's current and past patterns of physical activity and his or her preferred forms of activity. It should also identify goals and assess the risks. There should be a discussion with the participant about his or her beliefs regarding the benefits and risks of exercise, and an acknowledgement of any concurrent disease. Motivation and barriers should be considered together with the availability of social support throughout the programme. Finally, time and scheduling matters need to be agreed.

It is important to develop a realistic programme of physical activity and to monitor compliance and progress at regular intervals. The Par Q is an easy-to-complete questionnaire which can offer some guidance to potential health risks and is used widely in leisure centres for new and visiting members (see Appendix 4).

Type of Exercise

Exercise may have a variety of effects: it may strengthen a muscle, increase its flexibility, improve its endurance and refine its coordination ability, to mention a few. It may also fall into one of two categories or types: aerobic and anaerobic. Aerobic exercise consists of sustained rhythmic activity such as walking, swimming, cycling, jogging, distance running and dancing. It involves large muscle groups contracting in a repetitive manner at low-to-moderate levels of energy expenditure for long periods. This kind of exercise strengthens the cardiovascular system and increases overall strength and stamina. Anaerobic exercise, on the other hand, improves muscle strength and flexibility.

There are three kinds of anaerobic exercise: isotonic, isometric and calisthenic. The first two single out particular muscle groups for the purpose of building up their strength. Isotonics are exercises where the muscles contract against a resistant object with movement, as in weightlifting; this type of resistance exercise increases muscle bulk. Isometrics are exercises where the muscles contract against resistance but without movement as in squeezing a tennis ball; this increases strength without building bulk. Calisthenics are stretching exercises which increase flexibility and joint mobility. Examples include raising the arms above the head and other exercises to be found in Chapter 14.

Many forms of exercise achieve aerobic and strengthening effects, and both kinds have been found useful in the context of mental health. Stretching exercises are often used to warm up the muscles before starting the exercise.

Dosage of Exercise

A general principle of exercise prescription is that it should be introduced gradually and progress by small stages covering a period of several weeks. This is to ensure that the activity designed to benefit the body is matched by the body's capacity to tolerate the exercise. The chosen activity and setting should be attractive to the individual and one that they believe will be enjoyable. Personal preference should influence whether it is performed in a group or as an individual activity. Important aspects at the outset are fitness for

---

BOX 15.2
GRADES OF EXERCISE INTENSITY

VIGOROUS

Activity in which the individual exerts himself or herself to the point of getting out of breath and sweating. It includes squash, football, tennis, strong sustained swimming, long-distance running, cycling over difficult terrain and energetic aerobics (CMO 2011, Department of Health 2020).

MODERATE

Activity which makes the individual feel comfortably challenged (CMO 2011, Department of Health 2020). Less demanding activities such as golf, social dancing, table tennis, garden digging, long brisk walks, climbing stairs or gentle uphill gradients are included, performed at an intensity which causes breathing to be somewhat harder than normal and sweating to occur for some of the time.

LIGHT

Activity of an unchallenging nature which has little effect on the breathing. A few of the above activities such as golf, social dancing and table tennis are performed in a light manner; also included are fishing, darts, snooker, bowls, weeding, planting, light do-it-yourself activities and long walks at an average pace.

---

participation in the chosen activity and willingness to continue exercising in the future.

Dimensions of Exercise

It is conventional to describe exercise in terms of its three dimensions:

1. Intensity. Intensity, which can be vigorous, moderate or light (Box 15.2), has received particular attention from researchers. Although results have not been consistent, there seems to be a consensus that moderate-intensity activity produces the greatest benefit. 'Moderate', in this context, means that the exercise should be vigorous enough to create a physical effect but not so strenuous that the person feels unduly challenged. Extremely high intensities can have negative effects by inducing a degree of stress (Gauvin & Spence 1996).

2. Duration. The exercise may be taken either in one 30-minute period or broken up into multiple short periods. One advantage of the short, frequent exercise period is that it can be fitted into break times, which makes it ideally suited for people experiencing work stress. In setting the duration, much depends, first, on the nature of the exercise, in that lighter activities are easier to sustain for longer periods, and second, on the physical health and age of the individual, both of which will affect their exercise tolerance.

3. Frequency. On the matter of frequency, programmes vary in their specifications from three to seven times a week. Certainly a high frequency of practice is advocated, but whether seven times a week confers more benefit than five times a week has not been established. Most researchers suggest that daily exercising has merit.

The amount of energy expended during exercise relates to the balance between these three variables. Dunn and colleagues (2005) have been investigating the amount of energy expenditure required to gain health benefits in the relief of symptoms of depression. Their findings suggest that energy expenditure of 17 kcal/kg/week should be attempted. This can be achieved by exercising for at least 30 to 60 minutes a day (depending on intensity) for a minimum of 3 days a week. Alternatively, 30 minutes of moderate-intensity exercise, 5 days a week, will have the same effect.

PRECAUTIONS

In recommending exercise to participants, the health care professional/exercise instructor needs to be aware of its hazards. Exercise can be excessive and beyond the capacity of the individual. There have been instances of muscles and tendons being injured and even death occurring in the course of exercise. It is important, therefore, to keep the activity within safe limits. The following points should be borne in mind.

1. Exercise should not be seen as a substitute for medical help in the presence of disease or suspected disease. People with cardiovascular problems should first consult their doctor before taking up exercise.
2. Any programme of exercise should be introduced gradually and progress in small stages to

allow the organs to adapt to the new demands. Walking or swimming are useful ways to start. Unaccustomed strenuous activity is potentially hazardous.

3. All exercise should be preceded by some kind of 'warming up' activity to prepare the muscles for action (Reisman et al 2005, Safran et al 1989). Warming up takes the form of mild activity such as running on the spot, gentle contractions against resistance and balance exercises performed for 5 to 10 minutes. The effect of this procedure is to open up the blood vessels in the working part, thus protecting against ischaemia (inadequacy of local blood supply), which can occur in unprepared muscles.

4. Cooling down is also important. During vigorous or moderate exercise, a higher than normal proportion of the total blood volume circulates through the voluntary muscles. This state continues for some while after the exercise has come to an end and causes a lowering of the blood pressure. It is potentially hazardous in older adults but should be guarded against even in the very fit. As a remedy, the exercise can be slowly reduced in intensity or, alternatively, some lighter activity such as slow walking can be performed to bring about a gradual return of normal blood distribution (Hough 2001).

5. Exercise should not be too strenuous. To be safe, exercise should be well within the participant's capacity and performed regularly. Participants should never feel they are exercising to the limit of their strength. They should also know how to recognize signs of fatigue. Warnings of overwork in the form of chest pain or faintness, for example, should never be ignored.

6. Although team sports and marathons can be fun, they involve a spirit of competition which may be stressful. Non-competitive activities, on the other hand, impose less pressure on individuals, who can pace themselves in a way that takes account of their reactions.

7. The capacity of individuals to carry out exercise may be compromised by medical problems or by the drugs they are taking. It is advisable to check that these do not conflict with the effects of exercise. If individuals are in doubt about their health, they should seek advice before taking up exercise.

8. The cardiovascular benefit of jogging has to be balanced against the physical stress it imposes on the weight-bearing joints (Schnohr et al 2015, US Preventive Services Task Force 1989), although hard evidence of any association between running and the risk of osteoarthritis in weight-bearing joints is slight (Blair et al 1992, O'Connor & Wilder 2001). However, if there is a family history of joint problems, it may be advisable to consider an alternative form of aerobic exercise such as cycling or swimming.

9. Exercise is contraindicated during any kind of fever and should be avoided during viral infections such as influenza.

KEY POINTS

1. Regular physical activity offers protection from life-threatening diseases such as heart attack, stroke and some cancers and may offer protection from depression.

2. Exercise can be offered as a treatment in its own right for mild-to-moderate depression or as an adjunct to medication and/or cognitive–behavioural therapy.

3. Exercise may be helpful in managing state anxiety because it reduces the stress response.

4. The minimum requirement for general health benefits is 30 minutes of moderate activity on at least 5 days of the week.

5. Getting started in exercise where there are health problems should involve an appropriate assessment by a general practitioner, health care professional or exercise instructor. Previous medical and exercise history is important to ensure fitness to start exercising and to provide appropriate guidance on type, frequency, intensity and duration.

6. Support is needed in maintaining motivation. Goals should identify where support is being provided and indicate how feedback will be monitored.

Reflection

Describe how you carry out physical activity.

What physical activity do you do?

Why do you need to do physical activity?

How do you feel after physical activity?

What techniques/methods have you used?

What is your future action plan in terms of physical activity?

CASE STUDY LEARNING OPPORTUNITY

The key points and reflection provide the background and knowledge required in relation to the case study, Duncan, to help deepen understanding of how physical activities can help improve physical and mental well-being.

CASE STUDY

Low Back Pain: *Physical Activity Outcomes for Duncan*

Following on from Duncan's thoracic stretching exercises he was given three thoracic muscle-strengthening exercises as part of his ongoing treatment plan. The first thoracic strengthening exercise was competed with Duncan sitting in a chair. Once seated, Duncan was asked to hold a 3-kg weight in each hand, placing his arms behind his head. This was followed by a gentle backward arching and raising of his head. For the second thoracic muscle-strengthening exercise, Duncan was asked to lie on his back (supine), with his knees and hips held at 90 degrees. Duncan was then asked to hold a 3-kg weight in each hand, placing his arms behind his head and lifting his head and upper thoracic region off the ground, hold for a few seconds and then return to the starting position. For the third thoracic muscle-strengthening exercise, Duncan was asked to lie on his side, ensuring his hips, torso and shoulders were in line with each other. Duncan's feet and lower limbs were then held secure and he was asked to lift his torso off the ground, hold for a few seconds and then return to the starting position. In all three thoracic muscle-strengthening exercise it was ensured that the lumbar movement was limited.

Duncan was asked to perform these three thoracic muscle-strengthening exercises for a month, completing 10 sets of 10 repetitions a day. After a month, Duncan reported a visual analogue scale lower back pain score of 3, and and all his range of movement in the lumbar, flexion and rotation had increased by 5%. Duncan also reported that the anxiety he was experiencing had gone and he was able to travel further for work without having to take additional strops.

ACTIVITY

For the case study:

1. List the physical activities helping with the condition.
2. Write down the impact physical activity is having from a physical perspective.
3. Write down the impact physical activity is having from a psychological perspective.
4. Write down the impact physical activity is having from an emotional perspective.
5. Consider the effects of physical activity on overall quality of life.

This chapter concludes Section 2 on somatic approaches to relaxation. Chapter 16 will begin Section 3, focusing on cognitive approaches to relaxation, which includes nine cognitive approaches.

REFERENCES

Anderson, E., & Shivakumar, G. (2013). Effects of exercise and physical activity on anxiety. *Frontiers in Psychiatry, 4,* 1045–1055.

Babyak, M., Blumenthal, J. A., Herman, S., et al. (2000). Exercise treatment for major depression: maintenance of therapeutic benefit at 10 months. *Psychosomatic Medicine, 62,* 633–638.

Bernaards, C. M., Jans, M. P., van den Heuvel, S. G., Hendriksen, I. J., Houtman, I. L., & Bongers, P. M. (2006). Can strenuous leisure time physical activity prevent psychological complaints in a working population? *Occupational and Environmental Medicine, 63,* 10–16.

Biddle, S. J. H., Fox, K. R., & Boucher, S. H. (Eds.). (2000). *Physical activity and psychological well-being* (pp. 63–88). London: Routledge.

Biddle, S. J. H., & Mutrie, N. (2008). *Psychology of physical activity: Determinants, well-being and interventions* (2nd ed.). New York: Routledge.

Blair, S. N. (1995). Exercise prescription for health. *Quest, 47,* 338–353.

Blair, S. N., Kohl, H. W., Gordon, N. F., & Paffenbarger, R. S., Jr. (1992). How much physical activity is good for health? *Annual Review of Public Health, 13,* 99–126.

Blumenthal, J. A., Babyak, M. A., Doraiswamy, M., et al. (2007). Exercise and pharmacology in the treatment of major depressive disorder. *Psychosomatic Medicine, 69,* 587–596.

Blumenthal, J. A., Babyak, M. A., Moore, K. A., Craighead, W. E., Herman, S., & Khatri, P. (1999). Effects of exercise training on older patients with major depression. *Archives of Internal Medicine, 159,* 2349–2356.

Broocks, A., Bandelow, B., Pekrun, G., et al. (1998). Comparison of aerobic exercise, clomipramine and placebo in the treatment of panic disorder. *American Journal of Psychiatry, 155*(5), 603–609.

Bulley, C., Donaghy, M. E., Payne, A., & Mutrie, N. (2007). A critical review of the validity of measuring stages of change in relation to exercise and moderate physical activity. *Critical Public Health, 17*(1), 17–30.

Calogiuri, G., Evensen, K., Weydahl, A., et al. (2014). Green exercise as a workplace intervention to reduce job stress. *Work, 53,* 99–111.

Chaouloff, F. (1997). The serotonin hypothesis. In W. P. Morgan (Ed.), *Physical activity and mental health* (pp. 179–198). Washington, DC: Taylor and Francis.

Chang, Y. C., Lu, M. C., Hu, I. H., Wu, W. C. I., & Hu, S. C. (2017). Effects of different amounts of exercise on preventing depressive symptoms in community-dwelling older adults: a prospective cohort study in Taiwan. *BMJ Open, 7*(4), e014256.

Chief Medical Officers (CMO). (2011). Start Active, Stay Active: A report on physical activity for health from the four home countries.' Available at: https://assets.publishing.service.gov.uk/government/uploads/system/uploads/attachment_data/file/216370/dh_128210.pdf. Accessed September 2019.

Clow, A., & Edmunds, S. (2014). *Physical activity and mental health.* Campaign, IL: Human Kinetics.

Cooney, G. M., Dwan, K., Greig, C. A., et al. (2013). Exercise for depression. *Cochrane Database of Systematic Reviews, 9,* CD004366.

Cooper-Patrick, L., Ford, D. E., Mead, L. A., Chang, P. P., & Klag, M. J. (1997). Exercise and depression in midlife: A prospective study. *American Journal of Public Health, 87*(4), 670–673.

DeBoer, L. B., Powers, M. B., Utschig, A. C., Otto, M. W., & Smits, J. A. (2012). Exploring exercise as an avenue for the treatment of anxiety disorders. *Expert Review of Neurotherapeutics, 12*(8), 1011–1022.

Department of Health. (2004). *At Least Five a Week: Evidence on the Impact of Physical Activity and its Relationship to Health. A report from the Chief Medical Officer.* London: HMSO.

Department of Health. (2020). *Physical Activity Guidelines: UK Chief Medical Officers' report.* London: HMSO. Available at: https://www.gov.uk/government/collections/physical-activity-guidelines. Accessed April 2020.

DiClemente, C. C., Prochaska, J. O., & Gibertini, M. (1985). Self-efficacy and the stages of self-change of smoking. *Cognitive Therapy and Research, 9,* 181–200.

Donaghy, M. E. (2007). Exercise can seriously improve your mental health: Fact or fiction? *Advances in Physiotherapy, 9*(2), 76–89.

Dunn, A., Trivedi, M. H., Kampert, J., Clark, C. G., & Chambliss, H. O. (2005). Exercise treatment for depression: Efficacy and dose response. *American Journal of Preventive Medicine, 28,* 1–8.

Farmer, M., Locke, B., Moscicki, E., Dannenberg, A., Larson, D., & Radloff, L. (1988). Physical activity and depressive symptoms: The NHANES-1 epidemiological follow-up study. *American Journal of Epidemiology, 128,* 1340–1351.

Fremont, J., & Craighead, L. W. (1987). Aerobic exercise and cognitive therapy in the treatment of dysphoric moods. *Cognitive Therapy and Research, 11,* 241–251.

Gauvin, L., & Spence, J. C. (1996). Physical activity and psychological well-being: Knowledge base, current issues and caveats. *Nutrition Reviews, 54*(4), S53–S65.

Greist, J. H., Klein, M. H., Eischens, R. R., Faris, J. W., Gurman, A. S., & Morgan, W. P. (1979). Running as a treatment for depression. *Comprehensive Psychiatry, 20,* 41–54.

Haller, N., Lorenz, S., Pfirmann, D., et al. (2018). Individualized web-based exercise for the treatment of depression: randomized controlled trial. *JMIR Mental Health, 5*(4), e10698.

Harris, A., Cronkite, R., & Moos, R. (2006). Physical activity, exercise, coping and depression in a 10-year cohort study of depressed patients. *Journal of Affective Disorders, 93,* 79–85.

Hough, A. (2001). *Physiotherapy in respiratory care: An evidence-based approach to respiratory and cardiac management* (3rd ed.). Cheltenham, UK: Nelson Thornes.

Khalil, E., Callaghan, P., Carter, T., & Morres, I. (2012). Pragmatic randomised controlled trial of an exercise programme to improve wellbeing outcomes in women with depression: findings from the qualitative component. *Psychology, 3*(11), 979–986.

Klein, M. J., Griest, J. H., Gurman, A. S., et al. (1985). A comparative outcome study of group psychotherapy vs. exercise treatments for depression. *International Journal of Mental Health, 13,* 148–177.

La Forge, R. (1995). Exercise-associated mood alteration: a review of interactive neurobiological mechanisms. *Journal of Medicine, Exercise, Nutrition and Health, 4,* 17–32.

Lampinen, P., Hiekkinin, R. L., Kauppinen, M., & Hiekkinin, E. (2006). Activity as a predictor of mental well-being among older adults. *Ageing and Mental Health, 10,* 454–466.

Martinsen, E. W. (1990). Physical fitness, anxiety and depression. *British Journal of Hospital Medicine, 43,* 194–199.

Mental Health Foundation (2019). Up and running: exercise therapy and the treatment of mild or moderate depression in primary care. Available at: www.mentalhealth.org.uk/campaigns/mhaw/exercise-and-depression/. Accessed September 2019.

MIND Survey. (2001). Available at: http://news.bbc.co.uk/2/hi/health/1338145stm. Accessed September 2019.

Mikkelsen, K., Stojanovska, L., Polenakovic, M., Bosevski, M., & Apostolopoulos, V. (2017). Exercise and mental health. *Maturitas, 106,* 48–56.

Mitchell, R. (2012). Is physical activity in natural environments better for mental health than physical activity in other environments? *Social Science & Medicine, 91,* 130–134.

Mobily, K. E., Rubenstein, L. M., Lemke, J. H., O'Hara, M. W., & Wallace, R. B. (1996). Walking and depression in a cohort of older adults: The Iowa 65+ Rural Health Study. *Journal of Aging and Physical Activity, 4,* 119–135.

Motl, R. W., Birnbaum, A. S., Kubik, M. Y., & Dishman, R. K. (2004). Naturally occurring changes in physical activity are inversely related to depressive symptoms during early adolescence. *Psychological Medicine, 66*, 336–342.

Motl, R. W., Konopack, J. F., McAuley, E., Elavsky, S., Jerome, G. J., & Marquez, D. X. (2005). Depressive symptoms among older adults: Long term reduction after a physical activity intervention. *Journal of Behavioral Medicine, 28*, 385–394.

Mutrie, N., & Faulkner, G. (2003). Physical activity and mental health. In T. Everett, M. Donaghy, & S. Feaver (Eds.), *Interventions for mental health* (pp. 82–98). Oxford: Butterworth-Heinemann.

National Institute for Clinical Excellence (NICE). (2003). *Depression: NICE Guideline 2nd consultation.* London: NICE.

O'Connor, F., & Wilder, R. (2001). In S. E. Willick (Ed.), *Running and osteoarthritis* (pp. 387–394). New York: McGraw-Hill.

O'Donovan, G., Blazevich, A. J., Boreham, C., et al. (2010). The ABC of physical activity for health: A consensus statement from the British Association of Sport and Exercise Sciences. *Journal of Sports Science, 28*(6), 57391.

Otto, M., & Smits, J. (2011). *Exercise for mood and anxiety: proven strategies for overcoming depression and enhancing well-being.* New York: Oxford University Press.

Paffenbarger, R. S., Lee, I. M., & Leung, R. (1994). Physical activity and personal characteristics associated with depression and suicide in American college men. *Acta Psychiatrica Scandinavica, 89*(S377), 16–22.

Pedersen, B. K., & Fischer, C. P. (2007). Beneficial health effects of exercise – the role of IL-6 as a myokine. *Trends in Pharmacological Sciences, 28*(4), 152–156.

Rebar, A. I., & Taylor, A. (2017). Physical activity and mental health; it is more than just a prescription. *Mental Health and Physical Activity, 13*, 77–82.

Reisman, S., Walsh, L. D., & Proske, U. (2005). Warm-up stretches reduce sensations of stiffness and soreness after eccentric exercise. *Medicine & Science in Sports & Exercise, 37*(6), 929–936.

Safran, M. R., Seaber, A. V., & Garrett, W. E. (1989). Warm-up and muscular prevention. *Sports Medicine, 8*, 239–249.

Schnohr, P., O'Keefe, J. H., Marott, J. L., Lange, P., & Jensen, G. B. (2015). Dose of jogging and long-term mortality: The Copenhagen City Heart Study. *Journal of the American College of Cardiology, 65*(5), 411–419.

Scully, D., Kremer, J., Meade, M. M., Graham, R., & Dudgeon, K. (1998). Physical exercise and psychological well-being: A critical review. *British Journal of Sports Medicine, 32*, 111–120.

Scottish Intercollegiate Guidelines Network (SIGN). (2009). *Nonpharmacological Management of Mild to Moderate Depression.* Edinburgh: Scottish Intercollegiate Guidelines Network.

Strawbridge, W. J., Deleger, S., Roberts, R. E., & Kaplan, G. A. (2002). Physical activity reduces the risk of subsequent depression for older adults. *American Journal of Epidemiology, 156*, 328–334.

Tsatsoulis, A., & Fountoulakis, S. (2006). The protective role of exercise on stress system dysregulation and comorbidities. *Annals of the New York Academy of Sciences, 1083*, 196–213.

US Preventive Services Task Force. (1989). Exercise counselling. *Guide to clinical preventive services.* Baltimore: Williams and Wilkins, US Preventive Services Task Force.

van Gool, C. H., Kempen, G. I., Penninx, B. W., Deeg, D. J., Beekman, A. T., & van Eijk, J. T. (2003). Relationship between changes in depressive symptoms and unhealthy lifestyles in late middle aged and older persons: Results from the Longitudinal Ageing Study, Amsterdam. *Age and Ageing, 32*, 81–87.

Warburton, D. E. R., Nicol, C. W., & Bredin, S. S. D. (2006). Health benefits of physical activity: the evidence. *Canadian Medical Association Journal, 174*(6), 801–809.

Wegner, M., Helmich, I., Machado, S. E., Nardi, A., Arias-Carrion, O., & Budde, H. (2014). Effects of exercise on anxiety and depression disorders: review of meta-analyses and neurobiological mechanisms. *CNS & Neurological Disorders Drug Targets, 13*(6), 1002–1014.

Weyerer, S. (1992). Physical inactivity and depression in the community: Evidence from the Upper Bavarian Field Study. *Journal of Sports Medicine, 13*, 492–496.

World Health Organization (WHO). (2004). Global strategy on diet, physical activity and health. Available at: www.who.int/dietphysicalactivity/strategy/eb11344/strategy–english–web.pdf.

Section 3

COGNITIVE APPROACHES TO RELAXATION

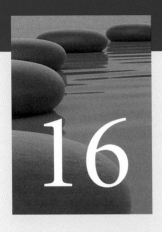

16

COGNITIVE–BEHAVIOURAL APPROACHES

DR CAROLINE BELCHAMBER

LEARNING OBJECTIVES

The aim of this chapter is to provide a broad understanding of cognitive–behavioural approaches and how they can be applied within a practical framework.

By the end of this chapter you will be able to:

1. Understand the theory behind cognitive-behavioural approaches.

2. Appreciate the evidence underpinning cognitive-behavioural approaches.

3. Understand what an individual assessment involves.

4. Recognize the format of cognitive restructuring.

5. Identify the relaxation component within cognitive-behavioural approaches.

6. Discern how this is applied in practice.

This chapter will conclude with key points and time for reflection, providing learning opportunities through a case study.

INTRODUCTION TO COGNITIVE-BEHAVIOURAL APPROACHES

Cognitive–behavioural interventions were first used clinically with mental health disorders such as anxiety and depression, acknowledging that mood is regulated through cognition and behaviour and the interaction between these systems. In recent years the application of cognitive–behavioural therapy (CBT) has been extended to areas where anxiety and depression are associated with other clinical conditions such as pain, fibromyalgia and chronic fatigue.

CBT is an approach designed to alleviate symptoms and to help people learn more effective ways of overcoming the problems and difficulties that contribute to their distress (Davidson 2008). It seeks to address individuals' difficulties from their point of view and to equip them with the information and confidence to become an active participant in the management of their condition (Marshall & Turnbull 1996). It thus lends itself to conditions such as anxiety, depression, psychotic disorders, eating disorders, chronic fatigue syndrome and chronic pain and is relevant in many other illnesses and dysfunctions. The theory behind CBT also has a major role to play in the field of prevention and is an evidence-based psychological therapy that has mainly been used and evaluated with individuals who have anxiety and depressive disorders (Cuijpers et al 2010, Hofmann et al, 2012, Stewart & Chambless 2009).

Although CBT is a psychological speciality, many of its techniques are highly accessible to the health care professional, and because health care professionals have been asked to broaden their approach by taking account of psychosocial aspects of assessment and treatment, they will find in CBT techniques a means of achieving this (Everett 2003, Johnstone et al 2002). CBT approaches now feature in occupational and physiotherapy treatment programmes, although relatively few studies of effectiveness in these professions have so far been carried out (Duncan 2003). Health care professionals can acquire CBT expertise from a variety of postgraduate courses, many of which are condition focused, such as CBT for chronic pain or cardiac rehabilitation. These programmes allow people to get a basic training but for further competence, supervision with an experienced cognitive–behavioural therapist is required.

CBT helps people to challenge their beliefs and thoughts and to develop positive coping strategies. Relaxation is taught to reduce the physiological symptoms and is a component of the cognitive–behavioural strategies used in many of the conditions mentioned in this chapter. The overall effect of CBT, however, goes far beyond the strict bounds of relaxation.

INTRODUCTION TO EVIDENCE

The effectiveness of CBT has been clearly demonstrated (Butler et al 2006, Roth & Fonagy 2005). It is now the most widely endorsed form of psychological therapy (Rachman 2003) and has broad application in both physical (Beltman et al 2010, NICE 2009) and mental health (DOH 2001). With the theoretical and practical integration of cognitive and behavioural strategies, CBT has become influential in terms of health service delivery. As a clinical intervention, research has demonstrated not only that CBT works but also how it works (Salkovskis 2002).

CBT has been found to be effective in the treatment and management of major mental health problems. A meta-analyses undertaken by Butler et al (2006) found large effect sizes for CBT in a range of mental health disorders including unipolar depression, anxiety, panic disorder (with or without agoraphobia), social phobia, posttraumatic stress disorder, and childhood depressive and anxiety disorders. Moderate effect sizes for CBT were found in the treatment of marital stress, anger, childhood somatic disorders and chronic pain. CBT was also found to be as effective as behaviour therapy in the treatment of adult depression and obsessive compulsive disorder and as effective as antidepressants for the initial treatment of moderate-to-severe depression (Hollon et al 2005).

A Cochrane review found that CBT was effective in the treatment of anxiety and more effective than psychodynamic therapy (Hunot et al 2007). Öst and Breitholtz (2000), comparing CBT with applied relaxation in a small study of 36 outpatients with generalized anxiety disorder, found no significant differences between the two methods, although both demonstrated improvements. There was, however, a lack of evidence for the longer-term effectiveness of CBT in treating generalized anxiety disorder (Hunot et al 2007).

Evidence for the effectiveness of CBT in patients with alcohol disorders consists of findings from meta-analyses and randomized controlled studies (Longabaugh et al 2005). The strongest evidence is linked to social skills training, community reinforcement approaches and relapse prevention (Miller & Hester 1995). In a large study comparing CBT with the twelve steps Alcoholics Anonymous programme and motivational enhancement therapy (Project MATCH 1998), all treatments were equally effective.

Many other clinical conditions have benefited from CBT. The literature is extensive, as the following studies indicate. A Cochrane review of CBT found it more effective than orthodox medical management or other interventions for adults with chronic fatigue syndrome; here, benefits were equal to those of graded exercise (Price & Couper 1999). CBT has also been found effective in reducing symptoms of pain, anxiety and fatigue in children with fibromyalgia (Degotardi et al 2006). Meta-analysis of studies of breast cancer found CBT effective in managing the distress and pain associated with this condition (Tatrow & Montgomery 2006).

Opinion suggests that cognitive–behavioural interventions are valuable in the treatment and management of chronic pain (Keefe et al 2004, Morley 2004, Vlaeyen & Morley 2005), an opinion which is based on published research trials and systematic reviews (Guzman et al 2001, Morley et al 1999, van Tulder et al 2000). The systematic review undertaken by Morley et al (1999) found CBT to be beneficial in exploring the components of the pain experience such as thoughts and feelings; it also improved social functioning.

Face-to-face CBT is now well established as a therapy of choice within the National Health Service for individuals with chronic physical illness (NICE 2009). However, while many of the cognitive–behavioural interventions currently in use contain elements which are transferable across conditions, research indicates that specific clinical problems require different approaches. For example, CBT in the treatment of depression is quite different from the treatment for obsessive compulsive disorder or the management of chronic pain. In recent years more innovative approaches have been researched, such as computerized CBT programmes for adults with mild-to-moderate depression and anxiety (Collins et al 2018) and religious cognitive–behavioural therapy for depression and anxiety in patients after coronary artery bypass graft surgery (Hosseini et al 2017).

THEORIES BEHIND COGNITIVE–BEHAVIOURAL APPROACHES

The origin of cognitive behavioural approaches lies in cognitive and behavioural theories (see Chapter 2). Cognitive theory is based on the premise that individuals constantly process information gathered from their surroundings and that problems arise as a result of the way the individual interprets a situation or event (Beck 1976, Beech 2000). Knowledge, previous experience and memories of situations or events all play a part, influencing these interpretations. An inaccurate or biased interpretation of an event or experience can lead to faulty patterns of thinking and unrealistic beliefs. This can cause symptoms of stress, anxiety and depression and can be linked to other physical and mental health problems (Donaghy et al 2008). Individuals need to recognize the negative content and bias in their thinking before they can learn ways of challenging it. This involves a re-evaluation of their

perception of vulnerability or danger, whether they are dealing with full-blown anxiety or day-by-day stress (Beck 1976, Greenberger & Padesky 1995).

Cognitive theory views the person as a self-determining agent in life, which means that, when receiving treatment, the individual needs to feel a degree of control over the management of his or her condition. This aspect makes the approach particularly applicable in the field of chronic disorder.

Behaviour theory, on the other hand, views human behaviour as a result of environmental conditioning and, when this behaviour is maladaptive, employs methods such as reinforcement, distraction and exposure to modify it. Positive and negative reinforcement are methods for increasing the likelihood of desired behaviours. Distraction (i.e., holding the attention elsewhere) can be a useful strategy particularly for people in chronic pain. Exposure (i.e., facing the anxiety-provoking situation itself) can be a useful tool for people who experience panic attacks or various forms of social anxiety.

The cognitive–behavioural approach combines both theories. Developed by Aaron Beck, it emphasizes the importance of thought processes while acknowledging that they can be influenced by reinforcement. This highlights the interrelationship of thoughts, feelings and behaviour, creating a unifying philosophy with a strong psychosocial emphasis (Marshall & Turnbull 1996). Therefore CBT is built on the theory of psychopathology, which recognizes the reciprocal interrelationship among the cognitive, behavioural, somatic and emotional systems (Beech 2000).

PROCEDURE

Individual Assessment

Central to the method is the collaborative relationship that is developed between the person and therapist (Ralston 2008). This begins with a first assessment to determine whether the person has the motivation and commitment to be an active participant, and also to determine whether CBT is the most appropriate path to follow. The approach can be illustrated in the handling of anxiety, for example, where a first step would be to discover the situation or event which triggers the anxiety and to review it alongside the various symptoms it provokes (i.e., physiological, cognitive, behavioural and emotional). The person is encouraged to articulate his or her beliefs and interpretations of that situation or event. Through dialogue with the therapist, individuals explore the factors which make the symptoms of anxiety better or worse and examine the ways in which they cope with them. This person-centred approach helps individuals to gain a sense of personal empowerment. Initially, they may need to be guided into active participation because they may not be aware that they have that power; they may not realize that any change in their symptoms will be the result of their own actions. With continued collaboration, however, information will emerge and be used in planning the treatment.

Cognitive Restructuring

Individuals are introduced to the format for each session, including agenda setting, shared goal setting and home-based tasks. In early sessions, general examples of links between thoughts, feelings, physical symptoms and behaviour are presented alongside examples specific to the person. It is important that the links among fear, anxiety and worry become evident because constant worrying intensifies anxiety and extends the associations which trigger it.

The next step is to help people recognize the negative content and bias in their thinking so that they can learn ways of challenging it. This process is termed cognitive restructuring. Both clinical dialogue and diary keeping are important in guiding the individual to recognize negative thinking. Between sessions, individuals will keep a note of any anxiety-provoking events, describing the situation, the emotion elicited and what was going through their mind at the time, whether it was a distressing image or a negative thought about themselves, their situation or the future.

With the information gathered from the interviews, negative thoughts, beliefs and assumptions are set out alongside the evidence that challenges them. For example, abdominal pain experienced with anxiety may be associated with the belief that they have cancer; people with cancer suffer pain. This negative thought can be challenged by different types of evidence, such as pain being confined to anxiety attacks, an absence of other symptoms or non-existent family history of cancer. Moreover, pain linked to anxiety can itself have a physiological explanation.

Learning about automatic negative thinking errors also helps people to understand that it is their thinking, not the event itself, which is causing their distress. In common with others who display negative thinking habits, people tend to overestimate danger and underestimate their own coping abilities.

Useful cognitive techniques to employ include the following: considering how other people would view the situation (an indication that other perspectives exist); reviewing past experiences where they have coped successfully; and considering what might happen if their worst fears came true. This helps people to see that their fears are unlikely to be realized. However, if the fear is plausible an action plan can be drawn up for use, should the event occur.

Yet another cognitive–behavioural approach is getting the person to confine worrying to previously agreed-on times. Specific worries are identified and a time and location set aside for addressing them. When worry occurs outside these times, the person is asked to note the item in the diary but not to dwell on it at that point. He or she is encouraged to wait until the prearranged 'worry time' when the person picks up the item and works on it with the use of the cognitive restructuring techniques outlined above.

A relaxation technique to deal with the physical symptoms can also be offered to individuals. It is helpful for them to learn brief relaxation techniques which can be used at times when panic or fear is experienced (see Chapter 24). People are also encouraged to face situations previously avoided, having first discussed them with the therapist. Such exposure is likely to be time limited, progressing in a phased manner. If managed appropriately, their beliefs and assumptions will change, their anxiety will be extinguished and they will experience the absence of any catastrophic outcome and begin to recognize their ability to cope with challenging situations.

In the case study presented at the end of the chapter homework includes a range of cognitive techniques which challenge Barbara's beliefs about cancer. One of these is thought stopping (see Chapter 24), a technique which intercepts the intrusive thoughts and replaces cancer fears with a vision of her two children, healthy and laughing. Six weeks from starting treatment, Barbara's symptoms of severe anxiety are extinguished and she is pain-free.

KEY POINTS

1. Cognitive–behavioural treatments combine a wide range of strategies drawn from both cognitive and behavioural approaches.
2. Treatment programmes are designed and carried out with the individual in the role of an active participant.
3. Self-management by the individual is a characterizing feature, particularly in chronic disease.
4. Although CBT is a psychological speciality, many of its techniques are highly accessible to the health care professional.
5. Strong evidence exists for the effectiveness of CBT.

Reflection

Describe your understanding of CBT.
How does CBT manage physical symptoms?
How does CBT manage psychological symptoms?
What approaches have you used/delivered? Were they successful?
What is your future action plan in terms of CBT?

CASE STUDY LEARNING OPPORTUNITY

The key points and reflection provide the background and knowledge required in relation to the case study, Barbara, to help deepen understanding of how cognitive–behavioural approaches can help improve physical and mental well-being.

CASE STUDY

Heightened Anxiety After the Birth of a Child: CBT Outcomes for Barbara

Barbara is a 28-year-old mother of two children under the age of 5. She describes having experienced feelings of heightened anxiety after the birth of her first child (a girl) 4 years ago. At that time she also developed pain in her neck and right shoulder and she associated the pain with a belief that she may have cancer (her friend had been diagnosed with a brain tumour 9 months previously). Barbara gradually recovered from her anxiety and from the pain with its associated beliefs but states that her self-confidence never returned to its level before the birth of her daughter. However, she managed to hold a job as manager in a large sports outlet, where she worked until the birth, 18 months ago, of her second child (a boy).

She had no anxious feelings after the birth of her second child and she has enjoyed her time as a mother, meeting other mothers and their children. However, in the last 10 weeks, Barbara has felt that her anxiety has returned and it seems to have been triggered by her daughter being hospitalized for 4 days with pneumonia.

Although the little girl has now fully recovered, Barbara's anxiety is not subsiding. Alongside this anxiety, she has again developed pain in her neck and shoulders. She referred herself to a physiotherapist, describing her symptoms as pain which intensifies as the day goes on.

After an initial assessment, Barbara explores with the physiotherapist her thoughts and beliefs about her pain and anxiety. They discuss how anxiety creates changes in the muscles, making them tense, and how this can cause pain. They discover that the pain is aggravated by lifting and carrying her son. Added to this, she is suffering from sleep disturbance and intense worry. Barbara also shares her thoughts about the possibility of having cancer, basing her thoughts on the experience of her friend with the brain tumour who had similar physical symptoms and died from the tumour 12 months ago. Barbara agrees to keep a diary and to note when anxiety afflicts her, what happens immediately before feeling anxious, what she is thinking, how it affects her pain, what helps reduce the anxiety/pain and what makes it worse. She learns to recognize a negative bias in her thinking and challenges it by reminding herself that she has never had a serious illness, that the chances of her getting cancer are very slim and that she has no other symptoms which might justify such a fear. She now appreciates that anxiety can trigger pain.

Together, Barbara and the physiotherapist develop a plan to help her relax by learning a relaxation technique which she agrees to practise every day. Using the information gathered from the interviews and diaries, the process of 'restructuring' her thoughts continues over a period of 4 weeks. Barbara also learns a brief relaxation technique for use during periods of anxiety when the worry about having cancer intrudes into her thoughts.

ACTIVITY

For the case study:
1. List the key aspects used in the CBT.
2. Consider why this approach was taken.
3. Write down the key areas associated with Barbara's anxiety.

4. Write down the impact CBT is having from a psychological perspective.
5. Write down the impact CBT is having from a physical perspective.
6. Write down the impact CBT is having from an emotional perspective.
7. Consider the outcomes of quality of life and overall well-being for Barbara.

Chapter 17 will focus on self-awareness, developing knowledge gained from cognitive–behavioural approaches.

REFERENCES

Beck, A. T. (1976). *Cognitive therapy and the emotional disorders.* New York: International Universities Press.

Beech, B. F. (2000). The strengths and weaknesses of cognitive behavioural approaches to treating depression and their potential for wider utilization by mental health nurses. *Journal of Psychiatric and Mental Health Nursing, 7*, 343–354.

Beltman, M. W., Voshaar, R. C. O., & Speckens, A. E. (2010). Cognitive–behavioural therapy for depression in people with a somatic disease: Metaanalysis of randomised controlled trials. *The British Journal of Psychiatry, 197*, 11–19.

Butler, A. C., Chapmen, J. E., Forman, E. M., et al. (2006). The empirical status of cognitive-behavioural therapy: a review of meta-analyses. *Clinical Psychological Review, 26*, 17–31.

Collins, S., Byrne, M., Hawe, J., & O'Reilly, G. (2018). Evaluation of a computerized cognitive behavioural therapy programme, MindWise (2.0), for adults with mild-to-moderate depression and anxiety. *British Journal of Clinical Psychology, 57*, 255–269.

Cuijpers, P., Smit, F., Bohlmeijer, E., Hollon, S. D., & Andersson, G. (2010). Efficacy of cognitive–behavioural therapy and other psychological treatments for adult depression: Meta-analytic study of publication bias. *The British Journal of Psychiatry, 196*, 173–178.

Davidson, K. (2008). Cognitive-behavioural therapy: origins and developments. In M. Donaghy, M. Nicol, & K. Davidson (Eds.), *Cognitive-behavioural interventions in physiotherapy and occupational therapy* (pp. 3–18). Butterworth-Heinemann: Edinburgh.

Degotardi, P. J., Klass, E. S., Rosenberg, B. S., Fox, D. G., Gallelli, K. A., & Gottlieb, B. S. (2006). Development and evaluation of a cognitive-behavioural intervention for juvenile fibromyalgia. *Journal of Paediatric Psychology, 37*, 714–723.

Department of Health (DOH) (2001). *Treatment choice in psychological therapies and counselling: Evidence based clinical practice guidelines.* London: DOH.

Donaghy, M. E., Nicol, M., & Davidson, K. (2008). *Cognitive behavioural interventions in physiotherapy and occupational therapy.* Edinburgh: Butterworth-Heinemann Elsevier.

Duncan, E. A. S. (2003). Cognitive-behavioural therapy in physiotherapy and occupational therapy. In T. Everett, M. E. Donaghy, & S. Feaver (Eds.), *Interventions for Mental Health: An Evidence-Based Approach for Physiotherapists and Occupational Therapists.*, Oxford, UK: Butterworth-Heinemann.

Everett, T. (2003). Chronic fatigue syndrome. In T. Everett, M. E. Donaghy, & S. Feaver (Eds.), *Interventions for Mental Health* (pp. 257). Oxford, UK: Butterworth-Heinemann.

Greenberger, D., & Padesky, C. A. (1995). *Mind over mood: Change how you feel by changing the way you think.* New York: Guilford.

Guzman, J., Ezmail, R., Karjalainen, J., Malmivaara, A., Irvin, B., & Bombadier, C. (2001). Multidisciplinary rehabilitation for chronic low back pain: systematic review. *BMJ: British Medical Journal, 322*, 1511–1516.

Hofmann, S. G., Asnaani, A., Vonk, I. J. J., Sawyer, A. T., & Fang, A. (2012). The efficacy of cognitive behavioural therapy: A review of meta-analyses. *Cognitive Therapy Research, 36*(5), 427–440.

Hollon, S. D., de Rubeis, R. J., Shelton, R. C., et al. (2005). Prevention of relapse following cognitive therapy vs medications in moderate to severe depression. *Archives of General Psychiatry, 62*, 417–422.

Hunot, V., Churchill, R., Teixeira, & Silva da Lima, M. (2007). Psychological therapies for generalized anxiety disorder. *Cochrane Database of Systematic Reviews, 1*(CD00), 1848.

Keefe, F. J., Rumble, M. E., Scipio, C. D., Giordano, L. A., & Perri, L. C. M. (2004). Psychological aspects of persistent pain: current state of the science. *Journal of Pain, 5*, 195–211.

Johnstone, R., Donaghy, M., & Martin, D. (2002). A pilot study of a cognitive-behavioural therapy approach to physiotherapy for acute low back pain patients who show signs of developing chronic pain. *Advances in Physiotherapy, 4*(4), 182–188.

Longabaugh, R., Donovan, D. M., Karno, M. P., et al. (2005). Active ingredients: How and why evidence-based alcohol behavioural treatment interventions work. Alcohol. *Clinical Experimental Research, 29*(2), 235–247.

Marshall, S., & Turnbull, J. (1996). *Cognitive-behaviour therapy: An introduction to theory and practice.* London: Baillière Tindall.

Morley, S., Eccleston, C., & Williams, A. (1999). Systematic review and meta-analysis of randomized controlled trials of cognitive behaviour therapy and behaviour therapy for chronic pain in adults, excluding headache. *Pain*, *80*, 1–13.

Morley, S. (2004). Process and change in cognitive behaviour therapy for chronic pain. *Pain*, *109*, 205–206.

Miller, W. R., & Hester, R. K. (1995). Treatment for alcohol problems: Towards an informed eclecticism. In R. K. Hester, & W. R. Miller (Eds.), *Handbook of alcoholism treatment approaches: Effective alternatives* (2nd ed., pp. 1–11). Needham Heights, MA: Allyn & Bacon.

National Institute for Health and Care Excellence (NICE). (2009). *The treatment and management of depression and adults with chronic physical health problems. CG91*. London: National Institute for Health and Clinical Excellence.

Öst, L. -G., & Breitholtz, E. (2000). Applied relaxation versus cognitive therapy in the treatment of generalized anxiety disorder. *Behavioral Research & Therapy*, *38*(8), 777–790.

Price, J. R., & Couper, J. (1999). Cognitive-behaviour therapy for chronic fatigue syndrome in adults. *The Cochrane Library*, *2*.

Project MATCH. (1998). Matching alcohol treatments to client heterogeneity: Project MATCH 3-year drinking outcomes. *Alcohol. Clinical Experimental Research*, *22*(6), 300–311.

Rachman, J. (2003). Eysenck and the development of cognitive-behavioural therapy. *The Psychologist*, *16*(11), 588–591.

Ralston, G. E. (2008). Cognitive behavioural therapy for anxiety. In M. Donaghy, M. Nicol, & K. Davidson (Eds.), *Cognitive behavioural interventions in physiotherapy and occupational therapy* (pp. 75–90). Edinburgh: Butterworth-Heinemann Elsevier.

Roth, A., & Fonagy, P. (2005). *What works for whom? A critical review of psychotherapy research* (2nd ed.). New York: Guilford Press.

Salkovskis, P. M. (2002). Empirically grounded clinical interventions: Cognitive-behavioural therapy progresses through a multi-dimensional approach to clinical science. *Behavioural and Cognitive Psychotherapy*, *30*, 3–9.

Stewart, R. E., & Chambless, D. L. (2009). Cognitive-behavioral therapy for adult anxiety disorders in clinical practice: A meta-analysis of effectiveness studies. *Journal of Consulting and Clinical Psychology*, *77*(4), 595–606.

Tatrow, K., & Montgomery, G. H. (2006). Cognitive behavioural therapy techniques for distress and pain in breast cancer patients: A meta-analysis. *Journal of Behavioral Medicine*, *29*(1), 17–27.

van Tulder, M. W., Ostelo, R. W. J. G., Vlaeyen, J. W. S., Linton, S. J., Morley, S. J., & Assendelft, W. J. J. (2000). Behavioural treatment for chronic low back pain (Cochrane Review). *The Cochrane Library*, *2*.

Vlaeyen, J. W. S., & Morley, S. (2005). Cognitive-behavioural treatments for chronic pain: What works for whom? Special Topic Series: Cognitive-behavioural Treatment for Chronic Pain. *Clinical Journal of Pain*, *21*, 1–8.

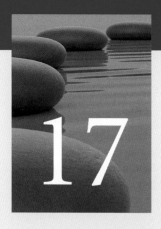

17

SELF-AWARENESS

DR CAROLINE BELCHAMBER

CHAPTER CONTENTS

LEARNING OBJECTIVES

The aim of this chapter is to understand how self-awareness exercises can be seen as relaxation techniques.

By the end of this chapter you will be able to:

1. Understand what is meant by self-awareness.

2. Appreciate the evidence underpinning self-awareness.

3. Define the theory behind self-awareness.

4. Recognize the impact of self-awareness deficits.

5. List different types of self-awareness exercises.

6. Describe how self-awareness exercises are applied in practice.

This chapter will conclude with key points and time for reflection, providing learning opportunities through a case study.

INTRODUCTION TO SELF-AWARENESS

'Being aware' or 'being conscious' convey similar ideas. Their use when applied to the self, however, is very different. Being aware of the self is defined as 'the tendency to focus attention on the private aspects of the self' (West 2016). This signifies a process of self-exploration, a getting to know oneself and, recognizing one's strengths and weaknesses. Being 'self-conscious', as we use the phrase in everyday language, on the other hand, implies the sense of being 'painfully aware of being observed by others' (Burnard 1991). A person who is self-conscious sees themselves as being critically scrutinized by other people. The result of self-consciousness is embarrassment; the result of self-awareness is self-knowledge.

Increased self-knowledge comes from listening to ourselves: to who we are, what we are and how we are (Tschudin 1991). It relates to questions such as 'Am I the person I want to be?' and if not, 'What is stopping me becoming that person?' or 'Why don't I allow myself to develop to my fullest?' The answers help us to understand ourselves. The better we know ourselves, the easier it is to make decisions which further our life plans. Without this knowledge, we may find decisions being made for us.

Self-awareness also puts us in touch with our outward behaviour and the way others may be responding to it. In this way, self-awareness can enhance our personal relationships.

The notion of self-awareness is fundamentally linked to the notion of living in the present, responding in the here-and-now and being aware of the present moment because that is where we express ourselves and make our impact on life. Of course, we need to take into account lessons learned from the past and goals set for the future, but it is all too easy to dwell on these and let the present take care of itself. This can lead to losing whatever control we had of it. Being aware of the self helps us perform in the present.

Greater control of our lives, enhanced relationships and improved self-knowledge all contribute to our peace of mind. Self-awareness exercises can thus be seen as relaxation techniques.

INTRODUCTION TO EVIDENCE

There is a body of literature supporting the view that subjective awareness of our true self is fundamentally connected to our mental health and well-being. Research has found that individuals who report higher levels of subjective true self-awareness also report increased feelings of self-actualization, vitality, positive affect, self-esteem and overall satisfaction with life (Kernis & Goldman 2006, Wood et al 2008). Other research findings indicate that high levels of subjective true self-awareness predicts lower levels of stress and anxiety. One study explored these findings further and found that individuals high in subjective true self-awareness report greater daily satisfaction with their lives and were protected from the negative longitudinal effects of daily interpersonal conflicts on their well-being (Wickham et al 2016). In addition, where individuals have higher levels of subjective true self-awareness there was a greater daily satisfaction of basic psychological needs (Heppner et al 2008) and increased reports of seeing life as meaningful (Schlegel & Hicks 2011). There is therefore considerable evidence to support the association between subjective awareness of our own true self and mental health well-being (Vess 2019).

Recent research has started to make important theoretical discoveries on the nature, experience and mechanisms that shape true self-awareness. Research has started to move away from the associated subjective true self-awareness and mental health well-being to exploring the basic psychological processes that influence individuals' sense of knowing who they truly are (Vess 2019). One such study found that the crossover of who people think they are and the way they behave had minimal impact on their sense of true self (Fleeson & Wilt 2010). Feelings of true self were instead linked to certain characteristics such as extraversion, even if individuals did not view those traits as revealing who they truly are. These findings imply that individuals' sense of being who they truly are may reflect a subjective feeling state facilitated by certain types of subjective experiences (Schmader & Sedikides 2018, Sedikides et al 2017), rather than a link between self-awareness and behaviour. Therefore research indicates that individuals' sense of connection to and awareness of their true self is strongly associated with mental health well-being and these feelings can be shaped by subjective or life experiences (Schmader & Sedikides 2018, Sedikides et al 2017). Thus within different environments self-awareness plays a significant role in maintaining safe and optimal participation in activities of daily living.

Certain clinical conditions result in deficits in self-awareness (Bloomfield et al 2016, Reich et al 2015, Robertson & Schmitter-Edgecombe 2015, Shany-Ur et al 2014), such as traumatic brain injury, stroke, dementia, Parkinson's disease and multiple sclerosis. Bach and David (2006) reviewed the literature on self-awareness deficits after acquired brain injury and found that lack of social self-awareness was a predictor of behavioural disturbance. These findings were independent of cognitive and executive function. Such deficits can persist for months, even years, after severe injury and greatly impede the rehabilitation process (Prigatano 2005). Equally, impaired self-awareness can affect functional recovery after stroke (Fleming et al 1996). As a result, after a stroke people are less likely to regain independence in self-care and mobility (Ekstam et al 2007, Hartman-Maeir et al 2002).

Self-awareness re-education may help to restore normality. Strategy training, which involves setting goals to address self-awareness deficits for people after a stroke, has been shown to improve overall ability to achieve activities of daily living (Skidmore et al 2015). Secondary analysis of the data was carried out to explore whether self-awareness influenced the persons' response to strategy training by measuring changes in independence over time (Skidmore et al 2018). The study concluded that people with self-awareness deficits achieved greater independence after strategy training compared with those who did not receive the training.

THEORIES BEHIND SELF-AWARENESS

Authors have structured self-awareness in different ways. Stevens (1971) divided it into three parts: an outer world of sensory information, one inner world of feelings (visceral and emotional) and a second inner world of mental activity (thoughts and images). Burnard (1997) sees the internal part as corresponding with Jung's four functions of the mind (thinking, feeling, sensing and intuiting), to which he adds a visceral component which includes muscle tension and body relaxation. The external part refers to what other people

see: our verbal and non-verbal behaviour together with other aspects of the way we present ourselves.

To Tschudin (1991), the inner world consists of thoughts and emotions and the outer world of people and environments, with a 'go-between' world relating to the senses. A further version of this categorization appears in the current development of Wellness Centres in Thailand (Pothongsunun 2006). These focus on an awareness of what has to be managed to maintain physical and mental health. Their key feature is self-image consisting, in this case, of sensation, feeling, thought and movement. Sensation includes the five senses plus a proprioceptive component which registers the body's orientation in space. It also includes perception of pain and the passage of time. Feeling covers the field of emotions such as joy, anger, grief and self-respect. Thinking embraces all cognitive functions: intellectual, intuitive, and moral as well as imagination and memory. Finally, movement includes all actions of the body, from breathing to athletics.

A composite view is presented in Fig. 17.1. The inner aspect covers thinking, intuition, emotions and body

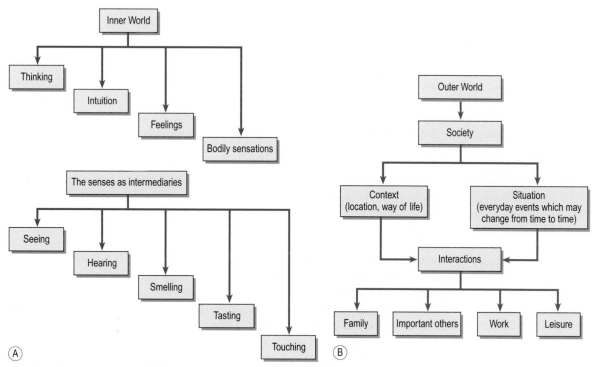

Fig. 17.1 ■ Aspects of the self. (A) represents the inner aspect and (B) represents the outer aspect.

sensations, which include those of muscle tension; the outer aspect refers to the way we relate to other people and to society in general. The social level refers to the context of our lives as well as the events which take place on a daily basis. On an individual level, it refers to the way we relate to our work, family and important others, including the way we spend our leisure time. Allowing us to experience the world are the five senses, which can be seen to play an intermediate role.

Self-awareness exercises are essentially of the mind, being concerned with the thoughts in the head. The approach is thus underpinned by cognitive theory; it also has a behavioural component. Exercises presented here are adapted from a variety of sources.

EXERCISES IN SELF-AWARENESS

Awareness of Thinking Style

We have different ways of thinking; sometimes we think in a vertical or focused way, as when doing arithmetic. At other times our thinking may be more inclined to a lateral style, as, for instance, when we are engaged in creative work. We also have our own personal styles of thinking: some people tend towards a cause–effect style, others to a broader canvas style.

Other modes of thinking relate to self-esteem. For example, thinking strategies which direct the individual into areas likely to lead to successful outcomes are associated with high self-esteem, whereas those which direct the person into areas with a low probability of success tend to be associated with low self-esteem (Fox 1997). Self-esteem can also be promoted by attributing successful outcomes to one's own efforts and poor outcomes to external factors over which one had no control (Blaine & Crocker 1993).

Or again, thinking can be influenced by the individual's health locus of control (see Chapter 1): an internal locus, with its accompanying sense of self-reliance, seems to be related to high self-esteem, whereas an external locus seems to be related to lower levels of self-esteem (Fox 1997). Although our self-esteem owes much to value systems set up by the culture and society we belong to, it is also governed by our use of self-serving strategies such as the way we present ourselves (Carless & Fox 2003). To Carless and Fox, low self-esteem is more a defect in the use of self-enhancement strategies than a reflection of any deep sense of disregard.

Individuals can review their own style in the following manner:

Take a few moments off to make a list of the thoughts that are going through your head and the dialogue that accompanies them. Write them down. Repeat this twice later in the day. Compare the items on your three lists and notice if a pattern emerges. Is some particular thought claiming your attention? If so, how do you approach it? Do you see it as a problem to be solved or do you let it dominate you? If you are trying to solve it, are you using a focused method or are you keeping your mind open and receptive to fresh ideas? Both approaches are useful. Do you have a tendency to favour one more than the other?

Do you tend to think in ways which enhance your self-esteem such as steering the self in directions likely to lead to success? Or do you tend to cling to areas where success is less likely to occur? Do you make a point of interpreting outcomes in ways which show yourself in the best possible light or do you let negative interpretations assert themselves?

Again, do you see most problems as being surmountable and, to some extent, within your control? Or do you, generally speaking, feel yourself to be a pawn in the hands of fate and a victim of events? This is an opportunity to examine your attitude towards yourself and to ask if it is serving you well.

Awareness of Intuitive Powers

Our glorification of the rational has all but eclipsed the imagination in everyday affairs. We distrust intuition or, at best, give it short shrift. Our belief in the undeniable value of logical thinking does not, however, mean we must stifle the imagination, and those who underestimate its power may do so at their peril for it communicates with the inner self.

Sit quietly and allow yourself to become relaxed. Follow your breathing, and next time you breathe out, release all your tension in a long sigh. Scan your body, checking that all your muscles are relaxed. Imagine yourself in a place of beauty and peace. Allow your thoughts to drift in and out. Focus on a matter that has been claiming your attention recently … keep it light … there's no compulsion to resolve it at this moment … just listen to yourself … tune into yourself … be receptive to any ideas that float into your head … listen to your gut feeling; you can judge its merits later … just be open to yourself … When you are ready, bring your visualization to an end.

Awareness of Feelings (Emotions)

The capacity to use our mental abilities is strongly influenced by the emotional state of the individual, whose thinking brain can be overwhelmed, even paralyzed by the emotional brain (Goleman 1996). Goleman emphasizes the importance of self-awareness in this area.

To focus on emotions need not be seen as self-indulgence. Rather, it is a form of self-examination which can provide us with insights and perhaps indicate useful paths of change. Although our emotions may be said to enrich our lives on the one hand, they give us trouble on the other; some feelings can be so strong that they cloud our judgement and others may be so uncomfortable that we repress the thought that gives rise to them. Anger and grief are two examples.

The handling of emotions requires skills which we have in varying degrees. In this connection Heron (1977) has picked out some salient points, which include the following:

The degree to which we are aware of our emotional patterns

Whether we are inclined to express ourselves in controlled or in spontaneous ways

Our tendency either to share our feelings with other people or to withhold them.

1. Awareness of Emotional Patterns

We need to recognize our feeling patterns and tendencies to react in certain ways. Only when we are aware of them can we see how they may be influencing our behaviour.

2. Control or Spontaneity

Many situations require us to hide our feelings, but there are other occasions when a more spontaneous response is called for. Whether we express our emotion or hold it back is governed not only by the circumstances but also by our general inclination. Some individuals have a tendency to respond in one way rather than another. If so, are they aware of it?

3. Sharing Our Feelings

Self-disclosure is part of the process of deepening a relationship and this applies whether the individual is making the disclosure or listening to another making theirs. Although the sharing of feelings involves taking a risk, the relationship is unlikely to develop without it. Most relationships are enriched by some degree of self-disclosure; the extent to which it occurs depends partly on the nature of the relationship and partly on the inclination of the individual. Are they inclined to share their feelings?

Awareness of the Body

From time to time, the body needs attention. In between, we spend periods of varying length without giving it a thought. Breathing, digestion, skin sensations can all be ignored; muscle tension also passes unnoticed. If we are interested in reducing muscle tension, it can be useful to make a point of listening to the body occasionally:

Allow your thoughts to focus on your body. Notice any sensations, such as stomach rumblings, joint discomfort, itches or the tendency to sigh … things you normally disregard as you concentrate on your work. Perhaps you are also ignoring feelings of tension in your muscles, in your back, your shoulders, your face or your writing arm … try focusing on those areas and releasing the tension … realize that you could just as easily increase it … try for a moment deliberately exaggerating the tension in the muscles … notice that you have the power to switch it on or off … simply by making a conscious effort you can increase or decrease those feelings of tension. Explore that idea for a few moments.

Awareness of the Environment

This aspect of the self is concerned with information from the five senses: sight, sound, smell, taste and touch. Much of this activity never gets through to our consciousness, which may be to our advantage if we are concentrating on a piece of work. However, it is through our senses that we experience our environment and are able to relate to the world.

Sit on your own. Allow the breath out to carry all your tensions with it. Bring your mind to focus on

what is happening around you: the sounds inside the building and outside … the smells of the kitchen/ office/shop/classroom/factory … the taste of the coffee you just drank … the arrangement of the furniture in the room … the colour of the decoration … the temperature of the room … the feel of the chair underneath you, the pen or the peeler in your hand … focus on each one separately for a few moments. If you are driving, notice the countryside. If you are waiting in a bus queue, pick out the different sounds in the street … if you are walking to the letterbox, notice the front gardens along the way …

Notice how the exercise has the effect of taking you away from your preoccupations and giving you an acute experience of the present moment.

Awareness of the Way We Relate to Others

People can only know about us from what we show of ourselves: our appearance, general demeanour and what we say. These are outer aspects of the individual and disclose much or little of the inner self, depending on the level of intimacy. All that can be known about a person is what they consciously or unconsciously reveal, thus what we reveal is important since it establishes our identity in the world. Our behaviour, whether verbal or non-verbal, creates us as individuals in other people's eyes.

Verbal behaviour refers to the actual words spoken. Non-verbal behaviour includes aspects of speech such as tone of voice, timing, emphasis, accent (paralinguistic features), as well as facial expression, eye contact, gesture, posture, physical proximity, clothes and appearance (Argyle 1994). The way we respond within the interaction provides a further level of behaviour: how we prompt, cut in and listen.

ASSERTIVENESS

We also define ourselves by our readiness to be assertive or not (see Chapter 2). Assertiveness involves knowing how to advance our life goals while respecting the interests of other people. Put another way, it means insisting on having our own interests respected while other people advance their goals. For example, are we able to refuse a request which we feel is unreasonable?

Do you find it easy to say 'No' to a request in a situation where saying 'Yes' makes you feel you are being taken advantage of? Can you think of an occasion when this occurred? How did you react? Were you happy with the outcome? If not, how did you feel? In your imagination, go back to the occasion. Recreate the scene and rescript your part with you saying 'No'. What effect does this have on the other person? What effect does it have on you? Now ask yourself why you said 'Yes' in the first place. How would you deal with a similar request in the future?

Promoting a relationship while retaining a feeling of self is one of the social skills. This feeling of self is tied up with our self-esteem – that is, the degree to which we feel we have worth. Low self-esteem is linked with non-assertive behaviour, high self-esteem with assertive behaviour. To increase assertiveness, individuals need to recognize their personal strengths and qualities; they have to question the appropriateness of the role they are playing and explore new possibilities. This will give them more rewarding personal experiences.

A script for an individual assessing his or her own assertiveness (or non-assertiveness) might run as follows.

Allow yourself to feel relaxed before you begin. Run through a relaxing procedure until you feel very calm and tuned in to yourself. Let your thoughts focus on a person you know … someone you are not close to … someone with whom you have had difficulties but are obliged to see from time to time …

Let your mind gently focus on this person … let them take shape … notice how they look: their expression … what they are wearing … spend a little time creating their presence … then see yourself also, including your expression, posture and clothes, as you, in your mind's eye, greet this person.

Observe your actions … do they strike the right note? … is the conversation balanced in the sense that neither person is acting aggressively to the other's submissive behaviour? … if it is unbalanced what, if anything, do you think you should do about it? … it may be that you feel your behaviour is appropriate … on the other hand, you may wish to modify your style, to make it more assertive … you will know best what is needed in the situation…

If you decide to modify your style, consider ways in which you might begin … test these out in your imagination … notice how your new behaviour feels … spend a few minutes mentally experiencing the scene …

BENEFITS OF SELF-AWARENESS EXERCISES

The exercises described can heighten our awareness of self and the way we relate to other people. We also, in the process, deepen our self-knowledge. Through self-awareness exercises we learn to 'listen' to the self in all its aspects and to tune in to its nuances. Self-awareness exercises, by their emphasis on 'exploring, experimenting, experiencing', thus lead us to a better understanding of ourselves (Stevens 1971). However, getting to know oneself can be a painful process, and changing oneself is difficult. Even so, our efforts are rewarded by the discovery that we have more power than we realized to control our lives, a thought which itself engenders a sense of calm.

As a relaxation technique, self-awareness might be said to be at the other end of the scale from distraction (the diversion of attention away from the self). Each is effective on its own but together they complement one another, self-awareness protecting the individual from the hazards of denial while distraction protects the person from too much introspection.

KEY POINTS

1. Awareness of the self leads to an increase in self-knowledge.
2. Self-awareness helps us to see ourselves as we really are. This insight helps enhance personal relationships.
3. Being aware of the self involves living in the present, responding in the here-and-now.

This helps the individual to achieve successful outcomes.
4. Exercises to raise self-awareness are broadly classified into inner world and outer world domains – the inner concerned with thinking and feelings, the outer with how we relate to other people.
5. Through these exercises we learn to 'listen' to the self and to others.
6. Self-awareness helps us discover sources of inner strength which enhance self-confidence and peace of mind.

Reflection

Describe your understanding of the techniques of self-awareness.
How do you feel about applying this technique to practice?
How aware are you of the self?
How can you develop your sense of self?
What is the main learning point you will take away from this chapter?

CASE STUDY LEARNING OPPORTUNITY

The key points and reflection provide background and knowledge required in relation to the case study, Helen, to help deepen understanding of how self-awareness can help improve physical and mental well-being.

CASE STUDY

Fear of Saying No: Self-awareness Outcomes for Helen

Helen works on a busy surgical ward and on a weekly basis she finds that certain colleagues ask her to do some of their duties. Helen finds it extremely difficult to say no. She feels that saying no will cause an argument and that she will come across as being unhelpful and rude. However, she also feels that her colleagues are taking advantage of her. As a consequence her workload is increasing and it is causing her stress levels to rise and her health to deteriorate.

Helen now dreads going to work, and the situation is affecting her overall self-esteem and confidence. Because of a number of absences in a short period of time, Helen's line manager asked her to be assessed by the Occupational Health department to establish a phased return to work.

After the assessment Helen was advised to seek support and was booked on to an assertiveness training course. At the course Helen assessed her own level of assertiveness or lack of, and through assertiveness training Helen learnt a number of techniques and coping strategies that she could apply to her everyday life and work life. The assertiveness training taught Helen that to say no to unmanageable tasks was not rude. It also taught her how to recognize that colleagues making requests of her time and effort were just trying to shift their own responsibilities, which was unfair to her. After the training Helen became much more self-aware, and now when she is asked to complete another colleague's task she doesn't feel guilty for saying no. Crucially, Helen has learnt that it is how you say no that is important, and she uses one of her pre-prepared phrases as a coping strategy: 'I would like to, but I have to...' instead of saying yes. Helen now finds she is able to go on and complete her own tasks at work with ease of mind, finding satisfaction in her working day. She no longer feel stressed

and therefore isn't taking time off work as a result of stress-related illness.

ACTIVITY

For the case study:

1. List the key aspects used in the assertiveness training course.
2. Consider why this approach was taken.
3. Consider the effects assertiveness training had on Helen's self-awareness.
4. Write down the impact that assertiveness training is having from a psychological perspective.
5. Write down the impact that assertiveness training is having from a physical perspective.
6. Write down the impact that assertiveness training is having from an emotional perspective.
7. Consider the outcomes on quality of life and overall well-being for Helen.

Chapter 18 will focus on imagery and how it can be applied to enhance the relaxation experience.

REFERENCES

Argyle, M. (1994). *The psychology of interpersonal behaviour* (5th ed.). London: Penguin.

Bach, L. J., & David, A. S. (2006). Self-awareness after acquired and traumatic brain injury. *Neuropsychological Rehabilitation, 16*(4), 397–414.

Blaine, B., & Crocker, J. (1993). Self-esteem and self-serving biases in reactions to positive and negative events: An integrative review. In R. F. Baumeister (Ed.), *Self-esteem: The puzzle of low self-regard* (pp. 55–86). New York: Plenum.

Bloomfield, J., Woods, D., & Ludington, J. (2016). Selfawareness of memory impairment in Parkinson's disease: A review of the literature. *Working With Older People, 20*(1), 57–64.

Burnard, P. (1991). *Coping with stress in the health professions: A Practical guide.* London: Chapman and Hall.

Burnard, P. (1997). *Know yourself! Self-awareness activities for nurses and other health professionals.* London: Wiley-Blackwell.

Carless, D., & Fox, K. R. (2003). The physical self. In T. Everett, M. Donaghy, & S. Feaver (Eds.), *Interventions in mental health.* Oxford, UK: Butterworth-Heinemann.

Ekstam, L., Uppgard, B., Kottorp, A., & Tham, K. (2007). Relationship between awareness of disability and occupational performance during the first year after a stroke. *American Journal of Occupational Therapy, 61*, 503–511.

Fleeson, W., & Wilt, J. (2010). The relevance of Big Five trait content in behavior to subjective authenticity: Do high levels of within-person behavioral variability undermine or enable authenticity achievement? *Journal of Personality, 78*, 1353–1382.

Fleming, J. M., Strong, J., & Ashton, R. (1996). Self-awareness of deficits in adults with traumatic brain injury: How best to measure. *Brain Injury, 10*, 1–15.

Fox, K. R. (Ed.). (1997). *The physical self: From motivation to well-being.* Leeds, UK: Human Kinetics.

Goleman, D. (1996). *Emotional intelligence: Why it can matter more than IQ.* London: Bloomsbury, London.

Hartman-Maeir, A., Soroker, N., Ring, H., & Katz, N. (2002). Awareness of deficits in stroke rehabilitation. *Journal of Rehabilitation Medicine, 34*, 158–164.

Heppner, W. L., Kernis, M. H., Nezlek, J. B., Foster, J., Lakey, C. E., & Goldman, B. M. (2008). Within-person relationships among daily self-esteem, need satisfaction, and authenticity. *Psychological Science, 19*, 1140–1145.

Heron, J. (1977). *Catharsis in human development human potential research project.* Guildford, UK: University of Surrey.

Kernis, M. H., & Goldman, B. M. (2006). A multicomponent conceptualization of authenticity: Theory and research. In *Advances in experimental social psychology* (Vol. 38, pp. 283–357). New York: Academic Press.

Pothongsunun, P. (2006). Wellness programmes in the community. *Journal of Physiotherapy, 92*(3), 133–134.

Prigatano, G. P. (2005). Impaired self-awareness after moderately severe to severe traumatic brain injury. *Acta Neurochirurgica, 93*(Suppl.), 39–42.

Reich, E., Arias, E., Torres, C., Halac, E., & Carlino, M. (2015). Anosognosia and self-awareness in multiple sclerosis. *Journal of the Neurological Sciences, 357*(1), e317.

Robertson, K., & Schmitter-Edgecombe, M. (2015). Self-awareness and traumatic brain injury outcome. *Brain Injury, 29*(7–8), 848–858.

Schlegel, R. J., & Hicks, J. A. (2011). The true self and psychological health: Emerging evidence and future directions. *Social and Personality Psychology Compass, 5*, 989–1003.

Schmader, T., & Sedikides, C. (2018). State authenticity as fit to environment: The implications of social identity for fit, authenticity, and self-segregation. *Personality and Social Psychology Review*, *22*, 228–259.

Sedikides, C., Slabu, L., Lenton, A., & Thomaes, S. (2017). State authenticity. *Current Directions in Psychological Science*, *26*, 521–525.

Shany-Ur, T., Lin, N., Rosen, H. J., Sollberger, M., Miller, B. L., & Rankin, K. P. (2014). Selfawareness in neurodegenerative disease relies on neural structures mediating reward-driven attention. *Brain*, *137*(8), 2368–2381.

Skidmore, E. R., Dawson, D. R., Butters, M. A., et al. (2015). Strategy training shows promise for addressing disability in the first 6 months after stroke. *Neurorehabilitation and Neural Repair*, *29*, 668–676.

Skidmore, E. R., Swafford, M., Juengst, S. B., & Terhorst, L. (2018). Brief report—self-awareness and recovery of independence with strategy training. *American Journal of Occupational Therapy*, *72*, 7201345010.

Stevens, J. O. (1971). *Awareness: Exploring, experimenting, experiencing*. Moab, UT: Real People Press.

Tschudin, V. (1991). *Beginning with awareness: A learner's handbook*. Edinburgh: Churchill Livingstone.

Vess, M. (2019). Varieties of conscious experience and the subjective awareness of one's "true" self. *Review of General Psychology*, *23*(1), 89–98.

West, M. A. (2016). *The psychology of meditation: Research and practice*. New York: Oxford University Press.

Wickham, R. E., Williamson, R. E., Beard, C. L., Kobayashi, C. L. B., & Hirst, T. W. (2016). Authenticity attenuates the negative effects of interpersonal conflict on daily well-being. *Journal of Research in Personality*, *60*(Suppl. C), 56–62.

Wood, A. M., Linley, A. P., Maltby, J., Baliousis, M., & Joseph, S. (2008). The authentic personality: A theoretical and empirical conceptualization and the development of the authenticity scale. *Journal of Counseling Psychology*, *55*, 385–399.

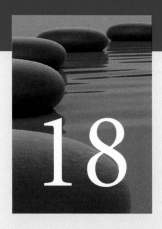

18

IMAGERY

DR CAROLINE BELCHAMBER

LEARNING OBJECTIVES

The aim of this chapter is to understand how the use of imagery can enhance the relaxation experience.

By the end of this chapter you will be able to:

1. Understand the theory behind imagery.

2. Appreciate the evidence underpinning imagery.

3. Recognize the different types of imagery.

4. Identify core aspects of the procedure in delivering imagery as a relaxation technique.

5. Understand the therapeutic effects of imagery.

6. Discern how imagery is applied in practice.

This chapter will conclude with key points and time for reflection, providing learning opportunities through a case study.

INTRODUCTION TO IMAGERY

This chapter is addressed to health care professionals who wish to use imagery to enhance the relaxation experience. It is different from the use of imagery in psychotherapy and other forms of counselling, where it may be used to get in touch with repressed thoughts and feelings. The aim of imagery, as represented in this chapter, is to encourage people to have positive emotions.

Imagery has already been mentioned during discussion of breathing, passive relaxation, the Alexander technique and self-awareness. Here imagery is considered in its own right.

Achterberg (2002) defines imagery as 'the thought process that invokes and uses the senses'. Sight, sound, smell, taste and touch modalities can all be involved in this activity, which may take place in the absence of any external stimulus. It could be said that imagery is thinking in pictures as opposed to thinking with words.

The importance of the image was underlined by Aristotle, who said that without it thought is impossible. Einstein also found imagery an essential component of thought. It is particularly associated with the creative aspect of thinking. However, we are forming images all the time, whether making plans for the future, remembering items from the past or creating fantasy in realms beyond our experience.

How can imagery relieve stress? A cognitive explanation was advanced by Dossey (1988), who suggested that imagery brought about a change in the individual's perceptions. Many researchers, on the other hand, consider that the mechanism lies in the distraction created by the pleasant imagery, which can divert the mind from intrusive thoughts. There are also physiological explanations; for example, McCance and Heuther (2014) proposed that pleasant images could trigger the release of endorphins and create an analgesic effect. This supports Melzack and Wall's (1983) theory whereby pain messages are blocked from consciousness by a 'gate' mechanism, which shuts them off when the neural pathways are loaded with other information (which may include imagery).

Imagery is a safe, non-invasive and inexpensive procedure that requires no elaborate equipment. It is often employed together with other mind–body techniques as an adjunct to medical and psychological treatment, and sometimes as sole therapy in the self-management of some mild conditions.

INTRODUCTION TO EVIDENCE

Imagery alone has rarely been studied as a treatment (Luskin et al 2000). It is usually combined with muscle relaxation techniques in the treatment of clinical conditions. For example, Cupal and Brewer (2001) found significantly less pain and re-injury anxiety after a course of relaxation and imagery among individuals undergoing rehabilitation after anterior cruciate reconstruction; and Johnson (2000) showed that the

mood levels of competitive adults with long-term injuries could be significantly raised by relaxation and guided imagery. Sordoni and colleagues (2002) discuss different kinds of imagery in relation to athletic injury (See Chapter 29).

Evidence supports the effectiveness of guided imagery in the relief of stress, anxiety and depression, and has therefore been used as a treatment strategy for these conditions. The use of guided imagery has been reported to decrease stress, anxiety and fatigue in self-reported measures and neuroendocrine measures of stress, such as cortisol in non-pregnant women (Jallo et al 2014, Watanabe et al 2006). Guided imagery has also been shown to be effective for the management of nausea and pain (Wood & Patricolo 2013).

Guided imagery is a form of mind–body technique which is often used in the care of patients with cancer. Roffe et al (2005) conducted a systematic review to determine the effectiveness of guided imagery in the treatment of symptoms resulting from chemotherapy, such as nausea and vomiting. The researchers in this case found no strong evidence to indicate effectiveness of the intervention, although they found some evidence to suggest that the imagery increased comfort and provided psychological support. However, a more recent study of people with prostate and breast cancer undergoing chemotherapy treatment were seen to benefit from progressive muscle relaxation and guided imagery (Charalambous et al 2015). Imagery training as an adjuvant therapy has also been found to reduce depression in community-dwelling cancer patients living in Sydney (Sloman 2002).

Halpin et al (2002) investigated the effects of guided imagery on cardiac surgery patients in a study in the USA, and found that patients who practised the method had a shorter length of hospital stay and took fewer pain-killers than patients who did not practise it. This supports the earlier work of Tusek and Cwynar (2000), who found that imagery enhanced the experience of hospital patients.

Pain is an area which has attracted much research. Here imagery has been used successfully in a wide range of conditions, including postoperative pain (Laurion & Fetzer 2003), fibromyalgia (Fors et al 2002) and osteoarthritis (Baird & Sands 2004). Imagery has also been found useful in studies with children. A randomized controlled trial compared a combination of imagery and progressive relaxation with breathing routines in children with abdominal pain. The results indicated significantly fewer days with pain in the imagery group than in the breathing group (Weydert 2006). In these and other conditions it has been shown to be an effective self-management strategy for reducing the intensity of pain.

Further evidence of the benefit of imagery may be found in Chapter 29 where reported trials involve the use of imagery and help to justify its widespread use in the clinical field.

THEORIES BEHIND IMAGERY

Although the precise mechanism of imagery is unknown, it is believed to involve the right cerebral hemisphere, which includes the theoretical concept of (1) laterality, (2) the unconscious mind and (3) the inner guide.

Laterality

The cerebral cortex is divided into two hemispheres, each of which has four lobes: frontal, parietal, temporal and occipital. Research indicates that the hemispheres have specialized roles (Fig. 18.1). The left hemisphere is believed to process logical thought and language. It is involved in linear, analytic and rational thinking, reading, writing and mathematical activity, and is normally the dominant hemisphere. The right hemisphere is seen as dealing with information of a non-rational nature, being concerned with creative thinking, fantasy, metaphor, imagery, dreams, analogies, intuition and emotion, including feelings of stress, and is normally

the non-dominant hemisphere. However, it is believed to acquire dominance during altered states of consciousness – that is, states of mental functioning which seem different to the individual from the ordinary pattern experienced by the person (Atkinson et al 1999). Deep relaxation is one such state. Others include dreaming, drug-induced states, hypnosis, meditation, daydreaming and guided imagery. During these states, the influence of the left brain is reduced, which allows material from the right hemisphere, normally hidden, to become accessible. Thus the altered state is seen as providing a path to the interior of the self.

Lyman et al (1980) claim to have found a connection between images and emotions, having shown experimentally that emotionally charged situations are more likely than neutral ones to be accompanied by imagery. They posit a direct relationship between the right hemisphere (which is associated with imagery) and the autonomic system (which governs the physiological responses associated with emotion).

The link between imagery and physiological processes can be demonstrated by imagining a lemon (Barber et al 1964).

> *Visualize its exterior shape, colour, scent and texture; then slice it across the middle, look at the pale, glistening flesh, squeeze it gently and watch the juice dripping from it; take the cut end to your mouth and lick it. Notice your mouth watering.*

Electromyographic recordings also demonstrate associations between visualization and physiological activity: positive imagery has been shown to lower muscle tension levels, and negative imagery to raise them (Jacobson 1938, McGuigan 1971).

In applying these findings, it is suggested that a useful approach to stress relief and relaxation is through methods which involve the right hemisphere (Davis et al 2000).

The Unconscious

Freud (1973) viewed the unconscious as a repository of repressed fears and unresolved emotions. It thus represented aspects of ourselves which we wished to forget. Its contents were only available in certain states, such as dreaming, when the conscious mind was less dominant. A Jungian view of the unconscious, however, saw it as also

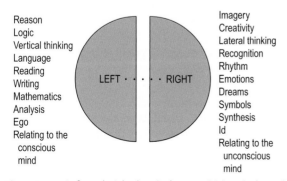

Reason
Logic
Vertical thinking
Language
Reading
Writing
Mathematics
Analysis
Ego
Relating to the conscious mind

LEFT · · · · RIGHT

Imagery
Creativity
Lateral thinking
Recognition
Rhythm
Emotions
Dreams
Symbols
Synthesis
Id
Relating to the unconscious mind

Fig. 18.1 ■ Left and right hemisphere activities. (Adapted from Shone 1996.)

containing the seed of infinite new possibilities deriving from insight, intuition and inspiration (Fordham 1966, Jung 1963). Thus, although Freud viewed it in negative terms, Jung's view was primarily positive.

Whatever their theoretical position, writers generally agree that the unconscious operates not with the language of logic, but through pictures, emotions, senses, symbols and imagery – that is, the concerns of the right hemisphere. Hidden and elusive, the unconscious does not lend itself to direct investigation, either from the scientist or from the self-analyzing individual. It is this quality of elusiveness that moves Jung to speak of the difficulty of penetrating one's own being. His archetypal figures (earth mother, wise man, persona, shadow, anima and animus) are the expression of attempts to find new ways of gaining access to the unconscious.

The Inner Guide

Arising out of these ideas is the concept of the 'inner guide', a mental construct that links the individual with their inner self. In its role as channeller of information from the unconscious, the inner guide may be seen as the personification of the intuitive self. It can take forms other than those of archetypal figures, and may appear as any person or animal whose attributes have appealed to the individual's imagination.

Typically the inner guide evolves in the mind during a session of deep relaxation, using an imagined setting of rich sensory quality. Oyle (1976) suggests a place of peace and beauty, such as a mountain lake or a natural grotto, whereas Ferrucci (1982) prefers an Alpine peak reached after an arduous climb. A figure is conjured up; it advances slowly. The visualizer welcomes the approaching figure, noticing everything about it: what it looks like, how it is dressed, who, if anyone, it resembles. A dialogue ensues. Ferrucci warns against the possibility of the guide being no more than a self-deceiving fantasy and suggests criteria for testing its authenticity.

- Does it bring answers which come from the self?
- Does it bring understanding?
- Does it carry a sense of rightness?
- Does its message make sense in the light of reason and morality?
- Will its advice stand up in real-life situations?

Even after acceptance of the guide as authentic, its advice should always be scrutinized and not blindly accepted. Although the guide is an aspect of the inner self, it may not be working in the individual's best interests. On the other hand, too sceptical an attitude will tend to generate fewer ideas than a trusting one.

The individual need not feel restricted to one guide and may find it useful to have one male and one female, each supplying complementary wisdom. A hazard of working with a number of inner guides, however, is that the personality may come to be seen as a collection of separate entities when the aim of the exercise is to achieve integration.

Any meeting with an inner guide should be rounded off with words of gratitude, respect and appreciation, as this helps strengthen the individual's respect for their inner self. Continuity also is important and may be established by a contract to meet on another occasion.

THERAPEUTIC EFFECTS OF IMAGERY

Imagery can be used in a therapeutic sense to promote the following:

- Self-development and psychological change: self-statements or affirmations. These effects are expanded in Chapter 19.
- Relaxation. Zahourek (1988), working in a nursing context, sees imagery as a therapeutic tool which can reinforce the message to relax and has been confirmed by Rankin (2003).
- Healing. This is an area not covered in the present work.

PROCEDURE OF A THERAPEUTIC IMAGERY SESSION

Relaxation

For the imagery to be effective, the individual should first be in a state of relaxation. Fanning (1988) regards relaxation as 'an absolute prerequisite' of effective imagery. The individual may use any method found to be helpful, but passive approaches are seen as being the most appropriate (Achterberg 2002). Thus relaxation is a precondition as well as a result of therapeutic imagery.

Introductory Remarks to Participants

As with other approaches, a short passage of explanation is necessary.

Imagery is about building pictures in the mind. The pictures can be pleasant or unpleasant. The first kind induce a feeling of calm, the second, of unease.

The relaxing effect of pleasant imagery is partly due to the distraction it creates from stressful thoughts. Day-dreaming is an example of this kind of imagery. However, the imagination can also bring us nearer to our inner selves, and this aspect of it is used to help people discover new possibilities within themselves, thereby enriching their lives. This kind of imagery is more structured than day-dreaming.

You'll find it helpful to make yourself relaxed before you begin.

Exercises in Imagery

Exercises which use different kinds of imagery are then presented. They may include any of the following:

- Single sense
- Imagery as symbol
- Imagery as metaphor
- Colour imagery
- Guided imagery

Termination

A session of imagery should be gradually brought to an end. First, the image is deliberately allowed to fade. Then the visualizer slowly brings the attention back to the room in which he or she is lying, and in time opens his or her eyes. In the next few minutes the participant gives the limbs a gentle stretch and then resumes normal activity.

EXPLORING SINGLE SENSES

Some people find it easier than others to conjure up images. Not only do people differ in the vividness and clarity of the images they create, but they also differ in their ability to control the image once formed (Finke 1989). Image making is thus a skill with more than one facet.

There is some evidence to suggest that image forming can be improved with practice, although the extent of any such improvement has not been determined (Kosslyn 1984, Lichstein 1988). Nevertheless, exercises are often used in the belief that they help to develop innate potential. A difficulty in imaging should not, however, be seen as a deficit, but rather as a manifestation of the many ways in which human beings differ from one another. People who report difficulty in forming images may also describe a sensation which fulfils the same function in their thought processes.

For those who wish to explore their capacity to create images, however, the following exercises are presented. They use the modalities of sight, sound, smell, taste, touch, temperature and kinaesthetic sense. A total of 15 to 20 seconds can be spent on each item.

Sight

Visualize:

- A shape: circle/triangle/square
- An oak tree
- A snail
- A sailing boat
- A button
- A strand of hair

Sound

Because auditory images tend to be less dominant than visual ones, it can be useful, when evoking the former, to surround oneself with an imaginary mist or darkness which swallows up any visual images and releases sounds in isolation. Imagine:

- The wind blowing through the trees/through river sedges/through sheets on a clothesline
- The ring of your telephone
- Different people calling your name
- Horses' hooves on different surfaces: cobblestone/tarmac/hard sand/deep mud
- Scales played on the piano
- Traffic starting off
- Water flowing along a rocky stream bed/lapping on a lakeshore/cascading from a height

Smell

Slowly conjure up, one by one, the following smells:

- Thyme trodden underfoot
- Petrol fumes
- Newly baked bread
- Hyacinth scent
- Chlorine
- New mown grass
- Vanilla

Taste

Imagine the taste of the following:

- Sprouts
- Figs
- Banana
- Mayonnaise
- Grapefruit
- Toothpaste

Touch

Let other sensory images fade as you turn your attention to those of touch. Evoke the following tactile images:

- Shaking hands
- Standing barefoot on loose/dry sand
- Running your fingers over satin/velvet/sacking
- Brushing past fur
- Holding a smooth pebble
- Threading a needle

Temperature

Imagine sensations of hot and cold:

- Drinking a hot liquid
- Sunlight falling on your arm
- Moving from a warm room to a cool one
- Holding an ice cube
- Stepping into a warm bath

Kinaesthetic Sense

This sense is the perception of body movement. Feel yourself engaged in a form of activity:

- Swimming
- Running on grass
- Sawing wood
- Throwing a ball
- Climbing a sand dune
- Hanging a coat on a peg
- Stirring syrup

Imagery Drawn From All Sense Modalities

Fanning (1988) suggests an exercise which draws on a variety of sense modalities.

Take a fruit that you like, say an orange. Feel its texture … weight … size … notice its shape … colour and surface markings … is it firm or soft? … smell it … then dig your nail into the peel and begin to tear it off. Listen to the faint sound of the tearing. As you peel the orange, notice how the flesh gets exposed here and there, releasing a new smell. Separate the segments and put one in your mouth … bite through its juicy flesh … feel the sensation of the juice running over your tongue … recognize the taste of orange …

From this exercise it can be seen that variety of sensory detail helps to build a vivid mental image. When we visualize a scene we usually draw on more than one sense modality, and we can make the scene still more vivid by adding further sensory information. Images of sight, sound, smell, texture, temperature and the sensation of body movement can all be used to enrich the mental picture. Guided imagery (See Page 214) develops these ideas.

SYMBOLIC IMAGERY

Jung (1963) writes that symbols serve to connect us with the unconscious; they are keys which can unlock the deeper parts of the psyche. Symbols also feature in the writings of Assagioli, where he notes the tendency for people to project meaningful ideas onto them. One of Assagioli's (1965) best-known examples is his visualization of a rose, paraphrased here:

Picture in your mind a rose bush … see its root … its stem … its leaves. Crowning the stem is a rose in tight bud. See it folded inside its protective sepals. As you watch, the sepals begin to roll back, revealing the closed flower, firmly and intricately packed … gradually, the petals begin to unfold and as they do, you may feel a blossoming also taking place within you … the rose continues to open and as you gaze at it, and smell its perfume, perhaps you can feel its rhythm resonating with your own rhythm … stay with the rose, and as it opens further, revealing its centre, allow an image to take shape – one that represents whatever is creative and meaningful within you … focus on the image … and let it speak to you …

The symbol is seen here as a phenomenon to be experienced rather than decoded. It is suggested that by identifying with the symbol, the individual can discover new aspects of themselves. This idea has been developed by Ferrucci, a student of Assagioli's. Two examples of Ferrucci's visualizations (1982) are presented next (in slightly altered form).

The Fount

Imagine a rocky cleft in which a natural spring rises. It is a warm summer day. See the bubbling jet of water sparkling in the sunlight … listen to its gurgling and splashing … the water is clear and pure … cup your hands and drink from it … imagine the liquid travelling down your throat and into your body … in your mind's eye step into the spring and feel the water flowing over you … your feet, legs and the whole of your body … imagine it also flowing through your thoughts … and through your emotions … feel the water cleansing you … let its purity unite with your purity … let its energy become your energy … and as the fount continues to renew itself, feel life within you also renewing itself …

The Bell

Picture a meadow on a warm day. Perhaps you are lying in the soft grass, surrounded by scented wildflowers. In a nearby village church, a bell begins to peal. The sound it makes is pure and clear, and as it reaches you, it seems to arouse within you a deep, hidden joy … the sound fades for a moment as the wind changes … then … it returns … carried back to you, this time with renewed force … filling the air

and echoing through the valley … and as you listen, the sound seems to vibrate inside you … resonating with your own melody … and awakening new possibilities within you …

THE USE OF METAPHOR

Imagery lies at the heart of metaphor. Metaphor itself, by describing one thing in terms of another, offers a fresh approach – a new and more telling interpretation.

Three items which illustrate the use of metaphor in relaxation imagery follow. In each one, the individual identifies with the image.

The Rag Doll

Sit in an armchair. Close your eyes. Take one deep breath low down in your chest. Then let your breathing set its own rhythm … listen to it … and as you listen to it, imagine a rag doll … see its soft floppy arms and legs … its lolling head … its slumped body … inert … immobile.

Now, try seeing yourself as that rag doll. Conjure up a feeling of being slumped … the weight of your arms dragging your shoulders down … your head rolling into the chairback … your face expressionless … your jaw relaxed … feel the passive quality of the rag doll … and as you continue to sit there … enjoy the feeling of being passive …

The Fragment of Seaweed

Lie down in a quiet place. Close your eyes. Breathe in deeply once … then relax into the rhythm of your natural breathing …

Picture a length of seaweed, rich, dark green, leafy seaweed, floating in the shallows. Air pockets keep it buoyant and allow it to bob up and down. As it floats, it changes shape, drawn this way and that as the currents swirl beneath it … pulling it … twisting it … stretching it … bunching it …

Now, picture yourself as that piece of seaweed … notice how limp your body feels … your outstretched arms and legs gently swept to and fro … imagine the wave passing underneath you … lifting you up as it rises, and lowering you as it dips, but always buoying you up … feel your body giving to the movement of the water …

The Jelly

Settle yourself in a peaceful place. Close your eyes and listen to your breathing … listen to it getting calmer with every moment that passes …

Imagine a jelly not quite set. It has been turned out of its mould and stands, holding itself together but not yet firm. Every time the plate is moved, it wobbles.

Now, think of yourself as that jelly. You are standing on a dish, and every time someone knocks the table, a ripple runs through you. You yourself are not able to initiate the movement; only others can do that by bumping into your table or moving your dish … and, every time this happens, you wobble. One bump, and you wobble several times … imagine you are about to be bumped into … feel your body limp … let all the tension go out of it … let yourself become a wobbly jelly …

Transformations

Images can also undergo transformations: harsh images can give way to smooth ones. Fanning (1988) shows how negative emotions, represented by harsh images, can be influenced to move in a more positive direction, when the harsh images are transformed into smooth ones.

Imagine the sound of discordant music … listen to its harsh tones … and as you do, let your painful thought express itself in terms of the dissonant notes … feel the mood of your difficulty resonating with the sound. Then gradually allow the image to undergo a transformation … follow the music as it slowly resolves into harmonies … and, as the harmonies fill the air, experience the beginnings of a change in your feelings …

Other examples of negative imagery resolving into more pleasant forms include the following:

- Sour lemon juice into sweet lemon sorbet
- Sandpaper into silky fabric

The previous two examples come from Fanning (1988). The next two are drawn from Davis et al (2008):

- A screaming siren into a woodwind melody
- The glare of a searchlight into the soft glow of a lamp

Four of the sense modalities (taste, touch, sound and sight) are represented in these examples. The fifth, smell, is illustrated in the transformation from burning rubber into smouldering pine logs.

These are simply examples. The most effective imagery is that which the individual creates for themselves, choosing the context to which they can best relate.

Distancing

The distress caused by unpleasant events can be overwhelming. Moreover, the intensity of the emotion aroused by them may cloud the individual's judgement. To gain a more objective view, they may find it useful to draw back from the scene mentally: in effect, to distance themself. Certain images promote the feeling of being able to put a distance between themselves and the situation:

- A leaf floating downstream
- Clouds moving across the sky
- Helium-filled balloons rising
- Bubbles being blown away
- A train receding along a straight track

COLOUR

People say they have favourite colours. Is this because certain colours make them feel good? And is this governed by the association that those colours have with pleasant events in their lives? It is generally believed that red is a stimulating colour and blue a soothing one, but to what extent is the preference for one over the other tied up with the mood of the moment? Such notions might help to explain why a person does not always choose the same colour. Or do they simply become sated with one colour and feel the need to replace it with another (as in decorations, clothes, etc.)? These are psychological considerations, although the aesthetic aspects of colour give the topic a further dimension.

However, in the present context we are concerned with psychological aspects. Certainly colours can create strong effects. Some of these can be explored through exercises in colour imagery. The following example is adapted from the work of an autogenic therapist, Kai Kermani (1990).

With your eyes closed let the word 'colour' float into your mind. The word may first evoke one particular colour, although others will quickly follow. Take the one that first appears. Stay with it. Let it develop in any way it wants to: flooding your field of vision, appearing in patches, little flecks or any other arrangement. Concentrate on the colour in a passive way, letting it speak to you. Does it remind you of anything? Does it trigger any special feelings or memories? If it has no effect on you, try 'stepping into' it and allowing it to surround you … notice any effect it now has on you …

After a few minutes, or when you are ready, allow the colour to draw itself away from you. In your mind's eye, watch it resuming the form it had in the beginning.

If colour can indeed influence our mood, then colour visualization could have particular value. We could mentally surround ourselves with single colours to gain specific effects, soothing our feelings when we are anxious and raising our mood when we are depressed. Single colours are again explored in the following two exercises.

Imagine finding yourself in a room decorated exclusively in a colour of your choice. See the entire room in this one colour, the walls, ceiling, paintwork, carpet, upholstery. If you have difficulty, try going through the motions of painting the walls and hanging the curtains. Totally immerse yourself in this colour and notice the effect it has on you … does it relax you or give you a lift? … why did you pick it? … what associations does it have for you? … stay with it long enough to absorb its full effect … then let it fade.

Now picture yourself in a room decorated in a colour you don't like … Surround yourself with this colour, let it permeate your consciousness (so long as it doesn't disturb you, in which case stop the exercise) … Ask yourself why you dislike this colour and what effect it is having on you … When you are ready, let the colour fade and be replaced by the colour of your choice before ending the visualization.

It is preferable to end colour imagery sessions with a colour that the visualizer feels comfortable with to carry away a rewarding sensation.

Ernst and Goodison (1981) present a sequence in which colour flows to and from the visualizer. It is reproduced here in modified form.

First relax yourself using any method you find works for you. Close your eyes if they are not already closed. Let your mind be as still as possible. Pick a colour that feels right for you. Pick it spontaneously and see it before your eyes. You can picture it as brushstrokes of paint, coloured cloth, tinted smoke or coloured atmosphere. Let it extend all round you. Notice its quality, its tone and be aware of any associations it has for you. Feel yourself relating to this colour, harmonizing with it, becoming infused with it. Imagine yourself absorbing the colour through every pore of your skin until your body is filled with it …

Now … let the colour begin to radiate from you … feel yourself releasing it … making it expand all round you until it gradually comes to fill the room you are in. As you continue to generate more colour, see if you can fill the building you are in … pause for a moment … then slowly begin to draw the colour back, first from the building … then from the room … watching it get more condensed … until it gathers in a cloud around you … feel yourself bathed in this colour … now … absorb it back into your being … into the very organs of your body … pause again … then watch it drawing itself away from all parts of you … feel yourself being emptied of the colour. Convert it back to the paint, cloth or smoke in which it started. Be aware of how you feel after doing the exercise. Notice any effect it had on you.

Chakras

In hatha yoga, vital energy is seen as being focused in specified areas of the body known as 'chakras'. These are situated at the following locations:

- Base of the spine
- Lower abdomen
- Navel
- Heart
- Throat
- Brow
- Crown of the head.

Each chakra is associated with one of the colours of the spectrum: the base of the spine with red, the lower abdomen with orange, the navel with yellow, the heart with green, the throat with blue, the brow with indigo and the crown of the head with violet.

Kermani (1990) presents a passage of healing imagery based on the chakras, which is reproduced here in slightly altered form.

See yourself lying in a natural setting of your choice. The sun is shining and it is warm and pleasant. Look around you … build the scene. What plants are growing? Do they have a scent? What sounds can you hear? Feel the sun on your body. Imagine its rays bringing warmth to all parts of you. Imagine, also, the light broken up into its component parts so that it lies in a coloured spectrum across your body: warm red rays falling on your legs and hips, relaxing and warming them; orange rays casting a gentle light over your lower trunk; a soft yellow light glowing across your stomach; green rays casting a soothing light over your heart; blue light bathing your throat and lower face, a cool indigo light falling on your brow and violet light around your head.

Picture a ray of blue light travelling from each eye … allow these twin rays to carry away any tension … carrying it into the vastness of space … as it recedes, feel yourself relaxing … finally, a silver light appears … let it gather up all the colours and … as it does, let it draw away any remaining tension from your body, dissolving it and leaving you in a state of deep calmness … imagine the silver light spreading around you to form a circle … allow the circle to include others who also wish to share this peace. They stay for a few moments and as they leave, you notice they have left a gift for you … it is a gift which you will recognize …

When you are ready, gently allow the scene to fade … slowly, bring your attention back to the room in which you are lying. Feel the floor beneath you as you open your eyes.

White Light

The Rosicrucians, a brotherhood formed during the Renaissance, regarded white light as a symbol of guidance, inspiration and healing. The idea has been developed by Samuels and Samuels (1975).

Take yourself in your mind's eye to a place that is special for you. Imagine it filled with brilliant white light … let that light flow through you … filling your body and your mind … healing you … strengthening you … renewing you.

GUIDED IMAGERY

Definition and Description

Guided imagery is a therapeutic technique which uses the imagination to achieve desirable outcomes such as decreased pain perception and reduced anxiety (Ackerman & Turkoski 2000). It has been described as an inner communication involving all the senses and is believed to form an emotional connection between the mind and the body (Jallo et al 2014, Tusek & Cwynar 2000). Typically the participant is led through a scene enriched by sensual descriptions in the belief that the state induced creates access to a deeper consciousness, which will release latent healing abilities. The method can be used in most situations of pain and distress and is a useful adjunct to conventional medical and psychiatric treatments (Tusek & Cwynar 2000, Wood & Patricolo 2013).

The visualizer conjures up a naturalistic scene, often of his or her own choosing, and moves around within it, noticing particularly its sensory content. A meadow, forest, beach or garden makes a suitable setting. Within this context, it is helpful to introduce a path, and for three reasons: it can suggest a goal, provide a passage for the inner guide or simply carry the visualizer through the scene.

Where imagery is being presented to a group, it is convenient for the trainer to decide on a particular scene and to suggest its basic structure. For example, if a meadow is decided on, the trainer can suggest other features such as a stream and a backdrop of distant hills. The time of year and the weather can make the scene more vivid. The visualizer is asked to notice the scents and sounds, as well as the appearance of the scene. It is left to the trainer as to how much information is offered. The participant fills in the detail.

The following paragraphs (adapted from Lichstein 1988) give the flavour of guided imagery.

Please get comfortable and close your eyes. As your mind becomes more peaceful, your body will also lose some of its tension. I am going to ask you to imagine a scene which you find pleasant and relaxing. Take a moment to choose the setting …

Let your scene take shape … do not force it in any way… just allow it to form by building its sensory detail … create it visually … making it as vivid as you can … imagine the sounds that accompany it … the scents that float in the air … the textures that surround you … feel the warmth of the sun on your skin … find a path and experience the sensation of moving through the scene … feel the tension leaving your body … feel it being carried away each time you breathe out … and enjoy the peace and calm of the scene you've created …

For those who are looking for more specific scenes, try a sunny beach, a country meadow or a scented garden. (If the trainee suffers from hay fever, the first item is the best choice.)

A Sunny Beach

Imagine a stretch of shoreline … make it rocky or smooth as you like … notice the ground underfoot, is the sand wet and hard or is it dry and soft? … if the sun is shining perhaps you can feel its warmth on your skin … and see the light dancing on the water … perhaps you can smell the sea air as it fills your nostrils … what sounds can you hear? … the gulls calling? … the waves breaking? … a motor chugging? … you may decide to take a walk along the beach and, as you travel, notice how the scenery changes … perhaps rocks begin to break up the surface of the beach, with pools beneath them … you might feel you want to dip your hand into one of them … and are surprised to find how warm this shallow water is …

A Country Meadow

Picture yourself in the country … perhaps you are in a field in early summer … notice how long the grass is … notice also how green it is … are there wildflowers growing in it? … which ones? … can you smell their scent rising up? … and is there a gentle breeze? … enough to rustle the leaves on the trees? … you may decide to wander along a narrow sheeptrack … and as you cross the ground, perhaps you can hear the sound of water … if it's a stream,

notice how it runs … whether smoothly or bubbling over rocks … and how soon does it swing out of sight? …

A Scented Garden

Let your mind conjure up the scene of a beautiful garden … notice the way it is laid out … the trees, shrubs and flower beds … perhaps it has just rained … a gentle summer rain … can you smell the air, warm and moist? … in your imagination notice the scents around you … is it honeysuckle? … or is it thyme? … or perhaps it's newly mown grass … you may decide to walk through the garden, along a path which perhaps carries you under some trees … notice how cool it is in their shade … and how warm when you step out into the sunlight again … notice also the trees which line the path … and the texture of their bark … in your mind's eye reach out to touch one of them … was it smooth or deeply incised? …

PRECAUTIONS

A cautious attitude is advised when using imagery. Therefore precautions to take for imagery and goal-directed visualization include the following.

1. Training in imagery and visualization should never be viewed as a substitute for medical treatment; wherever a disorder is present or suspected, medical help should be sought.
2. Imagery and visualization should only be used within the professional boundaries of the trainer.
3. People differ in their ability to form images. For those who find it difficult, a muscular approach might be more useful. On the other hand, because visualization is thought by some to be a learnable skill, practice may increase proficiency.
4. It is not the object of the exercise to create a hypnotic trance. Neither is it likely that one will occur. However, because some individuals are more susceptible than others, the possibility exists that the trainer may inadvertently create one. When a person is in a hypnotic trance, the power of suggestion becomes greater. That being so, the trainer needs to be aware of the phenomenon of posthypnotic suggestion.

Posthypnotic suggestion results in the individual blindly carrying out injunctions outside the trance situation. For example, a statement such as 'When you go home you will assert yourself' would be indiscriminately applied. This would leave no room for reassessment of the situation which might, in changing circumstances, call for a modified approach.

Any suggestion which could be applied inappropriately outside the relaxation session should be avoided. Generally speaking, however, posthypnotic suggestion is not a problem because individuals tend to resist any exhortation that runs counter to their personal goals and moral principles (Lynn & Rhue 1977).

Larkin (1988) has useful advice for the trainer who is offering imagery and is concerned to avoid hypnotizing the participant: suggestion should be indirect, incorporating words such as 'can', 'may', 'might' and 'perhaps'. Larkin emphasizes the importance of presenting the participant with options, so that the suggestion finally adopted comes from the participant themselves.

However, if trainers are in doubt as to the effect of their words, they can terminate the session with a cancelling statement (Shone 1996) along the lines of: 'Before you bring your visualization to an end, cancel any suggestion you do not wish to take effect in your waking life'.

As mentioned earlier, it is unlikely that unintentional hypnosis will occur.

5. Occasionally, participants have difficulty returning from their visualization. Repeating the termination procedure usually resolves the problem. Another device is to include in the termination procedure some reference to feeling alert and refreshed.

KEY POINTS

1. Imagery can enhance the relaxation experience.
2. Symbolic imagery, metaphor, transformation and distancing are different ways in which imagery can be employed.
3. Imagery should only be taught within the professional boundaries of the trainer.
4. Imagery is a safe, non-invasive and low-cost form of treatment.
5. Research suggests that this approach is potentially effective as an adjunct in some conditions.

Reflection

Describe your understanding of the techniques of imagery.

How do you feel about applying this technique in practice?

How does imagery help people to relax?

How does guided imagery differ from other types of imagery?

What is the main learning point you will take away from this chapter?

CASE STUDY LEARNING OPPORTUNITY

The key points and reflection provide background and knowledge required in relation to the case study, Anna, to help deepen understanding of how imagery can help improve physical and mental well-being.

CASE STUDY

Physiotherapy Student Anxiety: *Imagery Outcomes for Anna*

In the first year of studying a physiotherapy degree Anna found that the course requirements, such as assignments, tests, clinical experiences and placements, were creating an excessive amount of anxiety for her to progress her studies in a positive manner. Anna's high levels of anxiety were starting to interfere with her learning and her marks were dropping, heightening her anxiety levels further.

Anna's personal tutor noted that the stressors Anna was experiencing were lowering her productivity, and was concerned that this may cause a deterioration in Anna's overall well-being and mental health. A referral to the university's counsellor was made to support Anna. The counsellor suggested a course of imagery to help reduce the anxiety Anna was experiencing.

After a number of one-to-one imagery sessions Anna was provided with a recording to listen to for 15 minutes every day for 5 consecutive days, then three times a week for 3 weeks. There was no set time of day to complete this task, so it was at Anna's discretion as to when she listened to the tape.

After completing the course Anna reported an increased sense of well-being, improved ability to sleep, greater energy and improved self-confidence. Anna enjoyed the renewed sense of control over her life and planned on continuing to use the tape to manage her anxiety.

ACTIVITY

For the case study:

1. List the reasons for Anna's deteriorating performance at university.
2. Consider why this approach was taken.
3. Write down the impact that imagery is having from a psychological perspective.
4. Write down the impact that imagery is having from a physical perspective.
5. Write down the impact that imagery is having from an emotional perspective.

Chapter 19 will focus on goal-directed visualization and build upon the knowledge gained from imagery.

REFERENCES

Achterberg, J. (2002). *Imagery in healing: Shamanism and modern medicine*. Boston: Shambhala Publications.

Ackerman, C. J., & Turkoski, B. (2000). Using guided imagery to reduce pain and anxiety. *Home and Healthcare Nurse*, 18(8), 524–530.

Assagioli, R. (1965). *Psychosynthesis*. London: Turnstone Books.

Atkinson, R. L., Atkinson, R. C., Smith, E. E., Bem, D. J., & Nolen-Hoeksema, S. (1999). *Hilgard's introduction to psychology* (13th ed.). Fort Worth, TX: Harcourt Brace.

Baird, C. L., & Sands, L. (2004). A pilot study of the effectiveness of guided imagery with progressive muscle relaxation to reduce chronic pain and mobility difficulties of osteoarthritis. *Pain Management Nursing*, 5(3), 97–104.

Barber, T. X., Chauncey, H. M., & Winer, R. A. (1964). The effect of hypnotic and non-hypnotic suggestion on parotid gland response to gustatory stimuli. *Psychosomatic Medicine*, 26, 374–380.

Charalambous, A., Giannakopoulou, M., Bozas, E., & Paikousis, L. (2015). A randomized controlled trial for the effectiveness of progressive muscle relaxation and guided imagery as anxiety reducing interventions in breast and prostate cancer patients. Evidence-based commentary and Alternative Medicine.

Cupal, D. D., & Brewer, B. W. (2001). Effects of relaxation and guided imagery on knee strength, reinjury anxiety and pain following anterior cruciate ligament reconstruction. *Rehabilitation Psychology*, 46(1), 28–43.

Davis, M., Eshelman, E., & McKay, M. (2008). *The relaxation and stress reduction workbook* (6th ed.). Oakland, CA: New Harbinger.

Davis, M., Shellman, E., & McKay, M. (2000). *The relaxation and stress reduction workbook* (5th ed.). Oakland, CA: New Harbinger.

Dossey, B. M. (1988). Imagery: Awakening the inner healer. In B. M. Dossey, L. Keagan, C. E. Guzzetta, & L. G. Kolkmeier (Eds.), *Holistic nursing: A handbook for practice*. Rockville, MD: Aspen.

Ernst, S., & Goodison, L. (1981). *In our own hands: A book of self-help therapy*. London: Women's Press.

Fanning, P. (1988). *Visualization for change*. Oakland: CAL New Harbinger.

Ferrucci, P. (1982). *What we may be*. London: Mandala.

Finke, R. A. (1989). *Principles of mental imagery*. Cambridge, MA: Massachusetts Institute of Technology.

Fors, E. A., Sexton, H., & Gotestam, K. G. (2002). The effect of guided imagery and amitriptyline on daily fibromyalgic pain: A prospective randomized controlled trial. *Journal of Psychiatric Research*, 36(3), 179–187.

Fordham, F. (1966). *An introduction to Jung's psychology* (2nd ed.). London: Pelican.

Freud, S. (1973). *Introductory lectures on psychoanalysis (trans. Strachey J)*. Harmondsworth, UK: Penguin.

Halpin, L. S., Speir, A. M., Capobianco, P., & Barnett, S. D. (2002). Guided imagery in cardiac surgery. *Outcomes Management for Nursing Practice*, 6(3), 132–137.

Jacobson, E. (1938). *Progressive relaxation* (2nd ed.). Chicago: University of Chicago Press.

Jallo, N., Jeanne, R., Elswick, R. K., & French, E. (2014). Guided imagery for stress and symptom management in pregnant African American women. *Evidence-Based Complementary and Alternative Medicine*, 840923, 13.

Johnson, U. (2000). Short-term psychological intervention: a study of long-term injured competitive athletes. *Journal of Sport Rehabilitation*, 9(3), 207–218.

Jung, C. G. (1963). *Memories, dreams, reflections*. New York: Vintage Books.

Kermani, K. S. (1990). *Autogenic training*. London: Souvenir Press.

Kosslyn, S. M. (1984). *Ghosts in the mind's machine*. New York: WW Norton.

Larkin, D. M. (1988). Therapeutic suggestion. In R. P. Zahourek (Ed.), *Relaxation and imagery: Tools for therapeutic communication and intervention*. Philadelphia: WB Saunders.

Laurion, S., & Fetzer, S. J. (2003). The effect of two nursing interventions on the postoperative outcomes of gynecologic laparoscopic patients. *Journal of PeriAnesthesia Nursing, 18*(4), 254–261.

Lichstein, K. L. (1988). *Clinical relaxation strategies*. New York: John Wiley.

Luskin, F. M., Newell, K. A., Griffith, M., et al. (2000). A review of mind–body therapies in the treatment of musculoskeletal disorders with implications for the elderly. *Alternative Therapies in Health and Medicine, 6*(2), 46–56.

Lyman, B., Bernadin, S., & Thomas, S. (1980). Frequency of imagery in emotional experience. *Perceptual and Motor Skills, 50*, 1159–1162.

Lynn, S. J., & Rhue, J. W. (1977). Hypnosis, imagination and fantasy. *Journal of Mental Imagery, 11*, 101–113.

McCance, K., & Heuther, S. (2014). *Patho-Physiology: The biologic basis for disease in adults and children* (7th ed.). St Louis: Mosby.

McGuigan, F. J. (1971). Covert linguistic behaviour in deaf subjects during thinking. *Journal of Comparative and Physiological Psychology, 75*, 417–420.

Melzack, R., & Wall, P. D. (1983). *The challenge of pain*. London: Penguin.

Oyle, I. (1976). *Magic, mysticism and modern medicine*. Millbrae, CA: Celestial Arts.

Rankin, D. (2003). *Nurse's handbook of alternative and complementary therapies* (2nd ed.). Philadelphia: Lippincott Williams & Wilkins.

Roffe, L., Schmidt, K., & Ernst, E. (2005). A systematic review of guided imagery as an adjuvant cancer therapy. *Psychooncology, 14*(8), 607–617.

Samuels, M., & Samuels, N. (1975). *Seeing with the mind's eye: The history, technique and uses of visualization*. Toronto: Random House.

Shone, R. (1996). *Autohypnosis: A step by step guide to self-hypnosis*. Wellingborough, UK: Thorsons.

Sloman, R. (2002). Relaxation and guided imagery for anxiety and depression control in community patients with advanced cancer. *Cancer Nursing, 25*(6), 432–435.

Sordoni, C., Hall, C., & Forwell, L. (2002). The use of imagery in athletic injury rehabilitation and its relationship to self-efficacy. *Physiotherapy Canada, 54*(3), 177–185.

Tusek, D. L., & Cwynar, R. E. (2000). Strategies for implementing a guided imagery programme to enhance patient experience. *AACN Clinical Issues, 11*(1), 68–76.

Watanabe, E., Fukuda, S., Hara, H., Maeda, Y., Ohira, H., & Shirakawa, T. (2006). Differences in relaxation by means of guided imagery in a healthy community sample. *Alternative Therapies in Health and Medicine, 12*(2), 60–66.

Weydert, J. A. (2006). Evaluation of guided imagery as treatment for recurrent abdominal pain in children: A randomized controlled trial. *BMC Pediatrics, 6*, 29.

Wood, D., & Patricolo, G. E. (2013). Using guided imagery in a hospital setting. *Alternative and Complementary Therapies, 19*(6), 302–305.

Zahourek, R. P. (Ed.). (1988). *Relaxation and imagery: Tools for therapeutic communication and intervention*. Philadelphia: WB Saunders.

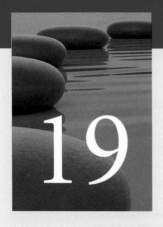

19 GOAL-DIRECTED VISUALIZATION

PROFESSOR TEENA CLOUSTON

LEARNING OBJECTIVES

The aim of this chapter is to provide a practical guide to basic concepts of goal-directed visualization.

By the end of this chapter you will be able to:

1. Describe the key principles and process of goal-directed visualization.

2. Understand how goal-directed visualization can motivate behaviour change in everyday life.

3. Recognize the importance of the individual's role and intention in goal-directed visualization.

4. Identify how goal-directed visualization can be used to promote health and well-being.

5. Carry out a goal-directed visualization session.

This chapter will conclude with key points and time for reflection, providing learning opportunities through case studies.

INTRODUCTION TO GOAL-DIRECTED VISUALIZATION

Goal-directed visualization is a form of imagery which requires purposeful thinking leading to the fulfilment of self-directed goals.

In their book *Seeing with the Mind's Eye*, Samuels and Samuels (1975) describe a technique using imagery which has two phases, receptive and programmed. In the receptive phase, individuals passively listen to their inner self, drawing on their own wisdom. In the programmed phase, the individual engages in an active and deliberate thought process for the purpose of improving a situation or resolving a problem in their life. This is based on the assumption that, by repeatedly experiencing an outcome in the imagination, we increase the likelihood of it taking place in real life.

The Samuels' work has been developed by Achterberg (1985), Simonton et al (1986) and others in areas of medicine and healing, and by Shone (1984) and Fanning (1988), among others, in areas of self-development and relaxation. Because in this book we are concerned with the latter area, the definitions of Fanning and Shone are appropriate. Fanning (1988), p8 describes this kind of imagery as 'the conscious, volitional creation of mental sense impressions for the purpose of changing oneself'; Shone refers to it as a mental experience which helps bring about desired outcomes. Implicit in both definitions is the notion of a goal.

How does this form of imagery differ from other forms? One answer is that it is more explicit than techniques which rely on metaphor and symbolism; it is also more purposeful than reverie states such as daydreaming. How is it different from talking to yourself, reflecting and giving yourself advice? It may not *be* very different, but it does seek to offer a structured, step-by-step approach and has a clearly formulated outcome or goal. It also taps into one's volition (i.e., self-determination or free will) and requires the individual to utilize their personal intention to change.

An interesting study by Munezane (2015) identified that using goal setting and visualization together was more effective than visualization alone in supporting Japanese students' willingness to speak English, thus suggesting that these two processes work well together to effectively motivate participation and promote behaviour change.

INTRODUCTION TO EVIDENCE

Evidence that goal-directed visualizations can be effective in motivating changes in health promoting behaviours is replete in the literature (Armitage & Reidy 2008; Conroy & Hagger 2017; Gollwitzer & Sheeran 2006; Kross & Grossman 2012; Libby et al 2007, 2009; Libby & Eibach 2011; Oettingen 2012; Rennie et al 2014, 2016; Schaeffer et al 2015).

Conroy et al (2015) and Hagger et al (2011, 2012) investigated the effectiveness of goal-directed visualization on alcohol consumption and found drinking decreased when it was used. Conroy et al's (2015) study identified that students (n = 211) who used visualization had a substantial decrease in alcohol consumption compared with the control group at 2-week and 4-week follow-ups. Hagger et al's (2011) study accessed employees in three different corporate

organizations and also found a significant effect on the number of units consumed. However, there was no apparent impact on the frequency of binge drinking. In a later study Hagger et al (2012) considered variables such as intention, motivation and nationality in terms of the rates of decreased alcohol consumption and binge drinking for undergraduate students from the UK, Finland and Estonia. They found significant reduction in alcohol consumption for the intention group from the UK and Estonia and a notable and significant reduction in binge drinking for the UK sample only; this suggests that intention and nationality have some part to play in the effectiveness of goal-directed visualizations for alcohol consumption and frequency of binge drinking.

Whereas outcomes from formal smoking cessation programmes have been shown to have varying degrees of success, those that used goal-directed visualizations have been shown to be comparatively more effective. Tindle et al (2006) conducted a randomized pilot trial to test the efficacy of guided imagery for smoking cessation in adults. Results showed that 36% of intervention participants compared with 18% of controls had abstained at 6 weeks. At 1-year follow-up, 24% of the intervention participants continued to be abstinent. Of those who attended the training classes in guided imagery, 94% reported that the technique was helpful. The authors concluded that a programme of guided imagery for smoking cessation was associated with a trend towards both quitting and abstinence. However, they also identified that quitting was one outcome and abstinence another: relapse rates were high, either because people lost their motivation or because they lacked the coping skills to continue. Nonetheless, the results showed that resolve can be strengthened by visualizations of improved health or behavioural strategies such as removing oneself from a scene where others are smoking. A study by Gordon et al (2019) is exploring the potential of guided visualization delivered by phone as a tool to support quitting for hard to reach groups. The findings aim to guide the efficacy of a future randomized controlled trial.

Ouellette et al (2005) explored the effectiveness of using visualization to increase participation in exercise, and Koka and Hagger (2017), physical activity more generally. Both found goal-directed visualization to be effective in that it motivated individuals to participate in physical activity, with Koka and Hagger's study noting this outcome was specific to low-activity adolescents. Finding similarly positive results, Knauper et al (2011) reported people could be motivated to change their behaviour in terms of diet and eating more fruit. Thus all these studies maintain that goal-directed visualizations can promote more beneficial and healthful behaviour patterns for certain groups of people.

Interestingly, a study by Rennie et al (2016) suggest that using the third person in goal-directed visualization can be more motivating, and thus more impactful in long-term behaviour change, than using a first person perspective. Using two studies, one with 153 undergraduate students and the second with 142 undergraduate students, they tested the use of first and third person visualizations in terms of increasing fruit and vegetable consumption and participation in 20 minutes of moderate exercise, respectively. They found that the third person perspective created significantly stronger intentions (i.e., personally motivated goals) and that this, in turn, created a greater likelihood of performing the required behaviour change.

These findings are supported by an earlier study by Libby et al (2007). Investigating the influence of third and first person visualizations in terms of voting at the 2004 American elections, they found that those using third person perspectives were more likely to actually vote (90% in the third person versus 72% in the first person). Theorizing reasons for this, they reasoned that third person constructs were more dispositional (i.e., personal traits, abilities and feelings), as opposed to situational (external factors), and thus more motivating.

A study by Vasquez and Behuler (2007) also found that students using third person perspectives were more motivated, in this case to study, than those using the first person. Drawing on construal level theory, they posited this was a consequence of third person visualizations facilitating more abstract rather than concrete construals. Simply put, the third person perspective seemed to create a stronger ability to predict, imagine or visualize a future self and the different ways one might move from the present to achieve that future self (Trope & Liberman 2010).

This would suggest that by making small changes to the way people approach goal-directed visualization – that is, by accommodating a third person

perspective – it could have a positive effect on the outcome and sustain any behaviour change over longer periods. However, these studies are tempered by the fact that the behaviours in question were reported as not complex or difficult to change; other studies have shown that where this is the case, third person visualization appears to be less successful in increasing the levels of motivation to change than the first person approach (Libby & Eibach 2011).

THEORIES BEHIND GOAL-DIRECTED VISUALIZATION

The mechanism of visualization as a method for enhancing well-being is incompletely understood. However, its success is often explained by the belief that the body cannot distinguish between the event as experienced and the event as imagined, a notion which is supported by a finding that the same physiological responses occur in each case (Dalloway 1992). As a result, new cognitive responses can be learned and practised in a safe environment, from which, it is proposed, they can later be transferred to the event in real life; and if not wholly transferred, at least the likelihood of this occurring is strengthened (Dalloway 1992).

Thus tasks perceived to be difficult can lose some of their threat after being visualized with a successful outcome. This is mental rehearsal, a procedure which allows the individual to familiarize themselves with the feared event and, in their imagination, to achieve their goal. Impending stressful events such as athletic competitions and performances of various kinds can be approached in this way (Farmer 1995).

KEY ASPECTS OF THE PROCEDURE

The method, which incorporates other techniques such as progressive relaxation and guided imagery (see Chapters 5 and 18, respectively), lends itself to a variety of conditions and situations, of which smoking cessation is one, and this topic is considered in some detail later. This section opens with a general description of the procedure for goal-directed visualization under the following headings:

- Position
- Preparatory relaxation

- Special place
- Receptive visualization
- Positive self-statements or affirmations
- Programmed visualization
- Termination
- An additional technique

Position

The visualizer lies down in a comfortable position in a dimly lit, warm room, free from noise and interruption. The eyes are closed.

Preparatory Relaxation

Imagery is preceded by a short session of relaxation because relaxation is generally regarded as a precondition as well as an effect of visualization. Its role here is to create a 'state of balance, quietude and peace, free of negativity' (Ryman 1994). It allows the mind to be receptive to new information and tends to enhance the formation of images (Tusek & Cwynar 2000). The technique employed can be chosen by the individual, although Achterberg (1985) suggests that passive forms of muscle relaxation are more appropriate than tense–release, which she claims is ineffective for imagery work. Slow, gentle abdominal breathing will also help to induce deep relaxation. The visualizer may recite appropriate phrases such as 'My mind is calm and clear', or 'I am open to images that will help me'.

Although this preliminary relaxation is common practice, there is little evidence to support its value as a facilitator of imagery (Lichstein 1988). Indeed, there are those who claim the opposite, that is, that a totally relaxed body is accompanied by a mind devoid of images (Jacobson 1938). If muscular relaxation clears the mind of images, how can it also promote them? Lichstein (1988) refers to this as a matter yet to be resolved. Perhaps the answer lies in finding a level of relaxation which is deep enough to release tension, but not so deep that images cannot form.

Special Place

Lying quietly, the visualizer builds an imaginary scene or 'special place' as a retreat for relaxation and guidance (Davis et al 2000). The scene is rich in sensory images of sight, sound, smell, taste, texture, and temperature, and gives a feeling of peace and tranquillity. A beach, meadow, lake or forest all offer possibilities.

The visualizer is encouraged to imagine how the body would feel in the special place, emphasizing sensations such as sinking into springy turf or soft sand. Some time is spent initially setting the scene so that it can easily be recreated in subsequent visualizations. Because imagery is a right hemisphere activity, the constraints of logic do not apply. Thus the special place may contain any figment of the imagination which the visualizer finds useful, such as a permanent sunset in the background, a viewing screen in a forest clearing or a crystal ball in a mountain spring. It is in such a scene that the inner guide could appear (see Chapter 18), and so there should be a clearly defined way in.

Some people prefer an indoor special place such as an attic room or a garden shed; others like to have both, using them on different occasions. There is no right or wrong way: whatever works for the individual is right.

Receptive Visualization

The visualizer imagines they are in their special place. This is where they can feel in tune with themselves and where they will be likely to gain insights. In this place they will be in a state of mind that allows them to listen to the part of themselves which is normally beyond conscious awareness. It is a passive state of mind which in some ways resembles daydreaming, but differs from the latter in that the visualizer is asking themselves specific questions (Samuels & Samuels 1975). Whether this is making a choice, sorting out a conflict, uncovering motivations or exposing automatic thoughts, the receptive visualization is a way of allowing intuitive insights to be released and inner wisdom to be revealed.

The visualizer should be advised that if uncontrollable or unpleasant feelings arise which they are not ready to deal with, they can walk away or distance themselves in some other manner. They can also end the visualization. Alternatively, they can quietly tune in to their unconscious. If ideas do not flow, the inner guide can be called and asked for advice (see Chapter 18).

An example of a receptive visualization script is given here. (Allow 10 to 15 minutes for it.)

Lie down. Get yourself comfortable and close your eyes. Run through a relaxing procedure until you feel very calm. Visualize yourself lying in your special place. Evoke its atmosphere by mentally experiencing its sights, sounds, smells and textures. Feel at home there. Let your attention gently focus on the item that preoccupies you … just keep an open mind … quietly listen to the thoughts that flow through it … if you are stuck, call on your inner guide … listen to the wisdom your inner guide brings … realize that it is your own wisdom, coming from your deeper self … spend a few minutes listening to yourself …

When you are ready, end your visualization and gently bring your attention back to the room.

Write down any ideas that came to you. Consider them. Have you gained any insights? Do you want to change your way of handling this situation? Are there more positive ways of dealing with it?

Receptive visualizations can be repeated as often as they continue to provide insights.

Positive Self-Statements or Affirmations

The positive self-statement, often referred to as an affirmation, helps visualizers to see themselves as being capable of realizing personal aspirations and achieving individual goals. Inherent in the affirmation is the suspension of self-doubt. Examples include the following:

- I believe in myself.
- I am in control of my life.
- I can achieve my aim.

Although these statements are of a general nature, additional affirmations relevant to the matter in question can also be composed. Thus, for a person wishing to become more relaxed, the following statements may be included:

- I feel calm.
- I am at peace.
- I can cope in stressful situations.

Positive self-statements need to be short, and are traditionally in the first person and in the present tense. The most effective tend to be those composed by the individual personally (Fanning 1988). When repeated, they act like self-hypnotic suggestions, influencing the individual's view of the self in a positive direction and adding force to the positive images of the programmed visualization (described later).

Programmed Visualization

In the programmed visualization phase, individuals may work on images that emerged during the receptive phase, turning them over and trying them out in different forms in their imagination. When the visualizers find the most effective solution to their problem, they visualize themselves as instrumental in achieving it. Actions are imagined which allow them to feel they are displaying the qualities they want to possess. Goals are mentally reached, with individuals operating as their own successful agent. By daily repetition, the new images they create start to blend with their actual self-image, tending to generate still more positive internal dialogue and, in the manner of a self-fulfilling prophecy, increasing the likelihood of the desired outcome in real life.

Sometimes, while in the programmed stage, the visualizer gets 'stuck'. In this case, returning to the receptive stage may help to clear the block.

On other occasions, the receptive and programmed phases may not be clearly separated. Not all visualization work falls neatly into receptive and programmed categories, and individuals should not feel under pressure to structure them separately if one continuous visualization seems more appropriate. There is no set pattern for the programmed visualization: the topic itself will determine the style.

Procedure for Programmed Visualization

The preliminaries are similar to those for receptive visualization; that is, individuals relax using cue-controlled relaxation (see Chapter 9) or passive muscular relaxation (see Chapter 8).

They then evoke the scene of the situation they want to resolve, whatever it might be; in this context, this is not the special place but a real-life situation. Again, rich sensory detail is essential to bring it to life. Time spent building the scene enables visualizers to experience it more keenly. The individuals then work on the item, experimenting with it until they find a good solution, which they then enact in their imagination, ensuring that the outcome is positive and successful.

The tone of the programmed visualization is demonstrated in the following passage.

Let your thoughts become quiet and bring your attention to focus on your goal. Believe in your capacity to reach it … don't dwell on the difficulties;

just think of the result. If there are problems, see them as a challenge ... feel an eagerness to achieve ... to be a person who has reached that goal ... feel yourself in the part ... imagine yourself as having arrived ... congratulate yourself for getting there ... enjoy it ...

Termination

When the visualization is over, the procedure is brought to an end with a termination on the following lines.

If you are ready, gradually bring your attention back to the room you are in ... slowly count one ... two ... three ... and, as you open your eyes, feel yourself alert and refreshed.

Goal-directed visualization thus consists of individuals opening themselves to their own wisdom (receptive phase) and then using it in their own imagination to bring about the desired outcome (programmed phase).

Additional Technique

'Distancing' – that is, drawing back from the scene to examine their actions – is a technique which allows visualizers to gain a more objective view. In an imaginary viewing screen or crystal ball the individuals watch their own behaviour patterns: how they cope with situations and relate to other people.

This approach may reveal maladaptive responses that individuals may be making. By observing these in this way, visualizers can reflect on them, then modify those responses and rerun the film or script in a way which leads to a successful outcome. The next move is for the individuals to use what they have learned, and through their imagination, step back into the scene to experience and practice in their mind's eye the more positive approach and outcome.

RELAXATION AND GOAL-DIRECTED VISUALIZATION

It can be seen that relaxation is related to goal-directed visualization in a variety of ways:

It is used as a preparatory measure to induce a state of mind conducive to visualization. Before individuals begin their visualization, they should first become relaxed.

It may be experienced as a secondary effect after mental rehearsal, in which the individuals see themselves as successfully coping with an activity which has hitherto been associated with stress.

A need for relaxation may be created while the goal is being achieved, such as during the struggle to withdraw from cigarettes or tranquillizers.

Goal-directed visualization is thus not a primary method of inducing relaxation, but it does have close links with it.

PRECAUTIONS

Goals, which should be set by the individual, need to be attainable. To set goals which are out of the individual's reach will only create additional stress. Goals may also be set too low to be constructive. These potential pitfalls and precautions should be considered alongside those found at the end of Chapter 18.

APPLICATION

Unlike most other methods described in this book, goal-directed visualization addresses the specific problems of a person. This feature is seen in both the receptive and the programmed components. Thus it is not possible to present a model script without a clear understanding of the background.

A key factor in the success of any plan is the motivation of the visualizer. Although for some individuals this is not a problem, others may need encouragement. One way of fostering motivation is to make the goals specific. For example, having a timescale for a smoking abstinence plan defines it more clearly. Creating subgoals or intermediate stages is another useful strategy because they act as steppingstones along the way. Clouston (2015, p137) calls these 'small moves'; that is, setting achievable goals that are attainable and thus can underpin success and stimulate motivation. This has the effect of making the ultimate goal seem easier to reach, as well as providing rewards at intervals. Smoking one less cigarette a day can constitute a subgoal, as can taking one more step to a person recovering from

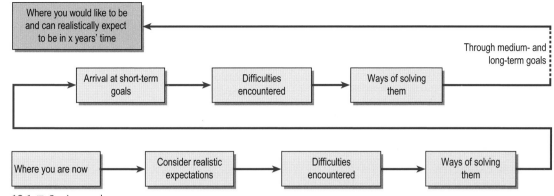

Fig. 19.1 ■ Setting goals.

leg injury. Difficulties can be considered in advance, and ways of solving them worked out (Fig. 19.1).

Samuels and Samuels (1975) advise individuals not to confide their visualization to anyone who may not share their faith in the wisdom of the goal and in their capacity to reach it. Unshaken belief is considered vital for success.

Of course, participants in some groups may be too demoralized to begin; they may feel they have little future; they may be angry or depressed. These are valid reactions which call for modification of the method and perhaps referral to a specialist agency. In general, however, the approach can be a useful one.

Although it is difficult to construct a model script without specific knowledge of the problem concerned, an attempt is made here to provide an example.

The reader is reminded of the principal items in the method:

Receptive visualization. Individuals tune in to their own wisdom.
Self-statements. Individuals reaffirm their intention through positive internal dialogue.
Programmed visualization. Individuals work on a plan for the future in which they see themselves surmounting obstacles, realizing possibilities and achieving goals. The keynote of this stage is seeing the self as succeeding.

When techniques are being learned and applied, one cannot count on instant success. As with any new skill, the most that can be expected is a trend in the desired direction. Frequent practice, however, strengthens this trend.

Visualizations for People Who Want to Give Up Smoking

It could be argued that smoking has more to do with relaxation than smoking abstinence has, and many people become smokers because they perceive cigarettes as being a source of mental calm. However, many such people may then wish to quit smoking. Quitting is associated with stress, which means that the same people may be seeking an alternative means of obtaining relaxation. Health care professionals increasingly find themselves faced with groups of people who are struggling to give up cigarettes and for whom relaxation training has been prescribed. Although any of the methods in this book might help, a method which directly addresses the problem would seem to have particular advantages.

Within a single group of people who wish to reduce their smoking habits, there may be a wide variety of aspirations: one person may want to cut down from 40 cigarettes a day to 20, another may want to give up altogether. They may also have different ideas as to how to go about it: one may want to reduce by one cigarette a day, another may want to make a more abrupt change, a third may want to kick an e-cigarette habit, which may or may not have been started to help with giving up nicotine. Or again, the group may consist of people who are looking for ways of avoiding relapse after having successfully given up smoking. The following visualization and sequel (adapted from Fanning 1988) are designed for people who have decided to give up altogether.

Receptive visualization

Lie or sit in a position which you find comfortable. Close your eyes. Allow yourself to unwind. (The instructor presents either passive relaxation or slow breathing.) As your body and mind become calm, let your special place take shape in your imagination. Notice the sights, sounds and smell of the place. Put out your hand and feel the textures: the grass, the rug, the pine needles, etc. … feel that you are there … lying peacefully … tuned in to yourself.

Gently bring your mind to focus on your smoking habit. Explore your feelings about it. Why do you smoke? Perhaps you hadn't thought about it before, just taken it for granted. In your mind's eye, take out a cigarette and light up … what does it do for you?

Run through different situations during the day when you feel the need of a cigarette … start with breakfast time … what prompts you to reach for the first cigarette? … then follow yourself to work … smoking on the journey … at work in your coffee break … after the midday meal … again in the afternoon … on the way home … to round off the evening meal … last thing at night … do you notice if you smoke for different reasons? … do you get different rewards from smoking? … when do you find you particularly want a cigarette? …

Bring your visualization to an end when you are ready …

Visualizers may feel they smoke for different reasons at different times. Some of the reasons why people smoke are to:

- feel reassured;
- relieve boredom;
- feel soothed;
- feel relaxed;
- give their hands something to do;
- give themselves a lift;
- reward themselves;
- keep their weight down.

Visualizers decide which of these applies and are then urged to think of alternative ways of meeting these needs. For example:

- For reassurance, they visualize they do not need a crutch.
- To relieve boredom, they get out a crossword puzzle, read a book, go for a run or play on their mobile phone.
- To feel soothed, they think of the love of their partner, make a cup of tea or invoke their special place.
- To feel relaxed, they run through a relaxation sequence or invoke their special place.
- To give their hands something to do, they carry a small, rounded pebble and roll this in their hand. The use of electronic cigarettes or 'vaping' is not recommended because the long-term health effects are unknown.
- To give themselves a lift, they remember the prize they won for cookery/essay writing/athletics last year.
- To reward themselves, they buy the salmon roll instead of the cheese roll.
- To keep their weight down, they eat an orange instead of chocolate pudding, or go for a walk/workout, etc.

Positive Self-Statements or Affirmations

The individual cultivates a view of the self as a healthy non-smoker by composing a few positive self-statements which they recite regularly. These are in the first person but can be modified:

- I am healthy.
- I am a non-smoker.
- I have the strength to control my habits.
- I value the time when I am not smoking.

Additionally, it is important to be gentle and accept the occasional breaking of the resolve.

- I can forgive myself for occasionally breaking my resolution.

Some people find it helpful to have one strong reason for changing their behaviour and to focus on this one idea whenever they feel in danger of weakening.

Programmed Visualization

This takes the form of a mental rehearsal of coping activities, which may focus on the goal itself (the end result) or on the means of achieving it (the process) (Ryman 1995). The following example is mainly concerned with the process.

At the start of the session the instructor can offer passive relaxation or relaxation through abdominal breathing.

Lie down and spend a few minutes relaxing quietly. Imagine yourself at the beginning of a normal day. Run through every moment when you think you might want to light up. Have an alternative way of dealing with every urge to smoke. Start with the moment when you would have the first cigarette of the day … evoke the scene using sensory detail to bring it to life … really live the moment in your imagination … feel yourself craving a cigarette, then promptly use your alternative strategy … and as you do so, encourage yourself with your positive self-statements …

Move on to the next moment when you would want to light up … and the next and so on … making each moment come alive by recreating the scene as vividly as you can … employing alternative strategies and encouraging yourself with positive self-statements … remind yourself of the benefits of giving up smoking: clear lungs, no cough, extra change in your pocket … and if you feel your resolution weakening, remind yourself why you made it in the first place.

Continue through the day, appreciating the experiences that not smoking opens up to you: the taste of your food … the garden scents … the fresh smell of your clothes … and the easy way you climb the hill. See yourself as someone who doesn't smoke …

At some point, feel your stress levels rising as something goes wrong at work … you weaken and take out a cigarette … but after a couple of puffs you stub it out … allow yourself to feel pleased that you could have a slight relapse but not let it interfere with your determination to conquer your habit … see yourself continuing to carry out your resolution and succeeding … see yourself

as someone who can cope without resorting to cigarettes …

When you are ready, bring your visualization to an end with a count of one … two … three … open your eyes … look around you … stretch your arms and legs … and in your own time prepare to resume normal activity.

Some visualization therapists include an aversion component as a further incentive to give up smoking. This could take the form of images of dirty ash trays, blackened lungs, stained fingers or, depending on the country or social stigma, thinking of the health of others, smoking outside in the cold and wet or creating smoky and unhealthy atmospheres. Aversive measures work for some people; other people simply switch off if the image becomes too unpleasant.

The benefits of programmed visualization come from daily practice: the constant repetition of a routine in which individuals see themselves as successful in the task that has been personally set. The previous example is offered as a guideline or starting point from which health care professionals may wish to develop their own script. Alternatively, participants can be encouraged to compose their own visualizations because the most effective ones are those designed by individuals for their own use (Fanning 1988).

Where motivation needs strengthening, the following additional visualization may be found useful.

Find a quiet moment. Relax yourself and close your eyes. Imagine the house in which you expect to be living 10/5/2 years from now. Go inside … explore it … what does it tell you about the occupant: yourself? … who else lives there? … try identifying with your older self … notice how it might feel to be that older self … at work … participating in your hobby … with your family … then, try looking back at yourself as you are now … do you have anything to say to yourself? …

When you are ready, allow your visualization to fade … slowly, bring yourself back to the present … counting one … two … three … as you open your eyes …

Evidence of effectiveness of imagery in changing smoking behaviour can be found in the introduction to the evidence section of this chapter.

OTHER APPLICATIONS

Goal-directed visualization can be used in a wide range of situations and conditions associated with stress. From insights gained during the receptive phase, a realistic solution can be worked out. This solution can then be mentally rehearsed during the programmed visualization, where a successful outcome is experienced in the imagination. A few examples follow:

- Alcohol and substance misuse
- Anger
- Anxiety
- Cancer
- Childbirth
- Injury
- Losing weight
- Pain
- Performance fear
- Phobia and panic disorder
- Problem solving and decision making
- Sport and athletics

Alcohol and Substance Misuse

In programmed visualization individuals mentally rehearse the successful achievement of their goal using positive self-talk and alternative strategies (See Page 229). They also find ways of relaxing during the period of managed withdrawal and beyond.

Anger

For individuals who wish to reduce their tendency to become angry, alternative and preferred courses of action can be mapped out (see Chapter 1). The programmed visualization is employed to familiarize the individual with their capacity to respond in these preferred ways. Relaxation and positive self-talk play a prominent part (Fanning 1988).

Anxiety

Generalized anxiety in terms of everyday responses to stressful situations can benefit from visualization. Some of these have been mentioned in the evidence section. In another example, Felix et al (2018) used guided imagery to support patients admitted for bariatric surgery with preoperative anxiety. Using the state-trait anxiety inventory and blood cortisol measurements, results showed the experimental group (n = 12) had a statistically significant reduction in anxiety scores and cortical levels.

Cancer

Imagery in this context can be used in a number of ways. In one, attention is focused on reversing the physiological changes produced by the tumour. Mental pictures of the cancer cells being attacked by white blood cells are created by the visualizer. The scene is made as vivid as possible by casting the cancer cells as villains. They can play any role which the visualizer chooses, such as, for example, enemy infiltrators. In this scenario, the white blood cells could be represented as a vast army which slowly and inexorably overpowers the intruders and destroys them. The scene is imagined in every detail and the exercise repeated at frequent intervals (Becker & Pentland 1996).

It has been shown that heightened immune responses can occur in patients with cancer who have practised relaxation and healing imagery compared with those who have not practised these techniques (Gregerson et al 1996).

Childbirth

Visualization is often taught to expectant mothers in preparation for childbirth. Polden and Mantle (1990) offer several examples of imagery for use during the first stage of labour. Ocean waves and mountain peaks are used as metaphors to help women withstand the intensity of the contractions. The following is adapted from one of their suggested pieces.

Imagine a beautiful day out at sea … with blue sky, still air and calm water. As the day wears on, the surface of the water begins to show the odd ripple. These ripples may be small, so that at first you hardly notice them. Gradually, the tiny ripples turn into small waves, waves which you feel you can ride quite easily. After a while the waves get higher, and as they get higher, they also get closer together. You are beginning to find them difficult to ride. Still higher and closer together … the waves seem almost to overwhelm you, but as they dip, you notice that they are carrying you nearer to the shore … nearer to the shore where your baby will be born.

Injury

Provided a patient is receiving all necessary medical attention, he or she may find it helpful additionally to introduce a healing visualization.

> *Close your eyes. Let your injured part occupy your attention. See it as a part of your body which is being looked after by organs which control its recovery: your heart, which is pumping out nutrients, the blood vessels, which are carrying them, the injury site, which is receiving them. These nutrients are helping to rebuild the injured tissues. Let your mind focus on this healing process. Feel your mind willing it to take place. Flow with it. Nurse it with your thoughts.*

Losing Weight

In the case of people wishing to lose weight, alternative strategies may be found to take the place of eating. These are incorporated into daily programmed visualizations in which individuals see themselves successfully carrying out the conceived plan (Fanning 1988). In the course of this, individuals build an image of themselves as someone who looks nice whatever their size, but has chosen to lose some weight. Any diet should be medically approved. Anorexia and other forms of eating disorders call for more specialized treatment where goal-directed visualization may be used as part of treatment programme.

Pain

Imagery is used as a therapeutic aid in some types of pain, where it may have an adjunctive role alongside conventional medical treatment. It should not be viewed as a substitute for medical treatment. It can, however, be a useful coping device for chronic pain and minor ailments, such as aches and pains, where it can sometimes help the individual get through difficult patches. In addressing pain, imagery is used in different ways. It can be a distraction, on the one hand, and on the other, it can provide a focus which undergoes transformation in a positive direction; for example, the pain can be identified as a mass of red which gradually has its intensity drained away to become light pink (see Chapter 18). Its use in some forms of intractable pain is a specialized area not covered in the present work.

Performance Fear

The programmed visualization can be used to take the individual through every moment of the event, whether it is a stage performance, a speech or similar activity. As the scene becomes familiar, individuals mentally experience all possible occurrences and develop coping strategies for dealing with them. Above all, they experience the successful achievement of their goal. This has the effect of building and maintaining personal confidence.

Phobia and Panic Disorder

Programmed visualizations allows individuals to see themselves overcoming fear and mastering the situation. They are often performed in a hierarchical fashion; that is, a list of situations from low to high threat is drawn up. Individuals start with the lowest and, taking each one in turn, mentally go through the experience of overcoming their fear, using slowed breathing, relaxation techniques and positive self-talk. This method is known as desensitization and was first introduced by Wolpe in 1958; it is only used under the expert guidance of psychologists, psychotherapists and other trained therapists.

Problem Solving and Decision Making

A receptive visualization can be used to collect ideas for solutions. After weighing them up, the unrealistic ideas are discarded, and the realistic ones retained. Possible results are then predicted both in the short term and in the longer term. These are then considered for their merits and disadvantages, which together form the basis of individuals' final choice. Having picked what they consider to be the best solution, individuals mentally put it into effect, experiencing its successful outcome in a programmed visualization. Fig. 19.2 illustrates the process from identification of the problem to adoption of the best solution.

Vissing and Burke (1984) found that when faced with problems, individuals who regularly practised visualization had more success at solving them than those who did not.

Sport and Athletics

Physical skills have a psychological dimension which is served by imagery in two ways, one cognitive, the other motivational (Paivio 1985). In the cognitive area,

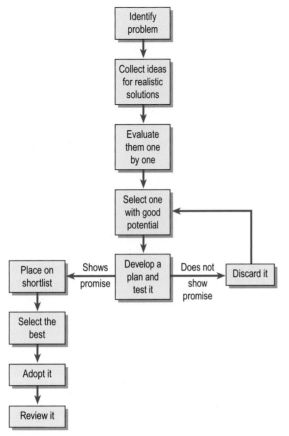

Fig. 19.2 ■ Problem solving.

players imagine successful routines in the game and rehearse appropriate strategies in their imagination. This leads to a strengthened integration between the physical and psychological elements of skill and helps refine performance. In the motivational area, attention is given to the feelings of arousal and affect which accompany performance. Players train the self to channel emotional energy in positive directions, such as imagining the experience of winning. In this way, the sensations of stress, pain and anxiety associated with the activity can be reduced.

A third type, healing imagery, is also practised by athletes after injury (Sordoni et al 2002) (see Chapter 29).

Visualization has been employed to great effect in the field of sport and athletics, with numerous research findings supporting its use. The classic study was performed by Richardson (1969), who showed that basketball players who spent 3 weeks simply visualizing their throws achieved almost the same level of improvement (23%) as players who spent the time practising throws with a ball and whose level of improvement was 24%. A control group whose members did neither showed no improvement.

KEY POINTS

1. Goal-directed visualization is a form of imagery which is structured to target particular behaviours.
2. The client plays an active role in the achievement of a desired outcome.
3. Affirmations are used to strengthen the resolutions.
4. In imagining the event or situation, the same biochemical changes may be stimulated as occur in reality.
5. As the visualization is repeated again and again, its message becomes stronger and more deeply embedded in the mind of the individual.

Reflection

Describe your understanding of the technique of goal-directed visualization.

How did you feel when you completed your own goal-directed visualization?

How do you think goal-directed visualization could be applied in practice?

What did you learn about the use of the third person perspective instead of the traditional first person approach?

What is the main learning point you will take away from this chapter?

What is your future action plan in terms of goal-directed visualization?

CASE STUDY LEARNING OPPORTUNITIES

The key points and reflection provide the background and knowledge required in relation to the case studies; Arian (Case Study 1) and Taran (Case Study 2) help to deepen understanding of how goal-directed visualization can be applied in practice.

CASE STUDY 1

Preparing for Childbirth: *Goal-Directed Visualization Outcomes for Arian*

Arian is pregnant with her second child. The first birth was difficult, and both she and the baby had become very distressed during labour. After several hours of struggling her baby was eventually delivered with forceps. It took Arian months to recover fully, both physically and psychologically, and now she is unsurprisingly anxious about giving birth to her second child. She is hoping that goal-directed visualization will help her with her fears, so she has joined your class.

In the first session you work with the group to learn relaxation techniques and visualize their 'special place'. You suggest to the class that this can be any place of their choice, a wooden glen or the beach with waves gently lapping at the shore; whatever works for them. All goes well and you progress to developing positive affirmations about expected outcomes. At the end of the class everyone seems positive about their achievements and you ask them to practise going to their special place and repeating their positive affirmations during the week.

In the second session you introduce your usual programmed visualization to the group, asking them to think about setting their goal for the successful birth of their baby, focusing on the outcome and not focusing on the difficulties and so on. As you progress through the class you introduce your usual imagery of the sea with the waves rising and crashing, representing the intensifying tide of the contractions. It is at this point that you notice that Arian is beginning to panic; she is hyperventilating and rushes out of the room. You signal to your students to continue the reading of the visualization and quietly leave to find and comfort Arian.

On discussion Arian explains that she has a fear of the sea after an unfortunate accident as a child, when she nearly drowned. She tells you that she had experienced some anxiety when you had suggested the beach as a possible special place the previous week, but she had not thought to mention this and had used a wooded glen anyway.

You realize that you had not asked the class if everyone would be happy with the imagery of water and apologize to Arian for this. On discussion with the group, all are happy to use the imagery of mountains as a metaphor for contractions; you also encourage each group member to ensure they continue to develop their own personalized visualization which they can practise with their birth partners.

Arian uses the mountain metaphor and personalized imagery with her partner to visualize giving birth to her baby successfully over the next few weeks. She feels it is helping her to prepare for the delivery.

You make a mental note to ensure that you always ask individuals about their levels of comfort with imagery you use in future.

CASE STUDY 2

Exam Stress and Anxiety: *Goal-Directed Visualization Outcomes for Taran*

Taran is a final year BSc (Hons) student. He has suffered from exam stress and anxiety since starting university, but it has been getting progressively worse. Now that he is in his final year, it is really impacting on his studies and he fears failure; or at least that his performance and thus marks will be affected adversely.

His general practitioner has prescribed medication, and he has joined relaxation and mindfulness meditation classes suggested by the student well-being services. To date he feels these have not really helped; the medication is making him feel drowsy, and he is finding he cannot concentrate in the classes because his thoughts and fears are fixated on failing the course.

Having listened to Taran, you suggest that he try goal-directed visualization in the hope that the active role he will have to take in the process will give him a greater sense of control over his own destiny; at the moment he feels he is at the mercy of his fears and anxiety.

You work through the process as described in this chapter. Taran locates and visualizes his special place easily. Drawing on imagery from his childhood he creates a beautiful garden filled with trees; it is night with a full moon, and it is calm, quiet and peaceful. In the receptive stage of the visualization, Taran focuses on the issue at hand: his anxiety. He calls on his inner guide, who appears in the shape an old and wise tawny owl; it tells Taran that his fear of failing is the problem and that if he can overcome this, then he can and will succeed.

After discussing his experiences with you, Taran composes four positive affirmations relevant to the matter at hand. These are: I believe in myself; I can achieve my aim and pass the exams; I can cope in exam situations and I feel calm and relaxed.

In the programmed visualization stage, Taran struggles to invoke a positive image of himself being in the exam room completing the paper; his feelings of panic are too strong. You suggest he take a step back and observe himself sitting at the desk rather than actually being present at the desk himself, or use a different image like watching himself successfully leaving the exam room or crossing the stage at his graduation ceremony.

This third person approach gives him some distance and allows him to watch himself at the desk objectively. As an observer, he feels great empathy and support for himself and finds he is able to find and direct positive energy towards himself at the desk. This is an encouraging step for Taran and he intends to build on using the third person perspective to help him 'see' himself more clearly and be more objective and reflective about his anxiety and ability to visualize success. He loves the image of watching himself leaving the exam room and crossing the stage at graduation; he gives himself a thumbs up on both occasions and finds this very motivating.

ACTIVITY

For each of the case studies:
1. List the key aspects used in the goal-directed visualization approach.
2. Consider why this approach was taken.
3. Write down the impact goal-directed visualization is having from a psychological perspective.
4. Write down the impact goal-directed visualization is having from a physical perspective.
5. Write down the impact goal-directed visualization is having from an emotional perspective.
6. Consider the outcomes on quality of life and overall well-being for both individuals.

Chapter 20 will focus on autogenic training. This method uses easy mental exercises to bring about a meditative state of mind and deep relaxation (Bird & Pinch 2002).

REFERENCES

Achterberg, J. (1985). *Imagery in healing: Shamanism and modern medicine*. Boston: New Science Library.

Armitage, C. J., & Reidy, J. G. (2008). Use of mental simulations to change theory of planned behaviour variables. *British Journal of Health Psychology, 13*, 513–524.

Becker, D. A., & Pentland, A. (1996). *Staying alive: A virtual reality visualization tool for cancer patients. AAAI Technical Report.* Cambridge, MA: AAAI.

Bird, J., & Pinch, C. (2002). *Autogenic therapy: Self-help for mind and body*. Dublin: Newleaf.

Clouston, T. J. (2015). *Challenging stress burnout and rust-out: Finding balance in busy lives*. London: Jessica Kingsley.

Conroy, D., Hagger, M. S. (2017). Imagery interventions in health behavior: A meta-analysis. Retrieved September 6, 2019 from https://osf.io/peyxs/.

Conroy, D., Sparks, P., & de Visser, R. (2015). Efficacy of a non-drinking mental simulation intervention for reducing student alcohol consumption. *British Journal of Health Psychology, 20*, 688–707.

Dalloway, M. (1992). *Visualization: The master skill in mental training*. Phoenix, AZ: Optimal Performance Institute.

Davis, M., Shellman, E., & McKay, M. (2000). *The Relaxation and stress reduction workbook* (5th ed.). Oakland, CA: New Harbinger.

Farmer, K. U. (1995). Biofeedback and visualization for peak performance. *Journal of Sport Rehabilitation, 4*, 59–64.

Fanning, P. (1988). *Visualization for change*. Oakland, CA: New Harbinger.

Felix, M. M. S., Ferreira, M. B. G., Oliveira, L. F., Barichello, E., Pires, P. S., & Barbosa, M. H. (2018). Guided imagery relaxation therapy on preoperative anxiety: A randomised control trial. *Revista Latino-Americana de Enfermagem, 26ce*, 3101. Retrieved November 26, 2019, from https://www.semanticscholar.org/paper/Guided-imagery-relaxation-therapy-on-preoperative-a-Felix-Ferreira/75012853311748e5f8ea5630b900e968bb73a9ca.

Gollwitzer, P. M., & Sheeran, P. (2006). Implementation intentions and goal achievement: A meta-analysis of effects and processes. *Advances in Experimental Social Psychology, 38*, 69–119.

Gordon, J. S., Giacobbi, P., Jr., Armin, J. R., Nair, N. R., Bell, M. L., & Povis, G. (2019). Testing the feasibility of a guided imagery tobacco cessation intervention delivered by a telephone quitline: Study protocol for a randomized controlled trial. *Contemporary Clinical Trials Communications*, *16*, 100437.

Gregerson, M., Roberts, I., & Amiri, M. (1996). Absorption and imagery locate immune responses in the body. *Biofeedback and Self-Regulation*, *21*, 149–165.

Hagger, M. S., Lonsdale, A., & Chatzisarantis, N. L. (2011). Effectiveness of a brief intervention using mental simulations in reducing alcohol consumption in corporate employees. *Psychology, Health & Medicine*, *16*(4), 375–392.

Hagger, M. S., Lonsdale, A., Koka, A., et al. (2012). An intervention to reduce alcohol consumption in undergraduate students using implementation intentions and mental simulations: A cross-national study. *International Journal of Behavioral Medicine*, *19*(1), 82–96.

Jacobson, E. (1938). *Progressive relaxation* (2nd ed.). Chicago: University of Chicago Press.

Knauper, B., McCollam, A., Rosen-Brown, A., Lacaille, J., Kelso, E., & Roseman, M. (2011). Fruitful plans: Adding targeted mental imagery to implementation intentions increases fruit consumption. *Psychology and Health*, *26*(5), 601–617.

Koka, A., & Hagger, M. S. (2017). A brief intervention to increase physical activity behaviour among adolescents using mental simulations and action planning. *Psychology, Health, & Medicine*, *22*(6), 701–710.

Kross, E., & Grossmann, I. (2012). Boosting wisdom: distance from the self enhances wise reasoning, attitudes, and behavior. *Journal of Experimental Psychology: General*, *141*(1), 43–48.

Libby, L. K., & Eibach, R. P. (2011). Visual perspective in mental imagery: A representational tool that functions in judgment, emotion, and self-insight. *Advances in Experimental Social Psychology*, *44*, 185–245.

Libby, L. K., Shaeffer, E. M., & Eibach, R. P. (2009). Seeing meaning in action: A bidirectional link between visual perspective and action identification level. *Journal of Experimental Psychology: General*, *138*(4), 503–516.

Libby, L. K., Shaeffer, E. M., Eibach, R. P., & Slemmer, J. A. (2007). Picture yourself at the polls: Visual perspective in mental imagery affects self-perception and behavior. *Psychological Science*, *18*(3), 199–203.

Lichstein, K. L. (1988). *Clinical relaxation strategies*. New York: John Wiley.

Munezane, Y. (2015). Enhancing willingness to communicate: Relative effects of visualization and goal-setting. *The Modern Languages Journal*, *99*(1), 175–191.

Oettingen, G. (2012). Future thought and behaviour change. *European Review of Social Psychology*, *23*(1), 1–63.

Ouellette, J. A., Gibbons, F. X., Reis-Bergan, M., & Gerrard, M. (2005). Using images to increase exercise behavior: Prototypes versus possible selves. *Personality and Social Psychology Bulletin*, *31*(5), 610–620.

Paivio, A. (1985). Cognitive and motivational functions of imagery in human performance. *Canadian Journal of Applied Sport Science*, *10*, 22S–28S.

Polden, M., & Mantle, J. (1990). *Physiotherapy in obstetrics and gynaecology*. Oxford, UK: Butterworth-Heinemann.

Rennie, L. J., Harris, P. R., & Webb, T. L. (2016). Short communication: visualizing actions from a third-person perspective: effects on health behavior and the moderating role of behavior difficulty. *Journal of Applied Social Psychology*, *46*(12), 724–731.

Rennie, L., Uskul, A. K., Adams, C., & Appleton, K. (2014). Visualisation for increasing health intentions: Enhanced effects following a health message and when using a first-person perspective. *Psychology & Health*, *29*(2), 237–252.

Richardson, A. (1969). *Mental imagery*. New York: Springer.

Ryman, L. (1994). Relaxation and visualization. In R. J. Wells, & V. Tschudin (Eds.), *Wells' supportive therapies in health care*. London: Baillière.

Ryman, L. (1995). Relaxation and visualization. In D. Rankin-Box (Ed.), *The nurses' handbook of complementary therapies*. Edinburgh: Churchill Livingstone.

Samuels, M., & Samuels, N. (1975). *Seeing with the mind's eye: The history, technique and uses of visualization*. Toronto: Random House.

Simonton, O. C., Matthews-Simonton, S., & Creighton, J. L. (1986). *Getting well again*. London: Bantam.

Schaeffer, E. M., Libby, L. K., & Eibach, R. P. (2015). Changing visual perspective changes processing style: A distinct pathway by which imagery guides cognition. *Journal of Experimental Psychology: General*, *144*(3), 534–538.

Shone, R. (1984). *Creative visualization*. Wellingborough, UK: Thorsons.

Sordoni, C., Hall, C., & Forwell, L. (2002). The use of imagery in athletic injury rehabilitation and its relationship to self-efficacy. *Physiotherapy Canada*, *54*(3), 177–185.

Tindle, H. A., Barbeau, E. M., & Davis, R. B. (2006). Guided imagery for smoking cessation in adults: a randomized pilot trial. *Complement. Health Pract. Rev*, *11*(3), 166–175.

Trope, Y., & Liberman, N. (2010). Construal level theory of psychological distance. *Psychological Review*, *117*(2), 440–463.

Tusek, D. L., & Cwynar, R. E. (2000). Strategies for implementing a guided imagery programme to enhance patient experience. *AACN Clinical Issues*, *11*(1), 68–76.

Vasquez, N. A., & Buehler, R. (2007). Seeing future success: Does imagery perspective influence achievement motivation? *Personality and Social Psychology Bulletin*, *3*(10), 1392–1405.

Vissing, Y., & Burke, M. (1984). Visualization techniques for health care workers. *Journal of Psychosocial Nursing and Mental Health Services*, *22*(1), 29–32.

Wolpe, J. (1958). *Psychotherapy by reciprocal inhibition*. Redwood City, CA: Stanford University Press.

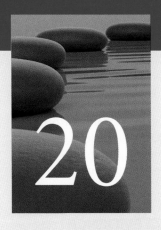

20

AUTOGENIC TRAINING

DR RUTH T NAYLOR

CHAPTER CONTENTS

LEARNING OBJECTIVES

The aim of this chapter is to offer health care professionals a practical and safe guide to the prescription of autogenic training (AT) practice for themselves and those in their professional care.

By the end of this chapter you will be able to:

1. Understand current explanations of how AT works as a prohomeostatic, self-normalizing psychophysiological process.

2. Describe in simple terms what daily practice of AT involves.

3. Recognize the many benefits of regular AT practice for people who are well, for the 'worried well' and for those who may be facing a variety of challenges.

4. Acknowledge safeguarding issues when working with participants.

5. Know about the evidence base for using AT for a variety of conditions.

The chapter will conclude with key points and time for reflection, providing learning opportunities through case studies.

INTRODUCTION TO AUTOGENIC TRAINING

AT is an easy-to-learn, drug-free, meditative-type method for inducing the relaxation response (Benson 1975) and allowing the organism to self-balance. It was developed between 1900 and 1925 by Dr Johannes H. Schultz. From observation, Schultz realized that heterohypnosis (hypnosis by an outsider) is only possible under a condition of autohypnosis, or self-suggested hypnosis. Schultz observed that when patients learned to put themselves, without the guidance and suggestions of another person, into a light trance by passively concentrating on sensing the heaviness and warmth which naturally exists in the musculoskeletal system, they seemed to benefit in terms of their mental and physical health. Schultz called this state 'autogenic'. He then proceeded to develop the therapeutic process further by teaching people how to quickly and safely emerge from the autogenic state, and by including other body parts in addition to musculoskeletal and associated circulatory systems. Since then, there have been numerous re-publications of his work in German and the volume has since been translated wholly or in part into English (1959), French (1958), Italian (1968), Japanese (1968), Portuguese (1967), and Spanish (1954); it is now taught and practised worldwide for performance improvement and for regaining and maintaining homeostatic and allostatic balance.

AT practice helps people 'Switch' quickly and easily out of a stressed state and into self-balancing state on cue (Schultz 1970) (Table 20.1). This switching is said by Schultz to 'break the circle of conditioning', naturally off-loading stress (allostatic load), thus, over time, normalizing and bringing the whole person back into balance. AT is at the heart of every other autogenic method, including autogenic meditation (Schultz & Luthe 2001), autogenic modification (Schultz & Luthe 2001), autogenic verbalization (Luthe 1979), autogenic neutralization (Luthe 2001a), autogenic feedback training (Cowings 1990, Cowings et al 2018, Luthe 1979) and autogenic behaviour therapy (Angers et al 1977; Benson 1975; Ikemi et al 1975; Luthe 1979, 1982a).

Autogenic modifications include specific, positive organ-related phrases and personally developed positive affirmations to add to standard AT practice. Autogenic meditation is learned after at least a year of AT practice and involves focusing on images of colours, objects, concepts and personalities. Autogenic verbalization is an introductory form of autogenic neutralization. It builds on the reactions and abreactions that develop during AT and is a more intensive, cathartic addition to standard AT practice. Autogenic feedback training was developed and used in NASA for more than 30 years to improve astronaut performance, and Schultz-type AT is taught by the US Veterans Administration (Fig. 20.1).

AT is accessible to almost anyone because it requires no special clothing or physical activities, it is a secular method, and the full method can be taught to people age 12 upwards. AT is a cost-effective intervention for primary care because it can be taught over the course of 8 to 10 weeks, either one to one or in groups of up to 10 people. Once learned, short or long versions of AT can be practised by most people almost any time and anywhere they wish to practise it. However, in almost every country where AT is practised, to acquire proficiency as a trainer it is necessary to join a course designed along the lines recommended by the International Committee of AT (ICAT) (see Appendix 2), which was founded by Dr Luthe in 1961. This chapter is included to inform the reader of the principles of AT itself, the safeguarding required, and the approved practitioner training courses, and to provide an introduction to the scope and contents of a standard AT course.

INTRODUCTION TO EVIDENCE

Over the course of 100 years, multiple physicians have contributed many studies of AT for a variety of conditions, and these can be found referenced in Schultz's original work (1932), in Schultz and Luthe's six volumes on Autogenic Therapy (1969, 1970, 1972) and in a compilation of work by members of the International Committee of Autogenic Therapy (ICAT), *Autogenic Training: Correlationes Psychosomaticae* (Luthe 1965). Schultz and Luthe argue that AT is more than a relaxation technique, and that profound relaxation may or may not co-occur with AT practice and is not the cause of AT's self-normalizing processes. Since then, qualitative and quantitative studies have been reported by many researchers in English.

Many benefits from practising AT have been reported in qualitative grounded theory studies of the method (Naylor 2013, Yurdakhul et al 2009), including being refreshed and recharged; returning to, finding and becoming themselves; having insights and epiphanies; discovering new meanings; increasing their resilience; and experiencing other positive psycho-spiritual and physiological benefits.

A meta-analytic study by Stetter and Kupper (2002) demonstrated that AT is effective in the treatment of anxiety, mild-to-medium depression and functional sleep disorders. Positive effects have also been observed in psychosomatic disorders such as tension headache, migraine, essential hypertension, coronary heart disease, asthma, Raynaud's disease and certain kinds of pain.

Krampen (1999) reports on a 3-year follow-up of a random allocation to conditions study, of 55 depressed outpatients who underwent psychotherapy only or in combination with learned AT. Findings show that the probability of success (significant reduction in

TABLE 20.1
The Concentrative (Authentic/True/Real Suggestive) Experience of the Switching Process   [*Das Konzentrative ('Echt Suggestive') Umschaltungs-Erlebnis*]

1. Passive Agreement

2. Centering

    Calmness, Through Body Scan

    'Closing Off Outer Distractions'

    'Critical Self Observation'

3. Closing the Eyes

    'Restricting the Visual Field'   Passiveness

    'Introversion – Turning to the Inside'   Deepening

4. Somatising

5. Quiet, Calm, Rest   All Is of Equal Value

6. Relaxation

7. Shift from Alert/Awake State of Consciousness

    Awareness of Sensory Stimulation* ↑

    Judging ↓ Spontaneity ↓

    'Introspection'

8. Slowing Down

9. Ego Detachment ('Not-Self')

    Receptivity ↑

    Knowing ↑

    Coherence Disintegrates

    Form Transforms & Disintegrates

    Meaning Changes and Disintegrates

    Ego Boundaries Shift

10. Affect

    Completely Self-Generated, Relaxation-Euphoria!

11. Switching   'Physiological'

    Breaking the Circle of Conditioning   Organismic

                                                                             'Psychological'

12. Experiencing an Evidence That Has a Quality of Redemption,† 'Visualised Comprehension', 'Seeing the Picture'

---

*Getting to the threshold situation, awareness of it from within, refer to autogenic discharges, the ability to be consciously aware of sensory stimulation increases.

†To be free, to have freed yourself – this is a healing release which arises from within the self, freeing from all kinds of connections and relationships and ties that bind metaphorically. The imaginary world (the inner world of entertaining possibilities) seems to be opened by the evidence.

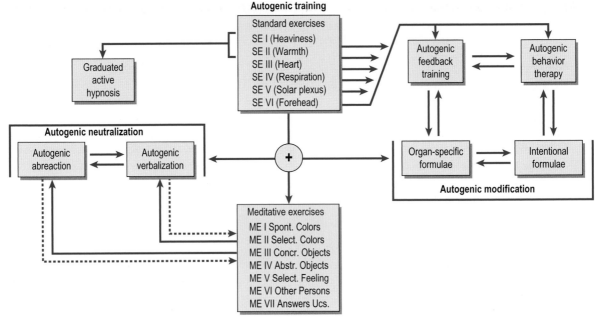

Fig. 20.1 ■ Autogenic methods, as of 1977. (Luthe, 1982b; Luthe, 1979)

depression relapse rates) with psychotherapy alone is 60%, whilst adding AT to the mix increases the probability of success to 91%. Psychosomatic complaints also reduced and the positive results were maintained over 3 years. Participants who underwent the psychotherapy- only intervention had a significant increase in Beck Depression Inventory (see Chapter 28) scores after 3 years and continued to have psychosomatic complaints. Extensive research has shown that psychotherapy plus AT has been shown to be six times more effective than psychotherapy alone.

Bowden et al (2011) carried out a prospective audit of the self-reported (see Chapter 28) experiences of 153 people learning AT at the AT Department of the Royal London Hospital for Integrated Medicine. A total of 73% of participants 'were identified as having sleep related problems'. The audit found that practice of AT improved sleep onset latency. People reported falling asleep more quickly after night waking and on awakening, feeling more refreshed and more energized, with well-being, anxiety and depression scores significantly improved.

Evidence has shown that AT can reduce anxiety, insomnia and panic attacks for many learners

(Bowden 2002, Bowden et al 2011). For example, nursing students' anxiety significantly reduced in simulated training situations (Holland et al 2017), and this was found to be generally consistent across nursing education (Kanji et al 2006). Posttraumatic stress disorder (PTSD) sufferers in the fire service also benefit from AT practice (Mitani et al 2006).

A case study of a psoriasis sufferer shows AT plus other biofeedback techniques clears this skin disorder, with gains maintained over 4 months (Kline & Peper 2013).

Takaishi's (2000) study of 120 anxious patients compared the uptake of AT with Jacobson's progressive muscle relaxation (PMR) (see Chapter 6) and found that AT was significantly superior to PMR in inducing muscle relaxation as measured by electromyography, and significantly superior by self-report in increasing mental calmness. Takaishi hypothesizes that these differences may be related to the simple facts that patients perceive AT as easier to learn and practise because it focuses on the autonomic nervous system and also includes the cognitive and emotion regulation phrases – positive personal affirmations and phrases relating to calmness.

Krampen and von Eye (2005) compared uptake and continuing practice of introductory courses for AT and PMR in German adolescents and adults in an outpatient, inpatient and preventative setting. Attrition rates for AT were 11% and for PMR 21%. Their study speaks to the ethical importance of matching the 'relaxation' intervention to the participant (Streifel 2004).

For coronary angioplasty patients, a randomized control trial comparing medical care only to medical care combined with AT found a significant difference between the two groups' anxiety levels, both at 2 months and again at 5 months, suggesting that AT is effective at reducing anxiety for these types of patients (Kanji et al 2004).

Kanji and Ernst (2000) studied the effectiveness of AT as a pain reliever in conditions such as childbirth, back, heart and cancer pain, and found AT practice to be useful. As a result, they proposed that AT be introduced into the treatment of a wide range of pain-related disorders where it could help to reduce the need for analgesic drugs. Furthermore, a randomized controlled trial with 152 university students suffering from headache pain found that AT plus cervical spine kinesiotherapy and posture training significantly decreased pain intensity and frequency of tension-type headaches (Álvarez-Melcón et al 2018).

Ajimsha and colleagues (2014) reported on a randomized controlled single-blind study of 67 Parkinson's patients who either learned AT in combination with physiotherapy or only received physiotherapy. Patients in the AT group 'performed better than the control group in weeks 8 and 12' (Ajimsha et al 2014) on the motor score subscale of the Unified Parkinson's Disease Rating Scale.

Other studies have shown the positive impact of AT practice on reducing anxiety and stress and improving coping, including Kanji and colleagues (2006), Lim and Kim (2014) and Golding, Kneebone and Fife-Schaw (2016).

THEORIES BEHIND AUTOGENIC TRAINING

Many people call the autogenic state an 'altered state of consciousness (ASC)', and some refer to it as being in a self-induced hypnotic trance. After studying brain responses using electroencephalogram (EEG) whilst people were practising AT, it was concluded that AT is not on the sleep–wake continuum, but is parallel to it (Luthe 2001b), so sleep appears to refresh people differently than AT practice does.

Some researchers hypothesize about how AT works. Data were gathered from 34 diaries and 19 interviews (335,110 words), which were provided by anxious individuals who learned and practised AT in England between 1985 and 2007 (Naylor 2013). Here is what some people said about how AT works for them (Naylor 2013):

- Opens lines of communication – identifying and naming feelings is part of the solution.
- AT continuously brings the unexpected to light in a safe and controlled way.
- Acts as a stress buffer, a mood-regulator.
- Restores good sleep along with confidence during the day.
- The practice integrates me, makes me feel whole.
- Brings calm mind, stability, and ability to put things into perspective.
- Self-hypnosis, auto-suggestion, dropping into deep relaxation.

Dr Schultz had an organismic (bionomic/psychophysiological) hypothesis for how AT may work. He proposed that switching into the 'autogenic state' daily and then repeatedly spending short bursts of time in this state facilitated the normalising action of all the regulatory systems in the body-mind (Schultz & Luthe 2001, Zannino 2017) (see Table 20.1).

Schultz had realized early on that AT was a form of psychotherapy, and he and his colleague, Dr Wolfgang Luthe, had extensive experimental evidence and clinical experience with people on waiting lists for psychotherapy. Their data and observations convinced them to call AT a 'small psychotherapy' (Luthe 1965, p174). This is because patients were able to get off the waiting list simply by practising the method, which allows all three levels of our brains (Zannino 2017), from our perceptual apparatus to our complex meaning making, to do their work. Zannino hypothesizes that AT re-establishes a flexible balance between the sympathetic and parasympathetic nervous systems, and this hypothesis is consistent with Schultz, Luthe and colleagues (2001).

Reptilian Brain

The first level is what we now call the 'reptilian brain'. This is the part of our brains telling us, for example, when there is a threatening environmental stressor. This part of our brain homeostatically prepares our body almost instantly to fight or flee (sympathetic response system) (see Chapter 1), or to freeze or faint (parasympathetic response system) (see Chapter 1). So AT is normally practised when people are free of external stressors and distractions.

Limbic Level

The second level of the brain that AT practice affects is the limbic level. When we are switching into the 'autogenic state', we are moving away from all kinds of attachments and judgements that are instigated at the limbic level. Turning off attachments and judgements and simply 'being' is beneficial for breaking cycles of thought, feeling and action that are 'stuck', such as in posttraumatic stress, chronic pain, anxiety and depression.

Neocortex

When we switch to the self-generated autogenic state, we are also letting go of awareness that arises from the third part of our brains, the neocortex. This is where our meaning making, along with our 'thinking' and feelings about these attachments, arise. As these processes are affected, people report epiphanies, changes of meaning and thought, increases in resilience and other positive psychospiritual benefits (Yurdakhul et al 2009).

These three levels of impact of AT practice are vital not only for off-loading internal stress and for maintaining allostatic balance (Ramsay & Woods 2014, Rosen & Schulkin 2004), but also for managing external stressors more efficiently and effectively.

KEY ASPECTS OF THE PROCEDURE

Unlike other relaxation techniques, such as PMR (see Chapter 8) and its short form (see Chapter 24), applied relaxation (see Chapter 9), both of which are about doing something 'to' the body in a striving way, AT procedures and guidance were and continue to be specifically designed to support dynamic and optimal self-regulation by simply 'being in' the body in the here and now in a structured, non-judgemental way.

AT practice enables the body and the mind to self-balance and maintain equilibrium. Participants experience this as switching off, being in flow, and being profoundly relaxed. AT practice is optimally done by:

1. Reducing external stimulation. If possible, participants are urged to practise in a quiet environment and to use specific postures which are not only comfortable but also reduce stimulation. Sitting in an armchair or on a stool or lying down on a floor or bed with neck and legs adequately supported are the three recommended postures (Fig. 20.2; also refer back to Chapter 3).
2. Developing an attitude of passive observation, concentration and acceptance. This is described by Schultz and Luthe (2001b) as a state of mind which is non-judgemental, non-striving and unconcerned with the end product. This means paying attention to the self and not forcing any

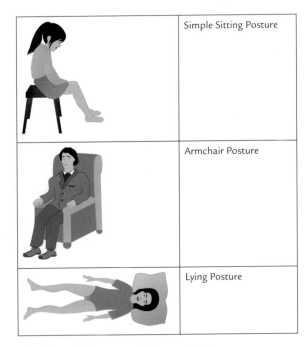

Fig. 20.2 ■ AT postures. (Coleman, 1986)

Simple Sitting Posture

Armchair Posture

Lying Posture

change, just letting the exercise work by taking an 'allowing' rather than a 'doing' approach (Naylor 2013). As and when distracting thoughts enter the mind, they are noticed, accepted and let go by gently turning back to the practice phrases about the body. Whilst on the surface the autogenic states of passive awareness, concentration and acceptance appear to be common to all forms of meditation, they differ in aim and method (Naylor 2010, Onda 1965). Discussion of these overlaps and differences are beyond the remit of this chapter.

3. Repeating subvocally six phrases focused on body systems in a proscribed order using what are called 'Standard Exercise' phrases or 'formulae':

   SE1: My arms and legs are heavy and warm

   SE2: My neck and shoulders are heavy

   SE3: My heart beats calmly and normally

   SE4: It breathes me

   SE5: My solar plexus is warm

   SE6: My forehead is cool

   PA: Personal affirmations and organ specific formulae may be added to practice as clinically appropriate and as developed between the participant and the AT practitioner. An example of a personal affirmation is 'I am confident', and an example of an organ specific formula is 'The lower part of my spine is warm' (Luthe & Schultz 2001).

4. Making mental contact with the body parts to which the phrases refer draws the person's attention away from the external environment and to their body as it is in the present moment. The first two SE phrases are often presented on their own by clinicians and researchers, and as necessary to tailor the training to the participant. It is not necessary to feel heaviness; some participants feel what is called 'paradoxical lightness', whereas others may feel twisting, forms of body dysmorphia or more heaviness on one side than the other, for example. Warmth is often felt before the SE2 Warmth phrase is introduced, as relaxation of muscles enables blood to flow more easily, thus warming the limbs. Heartbeat may be felt all over the body initially and in the form of pulses, although participants are

encouraged to feel their hearts beating by placing hand on heart to locate it and attend to it whilst subvocally saying the Heartbeat phrase. Warmth to the Solar Plexus, which is a complex system of radiating nerves, may be instantly felt by some participants. The SE phrases, 3, 4 and 5, are hypothesized to work in combination on one of the two vagal systems, the one which is associated with 'calm states and social behaviour (Porges 2007)'. Coolness of the forehead is a more localized experience, sometimes felt as a cool breeze.

Unlike heterohypnosis, central to AT practice is the principle of participant control. The trainer describes and demonstrates the technique and guides the participant to complete the process in the set way, and it is participants who carry it out as best as they are able in the moment.

To reinforce this notion, the phrases are styled in the first person at the start, although the possessive pronouns may be omitted to encourage loss of ego control and letting go after the technique is learned if the participant is comfortable doing so. About 30 seconds are assigned to each phrase, and a further 35 to 40 seconds for continued focusing of attention by the participant.

After working through the set of phrases, a cancellation procedure is carried out as a safeguard against a strong parasympathetic reaction (fainting) or a physiological disturbance, and to bring the participant back to a normal waking state of consciousness. The whole routine is then repeated, including the cancellation, three times in total, until the participant is trained to emerge from the autogenic state quickly and easily.

After these repetitions and cancellations, participants are comfortably seated so that the AT practitioner can gather feedback, which may be used to reduce or alter the set of phrases and the practice, depending on the participant's progress and reactions.

In the feedback session participants are asked to describe what happened and how they think and feel about their reaction. They are encouraged to write this in a journal and to bring this journal to the next training meeting as AT has a logotherapeutic aspect, too (Frankl 1969). There is also time set in feedback sessions to apply some basic cognitive–behavioural techniques (CBT) (see Chapter 16) as the AT practitioner thinks may be appropriate.

Schultz and Luthe (1969) worked slowly through the schedule, initially taking 6 months to complete for many people. The need to save time and money and to make the relaxation technique more widely available to people in community settings means it can now be completed in 8 to 10 weeks for participants who are able to tolerate and benefit from a faster pace. This is after an initial and complete clinical assessment and includes a follow-up meeting in 3 months.

The following version of the weekly procedures is adapted from Coleman (1986), Schultz and Luthe (2001) and the US Veterans Administration (2018). For safeguarding, it is important for health care professionals to note that practising as outlined here is not a substitute for learning AT for themselves from an autogenic practitioner trained in the technique; nor is it advised to try to guide others until after learning how to safely teach the technique.

Autogenic practitioners always start with a preparatory intake session to introduce themselves to the participant, and the participant to themselves and to the relaxation technique. Practitioners carefully assess whether AT is suitable for that participant in the first instance and to learn if there are any medical or psychological issues which may require the course to be tailored specifically to the participant from the outset. For example, for pregnancy Luthe and Schultz (2001) note that whilst AT practice is used prophylactically and therapeutically during prenatal stages (to prepare for effacement and dilation) and postnatal stages (to promote lactation and to reduce urinary retention), for safeguarding, SE5 is not used prenatally. It is added postnatally, however, and then with reduction in the number of repeats until the trainer and the mother agree the full set of repeats can be undertaken. Another example is this: for migraine sufferers SE6 is reduced or omitted entirely.

Preparatory Introduction for Participants

A short description introduces participants to the method or reminds them of the procedure. For this talk they can be seated.

AT practice has been shown to help people with a variety of conditions. Over time, practice of the exercises can help you to complete your internal stress cycle responses, to offload accumulated stress held in your body and mind, and to switch into a self-balancing state, which you may even find to be relaxing.

The technique consists of short phrases calling attention to naturally occurring sensations in the body, such as heaviness [gravity] and warmth [life, metabolism].

I'll be reading them out, and as I read them I'd like you to focus your attention on each one in turn, repeating the phrase in your mind without saying it aloud. Take your attention to concentrate passively on the body part(s) as completely and as passively as you can as I mention them.

Before we start, recall that AT modifies your state of mind, and for some people it may feel like self-hypnosis. Just like learning to drive a car or ride a bicycle, the first thing to learn is how to stop, as you will be moving from the state you are in now to a modified state of consciousness. So for your own safety it is important to know how to stop, how to return to your normal waking state all by yourself. It is important to know how to reinvigorate yourself – Here's how to do that [trainer demonstrates the cancelling or closing process].

Also, it's important that you are comfortable and safe [trainer demonstrates the postures participants can use]. And to check your comfort, I will teach you how to start with a very quick scan of your body. This body scan is not for relaxing. It is just for checking your comfort [trainer recites the body scan whilst participant listens with eyes closed and takes attention around the body in an orderly way for about 15 seconds].

AT is about passive observation of your body, passive concentration on specific parts, and passive acceptance of whatever happens when you do this observation and concentration as passively as you can. If other thoughts come into mind, gently bring your attention back to the phrase and your body. Focusing on the phrase keeps you in the present moment naturally and helps you to train your mind in concentrating on one thing at a time. Do not worry if you lose your place; just go back to whatever phrase you recall.

Now, let's begin with your dominant arm [practitioner then begins by asking participant to take a posture, recites the body scan and begins the practice … 'now, gently take your attention to your [right/left] arm…' and so on].

The Standard Exercises

Lesson 1 – Heaviness to Part of the Musculoskeletal System

After the body scan and beginning with your dominant side [example here is for right-handed participants]

   My right arm is heavy x3.
   My left arm is heavy x3
   Both arms are heavy x3.
   My right leg is heavy x3.
   My left leg is heavy x3.
   Both legs are heavy x3
   My arms and legs are heavy x3.

   Now open and close your hands at least three times; bring them up to your shoulders and down again. Do this at least three times. Bend and stretch your limbs. Take a few deep breaths, and at the top of a stretch, open your eyes. Let them scan the interior of the room. Check to see if you feel fresh and alert – if you want to, do the closing again.

This is followed by the second of three repeats of the full routine. When these come to an end there is a discussion and feedback session with the participant in a seated position. The autogenic practitioner then introduces the participant to Luthe's Checklist of Autogenic Reactions (Coleman 1986, pp110–114). This is a list of possible somatosensory experiences which may be felt during AT practice, such as tingling, lights, sounds, smells, pain in previously injured areas, sighing, awareness of heartbeat, anxiety, need to cry, sneezing and so on. Autogenic practitioners are unique in tracking these reactions, and they use them to help adjust the training programme to each individual participant (Carrington 1998). Participants are initially asked to tick all reactions that apply and to write further notes in their diaries.

Lesson 2 – Heaviness to the Whole Musculoskeletal System

This starts with the body scan and practice of the heaviness phrases, and ends with the addition of 'My Neck and Shoulders are Heavy' x3, along with a calming affirmation 'I am at Peace' x3, followed by the opening and closing of the hands.

Lesson 3 – Warmth to the Musculoskeletal System

   My right arm is heavy x1.
   My arms and legs are heavy x3.
   My right arm is warm x3.
   My left arm is warm x3.
   Both arms are warm x3.
   My right leg is warm x3.
   My left leg is warm x3.
   Both legs are warm x3.
   My arms and legs are warm x3.
   My neck and shoulders are heavy x3.
   I am at peace x3.

For safeguarding, it is important that no images, such as the image of lying on a warm beach or the image of weights attached to arms and legs, should be suggested by the autogenic practitioner or spontaneously adopted by the participant to induce any sensations suggested by any of the standard phrases (Schultz & Luthe 2001, p131).

Lesson 4 – Heartbeat

   My right arm is heavy x1.
   My arms and legs are heavy and warm x3.
   My heartbeat is calm and normal x3.
   My neck and shoulders are heavy x3.
   I am at peace x3.

The programme continues weekly and in a similar process to incorporate the remaining three standard exercises: SE3: It Breathes Me (breath); SE4: My (Upper/Lower) Abdomen (Solar Plexus) Is Warm, and My Forehead Is Cool. Intentional formulae (personal affirmations) and organ specific formulae may be added as required. There is a 3-month follow-up.

Each country uses culturally appropriate translations of the basic practice phrases and autogenic practitioners alter or add to the phrases as necessary depending on the participant's needs. For example, 'My forehead is cool' may become 'My forehead is pleasantly cool', 'My forehead is cool and light' or 'My forehead is slightly cool'. Choosing the phrase which works best is most important for people who suffer from headache or migraine.

HOME PRACTICE

Written handouts are given to participants so they can continue with home practice three times a day, when convenient for their lifestyle and starting around noon if possible. Home practice is essential, and builds up and conditions prohomeostatic normalizing responses and the skill of being able to respond readily to the phrases in most situations. Eventually, a single key phrase will have the capacity to switch on self-balancing and to induce a feeling of calmness and self-control in the present moment.

After several weeks of practice the participant is ready for the next stage, in which they introduce intentional formulae (personal affirmations), which help to lead in a positive direction. These are most effective when kept short, simple and positive; are expressed in the first person present tense; and are related to something in the participant's control. Affirmations may be designed to confirm the sense of self-worth or to counter negative thought patterns, for example: 'I accept myself as I am', 'I am calm and centred', and 'I have plenty of time for everything'. It may take discussion with the practitioner over more than one training session to develop together the affirmation that will be most helpful. Participants are then encouraged to write down in their diaries what happens, if anything, in relation to the affirmation, and to bring the journal to the next training session.

PRECAUTIONS

1. Autogenic training should be viewed as an adjunct to and not a substitute for medical treatment.
2. Depending on an individual's state of health, repetition of the standard phrases must be reduced, postponed or even omitted. A list of contraindications and adjustments are taught to autogenic practitioners, as participant safety is of paramount importance.
3. AT is not suitable for children younger than 5 years. There is a short form for children between the ages of 5 and 12.

APPLICATIONS

AT is useful as an adjunct to other medical, physical and psychological therapies and as a standalone technique for participants concerned with rebalancing, maintaining their health and well-being, increasing their resilience and performance in many areas of life, reducing the impact of pain, decreasing medications, reducing and eliminating pathological anxiety, and having a positive impact on other psychophysiological conditions.

AT is not, however, suitable for everyone. Health care professionals should be aware that although AT may be a suitable complementary treatment for participants who have these conditions – glaucoma, diabetes mellitus, hypoglycaemia, hyper- and hypotension, angina, ischaemic heart disease, tachycardia, bradycardia, arrhythmia, cardiac neurosis, asthma, hyperthyroidism, migraine, peptic ulcer, gastric or pancreatic disease and pregnancy – continued monitoring by a physician is required because medications may need to be reduced or other interventions applied, and the AT programme will need to be specifically tailored.

Furthermore, individuals who have mental incapacity to follow instructions or who have psychosis, schizophrenia, psychopathy and similar are not suitable for the full AT programme, although with the guidance of a trained psychologist or psychiatrist and with physician monitoring, a suitably tailored therapeutic programme may be developed for some individuals and may be beneficial.

KEY POINTS

1. Autogenic training (AT) requires persistence with practice of passively attending to, concentrating on, and accepting without judgement whatever happens in the present moment, whilst passively taking attention to parts of the body, always in the same specified order.
2. The method entails the subvocal repetition of standard phrases related to areas of the body, which are addressed in succession.
3. Practice of AT can be tailored to individuals, depending on their condition, including individually assigned affirmations.

4. After learning the method, participants become conditioned to associate the autogenic state with trigger phrases, such as 'My right arm is heavy' or 'My neck and shoulders are heavy'. Thus the autogenic state can be entered quickly and simply by thinking the trigger.
5. AT is often taught in combination with other therapies for more successful treatment.

Reflection

Describe your understanding of the techniques of AT.

How do you feel about applying this technique in practice?

How would you present AT to those whom you think would benefit from learning and practising the method?

How does recent literature offer insight into AT and its application to managing internal stress and external stressors?

What is the main learning point you will take away from this chapter?

What is your future action plan in terms of using AT?

CASE STUDY LEARNING OPPORTUNITIES

The key points and reflection provide background and knowledge required in relation to the case studies, Mike (Case Study 1) and Stella (Case Study 2), to help deepen understanding of how AT can help manage stress.

CASE STUDY 1

Drug Reaction: AT Outcomes for Mike

Mike faced a number of stressors at the age of 45 when he was diagnosed with cancer. This resulted in him being hospitalized at a psychiatric facility for violent behaviour at home and work after having been prescribed gabapentin for postoperative pain. He was suffering from a severe and rare drug reaction, which remained undiagnosed for approximately 3 weeks. After medication adjustment and behaviour stabilization, Mike was discharged from the psychiatric inpatient facility to home, to work in the transportation industry, and to his partner and family. He was on high doses of antianxiety and antidepressant medication. He tried cognitive–behavioural therapy and mindfulness as prescribed by his general practitioner (GP), with little relief from anxiety and depression. He then self-referred to autogenic training (AT), maintaining contact with his GP throughout the training course. The autogenic therapist also had telephone and written contact with his GP early

on. During intake for AT, Mike stated he wished to 'get back to myself' and to 'get off drugs'.

Mike learned AT one to one with a locally based AT therapist over the course of 6 months. There were difficulties with diary keeping and these were resolved by switching to email, which he sent almost daily over the first 2 months of learning AT. During these first 2 months of AT practice, learning the method proceeded slowly, with heaviness and warmth only, as many emotions were surfacing and Mike stated he needed time to 'get used to all these new emotions'. As his emotion vocabulary was limited and his 'new emotions' needed processing, Mike completed the entire AT training within 6 months.

At 1 year follow-up he stated he had been off antidepressants and anxiolytics and under the care of a new GP for a few months, saying 'thanks to AT, I'm off drugs entirely and I'm back to me'.

CASE STUDY 2

AT Training Course: AT Outcomes for Stella

Nine social workers and counsellors were trained in a group by an autogenic therapist. Some were posted daily to highly violent areas of the city, whereas others worked in middle class neighbourhoods. Each of them wanted to take the first steps to become autogenic therapists by learning for themselves. They thought this would also help them manage the daily stress of their work.

The standard autogenic training (AT) course was delivered with one adjustment. Sharon, one of the participants, was very heart conscious and said she could not consider doing Standard Exercise (SE) 3, My Heart beats Calmly and Normally (HCN), so for the whole group HCN was taught after SE4, It Breathes Me. This one week gave Sharon enough personal processing time and space for her to be able to start HCN in a reduced form, with only one repeat of the phrase the following week. She was able to gradually build up to three repeats over the next few weeks. Otherwise it was not necessary to make any further changes to the training schedule.

At the start of the course, participants were asked to write out a list of their hopes and fears on a sheet, which was then put into an envelope and sealed with their name on it. At the end of the course, participants were asked write a list of what they had achieved out of the course. Then they compared their lists.

At the start, one participant, Stella, described herself as a person who uses alternative therapy for her health and her moods. On precourse intake she said, 'I get angry quite quickly. I can go from 0 to 100 in 2 seconds – shouting – otherwise I am calm and patient. The trigger is when I am exhausted and I step into the house – my tolerance for noise is low and I get consumed with rageful anger. Maybe I have fibromyalgia; it's an unusual kind of tiredness, and I feel an emptiness – it takes me an hour to calm down'. Stella's list of reasons for taking the course were varied: 'As a person I would like to get an understanding of what AT is all about – how we put it into practice – how to self soothe – bring about shifts internally, deal with depression, anxiety, stress and how to teach AT to

clients'. By the end of the course her list of benefits was long. She wrote, 'I get a daily appointment with myself; AT is a stress release tool. I use it when I need to calm down and feel centred. I have acquired a tool that is accessible at any time and something I can facilitate on my own time. It has had an impact on me physiologically and emotionally – it feels like it has had an impact on my autonomic nervous system. I am calmer and have more joy. However, this is only the start'.

ACTIVITY

For each of the case studies:

1. List key aspects used in AT.
2. Consider why this approach was taken.
3. Write down the impact that AT is having from a psychological perspective.
4. Write down the impact that AT is having from a physical perspective.
5. Write down the impact that AT is having from an emotional perspective.
6. Consider the outcomes on quality of life and overall well-being for both individuals.

Chapter 21 will focus on meditation as a relaxation technique.

REFERENCES

Ajimsha, M. D., Majeed, N. A., Chinnavan, E., & Thulasyammal, R. P. (2014). Effectiveness of autogenic training in improving motor performances in Parkinson's disease. *Complementary Therapies in Medicine, 22*(3), 419–425.

Álvarez-Melcón, A. C., Valero-Alcaide, R., Atín-Arratibel, M. A., Álvarez-Melcón, A., & Beneit-Montesinos, J. V. (2018). Effects of physical therapy and relaxation techniques on the parameters of pain in university students with tension-type headache: A randomised controlled clinical trial. *Neurologia, 33*(4), 233–243.

Angers, P., Bilodeau, F., Bouchard, C., et al. (1977). Application of autogenic training an an elementary school. In W. Luthe, & F. Antonelli (Eds.), *Autogenic methods, applications, perspectives, conclusions and recommendations.* Rome: Edizioni Luigi Pozzi.

Benson, H. (1975). *The relaxation response.* New York: Morrow.

Bowden, A. (2002). *Autogenic training, a non-drug approach to anxiety, panic attacks and insomnia: Report on the introduction of autogenic training into a primary care group, Harrow East and Kingsbury PCG [now Harrow PCT].* The Royal London Homeopathic Hospital, Autogenic Training. London: The Royal London Homeopathic Hospital.

Bowden, A., Lorenc, A., & Robinson, N. (2011). Autogenic training as a behavioural approach to insomnia: A prospective cohort study. *Primary Health Care Research and Development,* 1–11.

Carrington, P. (1998). *The book of meditation: The complete guide to modern meditation.* Shaftesbury, UK: Element.

Coleman, J. (1986). *Cathartic autogenic training: A manual for therapists.* London: Jean Coleman.

Cowings, P. A., Toscano, W. B., Reschke, M. F., & Tsehay, A. (2018, September). Psychophysiological assessment and correction of spatial disorientation during simulated Orion spacecraft re-entry. *International Journal of Psychophysiology, 131,* 102–112.

Cowings, P. S. (1990). Autogenic-feedback training: A treatment for motion and space sickness. In *Motion and Space Sickness* (pp. 353–372). Boca Raton: CRC Press.

Frankl, V. (1969). *The will to meaning: Foundations and applications of logotherapy.* New York: Penguin Group.

Golding, K., Kneebone, I., & Fife-Schaw, C. (2016). Self-help relaxation for post-stroke anxiety: A randomised, controlled pilot study. *Clinical Rehabilitation, 30*(2), 174–180.

Holland, B., Gosselin, K., & Mulcahy, A. (2017). The effect of autogenic training on self-efficacy, anxiety, and performance on nursing student simulation. *Nursing Education Perspectives, 38*(2), 87–89.

Ikemi, Y., Nakagawa, T., Suematsu, H., & Luthe, W. (1975). The biologic wisdom of self-regulatory mechanisms of normalization in autogenic and oriental approaches in psychotherapy. *Psychotherapy and Psychosomatics, 25,* 99–108.

Kanji, N., White, A. R., & Ernst, E. (2006). Autogenic training to reduce anxiety in nursing students: randomized controlled trial. *Journal of Advanced Nursing, 53*(6), 729–735.

Kline, A., & Peper, E. (2013). There is hope: Autogenic biofeedback training for the treatment of psoriasis. *Biofeedback, 41*(4), 194–201.

Krampen, G. (1999). Long-term evaluation of the effectiveness of additional autogenic training in the psychotherapy of depressive disorders. *European Psychologist, 4*(1), 11–18.

Krampen, G., & von Eye, A. (2005). Treatment motives as predictors of acquisition and transfer of relaxation methods to everyday life. *Journal of Clinical Psychology, 62*(1), 83–96.

Lim, S. -J., & Kim, C. (2014). Effects of autogenic training on stress response and heart rate variability in nursing students. *Asian Nursing Research, 8*(4), 286–292.

Luthe, W. (Ed.). (1965). *Autogenic training: Correlationes psychosomaticae* (International ed.). New York: Grune Stratton.

Luthe, W. (1979). About the methods of autogenic therapy. In E. Peper, S. Ancoli, & M. Quinn (Eds.), *Mind/Body integration: Essential readings in biofeedback* (pp. 167–186). New York: Plenum Press.

Luthe, W. (1982, December 6a). Autogenic training and altered consciousness. In *Royal Society of Medicine: Lecture* (pp. 22). London: British Autogenic Society.

Luthe, W. (1982b). *Autogenic training: Complementary prohomeostatic approaches.* London: British Autogenic Society.

Luthe, W. (2001a). In W. Luthe (Ed.), *Autogenic therapy: Dynamics of autogenic neutralization* (Vol. V). London: British Autogenic Socity.

Luthe, W. (2001b). In W. Luthe (Ed.), *Autogenic therapy: Research and theory* (Vol. IV). London: British Autogenic Society.

Luthe, W., & Schultz, J. H. (2001). In W. Luthe (Ed.), *Autogenic therapy: Medical applications* (Vol. II). London: British Autogenic Society.

Mitani, S., Fujita, M., Sakamoto, S., & Shirakawa, T. (2006). Effect of autogenic training on cardiac autonomic nervous activity in high-risk fire service workers for posttraumatic stress disorder. *Journal of Psychosomatic Research*, 439–444.

Naylor, R. T. (2013). *Self-balancing sanctuarying: A grounded theory of relaxation and autogenic training.* Canterbury, UK: Canterbury Christ Church University. Unpublished doctoral dissertation.

Onda, A. (1965). Autogenic training and Zen. In W. Luthe (Ed.), *Autogenic training: corelationes psychosomaticae [Autogenic training: Psychosomatic correlations]* (Vol. International Edition, pp. 251–258). London: Grune & Stratton.

Porges, S. W. (2007). The polyvagal perspective. *Biological Psychology, 74*(2), 116–143.

Ramsay, D. S., Woods, S. C. (2014). Clarifying the roles of homeostasis and allostasis in Physiological regulation. *Psychology Review,* 121 (2), 225–47.

Rosen, J. B., Schulkin, J. (2004). Adaptive Fear, Allostasis and the Pathology of Anxiety and Depression. American Psychological Association. doi.org/10.1017/CB09781316257081.009

Schultz, J. H. (1970). Das autogene training *konzentrative selbstentspannung: Versuch einer klinisch-praktischen Darstellung [Autogenic training: Self-relaxation by/through concentration, a clinical – practical presentation].* (9th ed.). Stuttgart: Georg Verlag Thieme.

Schultz, J. H., & Luthe, W. (2001). In W. Luthe (Ed.), *Autogenic therapy: Autogenic methods* (Vol. I). London: British Autogenic Society.

Stetter, F., Kupper, S., 2002. Autogenic training: a meta-analysis of clinical outcome studies. *Application of Psychophysiological Biofeedback*, 27 (1), 45–98.

Streifel, S. (2004). Ethical issues in meditation. *Biofeedback, 32*(3), 5–7.

Takaishi, N. (2000). A comparative study of autogenic training and progessive relaxation as methods for teaching clients to relax. *Sleep and Hypnosis, 2*(3), 132–136.

Veterans Administration. (2018). *Whole Health For Life: Autogenic Training.* VA: US Department of Veterans Affairs. Retrieved from www.va.gov/PATIENTCENTEREDCARE/Veteran-Handouts/Autogenic_Training.asp.

Yurdakhul, L., Holttum, S., & Bowden, A. (2009). Perceived changes associated with autogenic trining for anxiety: A grounded theory study. *Psychology and Psychotherapy: Theory, Research and Practice, 82*(4), 403–419.

Zannino, L.-G. (2017). Bionomics, motivation and the Autogenic State. *International Journal of Autogenics Research, 1*(3), 1–16.

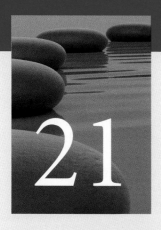

21 MEDITATION

DR CAROLINE BELCHAMBER - CASE STUDY DR RUTH T NAYLOR

CHAPTER CONTENTS

LEARNING OBJECTIVES

The aim of this chapter is to explore meditation and its benefits as a relaxation technique.

By the end of this chapter you will be able to:

1. Understand the background and theory that underpins meditation.

2. Describe the key elements of meditation.

3. Recognize the evidence that underpins meditation.

4. Identify different types of meditation.

5. Discern the effects of meditation.

This chapter will conclude with key points and time for reflection, providing learning opportunities through a case study.

INTRODUCTION TO MEDITATION

The word 'meditation' is used to describe varied states of inner stillness. It is also used to describe different methods of attaining those states. Again, the many schools of meditation all have their own interpretation. Thus, with no universally agreed meaning, attempts to define the word fail. Common to all interpretations, however, is the concept of emptying the mind of thought; that is, letting go of the preoccupations that make up the mind's chatter.

If there is a general aim in meditation, it might be described as non-attachment, although some writers, such as Fontana (1991), feel that to have an aim at all tends to destroy the result since any kind of goal setting calls on rational powers and left-brain activity (see Chapter 18).

Meditation could, therefore, be seen as an opening of the self to reveal its inner world, while at the same time conveying no hint of determination because that would be alien to the meditative state.

People come to meditation for many reasons:

- To find peace
- To achieve awareness
- To gain enlightenment
- To find themselves
- To empty the mind
- To experience true reality.

Because relaxation is one of the effects of all these pursuits, meditation is a relevant topic for inclusion in a book such as this.

Originating in the East, meditation is an integral part of the Hindu, Taoist and Buddhist religions. In the West, meditation has become a popular tool to reduce stress (Suchday et al 2014) and versions have been created which are simpler and these have, for the most part, evolved from Zen and yoga. The material presented in this chapter is of a non-religious form and comes from a variety of modern sources, notably the work of Fontana (1991, 2002).

Another approach is Transcendental Meditation (TM), the central feature of which is the contemplation and repetition of a Sanskrit mantra bestowed by Maharishi Mahesh Yogi who brought the movement to the West in 1959. As well as gathering many disciples, TM attracted a great deal of research: from several hundred studies it emerged that TM created significant physiological changes associated with relaxation. However, lack of controls and the use of self-selected (volunteer) participants weakened the validity of some of these findings.

INTRODUCTION TO EVIDENCE

To date scientific research has focused on neuropsychological and neurophysiological mechanisms of meditation (Chiesa 2010, Fox et al 2014, Sedlmeier et al 2012) as well as therapeutic benefits on people's physical and mental health and well-being (Shonin et al 2014).

Existing research revolves mainly around TM whose effects have been studied extensively across a variety of conditions. A systematic review of its efficacy in the field of medical illness concluded that the strongest evidence in its favour lay in the areas of epilepsy, premenstrual syndrome and menopausal symptoms. A somewhat lesser benefit was found for mood and anxiety disorders, autoimmune disease and emotional

disturbance in neoplastic disease (Arias et al 2006). However, perceived stress has been shown to benefit from meditation in a randomized controlled trial on a healthy population of hospital professionals. After a non-sectarian 8-week course, the researchers found significant reductions in stress levels which remained at that level 19 weeks later (Oman et al 2006).

Meditation is often offered to people with anxiety disorders because it helps to still the mind. However, very few studies are available. From those that exist, it can be seen that the effect of TM on anxiety is comparable with that of other relaxation approaches, as concluded in the systematic review of Krisanaprakornkit et al (2006). In a study to determine the effects of meditation on anxiety levels in people undergoing a colonoscopy, it was found that anxiety levels decreased when meditation was provided 10 to 15 minutes before the colonoscopy (Kartin et al 2017). However, a systematic review and meta-analysis of randomized controlled trials (RCTs) looked at meditation techniques to see if they reduced psychological stress. The study concluded that meditation had very little effect in reducing depression and anxiety (Goyal et al 2014). This study was criticized for its poor methodology because it excluded a number of studies relevant to the research question (Loucks 2014, Walach et al 2014), and it has since been recommended that future reviews of meditation should include cohort studies, random controlled trials (RCTs), controlled trials (CTs), comparing and reporting results for each level of evidence (Orme-Johnson & Barnes 2017). Following this framework the study concluded that TM is effective in reducing anxiety in participants receiving clinical treatment. A study looking at TM as an intervention for posttraumatic stress disorder (PTSD) concluded that TM reduced PTSD symptoms without the person reexperiencing trauma. It is therefore a promising alternative for treating PTSD (Herron & Rees 2018).

Another area of investigation is hypertension where trials have shown a favourable association with meditation (Canter 2003, King et al 2002). Barnes and colleagues (2001) demonstrated significant decreases in systolic blood pressure after a 2-month daily course of TM in an RCT of 35 American adolescents. However, methodological weaknesses characterize many trials exploring the effect of TM on blood pressure. This is the view of Canter and Ernst (2004), who in their systematic review were unable to draw conclusions about the effect of TM on blood pressure because of a lack of good-quality evidence. Conversely, in a recent systematic review and meta-analysis, meditation was seen to play a key role in decreasing blood pressure in people older than 60 years (Park & Han 2017). Even so, in a network meta-analysis looking at the effect of three different meditation exercises on hypertension it was found that there was no significant differences between meditation and other interventions on systolic blood pressure (Yang et al 2017). However, a review of the effects of TM on blood pressure in adults concluded that TM was a promising alternative therapy to reduce blood pressure but stated that future studies should consider RCTs over several months using a larger sample size (Schneider & Reangsing 2019).

In the case of heart disease, there is some evidence to suggest that risk factors such as high blood pressure, high cholesterol and psychosocial stress could be reduced and pathophysiological changes slowed or even reversed after a course of TM (Walton et al 2002, 2004). Results were found to resemble those of orthodox interventions.

It has been proposed that TM could improve cognitive function. Canter and Ernst (2003) conducted a systematic review to test this claim. They found that some trials did support it but the researchers attributed this result to an expectation effect and concluded that there was insufficient evidence to support the claim that meditation could improve cognitive function.

Cancer is another area where the effects of TM have been studied. Tacon (2003) proposed and designed a meditation programme for people experiencing different forms of this disease. Further research has explored meditation as a treatment intervention for people with head and neck cancer who experienced high levels of stress during radiotherapy. Meditation in this case was found to decrease anxiety, depression and emotional distress (Boxleitner et al 2017). A randomized controlled pilot study exploring the efficacy of a meditation intervention for people undergoing biopsy and breast cancer surgery also found that meditation improved psychological and physical well-being with the potential to improve health outcomes in the long term (Wren et al 2019).

A pilot study in older people with osteoarthritis of the knee, demonstrated a significant improvements in pain, physical function, mood and sleep after completion of an 8-week meditation programme (Selfe &

Innes 2013). After this pilot an exploratory randomized clinical trial indicated that meditation may be effective in reducing knee pain, dysfunction and stress while improving mood, sleep and quality of life for older people with osteoarthritis of the knee (Innes et al 2018).

Electroencephalographic changes during meditation suggest a state of decreased arousal in the cerebral cortex. This supports the view that mental activity is reduced. Certainly, meditation has been found to be effective in reducing tension and can often lead to deep states of physiological and phenomenological relaxation. However, it is unclear how much more effective it is than any other relaxation practice. Research findings are inconsistent; some point to the superior benefit of meditation, whereas others are unable to show that meditation is any more effective at lowering physiological arousal than ordinary rest. However, it is claimed that meditation helps quiet the mind and reduce the effect of stressful thoughts. It can thus contribute to a state of relaxation.

THEORIES BEHIND MEDITATION

A number of theories have been put forward to account for the effect of meditation on the individual. Of these, Banquet's (1973) shift in hemispheric dominance is widely accepted. His research suggests that during meditation the left cerebral hemisphere loses its dominance, resulting in a more influential right hemisphere than occurs in everyday life. As a result, linear, verbal thinking plays a less prominent part, allowing intuitive, wordless thinking to express itself. By this means the individual may come to know and understand themselves better and acquire a new peace of mind. In addition the relaxation response (see Chapter 22) originally described by Herbert Benson (1993) came from his research into the effects of meditation. The relaxation response is a model where meditation is used to stabilize the sympathetic nervous system, while activating the parasympathetic nervous system, enabling the physiological and psychological levels to operate together (Benson 1993, Chang 2004). Thus meditation is both a state and a method. As a state, it is one in which the mind is stilled and listening to itself. The meditator is relaxed but at the same time alert. As a method, it consists of focusing attention on a chosen stimulus. This concentration is sustained but effortless and has the effect of detaching the meditator from external life events on the one hand and from their own mental activity on the other. Thoughts may enter the person's head but instead of examining their content, the person allows them to drift away.

This attitude has been described as one of passive concentration and it implies that the meditator has a relaxed attitude while at the same time giving attention that is without criticism or judgement. Mental functions such as thinking and evaluating are inappropriate because they are processed by the left brain; rather, the meditator should cultivate what in Zen is called a 'don't know mind'; that is, a mind which is open and receptive to new, undreamed-of possibilities. Past and future associations are shed. The mind is emptied of all thought save awareness of the stimulus.

In common with hypnosis and daydreaming, meditation is an altered state of consciousness. Fontana (1991) distinguishes it from other altered states, seeing it rather as a rediscovery of normal consciousness because it takes the individual to the core of the self. The meditator does not fall into a trance, become drowsy or surrender control; on the contrary, the person is in a state of heightened awareness, alert, aware of their surroundings and securely focused on the present moment.

Passive concentration, referred to earlier, is also a feature of autogenic training (see Chapter 20) and receptive visualization, although not of programmed visualization which, because it is involved with the achievement of goals, is essentially a left-brain thinking activity and therefore remote from meditation. However, to say that meditation excludes the analytical thinking process does not imply that meditators consider left-brain activity to be of lesser value. Analytical thinking is an essential human function, but its tendency generally to dominate mental activity has the effect of devaluing its counterpart, the imagination. Meditation enables the individual to redress the balance.

A PROCEDURE FOR MEDITATION

Introductory Remarks to Participants

A few words describing the procedure are required before starting the first session.

Meditation is an ancient method of quietening the mind. The method you are about to experience is a non-religious form. It is concerned with focusing the

attention on different phenomena such as the breath, a visual object or a repeated phrase. The effect of the meditation will be to make you feel very peaceful. At no time will you lose consciousness or be controlled by any outside force. The state you reach will be entirely created by you. It is best to come to meditation without expectations; rather, to have an attitude which makes you content to be in tune with yourself.

A Meditation Session

A session may be seen to have four components:

1. Attention to position
2. A winding-down procedure
3. Concentration on a chosen stimulus
4. Return to everyday activity

Attention to Position

In an environment that is quiet and warm, the meditator takes up a sitting or a lying position. Sitting is preferred because some people tend to fall asleep when lying down. The individual may sit in a straight-backed chair, sit cross-legged on a cushion on the floor or take up the lotus position (cross-legged with each foot resting on the opposite thigh). This position can be very uncomfortable for people who are not used to it; even in the East it has never been obligatory if the novice found it unbearable.

Whichever sitting position is chosen, the hands rest on the thighs, with the fingers gently curled or arranged in traditional symbolic postures. The head should be held in a relaxed position directly above the spinal column to release the neck muscles from strain while the eyes may be closed or slightly open.

Winding-Down Procedure

Participants are asked to direct their thoughts inwards.

The meditation session is preceded by a check for muscle tension; that is, participants check all their muscle groups to make sure they are as relaxed as possible. It is often referred to as scanning and may be introduced in the following way.

I am going to ask you to check that your muscles are as relaxed as possible. Starting with your feet, notice any tension ... then move up to your ankles, shifting them slightly if they are not relaxed ... now your legs … and your hips … settle them into the chair or the floor. Continue up through your body to your shoulders, letting them drop down. Allow your arms to fall comfortably, with your fingers free of tension. And now your head: relax your jaw and let your tongue rest in your mouth … let all the muscles in your face feel smoothed out. Allow yourself to unwind, and as you unwind, feel in tune with yourself … listening to yourself … just being you … experiencing what it is to be you … being aware how it feels, without delving into reasons, explanations or even words …

Irritating sounds or bodily discomfort may interrupt the meditation. Davis et al (2000) suggest 'softening' them by purposely giving them attention for a few moments instead of pretending that they do not exist.

Concentrating on a Chosen Stimulus

'All meditations are built upon concentration and tranquillity' (Fontana 1992). The individual quietly focuses attention on the chosen stimulus which may take the form of breath watching, gazing at a visual object or chanting a mantra. The purpose of the stimulus is to hold the attention of the participant.

This may be difficult at first because the mind is used to being engaged in a constant stream of images, memories and associations, all competing with one another. It will not help individuals to fight these distractions, but if they can accept their presence and continue their concentration on the stimulus, the distractions will become weaker. Some people find it useful to regard intruding thoughts as clouds drifting by or leaves floating down a stream. The attention is then gently brought back to the item under focus.

The result of this meditation may be nothing more than a respite from stress for the individual. On the other hand, as the focused mind enters a state of clarity and tranquillity, a deeper part of the self may be reached whereby new insight is gained (Fontana 1991).

Grounding Strategy

Any hint of depersonalization may be counteracted by a process known as 'grounding' or bringing the individual back to the here and now. It involves encouraging the meditator to return their attention to some form of body awareness. Fontana (1991) suggests concentrating on the breathing, whereas Titlebaum (1988) emphasizes the value of feeling the ground. The following passage is adapted from Titlebaum (1988).

Be aware of the ground beneath you. Feel it taking the weight of your body. Feel it supporting you. Notice the parts of your body which touch the ground or are in contact with the chair, if you are sitting. Concentrate on the sensations you are getting from these contact points and feel safely tethered to the ground.

The duration of the session should depend on the experience of the meditator; 5 minutes is considered enough for the novice, 15 to 20 minutes for the experienced practitioner.

Return to Everyday Activity

The return to everyday activity, also known as arousal or termination, is a sequence which brings the meditation to a close.

When you are ready, let your meditation come to an end. If your eyes are open, remove your gaze from the point of focus. If your eyes are closed, allow the point of focus to fade until it disappears. Let it go with a feeling of gratitude towards it. Then turn your attention to your breathing, slowly counting three or four natural breaths.
To help your muscles regain their tone, try slowly moving the body round in small circles before you get up. A few gentle stretches will also enliven the muscles.

Home Practice

Regular practice enhances the benefits gained from meditation. Lichstein (1988), reviewing the evidence, refers to numerous studies which indicate a direct association between the number of hours spent practising and the beneficial effects of meditation.

FOCAL POINTS FOR MEDITATION

Items on which the attention may be focused cover a wide range of objects, sounds and other phenomena. Included in this section are the following:

- The breath
- Visual objects (i.e., circle, mandala, candle, china bowl)

- Parts of the body (i.e., space between the eyes, crown of the head, big toe)
- Mantras

Concentration on the breath is mentioned first for a number of reasons (Fontana 1991):

- It is constantly available.
- It has a rhythmical quality.
- It is directly linked to the autonomic system.
- It symbolizes the life force.

The Breath

The practice of counting the breaths, with one count for every outbreath, is commonly used as a stimulus to hold the attention. On reaching the count of 10, the meditator reverts to 1 again and continues the process for 5 minutes. The breaths should be natural and unhurried. Other forms of breathing meditation consist of focusing the attention on parts of the body involved in respiration such as the tip of the nose or the moving abdomen.

The Tip of the Nose

In the passage below, the meditator concentrates on the tip of the nose. It is assumed that the meditator has already gone through a winding-down procedure (see earlier). Plenty of time should be allowed between the sentences.

Let your attention focus on your breathing and in particular, on the tip of your nose, that curved piece of cartilage that separates your nostrils. If you like, touch it with your fingertips to increase your awareness of it … then concentrate on the feeling of air passing from the outside into your nostrils … notice how cool it is … notice also the warmth and moistness of the air that leaves your nostrils … allow your breathing rhythm to be completely natural as you focus your attention on the tip of your nose … feel the sensation of air being drawn in … sweeping through your nostrils and, in its own time, passing out again … if outside thoughts intrude, gently return to the sensation at the tip of the nose … continue to focus your attention on that point … feel your senses converging on that one spot.

On another occasion the meditator might wish to adopt a different focus, as in the next passage.

The Moving Abdomen

Here, a counting procedure is combined with focusing attention on the abdomen.

Gently turn your attention to your breathing. Begin by noticing it in a general kind of way, then slowly bring your mind to focus on the movement of your abdomen … keep your attention fixed on the movement of your abdomen … swelling as the air is breathed in and sinking as it is breathed out … allow the air to pass in and out quite naturally while you are concentrating on the abdominal movement. Do not try to influence the breathing rhythm but let yourself flow with it … if your mind wanders, gently bring it back to the swelling and sinking abdomen … counting the breaths helps to hold the attention … one count for every breath out … and when you get to 10 or lose count, start again. Please continue on your own.

Visual Object

Visual concentration on an object, sometimes referred to as gaze meditation, offers varied possibilities. Almost any object can become the focus of attention but typically the object is chosen for its symbolic value or its neutral associations: a geometric shape, a candle or a flower all have these characteristics.

The Circle

A circle has the following symbolic qualities:

- It has substance in that it may be solid.
- It has emptiness in that there may be nothing inside it.
- It has motion in that it can roll and spin.
- It has stillness in that it may come to rest.
- It has wholeness by virtue of enclosing all its parts within it.
- It has continuity in that any point along its circumference is both the end and the beginning.

If a circle is chosen as an object for meditation, the instructing meditator may produce one by drawing a thick-edged ring about 30 cm (1 foot) in diameter, emphasizing the centre with a dot and hanging it on the wall. It should be level with the eyes of the seated participants, who position themselves at a comfortable distance from it (Fontana 1991).

The following script can then be used.

Let your gaze fall on the centre of the circle and then remain there … consider the circle simply as a shape and let it speak to you in intuitive terms rather than in words … try to keep your gaze focused on the centre while at the same time absorbing the whole image … do not examine it but feel yourself experiencing it … maintain the visual experience without reacting to it … feel the image extending around your point of focus … be aware of its extremities as your mind flows from the centre to the edges and from the edges to the centre … if your attention should wander, gently bring it back to the centre point … spend several minutes gazing at the image.

The Mandala and the Yantra

The mandala and the yantra serve a sacred purpose in the Buddhist religion. Their complexity, beauty and harmony enrich their symbolic quality and make them the supreme focal object for visual meditation. Although created for use by devotees, they can be meditated on at any philosophical level, and examples are shown in Figs 21.1 and 21.2. The mandala generally contains representations of living things while the yantra is predominantly geometric.

Both enclose symbolic motifs arranged in concentric rings around a clearly defined central point. This point symbolizes the inner self on the one hand and divine consciousness on the other, whereas the enclosing circles represent the cycle of life and the notion of Nature forever renewing herself. Thus the mandala/yantra stands for the personal as well as the transpersonal, for change within permanence, for life both in the present and in eternity, while affirming the fundamental unity of all things.

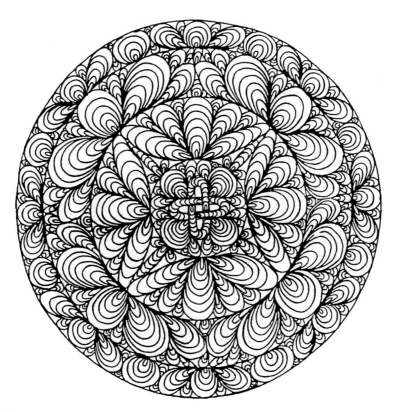

Fig. 21.1 ∎ A mandala.

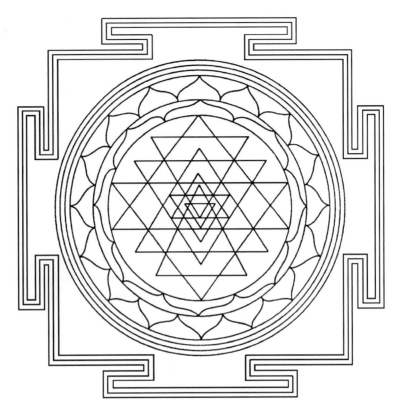

Fig. 21.2 ■ A yantra.

The Candle

As mentioned earlier, the visual image can be used in different ways to clear the mind of thought. For instance, while individuals are gazing at the object, they can intermittently close their eyes and allow the image to recreate itself in their mind, as in the following meditation on a candle burning in a darkened room.

Let the lighted candle hold your attention … settle your eyes on the upper part of the wax column rather than the flame itself … sit without moving while you gaze at it … focus on it in a relaxed but constant way, letting the image fill your mind … continue for at least a minute … Now close your eyes. Notice that the image of the candle prints itself in the darkness … hold the shape in your mind's eye, accepting any change of colour … if it slips to one side, gently bring it back … continue to focus on it until it fades … then open your eyes and resume your gaze on the candle … continue, repeating the sequence in silence for several minutes.

The image that appears behind the closed eyes is known as the 'after-image'

The After-Image

When the gaze is fixed on a particular point for about a minute and the eyes are subsequently closed, the phenomenon of the after-image occurs. This is the negative representation of the object stared at. It immediately begins to fade and after about 20 seconds or so has disappeared. It is a physiological reaction which occurs when the retinal cells get fatigued. Experiencing the after-image is quite different from recreating forms in the imagination, a practice which belongs more to visualization than to meditation.

If meditators are in doubt as to what is being seen behind closed eyes, there are two questions the person can ask themselves.

1. Does the image fade or disappear within 20 seconds? If so, it is likely to be an after-image.

2. Can they scan the image – that is, trace its outlines? If every time they move their eyes to trace the outline the image moves too, it is behaving like an after-image (Samuels & Samuels 1975).

A China Bowl

Certain objects lend themselves to a more exploratory approach. A flower or a piece of porcelain falls into this category. For instance, Davis et al (2000) suggest a china bowl.

Settle your gaze on the object … take it all in … after a few moments, allow your eyes to travel over the object, tracing its lines … noticing its colours … its decoration … and the way it glistens … do not dwell on who made it, how or for what purpose, but see it simply as a shape … experience its visual qualities as if you were seeing it for the first time … if your mind wanders, gently bring it back to the object …

Parts of the Body

Other body parts as well as the breathing organs can be used to provide a focus of attention. This kind of meditation is a feature of yoga, where energy centres (chakras) are represented by the base of the spine, the lower abdomen, the navel, the heart, the throat, the space between the eyebrows and the crown of the head. After meditating on the sites in this order, the physical energies are said to be transformed into spiritual energies.

Yoga is a separate subject and no attempt is made here to present it. However, the symbolic nature of the chakras makes them suitable sites for meditations outside yoga. Two examples are given here: the space between the eyebrows and the crown of the head.

The Space Between the Eyebrows

Behind closed lids, let your eyes turn upwards and settle on the space between your eyebrows … relate to it … recognize its closeness to your brain … feel its central position … imagine viewing it from the outside … then, imagine viewing it from the inside … continue to focus on that one spot … feel drawn to it … and consider that, as the space between your eyebrows is part of you, so you are part of that space.

(Pause)

If outside thoughts drift into your mind, mentally blow them away and return to your point of focus … to the space between your eyebrows.

The Crown of the Head

With your eyes closed, focus your attention on the crown of your head, concentrating on it in a passive way … let your inner eye be drawn to it and held there … see it from the outside, noticing how it appears … then imagine it from the inside, from under the dome of your head …

(Pause)

Symbolically as well as literally, it represents the highest part of you … if thoughts intrude, let them be carried away … let them drift away from you as you gently return your attention to the crown of your head … feel yourself identifying with it … experiencing it … feel yourself uniting with all that is highest within you.

On a simpler level, any part of the body can serve as the stimulus, for example, the big toe.

The Big Toe

With your eyes closed, your legs uncrossed and your muscles relaxed, draw your attention to your right big toe. See it in your mind's eye … move it gently to make its presence felt … notice how it feels when you move it … focus on the sensations you get from bending and stretching it … be aware of the feel of the sock or stocking over it, or of the shoe restricting it … think of it carrying the full weight of the body … think of its strength as well as its mobility … if unwanted thoughts intrude, gently bring your attention back to the toe … focusing on the toe …

Mantras

A mantra is a verbal stimulus which can be used to concentrate the attention. Traditionally it embodies an ancient, sacred truth whose meaning may reveal itself to the meditator during the process of concentration. A well-known example is the Sanskrit word 'om' which is said to represent the primal sound. Pronounced like 'home' without the 'h' (Smith & Wilks 1988), the sound can be intensified by stretching the syllable to form 'a … oo … mmmm' (Fontana 1991). It is the *sound* of the mantra that has articular value for the novice meditator, although its meaning may also be contemplated at a later stage. The following piece is adapted from a passage in Fontana (1991).

> *Breathe in gently and as you let the air out, recite the word 'om': a … oo … mmmm. Feel the sounds vibrating within your body: feel the 'a' ringing in your belly, feel the 'oo' resonating in your chest and the 'mmmm' resounding in the bones of your skull … let these sounds provide a focus for your attention … link them into your natural breathing rhythm … keep the breathing calm and slow and avoid any inclination to deepen it … after 10 breaths, gradually reduce the volume of the sound until the word is spoken under your breath … lower it further … keep your attention focused on the mantra … eventually, you will come to a point where your lips cease to move and the syllables lose their form so that you are left with just an idea … feel it clinging to your mind … united with it … if thoughts intrude, turn them into puffs of smoke and let them blow away.*

Many other sounds or words can act as mantras, e.g., 'peace', 'harmony', 'calmness' or phrases such as 'God is love' and 'here-and-now'. It does not matter if the word has a meaning, since constantly reciting it will tend to divest it of that meaning, although the word may still retain its aura. It is advisable, however, to choose a word that has no emotional associations for the user, and one that is unlikely to stir up their thoughts. While the main purpose of the mantra is to hold the meditator's attention, its rhythmic repetition also has a soothing effect.

On the other hand, a mantra may be picked expressly *for* its meaning. In this kind of meditation the mantra is not reflected on philosophically so much as experienced. It is identified with, rather than analysed.

Lichstein (1988) compares mantra chanting with dwelling on the muscles in progressive relaxation (see Chapter 5) and to the silent recitation of phrases in autogenic training (see Chapter 20) and points out

that in addition to their inherent relaxation properties, they all share the capacity to divert the attention from stressful thoughts.

Proponents of TM insist on the mantra being chosen with ceremony and in secrecy by a master teacher, although this practice has not been shown to be any more effective than one which uses simple words (Benson 1976) (see Chapter 22).

BENEFITS OF MEDITATION

Devotees of meditation claim that they benefit greatly from its practice. These are some of the advantages.

- A better understanding of the self is achieved through meditation. That is, through meditation individuals become more aware of themself and more receptive to the insights that arise from their deeper being.
- A new sense of relaxation and inner peace can be derived from meditation.
- The process itself promotes a clearer mind and improved powers of concentration. These extend outside the meditation session.
- Individuals, by discovering their inner self, are able to live more in harmony with themselves.
- By developing a sense of detachment, individuals come to accept that many of their unpleasant emotional reactions are no more than short-lived bodily sensations created by their thoughts.
- The emphasis on self-awareness helps individuals to live in the present and to value the here and now. When the mind is concentrated in the moment, it becomes keenly alert.

PRECAUTIONS

1. Training in meditation should never be viewed as a substitute for medical treatment; wherever a disorder is present or suspected, medical help should be sought
2. Meditation may not be suitable for people in acute psychotic states.
3. Although the central idea of meditation is to keep the mind focused and aware, it does occasionally happen that an individual loses the

sense of who and where he or she is or develops the feeling of being 'outside the body'. These are trance-like states of disorientation and depersonalization. In this event, a grounding strategy similar to the one referred to on page 253 may provide a remedy. The instructor can safeguard against disorientation and depersonalization by regularly reminding participants to keep their attention focused on the stimulus (Fontana 1991).

4. Meditation creates an altered state of consciousness. Novices will not know in advance how they will respond. It is therefore recommended that, to begin with, sessions be kept short, no more than 5 minutes in length. This can be increased to 15 or 20 minutes for those with experience but not exceeded, because it is possible to meditate too much and run the risk of getting out of touch with day-to-day life. Benson (1976) reports that none of the participants in his studies displayed ill effects after meditating for 20 minutes twice a day.

5. The breathing meditations in this chapter do not seek to interfere with the natural breathing rate or rhythm. However, the mere request to become aware of the breathing can result in a slight alteration of its rhythm. It is therefore suggested that, before attempting breathing meditations, the reader become familiar with the section on hyperventilation in Chapter 4.

6. Benson (1976) believed that it was better to practice meditation before a meal than directly after it. He considered that the process of digestion, by drawing the blood to the viscera, interfered with the physiological changes associated with meditation, and advised waiting for at least 2 hours after eating. More recent research investigating the distribution of blood during meditation supports Benson's view: Bricklin (1990) found that the blood flow to the brain during meditation increased dramatically, rising on average by 65% of its normal volume. It would not, therefore, be constructive to practise meditation at a time when other demands were being made on the vascular system.

7. Those who expect meditation to be a ready remedy for life's problems may become disillusioned. Meditation should be seen as a way of life, not as a panacea.

8. Guidance should be sought from an experienced teacher by those wishing to pursue more advanced forms of meditation because they are beyond the scope of this book.

KEY POINTS

1. Meditation can help to reduce an arousal state.
2. A meditation session begins with a winding-down procedure consisting of a scan of the voluntary muscle groups.
3. The session itself consists of focusing on an object such as the breath.
4. If distracting thoughts intervene, meditators should try to ignore them and bring their attention gently back to the breath or other focal point.
5. Mantras may be used to augment the concentration.
6. The effectiveness of meditation is unclear on account of the quality of much of the research. It is, however, widely used in a variety of conditions. Benefit is reported but does not appear to exceed that of other techniques.

Reflection

Describe your understanding of the techniques of meditation.

How do you feel about applying this technique in practice?

What other meditation techniques have you tried? How do they compare? What differences did you notice in your physical and mental state?

How do you feel after completing meditation?

What is the main learning point you will take away from this chapter?

What is your future action plan in terms of using meditation?

CASE STUDY LEARNING OPPORTUNITY

The key points and reflection provide background and knowledge required in relation to the case study, John, to help deepen understanding of how meditation can help reduce anxiety.

CASE STUDY

Emotional Turmoil: Meditation Outcomes for John

John had many stressors in his life: an unhappy marriage, a house move away from his family of origin, job changes and two young children. He had just graduated and was 'really unhappy' and 'looking for some peace of mind'. John stated that he was looking for a way to get out of the emotional turmoil he was suffering.

Soon after leaving university, John answered an advertisement in a newspaper, which read: 'Learn TM over four weekends'. After this he started to meditate on a daily basis, twice a day for a while, using the mantra a psychologist had given him. He stated he did not think of TM as a relaxing thing, although, he said, 'that's certainly what it was – it relaxed my body, mind and spirit. That was the result'. But he stopped regular meditation practice, and a few years later with his promiscuous wife expressing suicidal ideation, and with his own drinking getting excessive, he returned to meditation, having 'woken up' to an awareness of other people and their feelings and needs, and a realization that life wasn't all about him. He also went to counselling at this time.

Forty years later this is what John had to say about his ongoing meditation practice: 'When I meditate, I still today use a variation of TM. I do the deep breathing, I start to say a mantra, I close my eyes, and focus on a white light that is just inside my skull on my forehead, and that way I just clear my mind out of everything. There are no thoughts, or emotions, just a peaceful calm, centred on the light and my breathing. Pretty soon I stop noticing the breathing and the light, and everything is just blank. And it is peaceful, quiet, calm and serene. I can feel my body relaxing from the top of my head to the bottom of my feet. I feel all of my muscles letting go and relaxing. I do that for about 20 minutes, and then slowly bring myself out and say an affirmation at the end of it'.

The benefits of meditation spill over to John's hospice chaplaincy work as his practice has an effect on the rest of his day. He states he feels calmer, more centred, more alert to what is going on around him, and listens and empathizes better too.

ACTIVITY

For the case study:
1. List the key aspects used in meditation.
2. Write down the impact meditation is having from a psychological perspective.
3. Write down the impact meditation is having from a physical perspective.
4. Write down the impact meditation is having from an emotional perspective.
5. Consider the outcomes on quality of life and overall well-being.

Chapter 22 will focus on Benson's relaxation technique to bring another perspective on using meditation.

TM, Transcendental Meditation.

REFERENCES

Arias, A. J., Steinberg, K., Banga, A., et al. (2006). Systematic review of the efficacy of meditation techniques as treatments for medical illness. *Journal of Alternative and Complementary Medicine, 12*(8), 817–832.

Banquet, J. (1973). Spectral analysis of the EEG in meditation. *Electroencephalography and Clinical Neurophysiology, 35,* 143–151.

Barnes, V. A., Treiber, F. A., & Davis, H. (2001). Impact of transcendental meditation on cardiovascular function at rest and during acute stress in adolescents with high normal blood pressure. *Journal of Psychosomatic Research, 51*(4), 597–605.

Benson, H. (1976). *The relaxation response.* London: Collins.

Benson, H. (1993). The relaxation response. In: Goleman D, Gurin J, editors. *Mind Body Medicine: How to Use Your Mind for Better Health.* New York: Consumer Reports; pp. 233–257.

Boxleitner, G., Jolie, S., Shaffer, D., Pasacreta, N., Bai, M., & McCorkle, R. (2017). Comparison of two types of meditation on patient's psychosocial responses during radiation therapy for head and neck cancer. *Journal of Alternative and Complementary Medicine, 23*(5), 355–361.

Bricklin, M. (1990). Meditation: the healing silence. In: Bricklin, M. (Ed.), Positive Living and Health. Rodale Press: Emmaus, PA.

Canter, P. H. (2003). The therapeutic effects of meditation (leading article). *British Medical Journal, 326,* 1049–1050.

Canter, P. H., & Ernst, E. (2003). The cumulative effect of transcendental meditation on cognitive function: A systematic review of randomized controlled trials. *Wiener klinische Wochenschrift, 115*(21–22), 758–766.

Canter, P. H., & Ernst, E. (2004). Insufficient evidence to conclude whether or not transcendental meditation decreases blood pressure: Results of a systematic review of randomized clinical trials. *Journal of Hypertension*, *22*(11), 2049–2054.

Chang, H. K. (2004). Therapeutic application of meditation to the stress-related disorders. *Korean Journal of Health Psychology*, *9*, 471–492.

Chiesa, A. (2010). Vipassana meditation: Systematic review of current evidence. *Journal of Alternative and Complementary Medicine*, *16*, 37.

Davis, M., Shellman, E., & McKay, M. (2000). *The relaxation and stress reduction workbook* (5th ed.). Oakland, CA: New Harbinger.

Fontana, D. (1991). *The Elements of meditation*. Shaftesbury, UK: Element.

Fontana, D. (1992). *The meditator's handbook: A comprehensive guide to eastern and western meditation techniques*. Shaftesbury, UK: Element.

Fontana, D. (2002). *The meditator's handbook: A comprehensive guide to eastern and western meditation techniques*. London: Thorsons.

Fox, K. C. R., Nijeboer, S., Dixon, M. L., et al. (2014). Is meditation associated with altered brain structure? A systematic review and meta-analysis of morphometric neuroimaging in meditation practitioners. *Neuroscience and Biobehavioral Reviews*, *43*, 48–73.

Goyal, M., Singh, S., Sibinga, E. M. S., et al. (2014). Meditation programs for psychological stress and well-being. *JAMA Internal Medicine*, *174*, 357–368.

Herron, R. E., & Rees, B. (2018). The Transcendental Meditation Programe's impact on the symptoms of post-traumatic stress disorder of veterans: An uncontrolled pilot study. *Military Medicine*, *183*, e144–150.

Innes, K. E., Selfe, T. K., Kandati, S., Wen, S., & Huysmans, Z. (2018). Effects of mantra meditation versus music listening on knee pain, function and related outcomes in older adults with knee osteoarthritis: An exploratory randomized clinical trial (RCT). *Evidence-based Complementary and Alternative Medicine*, 7683897.

Kartin, P. T., Bulut, F., Ceyhan, O., et al. (2017). The effects of meditation and music listening on the anxiety level, operation tolerance and pain perception in people who were performed colonoscopy. *International Journal of Caring Sciences*, *10*(3), 1587.

King, M. S., Carr, T., & D'Cruz, C. (2002). Transcendental meditation, hypertension and heart disease: A review. *Australian Family Physician*, *31*(2), 164–168.

Krisanaprakornkit, T., Krisanaprakornkit, W., Piyavhatkul, N., et al. (2006). Meditation therapy for anxiety disorders. *Cochrane Database of Systematic Review*, *1*, CD004998.

Lichstein, K. L. (1988). *Clinical relaxation strategies*. New York: John Wiley.

Loucks, E. B. (2014). Meditation intervention reviews—comment. *JAMA Internal Medicine*, *174*, 1194–1195.

Oman, D., Hedberg, J., & Thoresen, C. E. (2006). Passage meditation reduces perceived stress in health professionals: A randomized controlled trial. *Journal of Consulting and Clinical Psychology*, *74*(4), 714–719.

Orme-Johnson, D. W., & Barnes, V. A. (2017). Comment on "Meditation Programs for Psychological Stress and Well-Being." *Journal of Alternative and Complementary Medicine*, *23*(1), 75–78.

Park, S.-H., & Han, K. S. (2017). Blood pressure response to meditation and yoga: A systematic review and meta-analysis. *Journal of Alternative and Complementary Medicine*, *23*(9), 685–695.

Samuels, M., & Samuels, N. (1975). *Seeing with the mind's eye: The history, technique and uses of visualization*. Toronto: Random House.

Schneider, J. K., & Reangsing, C. (2019). Effects of transcendental meditation on blood pressure in adults: A review. *Pacific Rim International Journal of Nursing Research*, *23*(3), 195–200.

Sedlmeier, P., Elberth, J., Schwartz, M., Zimmermann, D., Haarig, F., Jaeger, S. & Krunze, S. (2012). The psycholoical effects of meditation: a meta-analysis. *Psychological Bulletin*, *138*(6): 1139–1146. doi: 10.1037/a0028168

Selfe, T. K., & Innes, K. E. (2013). Effects of meditation on symptoms of knee osteoarthritis: A pilot study. *Alternative and Complementary Therapies*, *19*(3), 139–146.

Shonin, E., Gordon, W. V., Compare, A., Zangeneh, M., & Griffiths, M. D. (2014). Buddhist-derived loving-kindness and compassion meditation for the treatment of psychopathology: A systematic review. *Mindfulness*, *6*, 1161–1182.

Smith, E., & Wilks, N. (1988). *Meditation*. London: Optima.

Suchday, S., Mayson, S. J., Klepper, J., Meyer, H., Dziok, M., & Singh, N. N. (2014). Eastern and western perspectives on meditation. In N. N. Singh (Ed.), *Psychology of meditation* (pp. 45–64). New York: Nova Science.

Tacon, A. M. (2003). Meditation as a complementary therapy in cancer. *Family & Community Health*, *26*(1), 64–73.

Titlebaum, H. (1988). Relaxation. In R. P. Zahourek (Ed.), *Relaxation and imagery: Tools for therapeutic communication and intervention*. Philadelphia: WB Saunders.

Walach, H., Schmidt, S., & Esch, T. (2014). Meditation intervention reviews—comment. *JAMA Internal Medicine*, *174*, 1193–1194.

Walton, K. G., Schneider, R. H., Nidich, S., et al. (2002). Psychosocial stress and cardiovascular disease, part 2: Effectiveness of the transcendental meditation programme in treatment and prevention. *Behavioral Medicine*, *28*(3), 106–123.

Walton, K. G., Schneider, R. H., & Nidich, S. (2004). Review of controlled research on the transcendental meditation program and cardiovascular disease. Risk factors, morbidity and mortality. *Cardiology Review*, *12*(5), 262–266.

Wren, A. A., Shelby, R. A., Soo, S. M., Huysmans, Z., Jarosz, J. A., & Keefe, F. J. (2019). Preliminary efficacy of a lovingkindness meditation intervention for patients undergoing biopsy and breast cancer surgery: A randomized controlled pilot study. *Supportive Care in Cancer*, *27*, 3587–3592.

Yang, H., Wu, X., & Wang, M. (2017). The effect of three different meditation exercises on hypertension: A network meta-analysis. *Evidence-based Complementary and Alternative Medicine*, 9784271.

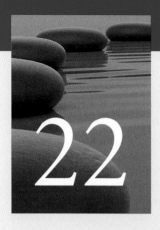

22

BENSON'S METHOD

DR CAROLINE BELCHAMBER

CHAPTER CONTENTS

LEARNING OBJECTIVES

The aim of this chapter is to explore what Benson's relaxation technique is, how it is taught in a non-religious setting, and its relevance to inducing the relaxation response.

By the end of this chapter you will be able to:

1. Understand the background and theory that underpins Benson's relaxation technique.

2. Describe the key elements of the relaxation response.

3. Recognize the evidence that underpins Benson's relaxation technique.

4. Identify the process and features of Benson's relaxation technique.

5. Discern the effects of Benson's relaxation technique.

This chapter will conclude with key points and time for reflection, providing learning opportunities through a case study.

INTRODUCTION TO BENSON'S RELAXATION TECHNIQUE

Benson's relaxation technique is known to reduce stress by focusing on the senses that affect a wide range of physical and psychological symptoms, including anxiety, depression, pain, mood and self-confidence (Smeltzer et al 2010). It does not involve muscle contraction, as this would increase blood pressure, pulse, respiration and consequently increase cardiac output (Van Dixhoorn & White 2005).

The development of Benson's relaxation technique came about in the 1970s, when the physiologist Herbert Benson was studying aspects of high blood pressure at Harvard's Thorndike Laboratory. Benson was approached by a group of transcendental meditators who believed that their meditations could lower their blood pressure. Unconvinced, Benson at first dismissed the idea but he later changed his mind. He and his colleagues then began to carry out a series of investigations which revealed that Transcendental Meditation (TM) was accompanied by marked physiological changes: there were reductions in the heart rate, breathing rate, oxygen consumption, blood lactate levels and, of particular interest to Benson, blood pressure. These changes reflected diminished activity in the sympathetic nervous system.

One study demonstrated drops in systolic and diastolic pressures from group averages of 146 and 93.5 mm Hg, respectively (borderline high pressure), to 137 and 88.9 mm Hg (within normal range) after several weeks of practising TM. Oxygen consumption was found to be reduced by 10% to 20% within the first 3 minutes of meditation (Benson 1976). It is interesting to compare this result with work on the sleeping state where the oxygen consumption was found to be reduced by only 8% and not before the person had been sleeping for 4 or 5 hours. These were impressive findings, particularly in the case of the blood pressure recordings which were not made during actual periods of meditation. The participants, however, were volunteers who had already applied to join a transcendental meditation course to reduce their blood pressure. This would suggest that their motivation was high.

Relaxation Response

Extensive study of other meditation practices led Benson to the belief that the effects described earlier were not confined to the practice of TM but were the result of certain key elements common to all meditation practices. From these findings Benson highlighted the value of détente (relaxing of tension), which he believed was central to care outcomes. He therefore set out to identify these elements, seeing them as responsible for eliciting what he called 'the Relaxation Response' or a state of decreased psychophysiological arousal. To Benson (1976), this was 'a natural and innate protective mechanism' that opposed the effects of the stress response. Viewed in these terms, the relaxation response appeared synonymous with parasympathetic nervous activity.

Benson's work (Benson 2000, Benson & Proctor 2010) acknowledged that the toxicity of the stress response (see Chapter 1) triggered the development of the relaxation response. Depression can arise from persistent long-term effects of stress and contribute to a number of stress-related physical and mental conditions that Benson (2000) identified could be improved by using this technique.

In identifying what Benson considered to be key elements in this relaxation technique, his purpose was not to create a rival approach but to devise a standardized technique which could be used in scientific investigation. Apart from that, his relaxation technique is very similar to TM except that the word 'one' replaces the Sanskrit mantra and the process is entirely secularized (Lichstein 1988).

The relaxation response consists of a diaphragmatic breathing pattern (see Chapter 4) and repetitive mental focus that distracts the person from everyday thoughts. The key elements that Benson and colleagues (1977) identified to induce relaxation were the following:

- A quiet environment
- A comfortable position
- A mental device such as a word to focus on
- A passive attitude

However, some research has questioned the importance of a quiet environment and a comfortable position. de Leon (1999) argued that the relaxation response could be elicited in a variety of locations even if they were noisy. It could also be elicited in a variety of positions even if they were uncomfortable. According to this researcher, it was the passive attitude and the mental device which were the essential ingredients of this approach, while Benson himself placed greatest value on the passive attitude.

The emphasis placed on 'passive attitude' recalls the 'passive concentration' of autogenic training (see Chapter 20). It is also not far removed from the quiet observation that characterizes progressive relaxation (see Chapter 5). It would seem that, underneath their varying procedures, the approaches are saying much the same thing (Lichstein 1988), and that in their psychophysiological effects, they are all evoking the relaxation response.

The Key Elements

Quiet Environment

In the ideal setting there is an absence of any background stimulus, pleasant or unpleasant.

Comfortable Position

Benson does not insist on any particular position because he feels that discomfort might draw the attention away from the mental device. Meditators should be allowed to choose their own position. They can, however, be too comfortable and tend to fall asleep; the orthodox lotus position (see Chapter 21) is thought to have been introduced partly to prevent that happening. For the same reason Benson does not recommend a lying position.

Mental Device

Because his studies had shown that TM was not unique in its ability to lower physiological arousal, Benson concluded that any repetitive, monotonous stimulus, capable of holding the attention, could fulfil the function of the Sanskrit mantra – that is, that any emotionally neutral object, sound or other phenomenon could be used as a focal point of attention. Benson chose the word 'one', which has similar qualities of resonance to the primal sound 'om', but he felt the choice of word or words was best made by the individual themselves. He refuted the idea that the mantra's meaning added to its effect.

Passive Attitude

Passive acceptance is an essential feature of the approach. A 'let it happen' attitude should be adopted. Benson regards the passive attitude as 'perhaps the most important element in eliciting the Relaxation Response'. Distracting thoughts may intervene but they should be ignored and the meditator's attention returned to the recited mantra.

INTRODUCTION TO EVIDENCE

Research suggests that when the relaxation response is carried out twice a day for about 10 to 20 minutes, it improves a number of stress-related conditions as well as anxiety, depression, hypertension and cardiac arrhythmias (Benson 2000). Therefore meditation appears to have a role to play in the field of coronary heart disease and hypertension, where the approach increasingly features in both prevention and treatment (King et al 2002). Among other cardiac conditions where benefit has been demonstrated is congestive cardiac failure. Veterans with this condition were trained in the relaxation response method and the effects compared with those of cardiac education and usual care. In terms of physical and emotional improvements, participants in the relaxation group experienced more benefit than those in the cardiac education group. No benefit was recorded in the usual care group, physically or emotionally. The authors concluded that the relaxation response may offer benefit to people experiencing congestive cardiac failure (Chang et al 2004).

Other research has examined many conditions, including pain management. Schaffer and Yucha (2004), in their review, found that non-pharmacological methods of pain management, such as Benson's relaxation response meditation, are able to reduce the emotional components of pain. Such methods can also strengthen coping abilities, give patients a sense of control, reduce fatigue and improve sleep. This is particularly so in the case of chronic pain and, to a lesser extent, in acute pain. One such painful condition is rheumatoid arthritis. Bagheri-Nesami et al (2006) conducted a pilot trial to investigate the effect of the relaxation response in this condition and found evidence to suggest a reduction in depression and anxiety and indications of a decline in the disease process (see Chapter 29).

A review of the evidence was undertaken by Wright (2006) to determine the effectiveness of the relaxation response in serious illness. Results showed a tentative positive effect. This is supported by the systematic review undertaken by Arias et al (2006) who found that meditation techniques improved the treatment of autoimmune illness. However, although both these reviews highlight the safety and potential benefits of meditation, the authors indicate that many of these studies are methodologically limited by non-randomization, lack of intention to treat analysis, single cohort design and inadequate follow-up data; further research is therefore required.

A pilot study carried out by Arcari (2008) involved 50 specialist nurses who took part in a course called 'Mind Body Strategies for Healing'. This course included the relaxation response as well as mindfulness and cognitive strategies. The results of the study indicated that the nurses who carried out these interventions on a regular basis reported increased competence and confidence in stress management, resilience and coping. Therefore Benson's relaxation response supports a holistic self-care, which encompasses aspects of the person's physical, emotional, mental and spiritual wellbeing. This links with several decades of research where the power of the individual's expectation and belief of wellness is seen when there is a mind–body connection towards self-healing (Benson & Proctor 2010). Benson (2000), Arcari (2008) and other researchers have translated this evidence base into practice offering stress-reduction programs to nurses (White 2013). A 2017 pilot study described the potential effects of relaxation response in nurse's self-care. The randomized, wait-list controlled quantitative study design measured the pre and post effects of the relaxation response over an 8-week period with 46 nurses. Findings indicated that the nurses had greater confidence in teaching the relaxation response, but there was no statistical significance in the reported level of anxiety, depression, well-being and work-related stress. Larger studies are needed to see if there are any significant reductions in workplace stress and anxiety (Calder Calisi 2017).

A randomized controlled clinical trial was carried out with 132 burns inpatients to investigate the Benson's relaxation technique, combined rose aroma–Benson's relaxation and control in managing, pain anxiety. This was performed over 3 consecutive days for 20 minutes each day before a daily dressing change. The Burn Specific Pain Anxiety Scale (BSPAS) was used to collect data and analysed using descriptive and inferential statistics. The researchers concluded that a combination of rose aroma and Benson's relaxation technique was more effective in reducing pain anxiety in burns patients than the intervention on its own. It is therefore recommended that health care providers deliver these interventions simultaneously because of their synergistic effect to help reduce pain anxiety before any painful interventions (Daneshpajooh et al 2019). As well as pain anxiety, Benson's technique has been shown to reduce death anxiety in a randomized controlled trial of 100 women with breast cancer (Moradipour et al 2019).

THEORY BEHIND BENSON'S RELAXATION TECHNIQUE

The theory underpinning Benson's relaxation technique is a unitary one in that the meditation creates a general, integrated calming effect. Although the participant is engaged in the cognitive activity of focusing on the mantra, the effect on the system is global. This led Benson to coin the phrase 'relaxation response' as described earlier. Benson writes that his relaxation technique carries little embellishment. Perhaps he made it too simple; in excluding all but the essentials, he may have overlooked the value of ceremony and ritual, which are important factors for some individuals (Carrington 1984, Lichstein 1988). By focusing the attention on a particular object, word or concept in a sustained and effortless way, meditators are able to detach themselves from daily events and induce a mental stillness. This stillness is reflected in reduced physiological responses – that is, diminished activity in the sympathetic nervous system (Benson 1976). Both cognitive and physical elements are present: the first relating to the focusing of attention on the mantra (or other stimulus) and the second, to the role of the breath.

PROCEDURE

Benson's relaxation technique is quick and easy to learn. It does not require expertise or equipment and is applicable to a range of age groups (Benson et al 1977).

Introductory Remarks to Participants

A few words explaining the relaxation technique are addressed to novices, who should be seated.

> *The relaxation technique you are about to learn is a non-religious version of meditation. It has a very simple form, requiring that you sit comfortably in a quiet place, that you focus your attention on the word 'one' and that you adopt an attitude which is accepting and unconcerned.*
>
> *These conditions will help you to experience what is called the relaxation response; a state which research shows is associated with reduced physiological activity. That means the heart rate will become slower and the blood pressure will fall. You'll notice that you feel calmer than usual and the whole sensation will be a pleasant one.*
>
> *At no time will you lose consciousness or be controlled by an outside force. The state you reach is one which you will have induced in yourself.*

The induction is short and simple.

Induction

When participants are ready, the induction sequence itself is carried out. The following version is adapted from Benson (1976). The '10 minutes' indicated can be extended to 20 as the meditator becomes more experienced.

> Settle comfortably in whatever position you have chosen, and close your eyes. Relax all your muscles, starting with your feet and ending with your face. Feel yourself deeply relaxed.
>
> Notice the rhythm of your breathing. Let the air in through your nose, allowing the breaths to take place quite naturally. Each time you exhale, recite the word 'one' under your breath. Repeat the word slowly every time you breathe out. If thoughts intrude, try to ignore them, and continue repeating the word 'one'.
>
> Avoid any inclination to judge how successful you are being. Keep your attitude passive, and allow relaxation to occur in its own time. Please continue for 10 minutes …
>
> When you are ready to end your meditation, continue to sit quietly for a few minutes with your eyes closed, then for a few minutes longer with them open.

In common with the authors of other relaxation techniques, Benson stressed the importance of regular practice, to be carried out once or twice a day. When practising at home, people are urged not to use an alarm but to guess when it is time to end the meditation.

PRECAUTIONS

Precautions can be found at the end of Chapter 21 (see Precautions).

KEY POINTS

1. The relaxation response is a form of meditation introduced by Herbert Benson.
2. Benson's relaxation technique is based on the belief that all forms of meditation elicit the same response, a reduction in sympathetic nervous activity.
3. Benson's relaxation technique is characterized by a simple formula consisting of four elements: (a) a quiet environment, (b) a comfortable position, (c) a mental device to hold the attention and (d) a passive attitude.
4. The induction procedure consists of gentle breathing which incorporates a soothing mantra.
5. Benson's relaxation technique is a widely used relaxation technique; however, robust evidence for its effectiveness is lacking.

Reflection

Describe how you would carry out Benson's relaxation technique.

What other meditation techniques have you tried? How do they compare? What differences did you notice in your physical and mental state?

How do you feel after completing Benson's relaxation technique?

What is your action plan following this reflection?

CASE STUDY LEARNING OPPORTUNITY

The key points and reflection provide the background and knowledge required in relation to the case study, David, to help deepen understanding of how Benson's relaxation technique can help reduce anxiety.

CASE STUDY

Generalized Anxiety Disorder: *Benson's Relaxation Technique Outcomes for David*

David was increasingly finding it hard to control his worries, which had started to affect his daily life and sleep. This was affecting his work, and his general practitioner (GP) discussed trying an intervention rather than medication in the first instant. David was referred by his GP to the Benson's relaxation technique facilitator to see if this technique would help him manage his worries. David was sceptical at first but decided to give it a go.

David was introduced to the Benson's relaxation facilitator, who explained what the intervention would involve. A quiet environment was then provided for David to sit in a comfortable position with his eyes closed. The facilitator asked David to avoid disturbing thoughts during the session and to select a word that provided him with tranquillity, such as 'one'. David was then asked to breathe deeply and regularly and to inhale and exhale while repeating his word, relaxing his muscles from the tip of his toes through all the muscles of his body to his head. This session lasted for 20 minutes, after which David was asked to open his eyes and to rest to achieve the desired effect of relaxation.

David was advised to stop the session whenever he wished if he felt uncomfortable. David at first was a bit self-conscious in saying his word out loud, but once he familiarized himself with the relaxation technique he began to find it beneficial. David repeated this session over 3 days with the facilitator, and in addition to this, David practiced the relaxation technique at home.

Over a period of 4 months David had got into a routine of using the Benson's relaxation technique on a daily basis and found that his worries were reducing and he felt more in control of his daily life. He had started to sleep better, which then enabled him to concentrate better at work.

ACTIVITY

For the case study:

1. List the effects of Benson's relaxation technique in managing David's worries.
2. Write down the impact Benson's relaxation technique is having from a psychological perspective.
3. Write down the impact Benson's relaxation technique is having from a physical perspective.
4. Write down the impact Benson's relaxation technique is having from an emotional perspective.
5. Consider the outcomes on quality of life and overall well-being for David.

Chapter 23 will focus on mindfulness-based meditation to bring another perspective on using meditation as a relaxation technique.

REFERENCES

Arcari, P. M. (2008). *Resiliency in nursing. Paper presented at the Spirituality and Healing in Medicine: The Resiliency Factor*. Boston, MA.

Arias, A. J., Steinberg, K., Banga, A., et al. (2006). Systematic review of the efficacy of meditation techniques as treatments for medical illness. *Journal of Alternative and Complementary Medicine, 12*(8), 817–832.

Bagheri-Nesami, M., Mohseni-Bandpei, M. A., & Shayesteh-Azar, M. (2006). The effect of Benson's relaxation technique on rheumatoid arthritis patients: Extended report. *International Journal of Nursing Practice, 12*(4), 214–219.

Benson, H. (1976). *The relaxation response*. London: Collins.

Benson, H., Kotch, J. B., & Crassweller, K. D. (1977). The relaxation response: A bridge between psychiatry and medicine. *Medical Clinics of North America, 61*(4), 929–938.

Benson, H. (2000). *The relaxation response*. New York: HarperCollins.

Benson, H., & Proctor, W. (2010). *Relaxation revolution: Enhancing your personal health through the sciences and genetics of mind/body healing*. New York: Scribner.

Calder Calisi, C. (2017). The effects of the relaxation response on nurses' level of anxiety, depression, well-being, work-related stress, and confidence to teach patients. *Journal of Holistic Nursing, 35*(4), 318–327.

Chang, B. H., Jones, D., Hendricks, A., et al. (2004). Relaxation response for veterans with congestive heart failure: Results from a qualitative study within a clinical trial. *Preventive Cardiology, 7*(2), 64–70.

Carrington, P. (1984). Modern forms of meditation. In R. L. Woolfolk, & P. M. Lehrer (Eds.), *Principles and practice of stress management*. New York: Guilford Press.

Daneshpajooh, L., Ghezeljeh, T. N., & Haghani, H. (2019). Comparison of the effects of inhalation aromatherapy using damask rose aroma and the Benson relaxation technique in burn patients: A randomized clinical trial. *Burns, 15*, 1205–1214.

de Leon, D. (1999). The relaxation response in the treatment of chronic pain. In M. S. Micozzi, & A. N. Bacchus (Eds.), *The physician's guide to alternative medicine* (pp. 335–337). Atlanta: American Health Consultants.

King, M. S., Carr, T., & D'Cruz, C. (2002). Transcendental meditation, hypertension and heart disease: A review. *Australian Family Physician, 31*(2), 164–168.

Lichstein, K. L. (1988). *Clinical relaxation strategies*. New York: John Wiley.

Moradipour, S., Soleimani, M. A., Mafi, M., & Sheikhi, M. R. (2019). Effect of Benson's relaxation technique on death anxiety among patients with breast cancer. *Journal of Hayat, 24*(4), 355–367.

Schaffer, S. D., & Yucha, C. B. (2004). Relaxation and pain management: The relaxation response can play a role in managing chronic and acute pain. *American Journal of Nursing, 104*(8), 75–76, 78–79, 81–82.

Smeltzer, S., Bare, B., Hinkle, J., & Cheever, K. (2010). Biophysical and psychological concepts in nursing practice. In *Brunner & suddarth's textbook of medical-surgical nursing* (12th ed., pp. 76–227). Philadelphia: Wolters Kluwer.

Van Dixhoorn, J., & White, A. (2005). Relaxation therapy for rehabilitation and prevention in ischaemic heart disease: A systematic review and meta-analysis. *European Journal of Cardiovascular Prevention & Rehabilitation, 12*(3), 193–202.

White, L. (2013). Mindfulness in nursing: An evolutionary concept analysis. *Journal of Advanced Nursing, 70*, 282–294.

Wright, L. D. (2006). Meditation: A new role for an old friend. *American Journal of Hospice and Palliative Medicine, 23*(4), 323–327.

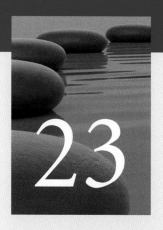

23

MINDFULNESS-BASED MEDITATION

DR HELEN BOLDERSTON

CHAPTER CONTENTS

LEARNING OBJECTIVES

The aim of this chapter is to explore what mindfulness meditation is, how it is taught in Western health settings, and its relevance to stress and psychological well-being.

By the end of this chapter you will be able to:

1. Understand what mindfulness is and how it differs from other practices.

2. Outline the main features of two mindfulness-based interventions commonly used in health settings.

3. Evaluate the empirical evidence for these interventions.

4. Identify the strengths and limitations of self-help approaches to practicing mindfulness.

5. Recognize when caution might be needed in relation to mindfulness.

This chapter will conclude with key points and time for reflection, providing learning opportunities through a case study.

INTRODUCTION TO MINDFULNESS

Buddhist principles of awareness and acceptance lie at the core of mindfulness. The practice has also been studied by psychologists working in the areas of stress, mental health, and cognition and this has led to the formation of a new structured approach to teaching mindfulness within health and other secular settings. Notable contributions have been made by Kabat-Zinn (e.g., 2013) and others working in the field of anxiety, stress management, and coping with chronic physical health conditions, while Segal and colleagues (2013), combining mindfulness with cognitive therapy principles, have investigated its application to relapse prevention in clinical depression.

A commonly used definition of mindfulness is 'the awareness that arises from paying attention in a particular way: on purpose, in the present moment, and non-judgementally' (Kabat-Zinn 1994, p4). The Buddhist monk, Thich Nhat Hanh, sees it as 'keeping one's consciousness alive to the present reality' (Hanh 1976), while Bishop (2002) sees it as a state in which the individual is highly aware of the reality of the present moment. Mindfulness is usually referred to as a type of meditation, but Shapiro and colleagues (2006) clarify that more precisely, mindfulness is a state of being or consciousness that is characterized by awareness of present moment experience. The meditation practices we tend to label as mindfulness are designed to cultivate the ability to be more mindful; they are the 'scaffolding' used to build the ability (Kabat-Zinn 2003).

Expanding on Kabat-Zinn's definition, mindfulness is cultivated by gently reminding oneself to be aware of what you are doing, whatever you happen to be doing; of being present in each moment with a sense of wakefulness, accepting and acknowledging your experience in the present moment as best you can without judgement, and with curiosity and kindness (Williams 2008). This is, of course, easier said than done, which is why courses designed to teach these abilities tend to last several weeks and involve regular practice.

For people experiencing raised levels of stress in their lives, it is very easy to repeatedly get caught up in fight, flight or freeze stress reactions to challenging life events, with all of the biological and psychological costs associated with such repetitive reactions. The mindful capacity to step back from this unhelpful reactivity and to 'unhook' attention from worry and rumination can prove effective when dealing with stress. The physical sensations of breathing are often used as a focus of attention in mindfulness meditation. This is not to avoid or suppress stressful thoughts and feelings but rather to provide a place to return to, a place to stabilize attention, each time the mind becomes unhelpfully busy or dominated by stress-related reactivity.

Awareness of the passing moment enables individuals to become fully engaged with it but at the same time somewhat separate from the thoughts and feelings triggered by it. This gives them space to question the usefulness of their immediate responses. They may see that they need not be enslaved by their reactions because such reactions are separate from and subordinate to a person's sense of self – the self who can psychologically step back and watch thoughts and feelings come and go.

Segal and colleagues (2013) distinguish between being and doing modes of mind. The doing mode is characterized by a focus on solving problems, achieving goals, and the use of these active strategies to avoid difficulty or discomfort. These strategies can be effective in the world outside our skin, but it is impossible to 'solve' painful thoughts and emotions or to consistently avoid them, and such efforts can result in the individual getting caught up in worry and rumination, leading to greater psychological distress. There is often a sense of drive or compulsion when we are in the doing mode of mind, and this drive to avoid uncomfortable thoughts, feelings and sensations can lead people to engage in unhelpful coping strategies such as drinking alcohol to excess and compulsive over-working.

Mindfulness programmes aim to help people shift more easily to a being mode of mind in which they can pay curious, kindly attention to their thoughts, feelings and sensations, and relate to them as passing experiences of the mind, without feeling driven to immediately having to react, solve or suppress. To be able to do this, mindfulness practices support the individual to step out of automatic pilot and into conscious, present moment awareness. An illustration of an exercise that supports this can be seen in Box 23.1. The raisin exercise is a brief, practical introduction to paying mindful attention to experience, and it is often the first mindfulness practice encountered in a structured, evidence-based, mindfulness course.

Kabat-Zinn, referring to his mindfulness-based stress reduction (MBSR) programme, describes the liberating feeling of treating thoughts as being outside the individuals and not part of them. In his words, 'to see that your thoughts are just thoughts and that they are not you or reality'. Recognizing thoughts in this way can free a person 'from the distorted reality they often create'. Thus, although mindfulness does not aim to change people's thoughts and feelings, it can change their relationship to them (Segal et al 2004). This has implications for people experiencing negative thoughts such as those that occur in anxiety and depression. This emphasis on changing our relationship to difficult experiences rather than getting rid of or changing the actual experience differentiates mindfulness-based approaches from more change-oriented approaches such as cognitive–behavioural therapy and progressive muscle relaxation.

BOX 23.1
THE RAISIN EXERCISE*

(The word 'PAUSE' indicates a 10-second silence; the three dots, a 3-second silence.)

The mindfulness teacher asks the individual to hold out one hand in which he or she places a raisin.

I have placed an object in your hand and I'd like you to imagine you have never seen it before. Look at it as if you have just arrived from another planet and are seeing this object for the very first time.

Holding the object at a distance that makes it comfortable to look carefully at it. Paying detailed attention ... seeing what there is to notice. PAUSE. Perhaps noticing its size ... its shape ... perhaps noticing colour ... variations in colour as you turn the object around between your fingers. PAUSE. Noticing how the light catches some parts of the object while others may be darker and in shadow. PAUSE.

Exploring the texture and temperature of the object with your fingertips as you move it around. What can you feel? PAUSE.

Exploring every part of the object with your eyes and fingers ... paying detailed attention, moment-by-moment. PAUSE.

If, while you are exploring the object, you realize your mind has wandered or you are having thoughts such as 'this is an odd thing to be doing' or 'this is unpleasant' or 'I don't see the point of this' just acknowledging this and then bringing your attentiveness back to the object. PAUSE.

In a moment, I am going to invite you to bring the object up to just below your nostrils ... if, in your mind, you have already moved it, seeing if it is possible to reconnect with the object where it actually is right now and then slowly and consciously raising the object up so that you are holding it right below your nostrils ... and then breathe ... with each in-breath, seeing what you can notice ... perhaps closing your eyes if it helps you to focus on your sense of smell. PAUSE.

And now, moving the object to your lips ... perhaps noticing what happens in your mouth as you do this ... and then making a conscious decision to place the object in your mouth and then doing that, without biting, and noticing what happens in the mouth ... then exploring the object with your tongue, noticing what you can feel as you move the object around your mouth. PAUSE.

When you are ready, make a conscious decision to bite, and then bite ... noticing in detail what happens ... what happens with taste ... with texture ... with saliva in the mouth ... chewing, slowly and deliberately, and as best you can, bringing detailed awareness to each moment. PAUSE.

Seeing if you can notice when you have the urge to swallow, then actually swallowing ... seeing if you can detect any sensations as the object moves down towards your stomach ... and also noticing how things are in the mouth now that the object has gone. PAUSE.

* Based on an exercise created by Kabat-Zinn (2005).

How Mindfulness Differs From Other Practices

Mindfulness practice differs from other forms of meditation such as concentration. Concentration implies a focused attention on a particular item to the exclusion of other stimuli, in contrast to mindfulness which involves a more flexible approach to paying attention. This includes practicing stepping back and observing thoughts, emotions, sensations and so on arising in and fading from a broad field of awareness. It also differs from creative thinking, such as occurs in visualization and problem solving where a deliberate intellectual effort is required and active solution-seeking skills called for. Conversely, mindfulness calls for a more observational approach, one that fosters a sense of curiosity and acceptance. Although mindfulness may lead to more effective problem solving, its primary concern is to develop a different relationship to experience and self. Its purpose is not to deal with

problems but to create the state of mind in which new insights can occur, which makes solutions possible (Gunaratana 2002). In this way, as suggested earlier, mindfulness is more about 'being' rather than 'doing' (Kabat-Zinn 2003, Segal et al 2013).

To deepen one's understanding of mindfulness, Langer (1989) finds it useful to consider the reverse condition: mindlessness. In this state a person's attention is on outcome rather than process, on the future or past instead of the present. The task in question is carried out in an automatic manner using goal-based thinking styles with no thought as to how it is performed. These automatic responses may in the past have provided a convenient quick path for individuals, but if they become a habit, people may unwittingly become trapped in a rigid world where new possibilities are unlikely to occur to them. Individuals have been wishing away the present moment because it stood in the way of carrying out the next task; they have been considering the end result at the expense of how to get there. This mindless approach has perhaps had the advantage of quickness and even a measure of effectiveness, but it may leave people in a stressful and exhausted state. They have been rushing through the day to get everything done when a quiet moment of awareness might have revealed another way of managing the tasks, one which led to a more satisfying and less stressful outcome. Thus mindlessness involves the doing mode of mind referred to earlier.

Fundamentally, mindfulness is not a technique primarily designed to reduce stress or induce a state of relaxation. Indeed, the view amongst mindfulness teachers and researchers is that if people feel stressed and strive to be more relaxed, this mismatch between how they feel and how they think they ought to feel, and the striving associated with it, can actually lead to more tension and stress. The paradox is that relaxation tends to come about through mindfulness when individuals let go of any pressing goal to be more relaxed and instead pay curious and accepting attention to how they actually are in this moment.

INTRODUCTION TO EVIDENCE

Empirical evidence suggests that mindfulness can decrease stress and increase a sense of relaxation and well-being. There are two mindfulness-based programmes that have substantial empirical support: MBSR and MBCT.

Mindfulness-Based Stress Reduction

Kabat-Zinn first developed MBSR to help patients with chronic and debilitating physical health diagnoses deal with associated stress and distress. There is a range of empirical evidence relating to this type of MBSR application. For example, chronic pain seems particularly to respond to the benefits of mindfulness. Focusing on this area is a system called Breathworks mindfulness-based pain and illness management. In this programme, a distinction is drawn between the pain itself (regarded as primary) and the individual's reaction to it, which includes all secondary responses such as anger, fear, anxiety, depression, avoidance and catastrophizing. The person is supported to accept the primary pain and to reduce the secondary, which he or she does through strategies such as breath and

body awareness and self-compassion practices. It is an approach which helps the individual to live with the pain without being dominated by it. Evaluation of the Breathworks programme (Burch et al 2006) revealed a clinically significant improvement in the health status of affected individuals, with effect sizes ranging from moderate to large.

Chronic pain is a significant aspect of fibromyalgia for which mindfulness might have something to offer. Astin and colleagues (2003) combined mindfulness meditation with qigong and tested their efficacy in the treatment of this condition. Their randomized controlled trial used an education and support group as control. They found that both groups made statistically significant improvements during training and these were maintained at follow-up 6 months later. However, there was no evidence that mindfulness meditation offered any advantage over education and support, and, with these types of combination interventions, it is difficult to judge the relative contribution of each element.

Cancer is an area where MBSR has been found to provide benefit in the form of improvements in mood and sleep quality (Carlson & Garland 2005, Matchim & Armer 2007, Ott et al 2006, Smith et al 2005). A study of patients with breast and prostate cancer indicated that participation in an MBSR training group was associated with decreased stress symptoms and enhanced quality of life as well as the physiological changes consistent with reduced stress (Carlson et al 2007). A 2011 review of the use of MBSR and MBCT (see next section) in relation to cancer care (Shennan et al 2011) concluded that these mindfulness-based approaches show promise in terms of reduction of a range of psychiatric symptoms, sexual dysfunction and stress hormone levels. However, the authors of the review argue that more rigorous tests of these interventions are needed, including larger, better-designed studies.

A common use of 8-week MBSR courses is to help members of the general public learn how to effectively manage non-clinical levels of stress. A 2015 meta-analysis (Khoury et al 2015) examined findings from 29 studies where MBSR had been tested with non-clinical populations. The results suggested that MBSR may have a large, positive effect on stress and more moderate effects on depression, anxiety and other forms of distress in the general population. This meta-analysis also included evidence of MBSR moderately improving quality of life.

MBSR has also been evaluated as an intervention for a range of health and social care professionals. Mindfulness programmes are seen as being relevant because of the high levels of stress and burnout reported by almost every health and social care professional group. As an example, Warnecke et al (2011) randomly assigned 66 medical students to either an 8-week MBSR programme wholly based on audio recordings (no in-person meetings) or to a usual care group who received the intervention at the end of the study. Those in the intervention condition showed a significant reduction in anxiety and a borderline significant reduction in stress, with these improvements being maintained at 8-week follow-up. Similarly, a review of studies testing the use of MBSR for work-related stress in nurses showed that such interventions can lead to lower levels of stress and burnout and improved mood, concentration and empathy. However, the author of the review points out the need for far more research in this area to increase clarity about the impact of 'dose' because MBSR courses included in the review ranged from 4 to 8 weeks in duration (Smith 2014).

Overall, MBSR interventions appear to offer benefit for individuals experiencing stress in a range of contexts, including chronic physical illness and in occupational settings. However, there are some inconsistencies in the evidence base, and relatively little is understood to date about effective dose and mechanisms of action.

Mindfulness-Based Cognitive Therapy

An early investigation into the efficacy of MBCT was conducted by Teasdale and colleagues (2000). This randomized, three-centre controlled trial compared MBCT with treatment as usual. Participants were a group of people with a history of major depression whose symptoms were in remission. The intervention period ran for 8 weeks, with participants then being monitored for 1 year. In the follow-up period it was found that for participants who had had three or more episodes of depression, relapse rates were significantly less for those who received MBCT (40% relapsed) compared with those who had not received MBCT (66% relapsed). MBCT did not reduce risk of relapse for people who had experienced fewer previous episodes of depression. Thus people with a history of multiple episodes of major depression derived benefit from a course of MBCT. A review and meta-analysis of MBCT for psychiatric conditions (Chiesa & Serretti 2011) supported the view that MBCT significantly reduces relapse in depression compared with usual care based on four relevant randomized controlled trials. Additionally, MBCT has been found to be as effective in preventing relapse in depression as a tapering dose of antidepressant medication, with relapse occurring later in the posttreatment follow-up period for those patients who received MBCT (Kuyken et al 2008).

In recent years, MBCT has begun to be adapted and tested as a treatment for other disorders. For example, MBCT has been used in the treatment of substance abuse with co-occurring mood disorders. Early findings suggest that this approach may be useful in reducing the likelihood of relapse (Hoppes 2006). MBCT has also shown promise as an intervention for people living with cancer. A cohort of 115 patients with mixed cancer diagnoses were randomized to an 8-week MBCT intervention or to a waitlist control. After intervention, patients who had received MBCT reported significantly lower levels of anxiety, depression, and distress compared with the control group (Foley et al 2010).

A recent review of the MBCT for depression literature (MacKenzie & Kocovski 2016) concluded that overall it appears to be a promising intervention. However, the authors point out that there is currently mixed evidence regarding whether MBCT outperforms good quality active control interventions (as opposed to poorer quality treatment-as-usual controls), and also, far more research is needed to clarify mechanisms of action.

THEORIES BEHIND MINDFULNESS

Several biological mechanisms of mindfulness have been hypothesized and tested. For example, in an early study, Davidson and colleagues (2003) demonstrated that participating in an 8-week MBSR course significantly increased activity in the left-sided anterior region of the brain, noting that such activity had been linked with positive emotion in previous research. They also found that the same mindfulness training led to improved immune system functioning as measured by antibody response to a flu vaccine.

Matousek et al (2010) reviewed the impact of MBSR on hypothalamus–pituitary–adrenal axis (HPA) activity, specifically focusing on the hypothesis that mindfulness has its beneficial impact on stress at least in part through a reduction in cortisol levels. The authors focused on this particular hormone because of strong evidence of its association with stress and because measurement of cortisol levels can be achieved relatively cheaply and non-invasively through the collection of saliva samples. They reviewed evidence from several studies showing MBSR to be associated with reduction in cortisol levels. However, they also reviewed studies that showed no significant change in cortisol level after mindfulness training. The authors outlined several complications affecting the accurate measurement of cortisol levels and concluded that although cortisol secretion may well be affected by mindfulness interventions, this can only be a part of a more complex picture involving several chemical mediators of stress.

Zeidan (2015) has argued for 'a stage-based account of the neurobiology of mindfulness meditation', with the impact on brain function and structure depending on the length of mindfulness training, ranging from less than one week of training through to expert meditators with over a thousand hours of meditation experience. He argues that current evidence suggests early stages of mindfulness practice are associated with higher-order brain mechanisms, whereas only extensive practice is associated with substantial changes in brain structure such as increases in grey matter in various regions of the brain including hippocampus and posterior insula.

Zeiden (2015) also outlines a range of behavioural mechanisms at different stages of training, and indeed there is a growing literature addressing psychological mechanisms of mindfulness. For example, beginning with Kabat-Zinn's (1994) definition of mindfulness (see Introduction to Mindfulness section earlier), Shapiro and colleagues (2006) hypothesized that the key active ingredients of mindfulness are intention (I), attention (A), and attitude (A): 'we propose a model of the potential mechanisms of mindfulness, which suggests that intentionally (I) attending (A) with openness and non-judgmentalness (A) leads to a significant shift

in perspective, which we have termed reperceiving'. Shapiro and colleagues (2006) cite evidence of the impact of intention in the form of a study (Shapiro 1992) in which participants' intentions regarding their mindfulness practice moved along a continuum over time 'from self-regulation, to self-exploration, and finally to self-liberation'. The study findings suggested that the impact of their meditation practice was related to the meditators' current intention.

In terms of the role of attentional processes in mindfulness, Tang and Posner (2014) reviewed current empirical evidence that showed mindfulness impacting a range of attentional processes and behaviours including increasing interoceptive awareness, increasing alerting attention and improving the ability to sustain attention. Overall, they concluded that mindfulness training does appear to improve the functioning of the executive attention network and that, at least in part, these changes play a mediating role in the benefits associated with mindfulness practice.

Various processes might be included in the 'attitude' aspect of the Shapiro et al model, including acceptance of experience and self, non-judgemental stance towards the same, and self-compassion. In a study designed to test potential mechanisms of MBCT when used to prevent relapse in major depressive disorder, Kuyken and colleagues (2010) found that both mindfulness and self-compassion mediated the impact of the intervention. The measure of mindfulness addressed both attentional and acceptance/non-judgemental aspects of mindfulness, suggesting that all these processes play a role. However, the researchers did not examine the relative impact of these various processes.

Other researchers have taken a more fine-grained approach to exploring mindfulness mechanisms. For example, Ainsworth et al (2017) used a laboratory-based experiment to test the impact of 10-minute mindfulness practices on intrusive thoughts and worry in students. They examined the effects of two different mindfulness practices, one that focused on attentional control and the other on acceptance. The researchers found that both forms of mindfulness practice were associated with significantly fewer negative intrusive worry thoughts than a progressive muscle relaxation control practice. However, the acceptance practice was associated with a greater protective effect, with students in the acceptance condition experiencing fewer intrusive worry thoughts than those in the attention condition.

Finally, in terms of models of mindfulness, it should be noted that some mindfulness interventions are rooted in models that address psychological processes beyond mindfulness. For example, MBCT is based on a cognitive model of relapse in recurrent depression that implicates the reactivation of networks of negative, depressogenic thoughts and feelings. As such, the attentional control, acceptance and self-compassion aspects of mindfulness are used in MBCT to form a different, more functional relationship to negative thoughts and feelings as they occur and thus to 'break-up associative networks and offset the risk of relapse' (Kuyken et al 2010, p1106). Therefore, in addition to measuring mindfulness and self-compassion as potential mechanisms of action for MBCT, the researchers also tested the role of cognitive reactivity. They found that MBCT had a significant, protective effect on the relationship between cognitive reactivity and outcome, posttreatment, but that antidepressant medication did not lead to the same positive effect.

PROCEDURE

Procedure for Mindfulness-Based Stress Reduction

MBSR is a time-limited, structured programme originally developed by Jon Kabat-Zinn to help patients with a range of chronic physical health problems to manage the stress and distress associated with their conditions (Bishop 2002). Although it is still used in this way, it is now also commonly offered to people in the general population experiencing stress. It has thus been seen as an approach that addresses general vulnerabilities rather than specific vulnerabilities such as the risk of relapse in people who have been depressed. That said, MBSR had been tailored to address specific problems such as distress associated with chronic pain.

MBSR courses typically consist of 8 weekly group sessions, often with an additional whole day of practice falling in the sixth week. The sessions are facilitated by a trained mindfulness teacher and include psychoeducational content focussed on the psychophysiology of

stress and adaptive ways of responding to stress. This teaching is woven into a programme of mindfulness practices of varying lengths. These practices include the body scan, which brings mindful attention to sensations in different parts of the body, gentle mindful movement or yoga-type practices, and sitting practices where attention is paid to the sensations of breathing (see Chapter 4). Through skilful guidance and facilitated reflection on personal experiences of stress, the mindfulness trainer supports the participants to become curious about their moment-by-moment experience rather than being avoidant and to gently respond to challenging experiences rather than react compulsively and stressfully.

In addition to attending the eight course sessions, participants are also strongly encouraged to meditate on a daily basis. This can amount to 45 minutes of practice a day which is a substantial commitment for anyone and particularly for people who may be stressed because of the many demands life is making of them. However, this amount of practice over 8 weeks is viewed as a key factor in bringing about changes in unhelpful habits of mind which many have been in place for decades.

Procedure for Mindfulness-Based Cognitive Therapy

In recent years mindfulness has been combined with aspects of cognitive therapy to form an approach called mindfulness-based cognitive therapy (MBCT). It differs from cognitive therapy proper (with its emphasis on *content* of thoughts and the reappraisal of problematic and inaccurate thoughts) by emphasizing *awareness* of and *relationship* to thoughts and other private experiences such as emotions (Segal et al 2004, p54). MBCT teaches the individual to step back from thoughts and to observe them with curiosity as passing events in the mind, rather than treating them as decisive events which must be closely inspected, believed and acted upon.

The programme was originally designed to prevent relapse in patients in remission from recurrent major depressive disorder. It aims to teach such people to become more aware of and to relate differently to their thoughts, feelings and body sensations. Clients are taught how to disengage from habitual negative thought patterns and the emotions associated with them, which together increase the risk of relapse.

A principal feature of both MBSR and MBCT is the idea of acceptance of experience, which in mindfulness does not imply liking necessarily; a person can dislike a particular memory or emotion but accept that they are experiencing it and cultivate a curious, stepped-back relationship to it, rather than becoming dominated by it or alternatively, attempting to suppress it. In mindfulness-based approaches such as MBSR and MBCT, this cultivation of acceptance and non-judgement of experience is extended to experience of self, and, indeed, self-compassion has been shown to be a mechanism of action in MBCT when used to prevent relapse in depression (Kuyken et al 2010).

Whereas MBSR is often used to address general vulnerabilities such as stress – something which anyone can experience, MBCT tends to be applied to more specific vulnerabilities such as relapse in depression or cancer-related fatigue and distress. It could be argued that MBCT combines an acceptance-based strategy (mindfulness) with a change-based strategy (cognitive therapy), and that this might be both theoretically and clinically problematic. However, cognitive therapy always attended to relationship to thoughts as well as content of thoughts (the process in cognitive therapy is referred to as decentering), but this was relatively underemphasized until the development of mindfulness-based approaches such as MBCT. MBCT's developers, Segal et al (2004), speak of bringing 'a kindly awareness' to depressogenic thoughts, rather than an active determination to modify such thoughts.

The MBCT programme is similar to the MBSR one. It includes all of the mindfulness practices from MBSR and follows the same 8-week structure. However, whereas MBSR includes psychoeducation about stress and group exploration of responding to stress more mindfully, MBCT for relapse prevention in depression includes cognitive therapy–based information on relapse warning signs and how to respond effectively to them. Both place emphasis on an attitude of acceptance, an awareness of the reality of the present moment and the relationship of individuals to their thoughts, emotions and body sensations. Both approaches tend to be taught in groups (though both programmes can be adapted for one-to-one use), with weekly group sessions typically lasting 2 to 2.5 hours. Daily home mindfulness practice is seen as essential to bring about positive outcomes in both programmes.

SELF-HELP APPROACHES

In recent years there has been a rapid increase in the availability of mindfulness resources marketed as self-development tools to help individuals cultivate the ability to be more mindful. These include self-help books, websites and mobile phone apps. The latter are understandably popular because of ease of accessibility and low cost to the public. They also often emphasize brief mindfulness practices, which again makes them popular. However, to date, little good quality research has been conducted to evaluate their effectiveness. There is a small amount of evidence in support of the Headspace app, but far more evaluation is needed.

It is worth noting that traditional 8-week MBSR and MBCT courses typically involve regular mindfulness practices that last at least thirty minutes. People engaged in practices of this length are very likely to have difficult experiences during the practices – boredom, physical discomfort, worries and so on – and it is thought that through the provision of appropriate support and guidance to respond to these difficulties mindfully, a fundamentally different and more functional relationship with a range of difficulties can be developed. Practices that last just 5 or 10 minutes can be associated with physiological indications of relaxation such as reduction in heart rate and blood pressure, but in such brief practices there are far fewer opportunities to try bringing mindful responding to difficult experiences. As such, engaging in brief practices with relatively little appropriate guidance may bring about some experience of relaxation, but is less likely to help people with difficulties such as anxiety and depression to change their experience of those difficulties.

In contrast, several mindfulness self-help books have been written by experts and are designed to help individuals engage with mindfulness in a relatively in-depth way, over several weeks. These books usually include access to mindfulness practice recordings which are often designed so that a series of short practices can be listened to one after the other to form a longer practice. Some books address specific vulnerabilities;

for example, *The Mindful Way Through Depression: Freeing Yourself from Chronic Unhappiness* (Williams et al 2007). Others are aimed at more generally experienced stress – for example, *Mindfulness: A Practical Guide to Finding Peace in a Frantic World* (Williams & Penman 2011). Some books cover the use of mindfulness to address both general stress and more specific difficulties: *Full Catastrophe Living (Revised Edition): How to Cope with Stress, Pain and Illness Using Mindfulness Meditation* (Kabat-Zinn 2013). Again, far more research is required to be confident that the use of these books is effective, but the examples given here are based on empirically supported MBSR and MBCT programmes, which perhaps increases the likelihood that the books might also bring about some benefits.

PRECAUTIONS

Mindfulness practice involves individuals paying detailed attention to their current experience. People whose current experience involves persistent self-critical thoughts, suicidal ideation, hallucinations and other disturbing symptoms are likely to find this challenging, and there is potential for mindfulness practice to be detrimental. Similarly, mindfulness practice often involves being in silence for substantial periods. Some patients, such as those with borderline personality disorder, who may have an impoverished sense of self, may find this aspect of mindfulness anxiety provoking.

This is not to say that mindfulness cannot be helpful for people with these kinds of diagnoses and symptoms. There is preliminary evidence that mindfulness is beneficial for people with psychosis (Chadwick et al 2009), and dialectical behaviour therapy (Linehan 1993), an empirically supported psychotherapy which reduces suicidality and other symptoms in borderline personality disorder, has mindfulness as a core component. However, with patients with these kinds of severe and potentially risky presentations, mindfulness practices are significantly adapted to make them tolerable and safe. This is work that should be carried out by a clinician with specialist experience.

KEY POINTS

1. Mindfulness meditation is an ancient practice which has been adopted by therapists wishing to help individuals reduce stress and increase well-being.
2. Mindfulness practice involves being awake to in-the-moment experience, rather than being on automatic pilot.
3. The meditator cultivates an attitude of non-judgemental acceptance towards their experience, which they observe with curiosity. This allows them to be aware of private experiences such as thoughts, emotions, and physical sensations with reduced reactivity and thus step back from those experiences. The individual is aware of uncomfortable thoughts without necessarily reacting to them in a habitual and automatic way.
4. The approach is sometimes combined with aspects of cognitive therapy where it has particular relevance to reducing relapse in clinical depression.

Reflection

Describe your understanding of the techniques of mindfulness meditation.

How do you feel about applying this technique to practice?

Have you had a recent experience of being on automatic pilot while you did something? Have you had a recent experience of being very present and in the moment while you did something?

What do you think you might find challenging about paying more mindful attention to your experiences, including your thoughts, emotions, and physical sensations?

How do you think you might benefit from being able to bring a more mindful approach to your life?

If you were going to try to be more mindful, what first step might you take?

CASE STUDY LEARNING OPPORTUNITIES

The key points and reflection provide background and knowledge required in relation to the case study, James, to help deepen understanding of how mindfulness-based meditation can help improve the person's experience of well-being

Major Depressive Disorder: MBCT Outcomes for James

James is a 40-year-old university lecturer who lives with his long-term partner. He has experienced recurrent episodes of major depressive disorder throughout his adult life, the first of which occurred when he was in his late teens and was beginning to deal with his own realization that he was gay, as well as very negative reactions from his family. He has been treated with several different antidepressant medications in the past, as well as with counselling and cognitive–behavioural therapy. His most recent episode of depression lasted 8 months and involved him being signed off work for almost 2 months. After treatment with a combination of behavioural activation and sertraline, his depression is currently in remission, but given the high risk of relapse, he was offered a place on an 8-week mindfulness-based cognitive therapy (MBCT) course.

Between the first and second MBCT sessions, James found it difficult to do the main home practice – a daily, 35-minute body scan meditation. He initially reported that this was due to not having enough time, but during a group exploration of experiences of the body scan at the start of session two, James realized that his attempts to pay attention to physical sensations during the practice were often being 'derailed' by self-critical thoughts. With a great deal of embarrassment, he reported that he had spent most of the in-session body scan practice caught up in these thoughts, rather than paying attention to sensations in the body, as per the mindfulness teacher's guidance. To his surprise, this turned out to be a common experience in the group. Also to his surprise, the mindfulness trainer guided James and the group to bring kindly curiosity to this process of mind wandering and negative thinking, rather than viewing the practice as a failure.

For the first few weeks of the course, James made repeated resolutions that his mind would not wander during the various meditation practices, but slowly he began to accept that mind-wandering is an inevitable part of having a human mind, rather than a personal failing. He began to learn how to notice when his attention had drifted and to gently refocus his attention without a great deal of self-criticism or other cognitive reactivity.

Around the midpoint of the MBCT course James felt he had a breakthrough. He came to realize that historically his main way of coping with aversive self-critical thoughts was to do everything he could to avoid them. This included trying to block them out by working – the one thing he felt he was reasonably good at. At times this led to him working very long hours and caused arguments with his partner. James also drank alcohol to excess to try and get away from his thoughts. During the MBCT course, James learned it is possible to turn attention towards painful thoughts and acknowledge them, without being overwhelmed by them. He began to see mindfulness practice as a place where he could notice and then step back from painful thoughts and feelings; a place where he could just *be* for a while, rather than always having to be busy trying to be perfect and to keep his self-critical thoughts at bay.

In the latter MBCT sessions, James identified early warning signs that might indicate he was becoming caught up in depressogenic patterns of thinking and behaviour, and he planned effective coping strategies with an emphasis on self-compassion. By the end of the eight-session course, James still experienced negative, potentially depressogenic patterns of thinking at times. However, he was more able to spot them early, before they could become too entrenched, and he found it possible to view these products of his mind in a kindly, stepped-back way. In this sense, through the MBCT course, he had developed a different, less reactive relationship with his thoughts and related feelings.

ACTIVITY

For the case study:
1. List key aspects used in MBCT.
2. Consider why this approach was taken.
3. Write down the impact that MBCT is having from a psychological perspective.
4. Write down the impact that MBCT is having from a physical perspective.
5. Write down the impact that MBCT is having from an emotional perspective.
6. Consider the outcomes on quality of life and overall well-being for James.

Chapter 24 will focus on brief relaxation techniques for inducing relaxation at short notice, which includes a brief version of a mindfulness-based stress reduction.

REFERENCES

Ainsworth, B., Bolderston, H., & Garner, M. D. (2017). Testing the differential effects of acceptance and attention-based psychological interventions on intrusive thoughts and worry. *Behaviour Research and Therapy*, 91, 72–77.

Astin, J. A., Berman, B. M., Bausell, B., et al. (2003). The efficacy of mindfulness meditation plus qigong movement therapy in the treatment of fibromyalgia: A randomized controlled trial. *Journal of Rheumatology*, 30(10), 2257–2262.

Bishop, S. R. (2002). What do we really know about mindfulness-based stress reduction? *Psychosomatic Medicine*, 64, 71–83.

Burch, V., Hennessy, G., & Fricker, S. (2006). *Exploring how different management and treatment approaches affect the subjective experience of long-term back pain sufferers: A qualitative analysis.* Manchester, UK: Breathworks.

Carlson, L. E., & Garland, S. N. (2005). The impact of mindfulness-based stress reduction on sleep, mood, stress and fatigue symptoms in cancer outpatients. *International Journal of Behavioral Medicine*, 12(4), 278–285.

Carlson, L. E., Speca, M., Faris, P., et al. (2007). One year pre-post intervention follow-up of psychological, immune, endocrine and blood pressure outcomes of mindfulness-based stress reduction in breast and prostate cancer outpatients. *Brain, Behavior, and Immunity*, 21(8), 1038–1049.

Chadwick, P., Hughes, S., Russell, D., Russell, I., & Dagnan, D. (2009). Mindfulness groups for distressing voices and paranoia: A replication and randomized feasibility trial. *Behavioural and Cognitive Psychotherapy*, 37(4), 403–412.

Chiesa, A., & Serretti, A. (2011). Mindfulness based cognitive therapy for psychiatric disorders: A systematic review and meta-analysis. *Psychiatry Research*, 187(3), 441–453.

Davidson, R. J., Kabat-Zinn, J., Schumacher, J., et al. (2003). Alterations in brain and immune function produced by mindfulness meditation. *Psychosomatic Medicine*, 65(4), 564–570.

Foley, E., Baillie, A., Huxter, M., Price, M., & Sinclair, E. (2010). Mindfulness based cognitive therapy for individuals whose lives have been affected by cancer: A randomized controlled trial. *Journal of Consulting and Clinical Psychology*, 78(1), 72–79.

Gunaratana, B. H. (2002). *Mindfulness in plain English.* Somerville, MA: Wisdom.

Hanh, T. N. (1976). *The miracle of mindfulness.* Boston: Beacon.

Hoppes, K. (2006). The application of mindfulness-based cognitive interventions in the treatment of co-occurring addictive and mood disorders. *CNS Spectrums*, 11(11), 829–851.

Kabat-Zinn, J. (1994). *Wherever you go there you are: Mindfulness meditation in everyday life.* New York: Hyperion.

Kabat-Zinn, J. (2003). Mindfulness-based interventions in context: Past, present and future. *Clinical Psychology Science and Practice*, 10, 144–156.

Kabat-Zinn, J. (2013). *Full catastrophe living (revised edition): How to cope with stress, pain and illness using mindfulness meditation.* London: Hachette UK.

Khoury, B., Sharma, M., Rush, S. E., & Fournier, C. (2015). Mindfulness-based stress reduction for healthy individuals: A meta-analysis. *Journal of Psychosomatic Research*, 78(6), 519–528.

Kuyken, W., Byford, S., Taylor, R. S., et al. (2008). Mindfulness-based cognitive therapy to prevent relapse in recurrent depression. *Journal of Consulting and Clinical Psychology*, 76(6), 966.

Kuyken, W., Watkins, E., & Holden, E. (2010). How does mindfulness-based cognitive therapy work? *Behavioral Research and Therapy*, 48(11), 1105–1112.

Langer, E. J. (1989). *Mindfulness. Cambridge.* UK: Da Capo.

Linehan, M. M. (1993). *Cognitive-behavioral treatment of borderline personality disorder.* New York: Guildford Press.

MacKenzie, M. B., & Kocovski, N. L. (2016). Mindfulness-based cognitive therapy for depression: Trends and developments. *Psychology Research and Behavior Management*, 9, 125–132.

Matchim, Y., & Armer, J. M. (2007). Measuring the psychological impact of mindfulness meditation on health among patients with cancer: A literature review. *Oncology Nursing Forum*, 34(5), 1059–1066.

Matousek, R. H., Dobkin, P. L., & Pruessner, J. C. (2010). Cortisol as a marker for improvement in mindfulness-based stress reduction. *Complementary Therapies in Clinical Practice*, 16(1), 13–19.

Ott, M. J., Norris, R. L., & Bauer Wu, S. M. (2006). Mindfulness meditation for oncology patients: A discussion and critical review. *Integrative Cancer Therapies*, 5(2), 98–108.

Segal, Z. V., Teasdale, J. D., & Williams, M. G. (2004). Mindfulness-based cognitive therapy: Theoretical rationale and empirical status. In S. C. Hayes, V. M. Follette, & M. M. Linehan (Eds.), *Mindfulness and acceptance: Expanding the cognitive behavioral tradition.* New York: Guilford Press.

Segal, Z. V., Williams, J. M., & Teasdale, J. D. (2013). *Mindfulness-based cognitive therapy for depression* (2nd ed). New York: Guilford Press.

Shapiro, D. H. (1992). A preliminary study of long term meditators: Goals, effects, religious orientation, cognitions. *Journal of Transpersonal Psychology*, 24(1), 23–39.

Shapiro, S. L., Carlson, L. E., Astin, J. A., & Freedman, B. (2006). Mechanisms of mindfulness. *Journal of Clinical Psychology*, 62, 373–386.

Shennan, C., Payne, S., & Fenlon, D. (2011). What is the evidence for the use of mindfulness-based interventions in cancer care? A review. *Psycho-Oncology*, 20(7), 681–697.

Smith, J. E., Richardson, J., Hoffman, C., et al. (2005). Mindfulness-based stress reduction as supportive therapy in cancer care: A systematic review. *Journal of Advanced Nursing*, 52(3), 315–327.

Smith, S. A. (2014). Mindfulness-based stress reduction: An intervention to enhance the effectiveness of nurses' coping with work-related stress. *International Journal of Nursing Knowledge*, 25(2), 119–130.

Tang, Y.Y., & Posner, M.I. (2014). Handbook of Mindfulness: Theory, Research, and Practice. In: Brown, K. W., Creswell, J. D. & Ryan, R. M., Eds. 81–89, Guildford Press.

Teasdale, J. D., Segal, Z. V., Williams, J. M. G., et al. (2000). Prevention of relapse recurrence in major depression by mindfulness-based cognitive therapy. *Journal of Consulting and Clinical Psychology*, 68, 615–623.

Warnecke, E., Quinn, S., Ogden, K., Towle, N., & Nelson, M. (2011). A randomised controlled trial of the effects of mindfulness practice on medical student stress levels. *Medical Education*, 45(4), 381–388.

Williams, M., & Penman, D. (2011). *Mindfulness: A practical guide to finding peace in a frantic world*. London: Piatkus.

Williams, J. M. G. (2008). Mindfulness, depression and modes of mind. *Cognitive Therapy and Research, 32*, 721–733.

Williams, J. M. G., Teasdale, J. D., & Segal, Z. V. (2007). *The mindful way through depression: Freeing yourself from chronic unhappiness*. New York: Guilford Press.

Zeidan, F. (2015). The neurobiology of mindfulness meditation. In: Handbook of Mindfulness Science: Theory, Research and Practice. K.W. Brown, J.D. Creswell & R.M. Ryan, Eds. 171–189. New York: The Guilford Press.

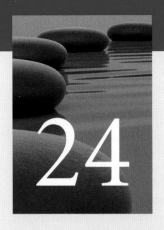

24

BRIEF RELAXATION TECHNIQUES

DR CAROLINE BELCHAMBER

CHAPTER CONTENTS

LEARNING OBJECTIVES

The aim of this chapter is to provide a resource of brief relaxation techniques that can be used to reduce the effects of a sudden stressor.

By the end of this chapter you will be able to:

1. Understand which relaxation techniques can be used in a brief form.

2. Know the evidence that underpins brief relaxation techniques.

3. Recognize that a deeper understanding of the parent relaxation technique is required before using a brief relaxation technique.

4. Discern the characteristics of brief relaxation techniques.

5. Identify the factors affecting the success of brief relaxation techniques.

6. Appreciate when and how to use brief relaxation techniques.

This chapter concludes Section 3 on cognitive approaches to relaxation techniques. Chapter 25 will begin Section 4 focusing on application to practice, which includes how relaxation techniques can help chronic long-term conditions, its place in supportive, palliative and end of life care and Covid-19.

INTRODUCTION TO BRIEF RELAXATION TECHNIQUES

The goal of most methods described in previous chapters has been the induction of deep relaxation, a slowly induced state which allows the individual to lose all tension. To achieve this, the person must detach themselves from environmental stimuli and focus all their attention on the relaxation technique. This approach is appropriate where total relaxation is required and where the environment is making no current demands on them.

The individual may, however, be looking for a shorter relaxation technique which works fast, a strategy to lighten the effect of a stressor suddenly imposed upon them. The aim here is not to release all tension but to lose superfluous tension. Far from being detached from the environment, the individual wants to be fully alert to deal with its challenges. Instead of eliminating stressors, the person wants to increase their tolerance of them. What they need is a relaxation technique which can be implemented at a moment's notice and still allow them to carry on with the task, whatever it might be.

Shortened forms of relaxation techniques have already been referred to. The rapid relaxation of Öst (1987) is one example (see Chapter 9), where the individual recites a cue word on exhalation while scanning the body for tension. Mitchell's (1987) 'key movements', which are capable of unlocking the body from tense postures (see Chapter 13), are another example.

Although the aim of brief relaxation techniques is to lose excess tension, retaining only what is necessary for the task, these relaxation techniques are not the same as differential relaxation (see Chapter 11). Differential relaxation is a principle to be applied throughout the day, regardless of activity. By contrast, brief relaxation techniques are designed to exert a momentary effect in the face of sudden threat.

A variety of techniques for inducing relaxation at short notice are presented in this chapter. They are derived from relaxation techniques already described, being, for the most part, abbreviated versions of them. They work best in individuals who have given the parent relaxation technique many hours of practice. It is practice that enables the individual to switch on the full effect at short notice. Thus brief relaxation techniques are shorthand versions of lengthier techniques previously learned.

There is a lack of research into the efficacy of brief relaxation techniques; however, there is growing body of evidence demonstrating that it is helpful in reducing stress and anxiety.

INTRODUCTION TO EVIDENCE

In 1973 Bernstein and Borkovec (1973a) developed a brief relaxation technique which produced the effects of relaxation following one session. This became known as the abbreviated progressive relaxation technique (APRT), which has become widely used in research (Masters et al 1987, Turner et al 1982). A review carried out in 1980 looked at psychophysiological effects of a single session of APRT across studies, which demonstrated that APRT consistently produced reductions in respiratory rate, heart rate,

blood pressure, muscle tension and skin conductance (King 1980). A literature meta-analysis of APRT also concluded that APRT was effective in reducing stress and generalized anxiety (Carlson & Hoyle 1993). Furthermore, an in vivo study with college students concluded that APRT of 20 minute duration significantly lowered self-reported stress and anxiety (Pawlow & Jones 2002), with overall results indicating a positive psychological, endocrinological and immunological change in normal healthy individuals. This study was followed by research into night eating syndrome, which is linked to stress and weight gain and involved two sessions of APRT 1 week apart, with daily practice in between the sessions. APRT was delivered in 20-minute sessions to 20 participants who were randomly assigned to either APRT or a control group. Stress, anxiety and relaxation were monitored by assessing salivary cortisol pre- and post-APRT. Mood and hunger ratings were also assessed on the first and eighth day. Results indicated a significant reduction in stress, anxiety and cortisol immediately after APRT. There was also evidence of reduced, stress, anxiety, fatigue, anger and depression on the eighth day (Pawlow et al 2003).

A brief relaxation technique, which included deep breathing, guided imagery and APRT, was used to explore the effect on psychological stress and impaired wound healing in people undergoing surgery. Participants were randomly assigned to usual care or usual care in combination with 45 minutes of brief relaxation technique. A relaxation CD was also provided for participants to take home to listen to 3 days before surgery and 7 days after surgery. Results indicated that brief relaxation technique before surgery reduced stress and improved wound healing (Broadbent et al 2012). Interestingly, a pilot study using the same brief relaxation technique combination of deep breathing, guided imagery and 10 minutes of APRT to manage cancer pain; participants reported greater improvements in pain, tension and confidence in managing their pain than those receiving usual care (Pollak et al 2015).

Brief relaxation techniques using cognitive–behavioural therapy (CBT) have been used to explore effectiveness in maintaining an improved physical functional status in people with fibromyalgia.

Participants were randomly assigned to usual care or usual care with six sessions of CBT. Of those receiving CBT 25% achieved clinically meaningful levels of long-term improvement in physical functioning compared with only 12% receiving usual care. However, there were no differences in relation to long-term pain ratings between the groups (Williams et al 2002).

A brief version of a mindfulness-based stress reduction has been explored and evaluated to ascertain its efficacy in managing stress in the nursing profession. Nurses were either assigned to a brief 4-week mindfulness intervention or to a control group. Nurses who completed the brief mindfulness-based intervention experienced significant reduction in burnout symptoms, improved relaxation and increased life satisfaction. It was concluded that this brief relaxation technique was a promising technique for managing stress in the nursing profession (Mackenzie et al 2006).

The efficacy of a brief relaxation technique which included psychoeducation and breathing retraining of 1-hour duration was explored in children with recurrent abdominal pain. Five children participated in the study receiving the brief relaxation technique at 1-week intervals, with a follow-up session 3 months later. Results indicated a reduction in abdominal pain in all of the children after the breathing re-training, as well as some of the children's general somatic symptoms (Bell & Meadows 2013).

There is therefore a growing body of evidence supporting the use of brief relaxation techniques for managing the effect of a variety of stressors and symptoms.

THEORIES BEHIND BRIEF RELAXATION TECHNIQUES

Please see the theories behind the parent relaxation technique because this will provide an understanding of the theory behind the abbreviated version.

CHARACTERISTICS OF BRIEF RELAXATION TECHNIQUES

In essence, brief relaxation techniques should be:

- portable: short enough and convenient enough to be used in most situations.

- unobtrusive: not attracting attention or interrupting ongoing work.
- capable of inducing moderate levels of relaxation. The object is not to induce deep relaxation but to enable the individual to carry on with the task, in as relaxed a state as possible.

FACTORS AFFECTING THE SUCCESS OF BRIEF RELAXATION TECHNIQUES

Not every strategy is going to succeed every time. A number of factors may influence the outcome.

1. *Situation.* The degree of inherent threat in a situation may vary. Situations of high threat tend to reduce the effectiveness of the relaxation technique.
2. *Sensitivity to internal cues.* People's ability to recognize their own physiological and psychological cues is important. As stress levels rise, the cues become more pronounced. The earlier people are able to pick them up, the more effective will be the relaxation technique that they apply.
3. *Level of skill attained by previous practice.* The capacity to 'switch on' relaxation whenever the individual feels under stress depends to a great extent on the level of skill attained in any one relaxation technique. This in turn depends on the amount of home practice that has been carried out.
4. *Personal preference in choice of relaxation technique.* Individuals have preferences for some techniques over others. The technique in which people feel most at ease will be likely to induce greater relaxation than a technique which feels alien to them.
5. *Diversionary content of the relaxation technique.* Diversion, such as the reciting of a mantra, is said to contribute to the effect of a relaxation technique. The stronger the diversionary element, the greater the power of the technique. It is a useful feature where all that is required is a reduction in stress levels, as in the condition of panic. Where successful coping relies on intellectual and verbal skills, distraction is less useful,

and a technique which leaves the mind free to focus on the issue is more appropriate.

THE EXERCISES

A brief relaxation technique may be picked from any of the following approaches:

- Physical actions
- Scanning
- Breathing
- Cognitive strategies

Physical Actions

When under stress, individuals tend to close up physically. It is an unconscious reaction to any kind of threat and has the effect of making them feel less exposed. Although the action may not be observable, the muscles involved may nevertheless be minutely contracting. To help release that tension, one of the following manoeuvres could be adopted:

- Key changes
- Posture
- Shaking a sleeve down
- Stretching

Key Changes

Certain physical actions may serve as keys to unlock body patterns of tension (Mitchell 1987) (see Chapter 13). The individual may find their personal key in one of the following four actions:

1. *Spreading the fingers.*
   The order is: fingers and thumbs long … hold them there for a moment … then stop … let them recoil into a gently curved position.
2. *Separating your teeth.*
   The order is: drag your jaw downwards … feel your jaw hanging down inside your mouth … then stop … feel your throat slack, your tongue loose and your lips gently touching.
3. *Pulling the shoulders towards the feet.*
   Feel a distance growing between your shoulders and your ears … and, stop pulling … let your shoulders rest where they are.

4. *Pushing the head back.*
   With your shoulders pulled down, lift your head; carry it up and back, keeping your chin pointing towards your feet. Stop. The resulting position should feel comfortable.

Posture

A mental impression of being at one's full height promotes a sense of ease and confidence. Reminders are contained in phrases such as the following:

- Think 'tall'
- Think 'up'

The second item is drawn from the Alexander technique (see Chapter 12).

Shaking a Sleeve Down

The 'shaking a sleeve down' action loosens the muscles in the arm and shoulder and has the added advantage of appearing a quite natural thing to do.

Stretching

Musculoskeletal benefit is derived from stretching (see Chapter 14). In the context of brief relaxation, they are aimed at structures which have been held in one position for some length of time, such as the spinal joints during long-distance motoring. A few examples are the following:

- Trunk twisting (Fig. 14.15)
- Back arching (Fig. 14.16)
- Crouching (Fig. 14.17)

Other stretching exercises may be found in Chapter 14.

Scanning

Scanning is a shortened version of passive relaxation. It involves a brief tour of the body during which the participant checks for unnecessary tension. Four approaches are described:

1. Relaxation by recall with counting
2. Behavioural relaxation checklist
3. Sweeping the body
4. The ripple

Relaxation by Recall With Counting

Bernstein and Borkovec (1973b) condensed their progressive muscular relaxation training programme into a release-only format for four groups of muscles: the arms, the head and neck, the trunk and the legs. In its most summarized form, it consists of a counting procedure: two counts are allotted to each body part as attention is focused on it and tension released (see Chapter 8).

> *One … two (arms relax) … three … four (head and neck relax) … five … six (trunk relax) … seven … eight (legs relax) … nine … ten (whole body relax) …*

Behavioural Relaxation Checklist

The behavioural relaxation checklist is based on the assumption that if individuals look relaxed, to some extent they will feel relaxed. A checklist (see Table 10.1 in Chapter 10), which can be memorized, covers 10 postures characteristic of relaxation (Poppen 1998).

- *Feet … resting with toes lying free*
- *Hands … fingers gently curled*
- *Body … without movement*
- *Shoulders … dropped and level*
- *Head … still, and facing forwards*
- *Mouth … teeth separated, lips unpursed*
- *Throat … loose*
- *Breathing … slow and gentle*
- *Voice … no sound*
- *Eyes … lightly closed behind smooth eyelids.*

Sweeping the Body

Kermani (1990) describes a routine used for releasing body tension. It involves sweeping the surface of the body with an imaginary large, soft paintbrush (see Chapter 8).

> *Starting at your feet, sweep the brush, in your mind's eye, up your legs and the front of your body as far as your shoulders … then down your arms to your fingertips … then, a long sweep up the full length of the back … continuing into the neck and scalp … over the brow … and down to the face and jaw.*

The Ripple

This is a single wave of relaxation which begins at the head and rolls down the body to the feet (Priest & Schott 1991) (see Chapter 8).

> *Starting at the top of your head, feel the relaxation rolling down your body in one continuous wave … feel it releasing tension as it descends … relaxing each part of your body in turn … until it reaches the tips of your toes. Try synchronizing the ripple with a slow breath out.*

Breathing

Stress is associated with physiological arousal. This arousal is brought about by the action of the sympathetic nervous system, and includes an increase in the respiratory rate. Slowed breathing is associated with parasympathetic activity. Thus, by consciously slowing the breathing rate, it may be possible to counteract the effects of the sympathetic nervous system and generally check the symptoms of arousal.

Three techniques are described. Each one has a greater chance of success if it is introduced before the state of stress becomes established.

1. Abdominal breathing
2. Using words as cues
3. A breathing cycle

Abdominal Breathing

Because sudden stress is associated with apical (upper costal) respiratory movements, and relaxation with abdominal respiratory movements, breathing which is focused on the abdomen will tend to have a quietening effect (see Chapter 4).

> *Let your attention focus on your abdomen. Feel it swelling as you breathe in and sinking as you breathe out. Keep the breathing light, gentle and slow.*

Using Words as Cues (Cue-Controlled Relaxation)

Repeated past associations of a word such as 'relax' with the relaxed state give the word the status of a cue. When subsequently recited on the outbreath, this word tends to bring about a state of relaxation (Öst 1987) (see Chapter 9).

Let your breathing be as natural as possible ... just before you begin to breathe out, think the word 'relax' ... slowly release the air as you focus on the word ... breathe in ... and, repeat the sequence ... keep the rhythm as gentle as you can ... avoid deliberately deepening the breaths ... continue for a few moments ...

A short version might run:

In ... relax and out slowly ... in ... relax and out slowly ...

or simply:

Relax.

A Breathing Cycle

A single breath cycle can be useful for helping to relieve stress in a crisis situation. It consists of a deeper than usual breath in, which is held for a few seconds before being slowly exhaled. Lichstein (1988) points out how each component of the exercise has value: the inbreath diverts attention from the distressing thoughts; the breath retention raises the PCO_2 level, inducing mild lethargy, and the slow outbreath helps reduce muscle tension. The cycle begins with an outbreath in the following exercise.

Breathe out a little more fully than usual. Let the air flow in to fill your lungs. Hold it for 5 seconds. Then exhale slowly. As you let the air out, feel the tension going with it. Then, let your breathing recover its normal rhythm.

Because deep breathing can increase the possibility of hyperventilation, immediate repetition of this exercise is not recommended.

Cognitive Strategies

These are methods which deal with stress by changing our thoughts. They include the following approaches:

1. Self-talk
2. Autogenic phrases
3. Imagery
4. Attention switching
5. Thought stopping
6. Thinking of a smile
7. Environmental markers
8. Additional strategies

Self-Talk

Because thoughts influence feelings, positive thoughts will tend to generate positive feelings. Phrases affirming the value of the self, repeated often, colour our view of ourselves, and in a positive direction (see Chapter 19). Feeling in control and feeling relaxed will tend to increase coping powers whatever the source of the stress.

Phrases tending to promote a sense of control over the situation include the following:

- I am competent.
- I can deal with this.
- I am in control.
- My coping powers are good.

Phrases tending to induce a relaxed state of mind include the following:

- I feel at peace.
- I am relaxed.
- I am calm.
- My thoughts are peaceful ones.

These phrases provide examples of positive self-talk; however, the most effective phrases are those which individuals have composed for themselves.

Autogenic Phrases

Training in autogenics (see Chapter 20) can result in relaxation occurring after recitation of a single phrase. It could be a heaviness phrase, a warmth phrase or one relating to feelings of peace. When recited, it can act as a key to switch on autogenic effects.

Imagery

Both single images and transformations can promote relaxation. Two examples of the former are the rag doll and the piece of seaweed (see Chapter 18). Identifying with the characteristics of an inert image can help to mitigate feelings of stress. Anger, panic and frustration may all respond to this kind of imagery.

'Transformations' refer to the mutation of one substance into another (see Chapter 18). The first substance is harsh, the second smooth, and they are linked by some sensory quality as in the following items (Fanning 1988):

- Sandpaper … to … silk
- Chalk squeaking on the blackboard … to … high musical notes
- Burnt toast fumes … to … baking bread
- Fluorescent orange … to … soft peach
- Sour gooseberries … to … sweet raspberries

Individuals focus attention on the harsh image, which they then resolve into the smooth one. The transformation becomes a metaphor for their own feelings, which are thereby helped to undergo a change from negative to positive.

Thought Stopping

Thought stopping (Quick & Quick 1984) intercepts stress-inducing thoughts and substitutes stress-neutralizing ones. The technique involves the word 'STOP', spoken or imagined, but in such a way that it momentarily blots out the disturbing thought. This is immediately replaced with an idea or an activity which diverts and holds the attention, such as counting games, puzzles or physical exercise.

Thinking of a Smile

Facial expression has been found to influence emotions. A positive expression tends to induce a positive feeling in that individual (see Chapter 10). Thus, if a person smiles, his or her feelings of stress will tend to be diminished. However, as it is not always appropriate to smile, it is enough to stay with the thought of it and simply to imagine the smile.

The Environmental Marker

Several writers suggest placing a mark on appliances which are potential sources of stress (Mitchell 1987, Öst 1987) (see Chapters 9 and 11). Coloured dots stuck, for instance, on to the telephone, wristwatch or steering wheel serve to remind the individual to maintain low levels of tension. Öst suggests changing the colour of the markers frequently because their effect dwindles as the eye gets habituated to the dot.

Additional Strategies

A range of techniques can be used to distract the attention, including images of strong light and memorized telephone numbers. In the case of 'strong light', individuals can be asked to imagine an intensely bright light beamed into their eyes from a dark background. With regard to the 'telephone number', they can be asked to look at a new number, concentrating so hard that they memorize it; when they close their eyes, they can then recite it several times.

KEY POINTS

1. Brief relaxation techniques are shortened forms of specific relaxation techniques.
2. The aim of brief relaxation techniques is to lose excess tension in a given situation.
3. The techniques are designed to exert a momentary effect in the face of a sudden threat.
4. These techniques can help increase the person's tolerance to a sudden stressor.
5. The techniques enable people to be fully alert to deal with their challenge and continue with their task in hand.
6. Different factors influence the outcome and success of the brief relaxation technique.

Reflection

Describe your understanding about brief relaxation techniques.

How do you feel about applying these techniques in practice?

How do brief relaxation techniques help people to manage sudden stressors?

How do brief relaxation techniques differ from the parent relaxation technique?

What brief relaxation techniques have you used? Were they successful?

What is the main learning point you will take away from this chapter?

What is your future action plan in terms of using brief relaxation techniques?

CASE STUDY LEARNING OPPORTUNITIES

The key points and reflection provide background and knowledge required in relation to the case study, Philip, to help deepen understanding of how brief relaxation techniques can help manage sudden stressors.

CASE STUDY

Sudden Anxiety and Panic: Brief Relaxation Technique Outcomes for Philip

Whenever Philip had to present to a group of people he became anxious; his body went tense, his mouth dry, his breathing rapid and he could feel his heart thumping in his chest. He felt frightened, out of control and wanted to flee from the situation. This became an issue as overtime the symptoms worsened and his mind went blank. In addition Philip's lack of confidence and abundance of nerves had been noted by his colleagues and line manager. Delivering presentations was part of Philip's job role, so he needed to overcome his fears and anxieties. Philip therefore sought help with the support of his line manager.

Philip was introduced to self-talk techniques as his negative thoughts were interfering with his ability to deliver in a confident manner. These affirmations included 'I am competent in presenting',' I can deal with this situation' and 'I am in control of my actions'. As sudden stress produced a negative effect on Philip's breathing, abdominal breathing was also taught to manage this symptom, focusing on the word 'relax' on breathing out. Philip was then asked to practice these brief relaxation techniques daily when he was calm so that he could use these strategies when he was asked to present to a group of people.

After a couple of months Philip was finding he was much more in control; the breathing helped with his anxiety and removed the tension from his body, which in turn enabled him to breath more normally. With positive affirmations he felt more confident, leading to a more competent performance, which then increased his overall confidence.

ACTIVITY

For the case study:

1. List key aspects used in the brief relaxation technique.
2. Write down the impact that the brief relaxation techniques are having from a psychological perspective.
3. Write down the impact that the brief relaxation techniques are having from a physical perspective.
4. Write down the impact that the brief relaxation techniques are having from an emotional perspective.
5. Consider the outcomes on quality of life and overall well-being for Philip.

This chapter concludes Section 3 on cognitive approaches to relaxation techniques. Chapter 25 will begin Section 4 focusing on application to practice, which includes how relaxation techniques can help chronic long-term conditions and its place in supportive, palliative and end-of-life care.

REFERENCES

Bell, K. M., & Meadows, E. A. (2013). Efficacy of a brief relaxation training intervention for paediatric recurrent abdominal pain. *Cognitive and Behavioural Practice, 20,* 81–92.

Bernstein, D. A., & Borkovec, T. D. (1973a). *Progressive relaxation training.* Champagne, IL: Research Press.

Bernstein, D. A., & Borkovec, T. D. (1973b). *Progressive relaxation training: A manual for the helping professions.* Champaign, IL: Research Press.

Broadbent, E., Kahokehr, A., Booth, R. J., et al. (2012). A brief relaxation intervention reduces stress and improves surgical wound healing response: A randomised trial. *Brain, Behavior, and Immunity, 26,* 212–217.

Carlson, C. R., & Hoyle, R. H. (1993). Efficacy of abbreviated progressive muscle relaxation training: A quantitative review of behavioral medicine research. *Journal of Consulting and Clinical Psychology, 61,* 1059–1067.

Fanning, P. (1988). *Visualization for change.* Oakland, CA: New Harbinger.

Kermani, K. S. (1990). *Autogenic training.* London: Souvenir Press.

King, N. J. (1980). Abbreviated progressive relaxation. *Progressive Behavior Modification, 3,* 147–182.

Lichstein, K. L. (1988). *Clinical relaxation strategies.* New York: John Wiley.

Mackenzie, C. S., Poulin, P. A., & Seidman-Carlson, R. (2006). A brief mindfulness-based stress reduction intervention for nurses and nurse aides. *Applied Nursing Research, 19,* 105–109.

Masters, J. C., Burish, T. G., Hollon, S. D., & Rimm, D. C. (1987). *Behavior therapy: Techniques and empirical findings* (3rd ed.). New York: Harcourt Brace Jovanovich.

Mitchell, L. (1987). *Simple relaxation: The Mitchell method for easing tension* (2nd ed.). London: John Murray.

Öst, L. -G. (1987). Applied relaxation: Description of a coping technique and review of controlled studies. *Behaviour Research and Therapy, 25,* 397–407.

Pawlow, L. A., & Jones, G. E. (2002). The impact of abbreviated progressive muscle relaxation on salivary cortisol. *Biological Psychology*, *60*, 1–16.

Pawlow, L. A., O'Neil, P. M., & Malcolm, R. J. (2003). Night eating syndrome: Effects of brief relaxation training on stress, mood, hunger and eating patterns. *International Journal of Obesity*, *27*, 970–978.

Pollak, K. I., Lyna, P., Bilheimer, A., & Porter, L. S. (2015). A brief relaxation intervention for pain delivered by palliative care physicians: A pilot study. *Palliative Medicine*, *29*(6), 569–570.

Poppen, R. (1998). *Behavioral relaxation training and assessment* (2nd ed.). Thousand Oaks, CA: Sage.

Priest, J., & Schott, J. (1991). *Leading antenatal classes: A practical guide*. Oxford, UK: Butterworth-Heinemann.

Quick, J. C., & Quick, J. D. (1984). *Organizational stress and preventative management*. New York: McGraw Hill.

Turner, S. M., Calhoun, K. S., & Adams, H. E. (1982). *Handbook of clinical behavior therapy*. New York: Wiley.

Williams, D. A., Cary, M. A., Groneer, K. H., et al. (2002). Improving physical functional status in patients with fibromyalgia: A brief cognitive behavioral intervention. *The Journal of Rheumatology*, *29*(6), 1280–1286.

Section 4

APPLICATION IN PRACTICE

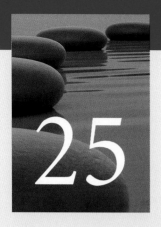

25

LONG-TERM CONDITIONS

DR CAROLINE BELCHAMBER

CHAPTER CONTENTS

LEARNING OBJECTIVES

The aim of this chapter is to provide an understanding of the application of relaxation techniques for people with long-term conditions.

By the end of this chapter you will be able to:

1. Recognize the different conditions which sit under the umbrella term of 'long-term conditions'.

2. Understand how long-term conditions affect the person's overall well-being.

3. Describe the physiological and psychological elements of long-term conditions.

4. Acknowledge the mental health needs of people with long-term conditions.

5. Identify relaxation techniques which can improve well-being and quality of life for people with long-term conditions.

The chapter will conclude with key points and time for reflection, providing learning opportunities through a case study.

INTRODUCTION TO LONG-TERM CONDITIONS

In England there are approximately 15 million people with long-term conditions (DOH 2012). Long-term conditions are also referred to as chronic diseases and illnesses, and include conditions such as chronic obstructive pulmonary disease (COPD), diabetes, arthritis and a variety of cardiovascular diseases, to mention a few (refer to Chapter 29 for more conditions). More recently certain cancers, the human immunodeficiency virus (HIV) and acquired immunodeficiency syndrome (AIDS) have been recognized as long-term conditions (Naylor et al 2012). Long-term conditions are those which currently have no cure but are managed through medication and non-pharmacological approaches. A 2012 Department of Health report estimated that the number of people with three or more long-term conditions would rise to 2.9 million people by 2018 (DOH 2012). In the United Kingdom approximately 1.8 million cancer survivors also have one or more long-term conditions (MCS 2015). These multiple co-morbidities often include mental health issues, such as anxiety and depression, which reduce the person's overall quality of life and prognosis (MCS 2015, Naylor et al 2012). Long-term conditions are therefore often described as complex conditions.

Complex Conditions

Scientific advancement means that we are living longer with complex conditions (Edelman et al 2005). An example is the improvements in cancer survival rates over the past decades resulting in a growing number of long-term survivors (Engert et al 2010, 2012). When they are diagnosed with a long-term condition, patients and their families will need to come to terms with this life-changing event. In addition, where there are prolonged health issues, mental 'unhappiness' can occur at any time. The National Institute for Health and Care Excellence (NICE 2011) confirms this with evidence demonstrating that people with long-term physical health conditions, such as cardiovascular disease and diabetes, often have a co-morbid mental health condition.

The underlying processes linking mental and physical health is complex and includes a combination of behavioural, environmental, biological and psychosocial elements (Prince et al 2007). Anxiety, depression, social isolation, loneliness, helplessness and hopelessness have commonly been reported (Levy 2000). Therefore the psychological impact of the diagnosis of a long-term condition is complex because people often experience a wide range of psychological conditions (Gunathilaka et al 2019, McLeod 2013), the most prevalent being anxiety and depression.

Anxiety and Depression

Studies that have followed up with people after a diagnosis of a long-term condition have reported significant increases in anxiety and depression, as well as relationship difficulties (Bohlmeijer et al 2010, Sarafino 2006). Depression has been reported as the most common psychological condition in people with end-stage renal disease (Finkelstein & Finkelstein 2000, Kimmel & Levy 2004). Diabetes and pulmonary conditions have also been associated with depression (Ali et al 2006) and anxiety, including cardiovascular conditions (Kinley et al 2015). It has been reported that rates of anxiety and depression are up to three times higher in those with cardiac conditions (Lane et al 2002), with major depression identified in 19.8% of survivors after acute myocardial infarction (Thombs et al 2006). Furthermore, evidence from a meta-analysis of chronic heart failure reported 11% to 45% with anxiety and 10% to 60% with depression (Yohannes et al 2010). Having a diagnosis of cancer is also a highly stressful event and is commonly linked to depression (prevalence 5% to 15%) and increased number of suicides (Misono et al 2008, Walker et al 2013).

COPD is a common long-term condition affecting more than 210 million people across the world (Global Initiative 2017). Because of continued exposure to risk factors and an aging population, COPD rates are projected to rise in the coming decades (Fraser et al 2016). Anxiety and depression are two of the main associated conditions of COPD, which can also include cardiovascular disease, skeletal muscle dysfunction, osteoporosis, metabolic syndrome and lung cancer, leading to a higher risk of exacerbations and reduced health status (Global Initiative 2020, Lipson et al 2018).

Anxiety and depression have multiple causes, including biological, social and behavioural factors (Pinnock et al 2011), and where two or more long-term conditions co-exist, people are seven times more likely to have depression (NICE 2009b). In general, the evidence indicates that at least 30% of all individuals with a long-term condition have mental health issues (Cimpean & Drake 2011) such as anxiety and depression. Anxiety and depression have therefore been classed as primary long-term conditions. People diagnosed with anxiety and depression have an increased likelihood of developing other long-term conditions, such as cardiovascular disease and diabetes (DOH 2012). Thus anxiety and depression have been linked to heightened morbidity and mortality rates (Frasure-Smith et al 2000). It is therefore paramount to understand the impact a diagnosis of a long-term condition has on a person.

Diagnosis

The diagnosis of a long-term condition presents individuals with challenges to their everyday lifestyle (Martz & Livneh 2007). Some people can make the required adjustments, but this still leaves the person more vulnerable to anxiety and depression over and above that of the general population (Clarke & Currie 2009, Moussavi et al 2007). For some people, the diagnosis and other key events relating to the onset of the condition are a traumatic experience (McLeod 2013). This experience has been described as a crisis reaction and involves initial shock and disbelief, followed by anxiety, anger, guilt and depression (Boulton et al 2001, Mehnert et al 2011, Uitterhoeve et al 2004). In each individual, new and challenging environmental information triggers different cognitive and physiological responses. These responses activate the sympathetic nervous system and hypothalamic-pituitary-adrenal axis, often affecting health and well-being (see Chapter 1). It can cause stress, which involves an increased heart rate, increased blood pressure and release of the stress hormone. Stress of diagnosis can therefore directly affect the body's responses – the 'fight or flight' response (see Chapter 1). When this response becomes constant, as is the case in long-term conditions, the physiological elements of the response create harmful consequences, such as increased blood pressure or exacerbation of the condition (Mayer 2000).

Thus the diagnosis of a long-term condition can be a very stressful life event, creating significant psychological issues. It can affect the person's quality of life and may affect not only their physical health but also their mental health, functional status and general well-being (Bakewell et al 2002, Blake et al 2000). In addition, anxiety and depression have been shown to affect adherence to treatment, often compromising treatment decision making, outcomes, self-efficacy and self-care, leading to an impaired health status and, as a consequence, increased use of health care services (Lane et al 2001, Strik et al 2003). It can also lead to several health risk behaviours and side effects (Lin et al 2004, NCCN 2012), so it is of great importance that the mental health needs of people with long-term conditions are met.

Mental Health Needs

A number of studies have indicated that the mental health needs of people with long-term conditions are not always being met. One study reported approximately 430,000 people with diabetes and depression were not receiving optimum care, which is a significant risk factor for cardiovascular disease (Knapp et al 2011).

For people with long-term conditions, the evidence base demonstrates a convincing connection between physical long-term conditions and psychological distress, manifesting in mental health issues such as anxiety and depression. This has led to a review of the National Health Service (NHS) provision for long-term conditions (DOH 2012). In addition, NICE has carried out several systematic reviews on the efficacy of different psychological interventions for anxiety and depression, publishing multiple clinical guidelines (NICE 2004a, 2004b, 2005a, 2005b, 2006, 2009a, 2009b, 2011). There is therefore a growing research interest in the application of psychological approaches as a treatment intervention for people with long-term conditions (Lambert et al 2017, Tsai 2004).

INTRODUCTION TO EVIDENCE

Various studies (Acros-Carmona et al 2011, Dayapoglu & Tan 2012, Demiralp et al 2010) have researched the efficacy of psychological interventions in long-term conditions, such as diabetes (Perfect & Elkins 2010) and multiple sclerosis (Dayapoglu & Tan 2012). Chapter 29 presents supporting evidence in the use of different relaxation techniques in several other long-term conditions; however, key research is discussed here.

Many studies have suggested that mindfulness-based stress reduction (MBSR) (see Chapter 23) may help people to manage a variety of long-term conditions, including chronic pain (Grossman et al 2004). Reibel and colleagues' (2001) heterogeneous study demonstrated that MBSR improved health-related quality of life, pain, anxiety and social functioning for people with long-term conditions. In another study, MBSR had positive effects on the immune profile of people living with cancer (Carlson et al 2003). Furthermore, a systematic review and meta-analysis investigated the outcomes of MBSR for people with long-term mental health conditions, which included psychological distress, anxiety and depression. Eight randomized controlled trials were analyzed. The researchers concluded that MBSR only had a minimal effect on psychological distress, anxiety and depression and suggested that integrating MBSR with behavioural therapy may increase the efficacy of this intervention (Bohlmeijer et al 2010). Another study, however, reported MBSR as being successful in reducing psychological distress in people with type 2 diabetes (Hartmann et al 2012). A number of studies have also evaluated mindfulness in relation to the management of cancer-related depression and stress (Mehta et al 2019) (see Chapter 23), and a study which combined progressive relaxation technique and guided imagery over a 6-week period demonstrated an improvement in chronic non-malignant pain (Chen & Francis 2010).

Rehabilitation programmes, which include group-based exercise for people with long-term conditions, have reported positive outcomes (Balducci et al 2010, Belchamber 2009, Nicholas et al 2013, Taylor et al 2009). A rehabilitation programme which supported self-management through health coaching included MBSR and supervised group exercise. Seventeen people with long-term conditions completed the rehabilitation programme. Findings from this study indicated improved self-reporting and performance outcomes; however, a randomized controlled trial would be needed to establish the effectiveness of this rehabilitation programme (Dufour et al 2014).

Numerous research trials support the hypothesis that relaxation techniques reduce anxiety and depression and improve quality of life in people with long-term conditions (Clarke & Currie 2009, Crepaz et al 2008, Fekete et al 2007, Galway et al 2012, Osborn et al 2006). Relaxation techniques have also been shown to increase self-efficacy (Diezeman 2011), reduce psychological distress (Yu et al 2007), increase positive attitudes (Oldenbury et al 1985) and improve pain management (Kwekkeboom et al 2010). Furthermore, interventions such as cognitive–behavioural therapy (CBT) have been shown to improve adherence to treatment, enabling psychosocial adjustment and improving coping strategies and overall quality of life for people with long-term conditions (Spurgeon et al 2005, Thompson et al 2011). However, there is a lack of research focusing on the effect of Benson's relaxation technique in long-term conditions, such as end-stage renal disease (Rambod et al 2013).

It has been evidenced that through releasing muscle tension and promoting positive thinking, relaxation techniques can help people with long-term conditions cope with stressful situations (Yu et al 2010). Therefore with an increased demand on both prevention and management of multiple conditions, rather than single conditions (Barnett et al 2012), national and international bodies have recommended psychological approaches such as relaxation techniques to be an integral part of care for people with long-term conditions (NCCINBC 2003, NICE 2004c). However, understanding the theory behind these psychological interventions is a prerequisite to the application of relaxation techniques for long-term conditions.

THEORIES BEHIND RELAXATION TECHNIQUES FOR LONG-TERM CONDITIONS

Although there are many variations in the theoretical background, content and mode of delivery of relaxation techniques, they fundamentally focus on the behavioural and psychological processes that predict maladjustment by providing coping strategies (Fekete et al 2007). Theories behind the effects of various relaxation techniques have been discussed throughout the chapters of this book, but there are also some theories specific to the effects of relaxation techniques for long-term conditions.

In people with long-term conditions, it is thought that relaxation techniques enable muscular stabilization and a distraction from pain (Diezemann 2011), whereas improvement in quality of life is thought to be related to spiritual or existential issues. For example, mindfulness-based relaxation techniques may significantly improve existential well-being (Foley et al 2010, Pagnini et al 2011).

The stress response (see Chapter 1) is known to activate chronically raised and sustained release of catecholamines and glucocorticoids (Powell & Sheridan 2013). This impairment in the long-term has an immunosuppressive effect, influencing the progression of the condition and tumour growth (Volden & Conzen 2013). Initial evidence, however, proposes that these neuroendocrine stress-sensitive systems are receptive to relaxation techniques in both early and advanced stages of cancer (Black et al 2017, Carlson et al 2013, Witek-Janusek et al 2008).

The theories behind relaxation techniques and the supporting evidence have been noted by key stakeholders and guidelines developed accordingly. This has enabled implementation of psychological interventions such as relaxation techniques to be integrated into practice. An example of this is the application and integration through rehabilitation programmes.

REHABILITATION PROGRAMMES

The King's Fund for Mental Health (2012) states that mental health interventions can be adapted and integrated within rehabilitation programmes designed to help people with long-term conditions manage their symptoms. A growing body of evidence indicates that this integrated way of working offers the best way of improving outcomes (Yohannes et al 2010).

A national programme, Improving Access to Psychological Training (IAPT), was created after the publication of 'Our Health, Our Care, Our Say' (DOH 2006). The programme aimed to widen access to evidence-based psychological interventions for the management of anxiety and depression within the NHS (Clark 2011). This programme was one of 15 long-term conditions pathfinder sites set up by the Department of Health to evaluate its feasibility. Between 2008 and 2014, approximately 6000 new psychological therapists were trained. This was to ensure services had enough therapists to provide treatment for a target of 15% of people with anxiety or depression in the community (Clark 2011).

After the successful roll out of IAPT, a guidance document, 'Commissioning Talking Therapies for 2011/12' (DOH 2011), was published by the Department of Health, highlighting the cost effectiveness and value of extending the IAPT programme to long-term conditions such as cardiovascular disease, diabetes and COPD. The NICE guidelines and IAPT provide compelling evidence in support of psychological interventions for anxiety and depression, one of which is CBT (see Chapter 16). CBT has since been used to successfully manage anxiety and depression as part of cardiac rehabilitation programmes (Child et al 2010, Clark 2011, Elliot et al 2014).

Rehabilitation programmes often have a physical activity component, which is another important element for successfully managing long-term conditions.

Physical Activity

Physical activity is a risk factor which can be modified through exercise for a number of long-term conditions such as COPD, cardiovascular disease, diabetes, cancer, osteoarthritis, rheumatoid arthritis and depression, to name but a few (Warburton et al 2006). For example, a sedentary lifestyle has been linked to increased insulin resistance, proinflammatory cytokines and adiposity (Yates et al 2010). Therefore, as discussed in Chapter 15, physical activity has many benefits, one of which is improved physical function, quality of life and cardiovascular status (Conn et al 2009), as well as primary and secondary prevention of long-term conditions (Warburton et al 2006).

The International Classification of Functioning, Disability and Health (ICF) is an established framework of health that can support, facilitate and guide clinical decision making in a number of populations, including those with long-term conditions (Hunt et al 2008, Stucki et al 2008). Application of the ICF in practice can increase accuracy in categorizing disability with regard to predicting secondary complications and death (Dale et al 2012). Functional data in relation to the ICF is described in Chapter 28, Measurement, under Assessment Tools. Furthermore, to improve understanding of long-term conditions and function, it has been suggested that the ICF is used alongside the International Classification of Diseases (ICD) (Escorpizo et al 2013). These frameworks should therefore be used by health care professionals to develop individually tailored rehabilitation programmes. Examples include cardiac and pulmonary rehabilitation for people with long-term conditions.

CARDIAC REHABILITATION

Cardiac rehabilitation programmes contain the following therapeutic components: physical activity, exercise, education, diet, weight management, medical management and psychological support. The cardiac rehabilitation care pathway in the UK consists of six stages (DOH 2010). A growing body of evidence suggests that adding enhanced psychological support to the rehabilitation care pathway improves overall outcomes.

Evidence from research (see Chapter 29) indicates that applying psychological interventions into practice for people with cardiovascular disease can enhance their quality of life by improving premorbid levels of psychosocial functioning. Research demonstrates that cardiac rehabilitation without the addition of this psychological care fails to meet the mental health needs of this group of people (Dusseldorp et al 1999, Linden et al 1996).

Where anxiety and depression have been identified as a mental health need for people with cardiovascular disease, key national guidelines such as NICE (2013) recommend following guidelines related to anxiety and depression (NICE 2009a, 2009b, 2011; DOH 2011). These recommendations are increasingly being incorporated into cardiac rehabilitation in two ways: (1) screening for anxiety and depression; (2) the inclusion of psychological interventions. An example of such a programme is Heart2Heart. Heart2Heart combined cardiac rehabilitation with psychological interventions for people with cardiovascular disease. This programme built upon the IAPT stepped-care approach (Clark 2011) and aimed to provide the basic care required to meet the mental health care needs of people with cardiovascular disease. CBT was used and a high level of patient satisfaction reported, as well as significant improvements in anxiety, depression and quality of life (Elliot et al 2014).

Pulmonary Rehabilitation

Pulmonary rehabilitation programmes vary in their delivery and may include a number of different therapeutic components, such as education for the person and their family, exercise reconditioning, breathing techniques, relaxation techniques, psychosocial therapy, vocational rehabilitation, treatment of chest infections and medicine management including oxygen therapy.

A growing body of evidence suggests that relaxation techniques, physical activity and exercise reconditioning as part of the pulmonary rehabilitation programme can help to reduce various mental health issues associated with COPD. For example, research indicates that anxiety and depression may be reduced through participation in pulmonary rehabilitation (Gordon et al 2019), with the evidence base demonstrating the benefits of physical exercise on depression (Bolton et al 2013, Coventry et al 2013). Behavioural lifestyle physical activity has also been shown to have a positive effect for people with moderate-to-severe COPD (Coultas et al 2018). Therefore adding a psy-

chological component to pulmonary rehabilitation has been shown to improve completion rates and reduce readmissions for people with COPD (Abell et al 2008). In addition, the National Institute for Health Research (NIHR) recently conducted a systematic review and meta-analysis of pulmonary rehabilitation, concluding that it modestly improves psychological symptoms, such as anxiety and depression, in people with COPD (NIHR 2019). This research supports the recommendations from NICE (2019) guidelines, advising personalized pulmonary rehabilitation programmes. However, this requires health care professionals to be trained in psychological interventions.

Health Care Professional Training Programmes

The Department of Health (DOH 2012) proposed training programmes for health care professionals to deliver psychological interventions such as CBT.

Health care professionals that have been trained to provide personalized CBT as part of pulmonary rehabilitation programmes reported enhanced outcomes for people with long-term conditions and include improved self-management, decreased anxiety, reduced exacerbations and, consequentially, reduced hospital admissions (NICE 2009b). However, with all interventions health care professionals need to be aware of key precautions.

PRECAUTIONS

Evidence suggests that the majority of people will benefit from the relaxation response; however, a minority of people may have undesirable or troublesome outcomes from relaxation techniques. For example, when people are very distressed relaxation training may induce a contradictory outcome, such as increased agitation if the person is unable to manage the distress stimulation (Pagnini et al 2013). Caution should therefore be taken when offering relaxation training to people with long-term conditions who are extremely distressed after diagnosis.

There are numerous types of relaxation techniques available, as discussed throughout this book, and extensive clinical skill may be needed to ensure people are given the most appropriate relaxation technique to manage their anxiety and depression. A combination of relaxation techniques may also be more beneficial (see Chapter 30) to the person rather than a single relaxation technique, which should be carefully considered.

KEY POINTS

1. In England there are approximately 15 million people with long-term conditions.
2. Long-term conditions are those which currently have no cure but are managed through medication and non-pharmacological approaches.
3. The psychological impact of the diagnosis of a long-term condition is complex as people often experience a wide range of psychological conditions, the most prevalent being anxiety and depression.
4. Where two or more long-term conditions coexist, people are seven times more likely to have depression.
5. Anxiety and depression have been classed as primary long-term conditions, and those identified with anxiety and depression have an increased likelihood of developing other long-term conditions, such as cardiovascular disease and diabetes.
6. Numerous research trials support the hypothesis that relaxation techniques reduce anxiety and depression and improve quality of life in people with long-term conditions.

Reflection

Describe your understanding of long-term conditions.

What changes will you make to your personal life and practice?

What is the main learning point you will take away from this chapter?

What is your future action plan in terms of using relaxation techniques for long-term conditions?

CASE STUDY LEARNING OPPORTUNITY

The key points and reflection provide background and knowledge required in relation to the case study, Rachel, to help deepen understanding of how relaxation techniques can help reduce anxiety and depression in long-term conditions.

CASE STUDY

Pulmonary Rehabilitation: Pulmonary Rehabilitation Outcomes for Rachel

Rachel is in her 50s and has chronic obstructive pulmonary disease (COPD). She struggles to breathe most of the time. Breathlessness is Rachel's most debilitating symptom, reducing her mobility and physical activity and producing a vicious cycle of breathlessness and ever decreasing activity. As a consequence Rachel's level of fitness is rapidly deteriorating. Rachel's fear of breathlessness and her inability to carry out normal activities of daily living (ADLs) is reducing her overall well-being and quality of life. To add to this, Rachel, who is an ex-smoker, feels guilty because she believes she has brought this condition upon herself and her family and she is to blame.

Rachel has made sporadic visits to the local doctor, followed sometimes by changes in her inhalers and medication, with the addition of steroids and antibiotics for exacerbations. However, this has done little to improve Rachel's symptoms and function. As a consequence, Rachel is starting to get anxious and have panic attacks, which are affecting her confidence to go out, leading to social isolation, depression and a feeling of being out of control. This has led to a number of hospital admissions.

At the last hospital admission it was decided that Rachel required a team approach with rehabilitation principles to successfully manage her long-term condition. Therefore, on discharge, Rachel was referred to pulmonary rehabilitation. After an in-depth phys-iotherapy assessment Rachel attended 20-minute exercise sessions on a weekly basis over a 12-week pe-riod. This was supported with a home-based exercise plan to achieve maximum benefit. Rachel also received psychosocial support, which included pro-gressive muscular relaxation and CBT. From week 6 Rachel started to feel the benefits of the programme; her panic attacks had reduced and her overall fitness levels increased, she was managing more of her ADLs and she felt less anxious and depressed and more in control. By week 12 Rachel was able to go out and socialize with confidence, improving her overall well-being and quality of life.

ACTIVITY

For the case study:

1. List key aspects used in pulmonary rehabilitation.
2. Write down the impact pulmonary rehabilita-tion is having from a psychological perspective.
3. Write down the impact pulmonary rehabilita-tion is having from a physical perspective.
4. Write down the impact pulmonary rehabilita-tion is having from an emotional perspective.
5. Consider the outcomes quality of life and over-all well-being for Rachel.

Chapter 26 will focus on supportive, palliative and end-of-life care, building on the knowledge gained in this chapter on long-term conditions.

REFERENCES

Abell, F., Potter, C., Purcell, S., et al. (2008). The effect of inclusion of a clinical psychologist in pulmonary rehabilitation on comple-tion rates and hospital resource utilisation (hospital admissions and bed days) in chronic obstructive pulmonary disease (COPD). *Thorax, 63*(VII), A74–A160.

Acros-Carmona, I. M., Castro-Sanchez, A. M., Mataran-Penarrocha, G. A., Gutierrez-Rubio, A. B., Ramos-Gonzalez, E., & Moreno-Lorenzo, C. (2011). Effects of aerobic exercise program and relax-ation techniques on anxiety, quality of sleep, depression and qual-ity of life in patients with fibromyalgia: A randomized controlled trial. *Medicina Clinica, 137*(9), 398–401.

Ali, S., Stone, M. A., Peters, J. L., Davies, M. J., & Khunti, K. (2006). The prevalence of co-morbid depression in adults with type 2 dia-betes: A systematic review and meta-analysis. *Diabetes Medicine, 23*, 1165–1173.

Bakewell, A. B., Higgins, R. M., & Edmunds, M. E. (2002). Quality of life in peritoneal dialysis patients: decline over time and associa-tion with clinical outcomes. *Kidney International, 61*(1), 239–248.

Balducci, S., Zanuso, S., Nicolucci, A., et al. (2010). Effect of an in-tensive exercise intervention strategy on modifiable cardiovascu-lar risk factors in subjects with type 2 diabetes mellitus. *Archives of Internal Medicine, 170*, 1794–1803.

Barnett, K., Mercer, S. W., Norbury, M., Watt, G., Wyke, S., & Guth-rie, B. (2012). Epidemiology of multimorbidity and implications for health care, research, and medical education: A cross-sectional study. *Lancet, 380*(9836), 37–43.

Belchamber, C. A. (2009). Participants' perceptions of groupwork in the management of cancer symptoms in older people. *Groupwork, 19*(2), 79–100.

Black, D. S., Peng, C., Sleight, A. G., Nguyen, N., Lenz, H. J., & Figueiredo, J. C. (2017). Mindfulness practice reduces cortisol blunting during chemotherapy: A randomized controlled study of colorectal cancer patients. *Cancer, 123*, 3088–3096.

Blake, C., Codd, M. B., Cassidy, A., & O'Meara, Y. M. (2000). Physi-cal function, employment and quality of life in end-stage renal disease. *Journal of Nephrology, 13*(2), 142–149.

Bohlmeijer, E., Prenger, R., Taal, E., & Cuijpers, P. (2010). The effects of mindfulness-based stress reduction therapy on mental health of adults with a chronic medical disease: A meta-analysis. *Journal of Psychosomatic Research, 68*, 539–544.

Bolton, C. E., Bevan-Smith, E. F., Blakey, J. D., et al. (2013). British Thoracic Society guidelines on pulmonary rehabilitation in adults. *Thorax, 68*(2), ii1–30.

Boulton, M., Boudioni, M., Mossman, J., Moynihan, C., Leydon, G., & Ramirez, A. (2001). 'Dividing the desolation': Client views on the benefits of a cancer counselling service. *Psychological Oncol-ogy, 10*, 124–126.

Carlson, L. E., Speca, M., Patel, K. D., & Goodey, E. (2003). Mind-fulness-based stress reduction in relation to quality of life, mood, symptoms of stress and immune parameters in breast and pros-tate cancer outpatient. *Psychosomatic Medicine, 65*, 571–581.

Carlson, L. E., Doll, R., Stephen, J., et al. (2013). Randomized con-trolled trial of mindfulness-based cancer recovery versus support-ive expressive group therapy for distressed survivors of breast can-cer (MINDSET). *Journal of Clinical Oncology, 31*(25), 3119–3687.

Chen, Y. L., & Francis, A. J. (2010). Relaxation and imagery for chronic, nonmalignant pain: Effects on pain symptoms, qual-ity of life, and mental health. *Pain Management Nursing, 11*(3), 159–168.

Child, A., Sanders, J., Sigel, P., & Hunter, M. S. (2010). Meeting the psychological needs of cardiac patients: an integrated stepped-care approach within a cardiac rehabilitation setting. *British Jour-nal of Cardiology, 17*(4), 175–179.

Cimpean, D., & Drake, R. E. (2011). Treating co-morbid medical conditions and anxiety/ depression. *Epidemiology and Psychiatric Sciences, 20*(2), 141–150.

Clarke, D. M., & Currie, K. C. (2009). Depression, anxiety and their relationship with chronic diseases: A review of the epidemiology, risk and treatment evidence. *Medical Journal of Australia, 190*, S54–60.

Clark, D. M. (2011). Implementing NICE guidelines for the psycho-logical treatment of depression and anxiety disorders: The IAPT experience. *International Review of Psychiatry, 23*(4), 318–327.

Coultas, D. B., Jackson, B. E., Russo, R., et al. (2018). Home-based physical activity coaching, physical activity and health care utilization in chronic obstructive pulmonary disease. Chronic obstructive pulmonary disease self-management activation research trial secondary outcomes. *Annals of the American Thoracic Society*, *15*(4), 470–478.

Coventry, P. A., Bower, P., Keyworth, C., et al. (2013). The effect of complex interventions on depression and anxiety in chronic obstructive pulmonary disease: Systematic review and meta-analysis. *PloS One*, *8*(4), e60532.

Crepaz, N., Passin, W. F., Herbst, J. H., et al. (2008). Meta-analysis of cognitive-behavioural interventions on HIV-positive person's mental health and immune functioning. *Health Psychol*, *27*, 4–14.

Dale, C., Preito-Merino, D., Kuper, H., et al. (2012). Modelling the association of disability according to the WHO International Classification of Functioning, Disability and Health (ICF) with mortality in the British Women's Heart and Health Study. *Journal of Epidemiology and Community Health*, *66*, 170–175.

Dayapoglue, N., & Tan, M. (2012). Evaluation of the effect of progressive relaxation exercises on fatigue and sleep quality in patients with multiple sclerosis. *Journal of Alternative and Complementary Medicine*, *18*(10), 983–987.

Demiralp, M., Oflax, F., & Komurucu, S. (2010). Effects of relaxation training on sleep quality and fatigue in patients with breast cancer undergoing adjuvant chemotherapy. *Journal of Clinical Nursing*, *19*(7–8), 1073–1083.

Department of Health (DOH). (2012). *Long-term conditions: Compendium of information* (3rd ed.). London: DOH.

Department of Health (DOH). (2006). Our health, our care, our say: A new direction for community services. Retrieved February 2020 from https://assets.publishing.service.gov.uk/government/uploads/system/uploads/attachment_data/file/272238/6737.pdf. [Accessed May 2020]

Department of Health, Strategic Commissioning Development Unit. Cardiac Rehabilitation Commissioning Pack. London: UK Department of Health 2010. Retrieved February 2020 from http://www.cardiacrehabilitation.org.uk/resources.htm#dhc. [Accessed May 2020].

Department of Health (DOH). (2011). Commissioning talking therapies for 2011/12. Retrieved February 2020 from https://www.iapt.nhs.uk.

Department of Health (DOH). (2012). *Long-term conditions: Compendium of information* (3rd ed.). London: DOH. Retrieved February 2020 from https://www.gov.uk/government/publications/long-term-conditions-compendium-of-information-third-edition. [Accessed May 2020]

Diezemann, A. (2011). Relaxation techniques for chronic pain. *Schmerz*, *25*(4), 445–453.

Dufour, S.P., Graham, S., Friesen, J., Rosenblat, M., Rous, C., Richardson, J. (2014). Physiotherapists supporting self-management through health coaching: A mixed methods program evaluation.

Dusseldorp, E., van Elderen, T., Maes, S., et al. (1999). A meta-analysis of psychoeducational programs for coronary heart disease patients. *Health Psychology*, *18*(5), 506–519.

Edelman, S., Lemon, J., & Kidman, A. (2005). Group cognitive behavioural therapy for breast cancer patients: A qualitative evaluation. *Psychology, Health & Medicine*, *10*, 139–144.

Elliot, M., Salt, H., Dent, J., Stafford, C., & Schiza, A. (2014). Heart-2Heart: An integrated approach to cardiac rehabilitation and CBT. *British Journal of Cardiac Nursing*, *9*(10), 501–507.

Engert, A., Haverkamp, H., Kobe, C., et al. (2012). Reduced-intensity chemotherapy and PET-guided radiotherapy in patients with advanced stage Hodgkin's lymphoma (HD15 trial): A randomised, open-label, phase 3 non-inferiority trial. *Lancet*, *379*(9828), 1791–1799.

Engert, A., Plutschow, A., Eich, H. T., et al. (2010). Reduced treatment intensity in patients with early-stage Hodgkin's lymphoma. *New England Journal of Medicine*, *363*(7), 640–652.

Escorpizo, R., Kostanjsek, N., Kennedy, C., Nicol, M. M., Stucki, G., & Ustun, T. B. (2013). Harmonizing WHO's International Classification of Diseases (ICD) and International Classification of Functioning, Disability and Health (ICF): Importance and methods to link disease and functioning. *BMC Public Health*, *13*, 742.

Fekete, E. M., Antoni, M. H., & Schneiderman, N. (2007). Psychosocial and behavioural interventions for chronic medical conditions. *Current Opinion in Psychiatry*, *20*, 152–157.

Finkelstein, F. O., & Finkelstein, S. H. (2000). Depression in chronic dialysis patients: Assessment and treatment. *Nephrology, Dialysis, Transplantation*, *15*(12), 1911–1913.

Foley, E., Baillie, A., Huxter, M., Price, M., & Sinclair, E. (2010). Mindfulness-based cognitive therapy for individuals whose lives have been affected by cancer: A randomized controlled trial. *Journal of Consulting and Clinical Psychology*, *78*(1), 72–79.

Frasure-Smith, N., Lespérance, F., Gravel, G., et al. (2000). Social support, depression and mortality during the first year after myocardial infarction. *Circulation*, *101*(16), 1919–1924.

Frazer, K., Callinan, J. E., Mchught, J., et al. (2016). Legislative smoking bans for reducing harms from secondhand smoke exposure, smoking prevalence and tobacco consumption. *Cochrane Database of Systematic Reviews*, *2*, CD005992.

Galway, K., Black, A., Cantwell, M., Cardwell, C. R., Mills, M., & Donnelly, M. (2012). Psychosocial interventions to improve quality of life and emotional well-being for recently diagnosed cancer patients. *Cochrane Database of Systematic Reviews*, *11*, CD007064.

Global Initiative for Chronic Obstructive Lung Disease. (2017). *Global strategy for the diagnosis, management and prevention of chronic obstructive pulmonary disease: 2017 report*. Retrieved February 2020 from https://goldcopd.org/gold-reports/. [Accessed May 2020].

Global Initiative for Chronic Obstructive Lung Disease. (2020). Global strategy for the diagnosis, management and prevention of chronic obstructive pulmonary disease: 2020 report. Retrieved February 2020 from https://goldcopd.org/wp-content/uploads/2019/12/GOLD-2020-FINAL-ver1.2-03Dec19_WMV.pdf. [Accessed May 2020]

Gordon, C. S., Waller, J. W., Cook, R. M., Cavalera, S. L., Lim, W. T., & Osadnik, C. R. (2019). Effect of pulmonary rehabilitation on symptoms of anxiety and depression in COPD: A systematic review and meta-analysis. *Chest*, *156*(1), 80–91.

Grossman, P., Niemann, L., Schmidt, S., & Walach, H. (2004). Mindfulness-based stress reduction and health benefits. A meta-analysis. *Journal of Psychosomatic Research*, *57*, 35–43.

Gunathilaka, H. J., Vitharana, P., Udayanga, L., & Gunathilaka, N. (2019). Assessment of Anxiety, depression, stress and associated psychological morbidities among patients receiving Ayurvedic treatment for different health issues: First study from Sri Lanka. *BioMed Research International, 2019,* 2940836.

Hartmann, M., Kopf, S., Kircher, C., et al. (2012). Sustained effects of a mindfulness-based stress reduction intervention in type 2 diabetic patients. *Diabetes Care, 35,* 945–947.

Hunt, M. A., Birmingham, T. B., Skarakis-Doyle, E., & Vandervoort, A. A. (2008). Towards a biopsychosocial framework for osteoarthritis of the knee. *Disability and Rehabilitation, 30,* 54–61.

The King's Fund (2012). Long Term Conditions and Mental Health: the cost of co-morbidities. Retrieved May 2020 from: https://www.kingsfund.org.uk/publications/long-term-conditions-and-mental-health. [Accessed May 2020].

Kinley, D. J., Lowry, H., Katz, C., Jacobi, F., Jassal, D. S., & Sareen, J. (2015). Depression and anxiety disorders and the link to physician diagnosed cardiac disease and metabolic risk factors. *General Hospital Psychiatry, 37,* 288–293.

Kimmel, P., & Levy, N. B. (2004). Psychology and rehabilitation. In J. T. Daugirdas, P. G. Blake, & T. S. Ing (Eds.), *Handbook of dialysis* (3rd ed., pp. 413–419). Philadelphia: Lippincott Williams & Wilkins.

Knapp, M., McDaid, D., & Parsonage, M. (2011). *Mental health promotion and prevention: The economic case.* London: Personal Social Services Research Unit, London School of Economics and Political Science.

Kwekkeboom, K. I., Cherwin, C. H., Lee, J. W., & Wanta, B. (2010). Mind-body treatments for pain-fatigue-sleep disturbance symptom cluster in persons with cancer. *Journal of Pain and Symptom Management, 39*(1), 126–138.

Lambert, S. D., Beatty, L., McElduff, P., et al. (2017). A systematic review and meta-analysis of written self-administered psychosocial interventions among adults with a physical illness. *Patient Education and Counseling, 100,* 2200–2217.

Lane, D., Carroll, D., Ring, C., et al. (2001). Mortality and quality of life 12 months after myocardial infarction: Effects of depression and anxiety. *Psychosomatic Medicine, 63*(2), 221–230.

Lane, D., Carroll, D., Ring, C., et al. (2002). The prevalence and persistence of depression and anxiety following myocardial infarction. *British Journal of Health Psychology, 7*(Pt 1), 11–21.

Levy, N. B. (2000). Psychiatric considerations in the primary medical care of the patient with renal failure. *Advances in Renal Replacement Therapy, 7*(3), 231–238.

Lin, E. H., Katon, W., Von Korff, M., et al. (2004). Relationship of depression and diabetes self-care, medication adherence and preventive care. *Diabetes Care, 27,* 2154–2160.

Linden, W., Stossel, C., & Maurice, J. (1996). Psychosocial interventions for patients with coronary artery disease: A meta-analysis. *Archives of Internal Medicine, 156*(7), 745–752.

Lipson, D. A., Barnhart, F., Berealey, N., et al. (2018). Once-daily single-inhaler triple versus dual therapy in patients with COPD. *New England Journal of Medicine, 378*(18), 1671–1680.

Martz, E., & Livneh, H. (2007). *Coping with chronic illness and disability: Theoretical, empirical and clinical aspects.* New York: Springer Science + Business.

Macmillan Cancer Support (MCS). (2015). *The burden of cancer and other long-term conditions.* London: MCS.

Mayer, E. A. (2000). The neurobiology of stress and gastrointestinal disease. *Gut, 47,* 861–869.

McLeod, J. (2013). Process and outcome in pluralistic transactional analysis counselling for long-term health conditions: A case series. *Counselling and Psychotherapy Research, 13*(1), 32–43.

Mehnert, A., Vehling, S., Hocker, A., et al. (2011). Demoralisation and depression in patients with advanced cancer: validation of the German version of the demoralisation scale. *Journal of Pain Symptom Management, 42,* 768–776.

Mehta, R., Sharma, K., Potters, L., Wernicke, A. G., & Parashar, B. (2019). Evidence for the role of mindfulness in cancer: Benefits and techniques. *Cureus, 11*(5), e4629.

Misono, S., Weiss, N. S., Fann, J. R., Redman, M., & Yueh, B. (2008). Incidence of suicide in persons with cancer. *Journal of Clinical Oncology, 26,* 4731–4738.

Moussavi, S., Chatterji, S., Verdes, E., Tandon, A., Patel, V., & Ustun, B. (2007). Depression, chronic diseases and decrements in health: Results from the World Health surveys. *Lancet, 370,* 851–858.

National Cancer Control Initiative, National Breast Cancer Centre (NCCINBC). (2003). *Clinical practice guidelines for the psychosocial care of adults with cancer.* Camperdown, NSW, Australia: National Breast Cancer Centre.

National Comprehensive Cancer Network (NCCN). (2012). *Distress management clinical practice guidelines. Plymouth Meeting.* PA: NCCN.

National Institute for Health and Care Excellence (NICE). (2004a). *Anxiety: Management of anxiety (panic disorder, with and without agoraphobia, and generalised anxiety disorder) in adults in primary, secondary and community care. Clinical Guideline 22.* London: NICE. Retrieved February 2020 from https://www.nice.org.uk/guidance/cg22/documents/cg22-anxiety-nice-guideline-marked-up-with-proposed-amendments2. [Accessed May 2020]

National Institute for Health and Care Excellence (NICE). (2004b). *Depression: Management of depression in primary and secondary care. Clinical Guideline 23.* London: NICE. Retrieved February 2020 from https://www.nice.org.uk/guidance/cg23. [Accessed May 2020]

National Institute for Health and Care Excellence (NICE). (2004c). *Guidance on cancer services: Improving supportive and palliative care for adults with cancer.* London: NICE.

National Institute for Health and Care Excellence (NICE). (2005a). *Obsessive-compulsive disorder: Core interventions in the treatment of obsessive-compulsive disorder and body dysmorphic disorder. Clinical Guideline 31.* London: NICE. Retrieved February 2020 from https://www.nice.org.uk/guidance/cg31/evidence/cg31-obsessivecompulsive-disorder-full-guideline2. [Accessed May 2020]

National Institute for Health and Care Excellence (NICE). (2005b). *Post-traumatic stress disorder (PTSD): The management of PTSD in adults and children in primary and secondary care. Clinical Guideline 26.* London: NICE. Retrieved February 2020 from https://www.nice.org.uk/guidance/cg26. [Accessed May 2020]

National Institute for Health and Care Excellence (NICE). (2006). *Computerized cognitive behaviour therapy for depression and anxiety. Technology Appraisal 97.* London: NICE. Retrieved February 2020 from https://www.nice.org.uk/guidance/ta97. [Accessed May 2020]

National Institute for Health and Care Excellence (NICE). (2009a). *Depression in adults: The treatment and management of depression in adults.* NICE Clinical Guideline 90. Retrieved February 2020 from https://www.nice.org.uk/guidance/cg90.

National Institute for Health and Care Excellence (NICE). (2009b). *Depression in adults with a chronic physical health problem: Treatment and management.* CG91 Full Guideline. Retrieved February 2020 from https://www.nice.org.uk/guidance/CG91/chapter/introduction. [Accessed May 2020]

National Institute for Health and Care Excellence (NICE). (2011). *Common mental health disorders: Identification and pathways to care.* NICE Clinical Guideline 123. Retrieved February 2020 from https://www.nice.org.uk/guidance/cg123. [Accessed May 2020]

National Institute for Health and Care Excellence (NICE). (2013). *MI – secondary prevention: Secondary prevention in primary and secondary care for patients following a myocardial infarction.* NICE Clinical Guideline 172. Retrieved February 2020 from https://www.nice.org.uk/guidance/cg172. [Accessed May 2020]

National Institute for Health and Care Excellence (NICE). (2019). *Managing COPD pathway.* London: NICE. Retrieved February 2020 from https://pathways.nice.org.uk/pathways/chronic-obstructive-pulmonary-disease#path=view%3A/pathways/chronic-obstructive-pulmonary-disease/managing-copd.xml&content=view-index. [Accessed May 2020]

National Institute for Health Research (NIHR) Signal. (2019). *Pulmonary rehabilitation may modestly improve anxiety and depression in adults with chronic obstructive pulmonary disease.* Retrieved February 2020 from https://discover.dc.nihr.ac.uk/content/signal-000794/copd-rehabilitation-may-improve-anxiety-and-depression. [Accessed May 2020]

Naylor, C., Parsonage, M., McDaid, D., Knapp, M., Fossey, M., & Galea, A. (2012). *Long-term conditions and mental health: The cost of co-morbidities.* London: The King's Fund and Centre for Mental Health.

Nicholas, M. K., Asghari, A., Blyth, F. M., et al. (2013). Self-management intervention for chronic pain in older adults: A randomized controlled trial. *Pain, 154,* 824–835.

Oldenbury, B., Perkins, R. J., & Andrews, G. (1985). Controlled trial of psychological intervention in myocardial infarction. *Journal of Consulting and Clinical Psychology, 53*(6), 852–859.

Osborn, R. I., Demncada, A. C., & Feuerstein, M. (2006). Psychosocial interventions for depression, anxiety and quality of life in cancer survivors: Meta-analyses. *International Journal of Psychiatry in Medicine, 36,* 13–34.

Pagnini, F., Lunetta, C., Rossi, G., et al. (2011). Existential well-being and spirituality of individuals with amyotrophic lateral sclerosis is related to psychological well-being of their caregivers. *Amyotrophic Lateral Sclerosis, 12*(2), 105–108.

Pagnini, F., Manzoni, G. M., Castelnuovo, G., & Molinari, E. (2013). A brief literature review about relaxation therapy and anxiety. *Body, Movement and Dance in Psychotherapy: An International Journal of Theory, Research and Practice, 8*(2), 71–81.

Perfect, M. M., & Elkins, G. R. (2010). Cognitive-behavioural therapy and hypnotic relaxation to treat sleep problems in an adolescent with diabetes. *Journal of Clinical Psychology, 66*(11), 1205–1215.

Pinnock, H., Kendall, M., Murray, S. A., et al. (2011). Living and dying with severe chronic obstructive pulmonary disease: Multi-perspective longitudinal qualitative study. *BMJ, 342,* d142.

Prince, M., Patel, V., Saxena, S., et al. (2007). No health without mental health. *Lancet, 370*(9590), 859–877.

Rambod, M., Pourali-Mohammadi, N., Pasyar, N., Raffi, F., & Sharif, F. (2013). The effect of Benson's relaxation technique on the quality of sleep of Iranian hemodialysis patients: A randomized trial. *Complementary Therapies in Medicine, 21,* 577–584.

Reibel, D. K., Greeson, J. M., Brainard, G. C., & Rosenzweig, S. (2001). Mindfulness-based stress reduction and health-related quality of life in a heterogeneous patient population. *General Hospital Psychiatry, 23,* 183–192.

Sarafino, E. P. (2006). *Health psychology: Biopsychosocial interactions* (5th ed.). New York: Wiley.

Spurgeon, P., Hicks, C., Barwell, F., Walton, I., & Spurgeon, T. (2005). Counselling in primary care: A study of the psychological impact and cost benefits for four chronic conditions. *European Journal of Psychotherapy and Counselling, 7*(4), 269–290.

Strik, J. J., Denollet, J., Lousberg, R., & Honig, A. (2003). Comparing symptoms of depression and anxiety as predictors of cardiac events and increased health care consumption after myocardial infarction. *Journal of the American College of Cardiology, 42*(10), 1801–1807.

Stucki, A., Cieza, A., Michel, A., et al. (2008,). Developing ICF core sets for persons with sleep disorders based on the International Classification of Functioning, Disability and Health. *Sleep Medicine, 9,* 191–198.

Taylor, D., Fletcher, J., & Tiarks, J. (2009). Impact of physical therapist-directed exercise counselling with fitness centre based exercise training on muscular strength and exercise capacity in people with type 2 diabetes: A randomized clinical trial. *Physical Therapy, 89,* 884–892.

Thombs, B. D., Bass, E. B., Ford, D. E., et al. (2006). Prevalence of depression in survivors of acute myocardial infarction. *Journal of General Internal Medicine, 21*(1), 30–38.

Thompson, R. D., Delaney, P., Flores, I., & Szigethy, E. (2011). Cognitive-behavioural therapy for children with comorbid physical illness. *Child and Adolescent Psychiatric Clinics of North America, 20*(2), 329–348.

Tsai, S. L. (2004). Audio-visual relaxation training for anxiety, sleep and relaxation among Chinese adults with cardiac disease. *Research in Nursing & Health, 27*(6), 458–468.

Uitterhoeve, R. J., Vernooy, M., Litjens, M., et al. (2004). Psychosocial interventions for patients with advanced cancer – a systematic review of the literature. *British Journal of Cancer, 91,* 1050–1062.

Walker, J., Holm Hansen, C., Martin, P., et al. (2013). Prevalence of depression in adults with cancer: A systematic review. *Annals of Oncology, 24,* 895–900.

Warburton, D. E., Nicol, C. W., & Bredin, S. S. (2006). Health benefits of physical activity: The evidence. *Canadian Medical Association Journal, 174,* 801–809.

Witek-Janusek, L., Albuquerque, K., Chroniak, K. R., Chroniak, C., Durazo, R., & Mathews, H. L. (2008). Effect of Mindfulness based stress reduction on immune function, quality of life and coping in women with newly diagnosed with early stage breast cancer. *Brain, Behavior, and Immunity, 22*(6), 969–981.

Yates, T., Davies, M. J., Gray, L. J., et al. (2010). Levels of physical activity and relationship with markers of diabetes and cardiovascular disease risk in 5474 white European and South Asian adults screened for type 2 diabetes. *Preventative Medicine*, *51*, 290–294.

Yohannes, A. M., Willgoss, T. G., Baldwin, R. C., & Connolly, M. J. (2010). Depression and anxiety in chronic heart failure and chronic obstructive pulmonary disease: Prevalence, relevance, clinical implications and management principles. *International Journal of Geriatric Psychiatry*, *25*(12), 1209–1221.

Yu, D., Lee, D. T., & Woo, J. (2007). Effects of relaxation therapy on psychologic distress and symptom status in older Chines patients with heart failure. *Journal of Psychosomatic Research*, *62*(4), 427–437.

Yu, D. S., Lee, D. T., & Woo, J. (2010). Improving health-related quality of life of patients with chronic heart failure: effects of relaxation therapy. *Journal of Advanced Nursing*, *66*(2), 392–403.

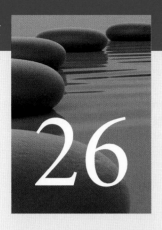

26

PALLIATIVE, SUPPORTIVE AND END OF LIFE CARE

DR CAROLINE BELCHAMBER

CHAPTER CONTENTS

LEARNING OBJECTIVES

The aim of this chapter is to provide a practical guide to palliative, supportive and end-of-life care.

By the end of this chapter you will be able to:

1. Describe palliative, supportive and end-of-life care.

2. Recognize how spiritual and psychological distress impacts on the person's overall well-being.

3. List key triggers and outcomes to family caregivers' and health care professionals' stress.

4. Understand the evidence base and theories behind relaxation techniques in palliative, supportive and end-of-life care.

5. Apply relaxation techniques within a palliative, supportive and end-of-life rehabilitative framework.

The chapter will conclude with key points and time for reflection, providing learning opportunities through a case study.

INTRODUCTION TO PALLIATIVE, SUPPORTIVE AND END-OF-LIFE CARE

Palliative, supportive and end-of-life care are key elements in the management of people with long-term conditions. As our life expectancy increases, more and more people with long-term conditions will be referred to these services, with palliative and supportive approaches being essential elements of care, culminating in end-of-life care.

Palliative Care

'Palliative care' is an umbrella term that encompasses different approaches to symptom control and management. It begins at diagnosis and is integral to the person's care and well-being and a valuable part of the person's therapy and treatment (Belchamber 2010). Palliative care can therefore be the main goal of care, or it may be delivered in tandem with curative treatments.

303

The aim of palliative care is to prevent and ease anguish, distress and pain from a physical, psychological, spiritual and social perspective (Rabow & Knish 2015). It also provides support to enable the best quality of life possible for people with long-term conditions and their families, irrespective of the current phase of their condition or requirement for other treatments (Pan et al 2000, WHO 2020). This is delivered in the form of supportive care, which is fundamental in managing symptoms and disabilities.

Supportive Care

Supportive care endeavours to maximize a person's function after disabilities that have arisen as a consequence of a long-term condition or its treatment. The multidisciplinary team (MDT) plays a key role in the supportive care of people living with palliative care needs. Interventions such as rehabilitative approaches, non-pharmacological approaches, psychological support and relaxation techniques provide a supportive care framework. However, for these interventions to be effective, they need to be delivered in a co-ordinated MDT approach so that the person's quality of life is enhanced until the end of life (Belchamber 2016). Supportive care therefore provides a feeling of support and ability to cope for both people with terminal illness and their family and caregivers, providing a robust foundation for end-of-life care.

End-of-Life Care

End-of-life care and bereavement are seen as the mainstay of hospice care provision; however, over the last decade this care has extended dramatically to encompass palliative and supportive care (Gomes & Higginson 2008). Equally, palliative, supportive and end-of-life care is now being delivered across a number of other settings, such as nursing care homes, to manage the increasing demand of an aging population. There are approximately 200,000 people with long-term conditions in the United Kingdom who are supported by hospice care (Hospice UK 2016), and this is expected to rise by 25% to 47% by 2040 (Etkind et al 2017). In addition, there are roughly 450,000 people in the UK who may well benefit from expert end-of-life care (Murtagh et al 2014). Therefore the demand on hospice care will rise significantly within the next two decades (Bone et al 2018) as people survive and live

longer with complex conditions (see Chapter 25). This shift in care and advances in treatment has seen the development of a palliative rehabilitative approach for people with long-term conditions to manage complex conditions and symptoms within a biopsychosocial-spiritual model (Belchamber 2004, 2009, 2010, 2016; Belchamber & Ellis-Hill 2013).

SYMPTOMS

People diagnosed with a terminal illness can experience a number or symptoms caused by the condition itself or the treatment. Of these, three types of suffering have been identified (Dezutter et al 2015, Frankl 2006, Saunders, 1964):

1. Spiritual – lack of a meaningful life, moral dilemmas
2. Psychological – emotional hardship, psychological disorders
3. Physical – pain, somatic diseases

Spirituality is a key dimension of quality of life; hence spiritual well-being is a fundamental component of palliative, supportive and end-of-life care and a key factor of high-quality, comprehensive care (Ferrell et al 2007, NCHPC 2018, Puchalski et al 2009). Spiritual well-being has been associated with symptoms such as anxiety, depression and pain (Bekelman et al 2010, Kandasamy et al 2011, Rawdin et al 2013); therefore, if palliative care needs are not adequately addressed, spiritual distress (e.g., guilt or enduring meaninglessness) and psychological distress (e.g., anxiety and depression) can lead to physical suffering and uncontrolled pain (Puchalski et al 2009).

SPIRITUAL DISTRESS

Spiritual distress has been identified in people with long-term conditions, and with a diagnosis of a terminal illness the person may face deep existential challenges, including issues of identity, meaning and control (Alcorn et al 2010, Rego & Nunes 2019, Sulmasy 2006, Winkelman et al 2011).

Finding meaning in illness is an element of spiritual well-being that promotes personal growth and may increase the likelihood of positive outcomes (Belchamber & Ellis-Hill 2013, Moreno & Stanton 2013). For example, existential well-being has been associated with survival (O'Mahony et al 2010) and spiritual care, with increased quality of life in the near-death period (Balboni et al 2010). In addition, early observations assessing distress in people with terminal illness using the Patient Dignity Inventory found an inverse relationship between 'sense of meaning' and 'intensity of distress' (Chochinov et al 2009, Thompson & Chochinov 2010).

It has been documented that people who are able to hold on to their sense of meaning are able to maintain their psychological and physical resilience (Frankl 2006). This theory is supported by longitudinal research demonstrating that people with enhanced levels of meaning in their lives are less at risk for pain (Dezutter et al 2015). Limited research around spirituality is therefore starting to show the importance of spiritual and existential issues and, in particular, the links among spiritual, psychological and social well-being in people with a terminal illness.

PSYCHOLOGICAL DISTRESS

Extreme psychological distress is often accompanied by the diagnosis of a terminal illness (Braun et al 2007, Reeve et al 2007, Wilson et al 2007) and most commonly includes anxiety and depression. This can be due to the primary disease, associated physical conditions, poor pain management, side effects of medication, or all four of these factors combined (Paice 2002). There is also convincing evidence that anxiety, depression and distress linked with uncertainty and hopelessness (spiritual distress) interact with pain, where unrelieved pain can increase the desire to hasten death (Syrjala et al 2014).

Unrelieved pain is one of the most frequently experienced and feared symptoms for those in the last months of their life (Potter & Higginson 2004), as people with advanced disease often experience pain which is more severe and occurs in more areas than people with early-stage disease (Keefe et al 2005). Also, in advanced cancer, pain is frequently seen as a continuous reminder of disease progression, uncertainty and death (Turk 2002). Therefore, in order to provide high quality palliative, supportive and end-of-life care, these psychological conditions need to be understood and managed appropriately. This should include a thorough assessment to highlight any history of mental health issues, such as panic disorder (see Chapter 1), generalized anxiety disorder (GAD) (see Chapter 1), posttraumatic stress disorder (PTSD) (see Chapter 1), or other types of anxiety which may be intensified by the diagnosis of a terminal illness.

Posttraumatic Stress Disorder

The diagnosis of a long-term condition is not a time-limited stressor but is associated with a multitude of prolonged traumatic experiences, which distinguishes it from a number of other stressors that can lead to PTSD. For example, around one third of people diagnosed with cancer experience symptoms of posttraumatic stress, with up to 22% developing PTSD (Smith et al 2011, Stuber et al 2010). PTSD can be triggered by the constant threat of reemergence of the disease, and it has been reported that untreated cancer-related PTSD increases pain and non-adherence to treatment, disability and the desire to die (Gold et al 2012). Therefore health care professionals need to be able to identify and address trauma associated with diagnosis and treatment to ensure high-quality supportive, palliative and end-of-life care, and understand how anxiety and depression can present themselves.

Anxiety and Depression

Anxiety and depression can encompass a wide range of moods, of which sadness and grief are normal emotions, after a diagnosis of terminal illness. However, the distress experienced from this devastating news can vary from mild to severe. In addition, delirium can sometimes be confused with depression, which is perhaps why anxiety and depression are often underdiagnosed and undertreated in this group of people (Block 2000, Chochinov 2004, Roth et al 2013, Wilson et al 2000).

A number of factors relating to long-term conditions can trigger depression, such as uncontrolled pain, fatigue, constipation, anorexia, anaemia, hypercalcemia, hypothyroidism and sepsis. Certain medications and treatments can also contribute to depression – for example, corticosteroids and some chemotherapeutic agents (Paice 2002). In addition, other external triggers can increase the likelihood of anxiety and depression, including social and financial concerns, age and previous history of anxiety and depression (see Chapter 25).

Major depression is prevalent in approximately 15% of people with palliative care needs and a number of others affected by mental health issues including depressive symptoms (Hotopf et al 2002). For example, anxiety and depression are commonly reported in people with cancer (Lovejoy et al 2000, Wise & Taylor, 1990), with 38% of people surviving cancer suffering from mood disorders (Mitchell et al 2011) and a number of other psychological responses linked to cancer pain (Porter & Keefe 2011, Rief et al 2011). A survey of people with cancer in the terminal stages of their disease receiving palliative care reported anxiety (42.5%) and depression (68.5%) (O'Connor et al 2010). There is therefore an increased risk of mental health issues in people with cancer (Park et al 2018).

In the final months of life anxiety and depression are common, with increasing burden from the deteriorating long-term condition reducing overall quality of life (Laird & Mitchell 2005, Robinson & Crawford 2005). At this stage the person may experience transitional withdrawal rather than social withdrawal, often associated with depression. In transitional withdrawal the person becomes extremely weak and more and more drowsy, with reduced appetite. There may also be some disorientation or the person may have a particularly short attention span (Paice 2002). Social withdrawal on the other hand tends to arise from internal factors, such as anxiety and depression, where the person actively chooses to reduce social interaction, with increased withdrawal from family and friends. This can be due to the effects of fatigue and overall coping ability on quality of life.

The majority of people with a long-term condition develop delirium at some point, but particularly so during the final weeks of their life (Lawlor et al 2000). Early symptoms of delirium, such as emotional lability, altered perception, impaired memory, incoherent speech, hallucinations and disorientation to time and place can often be mistaken for anxiety and depression. To help distinguish between the two, delirium has been divided into hyperactive delirium and hypoactive delirium according to the level of psychomotor activity. In hyperactive delirium the person becomes agitated and hyperaroused and experiences hallucinations and delusions, whereas in hypoactive delirium the person often appears lethargic and withdrawn (Breitbart & Cohen 2000), which can be confused with depression. Making the right clinical diagnosis can be achieved by observing if the person is crying or expressing feelings of hopelessness, along with completing cognition tests such as the Mini-Mental Status Examination. It is also important that a thorough assessment of the onset of symptoms is carried out with family caregivers, which can help to distinguish delirium from depression.

Caregiver Stress

Family Caregiver Stress

A number of studies have identified the importance of family caregivers for people who are seriously ill or dying (Cora et al 2012, Ross et al 2010); however, providing care for a family member can be a source of stress, especially when there is a terminal diagnosis. Until recently, research into the psychological aspects of palliative, supportive, and end-of-life care has focused on the person with the long-term condition. Conversely, long-term conditions are now known to be a key stressor, not only for people with the condition, but also for their family, especially the family caregiver (Park et al 2018). This is due to major readjustments that the family caregiver needs to make in their social, working and family life. Stress increases as physical and emotional support becomes the responsibility of caregivers, with many having additional financial and legal issues. This leads to a decrease in their own health, with a greater risk of anxiety and depression (Cora et al 2012, Haley et al 2001, Moody & McMillan 2003).

A study of people with cancer coming towards the end of their life reported family burden (time given to daily care by family caregivers), emotional distress (relating to the family's anxiety and depression) and cardiovascular risk, which was shown to increase, whereas quality of life decreased (Cora et al 2012, Ullrich et al 2017). Caring for a loved one who is in pain and dying is therefore deemed one of the most stressful experiences that family caregivers can go through (Keefe et al 2003), with concern about pain being the second most common issue reported by family caregivers (Tsigaroppoulos 2009). When caregivers struggle to express their emotions, this can affect their loved one's reactions reporting increased levels of pain and pain behaviour. However, caregiver stress is reduced and mood is improved when caregivers are confident that they are able to help their loved one manage pain (Keefe et al 2003).

Family caregivers often provide extensive and challenging levels of care over a prolonged period. This leads to increased stress, which ultimately affects the caregivers' quality of life (Chentsova-Dutton et al 2000). However, even if they have acknowledged their high levels of stress and need for help, the majority of caregivers are disinclined to accept care because all their attention and energy is spent on caring for their loved one (Walsh & Schmidt 2003). It is, therefore, paramount that the risks and needs of family caregivers are identified, so that the right support is put in place as a standard measure of palliative care (Choi 2010). In addition, the needs of the health care professionals need to be addressed because they are also at risk of the detrimental effects of stress (Berman et al 2007, Pereira et al 2011).

HEALTH CARE PROFESSIONAL STRESS

Health care professional stress can lead to increased medical errors, reduced productivity and absenteeism (West et al 2006, Sanchez-Reilly et al 2013). Stress is also thought to play a role in the quality of care provided, with increased stress leading to poor communication and teamwork (Berman et al 2007, Sanchez-Reilly et al 2013). Stressors include continual exposure to death and bereavement, increasing demands on workload (see Chapter 1), unpredictable schedules, time pressures and competing role demands (Kerney et al 2009, Perez et al 2015, Rokach 2005). Emotional demands can also add to stress levels through absorption of negative emotional responses, such as breaking bad news and feelings of helplessness when there is no cure, as well as challenges to personal belief systems and emotional conflicts (Breen et al 2014, Rokach 2005, White et al 2004), all of which can eventually affect the health care professional's emotional management and well-being (Uren & Graham 2013). It is estimated that at least 50% of health care professionals working in palliative, supportive and end-of-life care are at risk of poor psychological outcomes due to a lack of resilience and coping strategies and mechanisms to manage these demands (Kamau et al 2014).

RESILIENCE

In recent years there has been an increased interest in health care professional wellness and resilience (the ability of an energetic and flexible system to endure challenges to its viability, stability or development), especially within palliative, supportive and end-of-life care settings (Mehta et al 2016).

In 2016 a systematic review was carried out to investigate the effectiveness of psychosocial interventions to manage the psychological well-being of staff working in this area of care. This study identified 1786 potential studies, but only 9 met the study criteria following screening and quality assessment. The interventions included relaxation techniques, cognitive training, education and support to manage stress, depression, fatigue, burnout and satisfaction levels. Results were varied, with some improvement in staff well-being in two of the studies, but the methodology was deemed weak. No improvement was identified in the randomized controlled trials (RCTs) reviewed, and the study concluded that high-quality research was required to address this urgent need within the UK health care system (Hill et al 2016). This is of vital importance as health care professionals' well-being affects quality of care and patient outcomes (DOH 2009, Maben et al 2012). Therefore for palliative, supportive and end-of-life care to be successful in delivering high-quality care, it is reliant on the cohesion and well-being of all the health care professionals within the multidisciplinary team.

Extensive research has been undertaken on the psychological well-being and quality of life of people with long-term conditions and their family caregivers (Harding 2012, Jaiswal et al 2014); however, evidence on the effectiveness of psychological interventions for the well-being of health care professionals remains scarce (Hill et al 2016).

INTRODUCTION TO EVIDENCE

A mind-body program known as the Relaxation Response Resiliency Program (3RP), developed to encourage resiliency (Park et al 2013), has been shown to decrease stress and increase resiliency in a wide range of populations (Bhasin 2013, Duseck et al 2008, Jacquart et al 2014, Vranceanu et al 2014). Mehta and colleagues

(2016) carried out a pilot study to test the feasibility of the 3RP for health care professionals working in palliative care. The intervention was delivered in five sessions over a 2-month period. Data were collected pre- and post-3PR and non-parametric statistical tests investigated changes in self-efficacy, optimism, satisfaction with life, perceived stress, perspective taking, and positive and negative affect. Results indicated that the modified 3RP for health care professionals working in palliative care was feasible and may encourage resiliency and protect against the harmful effects of stress in this setting.

There is a growing body of evidence that psychological factors such as distress (psychological and spiritual) and pain catastrophizing can increase the severity and impact of pain in people with advanced disease (Syrjala et al 2014). Evidence of successful relaxation treatments for cancer-related PTSD is starting to be published, but the impact on pain is lacking (Kangas et al 2013). Interventions such as CBT and relaxation with imagery have been shown to be effective in teaching people with long-term conditions skills in managing pain at the end of their life. In a meta-analysis 37 studies were investigated, where 26 of the studies included samples with more than half of the participants in advanced stage of their disease. The findings indicated that skills-based interventions improved pain severity and pain interference (Sheinfeld et al 2012).

Findings from a number of meta-analyses (Johannsen et al 2013, Sheinfeld et al 2012, Tatrow & Montgomery 2006) and high-quality RCTs indicate that psychological and cognitive–behavioural interventions can reduce the severity of pain and interference of function from initial diagnosis of a long-term condition through treatment and palliative, supportive and end-of-life care. Relaxation techniques which have been shown to be effective include hypnosis, exercise, cognitive–behavioural approaches, relaxation with imagery, and education which includes coping strategies (see Chapter 29). Hypnosis and exercise have shown promise in controlling pain in advanced disease, but there is a lack of research around their effect in managing pain in end-of-life care (Syrjala et al 2014). However, a number of RCTs of self-hypnosis with supportive-expressive group therapy

for female participants with metastatic breast cancer found that over the year of therapy, increases in pain were reduced (Butler et al 2009, Johannsen et al 2013, Osborn et al 2006).

A review of the literature indicates that relaxation techniques are effective in the management of both distressing side effects of cancer treatments (Leubbert et al 2001) as well as common symptoms associated with advanced cancer (Hanratty & Higginson 1994). It has also been recorded that relaxation techniques have a positive psychological effect on depression (Sloman 2002), including anxiety management and stress reduction (Decker et al 1992), improving overall quality of life (Cheung et al 2003). In addition, relaxation techniques have been reported in the literature as efficacious in the management of side effects of the condition, drugs and surgical interventions, such as cancer- and treatment-related pain (Syrjala et al 1995), nausea and vomiting (Carty 1997), breathlessness (Cooper 1997), anxiety and stress (Leubbert et al 2001) (see Chapter 29).

A study compared the effects of progressive muscle relaxation (PMR) and guided imagery on anxiety, depression and quality of life in 56 people with advanced cancer. Participants were randomly assigned to either PMR, guided imagery, PMR and guided imagery or a control group. Outcome measures included the Hospital Anxiety and Depression Scale (see Chapter 28) and the Functional Living Index–Cancer Scale. Findings indicated a significant improvement in depression and quality of life, but no significant improvement in anxiety (Sloman 2002). This study was limited by a small sample size, but the statistical analysis is promising for these relaxation techniques. Several studies have also explored the effect of music and PMR on caregivers' stress, which have indicated positive outcomes in managing anxiety and reducing stress by decreasing muscle tension and improving quality of sleep (Robb 2000).

Theories Behind Relaxation Techniques in Palliative, Supportive and End-of-Life Care

Providing psychological support through relaxation techniques and psychological interventions enables people with a terminal illness to find meaning in their lives. This is achieved by empowering individuals to gather meanings, values and beliefs through activities such as narratives (life history). Empathetic listening to narratives provides therapeutic benefits permitting a more rounded understanding of the meaning of 'total pain' (Saunders 1963, Moore et al 2015, Mundle 2015). The concept of 'total pain' was first coined by Dame Cicely Saunders, who described it as the all-encompassing suffering of an individual's psychological, physical, emotional, spiritual and social distress (Saunders 1964). The understanding that pain is multifaceted was first documented by Dame Saunders in 1959, when she observed that pain could not be fully relieved by analgesics alone (Saunders 1959, Wachholtz et al 2016). She also noted that alleviating physical symptoms often improved psychological pain (Saunders 1963). Through various imaging technology, accumulating evidence now demonstrates that two regions in the brain, the anterior insula and the dorsal anterior cingulate cortex, share the same neurological substrates for social and physical pain. This explains the overlap of painful emotions experienced by social rejection or loss and physical pain (Eisenberger 2012). Psychological well-being is therefore thought to facilitate health outcomes and spirituality, which has a stress-buffering effect of meaning, beliefs and goals (Piko & Brassai 2016).

There is a prevalence of mental health issues within palliative, supportive and end-of-life care and a lack of specialist mental health workers (Price et al 2006). It is therefore imperative that palliative care teams are able to manage mental health issues and health care professionals feel supported to learn, with systems put in place to support efficient and effective palliative, supportive and end-of-life care (NCPC 2013). Dame Saunders stated that mental distress is possibly the most difficult pain of all and requires specific clinical skills to manage (Saunders 1963). Therefore having an overall understanding of different relaxation techniques and how to implement them into practice can help with this skill gap and help with symptom control.

Symptom Control

Within the field of palliative, supportive and end-of-life care there is an increasing prevalence of the use of non-pharmacological interventions to support conventional treatments for symptom control (Shen et al 2002).

NON-PHARMACOLOGICAL APPROACHES

Symptoms such as anxiety and depression experienced by people with long-term conditions can be improved through non-pharmacological interventions. However, this will require differentiating between preexisting anxiety and inadequately managed or untreated anxiety, from anxiety triggered by the diagnosis of a long-term condition, or other related factors such as treatment or symptom related causes (Paice 2002). The type of relaxation technique will also need to be considered carefully; for example, relaxation and guided imagery require concentration, energy and social interaction, which may be beyond the ability of people coming towards the end of their life. In addition to this, addressing the fears of caregivers is fundamental because these fears can often intensify the anxiety of the person they are caring for. Relaxation techniques as a treatment intervention should therefore be considered as part of the multidisciplinary team approach for both people with long-term conditions and their family caregivers.

The non-pharmacological approach to breathlessness helps manage the multidimensional nature of this symptom (Belchamber et al 2017, Corner et al 1996, Hately et al 2003, NICE 2005, Thomas et al 2011). This intervention incorporates narrative (Fig. 26.1), positioning (see Chapters 3 and 4), relaxation techniques (progressive relaxation) (see Chapter 5), tense–release script (see Chapter 7) and passive muscular relaxation (see Chapter 8), applied relaxation (see Chapter 9), physical activity (pacing, reconditioning and increasing exercise tolerance within the limitations of the condition) (see Chapter 15), cognitive–behavioural approaches (see Chapter 16) and breathing techniques (see Chapter 4), as well as the calming hand (Fig. 26.1) to improve the overall feeling of well-being and sense of control.

Relaxation techniques and management encourages a person-centred, educational approach, which

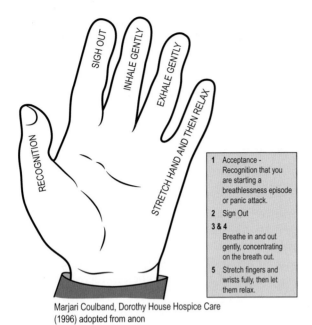

Marjari Coulband, Dorothy House Hospice Care
(1996) adopted from anon

Fig. 26.1 ■ Calming hand. (From Hanks et al 2010.)

facilitates the person's recognition of potential stressors (Ewer-Smith & Patterson 2002). Therefore relaxation techniques are seen as a key component and an essential element of palliative rehabilitation.

PALLIATIVE REHABILITATION

Palliative rehabilitation is an interdisciplinary (IDT) approach involving allied health professionals, nurses, psychosocial practitioners and doctors (Hospice UK 2015), where treatment is delivered by an MDT. The aim of palliative rehabilitation is to achieve the best quality of life for people living with life-limiting and terminal conditions (Pan et al 2000, WHO 1990). Palliative rehabilitation should therefore be implemented from diagnosis of a life-limiting or terminal illness, and support given in collaboration with the IDT, family and health care professional caregivers to realize the person's personal goals until the end of his or her life.

A sense of hope is key to enhancing quality of life in people with a diagnosis of a terminal illness and integral to their psychosocial well-being (Belchamber & Ellis-Hill 2013, McClement & Chochinov 2008).

Palliative rehabilitation enables people with a terminal illness to create new meaning, as well as hope and learn how to manage their symptoms (Belchamber & Ellis-Hill 2013).

The following have been identified as key components of palliative rehabilitation (Belchamber 2004):

- Evaluation/assessment of the person's symptoms and referral to the appropriate members of the MDT
- Physical care, such as therapeutic interventions and non-pharmacological approaches
- Coordinated care
- Psychological care
- Supportive care
- Spiritual care
- Group work, incorporating social care
- Exercise
- Relaxation
- Aromatherapy
- Diversional therapy

Group work and physical activity are key components of palliative rehabilitation because they improve functional capacity and activities of daily living, increasing independence and ability (Belchamber 2009, Williams 1994).

GROUP WORK AND PHYSICAL ACTIVITY

Group work encourages connectivity among people with similar conditions and disabilities, enabling socialization and relaxation. This is thought to have a positive effect on psychological well-being as well as treatment compliance or adherence (Belchamber 2004, Lord et al 1993, Rogind et al 1998). Evidence suggests that physical activity can improve levels of stress and depression in people with palliative care needs (Kumar & Jim 2010), with physical activity slowing down or maintaining functional decline (Lowe et al 2009, Oldervoll et al 2006). A qualitative study exploring social, exercise and diversional therapy group work within palliative rehabilitation identified best practice for the management of three distressing symptoms: pain, dyspnoea and fatigue in people with advanced cancer. The main factors identified included environmental, mobilization and normalization. The normalization process was described as coming to terms with the person's diagnosis and disability and, in particular, the person's needs (Belchamber 2009). There is therefore evidence that group exercise, frequent physical activity, energy conservation techniques, relaxation techniques and psychological techniques (see Chapters 15 and 25) can be beneficial in managing symptoms of fatigue, breathlessness, pain, anxiety and depression experienced by people living with a terminal illness (Belchamber 2004, 2010, 2016). Group interventions have also been studied and found to enhance resilience in health care professionals, resulting in improvements in several domains of well-being (Krasner et al 2009, Pipe et al 2012). In addition, physical activity is deemed to improve a person's resilience to emotional stress (see Chapter 15).

A key component in determining quality of life and life expectancy in people with palliative, supportive and end-of-life needs is their physical fitness levels (Eyigor & Akdeniz 2014). This can be achieved through physical activity because it is perceived to empower people to manage their condition (see Chapter 25), providing social support and a sense of connection and belonging, while distracting people from concerns associated with their condition and ultimately improving physical ability, which achieves an overall positive outcome and sense of normality (Belchamber 2004, 2009, 2010; Malcolm et al 2016).

However, to successfully change and sustain physical activity behaviour it has been recommended that a physical activity care pathway is implemented that includes assessment of the person's physical activity levels, personalized prescription, advice and education with guidance on physical activity opportunities (Burke et al 2020).

2. This shift in care and advances in treatment has seen the development of palliative rehabilitation and increasing use of non-pharmacological approaches.
3. Three types of suffering (spiritual, psychological and physical) have been identified in people with a terminal illness.
4. A number of factors related to long-term conditions can trigger depression, such as uncontrolled pain, fatigue, constipation, anorexia, anaemia, hypercalcemia, hypothyroidism and sepsis.
5. Extreme psychological distress most commonly presents itself as anxiety and depression.
6. Caring for a loved one who is in pain and dying is deemed one of the most stressful experiences that family caregivers can go through. Stress is also thought to play a role in the quality of care provided by health care professionals, with increased stress leading to poor communication and teamwork.

Reflection

Describe your understanding of palliative, supportive and end-of-life care.

What effects can psychological and spiritual distress have on an individual?

What changes will you make to your personal life or practice?

What is the main learning point you will take away from this chapter?

What is your future action plan in terms of using group work and physical activity to help caregivers who are supporting loved ones with a terminal illness?

KEY POINTS

1. Palliative, supportive and end-of-life care are key elements in the management of people with long-term conditions, which is now being delivered across a number of health care settings to manage the increasing demand of an ageing population.

CASE STUDY LEARNING OPPORTUNITY

The key points and reflection provide background and knowledge required in relation to the case study, Harry, to help deepen understanding of how palliative rehabilitation can help improve quality of life in people with a life-limiting condition or terminal illness.

CASE STUDY

Non-pharmacological Approach to Breathlessness: Non-Pharmacological Outcomes for Harry

Harry is a 54-year-old teacher who was diagnosed with squamous cell lung cancer in his left lung a year ago and, after diagnosis of an inoperable tumour, went on to have three courses of palliative chemotherapy. Until recently, Harry was coping well at home, but he is now feeling very low and finding it difficult to walk upstairs without getting short of breath. Investigations revealed new lesions in his right lobe, and Harry was told that his disease had progressed. The fear and anxiety of becoming more breathless were making Harry feel out of control, leading to panic attacks. This was also making his wife feel extremely anxious and helpless. Harry was therefore referred to a breathlessness clinic to help him manage his symptoms and improve his quality of life.

Harry attended the clinic alone. He was breathless, exhibiting shallow breathing with shoulders elevated. Through narrative Harry became tearful as he spoke of his fears and anxieties. A referral was made for him to see the appropriate members of the team for further exploration of his psychological and spiritual distress. Harry was also encouraged to bring his wife along to the following clinic appointments. A thorough assessment of Harry's respiratory, functional status and fitness levels were then carried out and vital signs monitored. Outcome measures indicated Harry had moderate-to-severe breathlessness, with a heightened perception of breathlessness causing him to hyperventilate.

Harry attended three clinic appointments in total, with 2 weeks between each appointment to practice positioning, relaxation techniques, breathing techniques and prescribed exercises, as well as other coping strategies, such as the calming hand (see Fig. 26.1) to manage his breathlessness. After 6 weeks Harry reported being more in control of his breathlessness, he was able to manage stairs using controlled and pursed lipped breathing, and his overall fitness levels had improved. His wife's fears and anxieties were also addressed, and she no longer felt helpless, having learned the coping strategies and techniques alongside Harry.

ACTIVITY

For the case study:

1. List key aspects used in the non-pharmacological approach to breathlessness.
2. Write down the impact the non-pharmacological approach to breathlessness is having from a psychological perspective.
3. Write down the impact the non-pharmacological approach to breathlessness is having from a physical perspective.
4. Write down the impact the non-pharmacological approach to breathlessness is having from an emotional perspective.
5. Consider the effects of the non-pharmacological approach to breathlessness on Harry's overall quality of life.

Chapter 27 will focus on COVID-19, which will be key to understanding how digital delivery of psychological interventions and relaxation techniques benefits individuals in COVID-19 crisis, recovery and rehabilitation.

REFERENCES

Alcorn, S. R., Balboni, M. J., Prigerson, H. G., et al. (2010). "If God wanted me yesterday, I wouldn't be here today": Religious and spiritual themes in patients' experiences of advanced cancer. *Journal of Palliative Medicine, 13*(5), 581–588.

Balboni, T. A., Paulk, M. E., Balboni, M. J., et al. (2010). Provision of spiritual care to patients with advanced cancer: Associations with medical care and quality of life near death. *Journal of Clinical Oncology, 28*(3), 445–452.

Belchamber, C. A., & Gousy, M. H. (2004). Rehabilitative care in a specialist palliative day care centre: A study of patients' perspectives. *International Journal of Therapy and Rehabilitation, 11*, 425–434.

Belchamber, C. (2009). Participants' perceptions of groupwork in the management of cancer symptoms in older people. *Groupwork, 19*(2), 79–100.

Belchamber, C. A. (2010). *A rehabilitative care approach for people living with cancer: People with cancer's views of a rehabilitative care approach within a specialist palliative day care centre.* Lambert Academic Publishing.

Belchamber, C. A., & Ellis-Hill, A. C. (2013). Fostering hope through palliative rehabilitation. *European Journal of Palliative Care, 20*(3), 136–139.

Belchamber, C. A. (2016). *Physiotherapy palliative cancer care: A case study approach.* Doctoral dissertation, Bournemouth University.

Belchamber, C. A., Rosser, E., & Ellis-Hill, C. (2017). P-90 Practice improvement project: Palliative care service provision for people with dyspnoea. *BMJ Supportive & Palliative Care, 7*(Suppl. 1), A33.

Berman, R., Campbell, M., Makin, W., & Todd, C. (2007). Occupational stress in palliative medicine, medical oncology and clinical oncology specialist registrars. *Clinical Medicine, 7*, 235–242.

Bekelman, D. B., Parry, C., Curlin, F. A., Yamashita, T. E., Fairclough, D. L., & Wamboldt, F. S. (2010). A comparison of two spirituality instruments and their relationship with depression and quality of life in chronic heart failure. *Journal of Pain and Symptom Management, 39*(3), 515–526.

Bhasin, M. K., Dusek, J. A., Chang, B. H., et al. (2013). Relaxation response induces temporal transcriptome changes in energy metabolism, insulin secretion and inflammatory pathways. *PloS One, 8*, e62817.

Block, S. D. (2000). Assessing and managing depression in the terminally ill patient. ACP-ASIM End-of-Life Care Consensus Panel. American College of Physicians-American Society of Internal Medicine. *Annals of Internal Medicine, 132*(3), 209–218.

Bone, A. E., Gomes, B., Etkind, S. N., et al. (2018). What is the impact of population ageing on the future provision of end-of-life care? Population-based projections of place of death. *Palliative Medicine, 32*(2), 329–336.

Braun, M., Mikulincer, M., Rydall, A., Walsh, A., & Rodin, G. (2007). Hidden morbidity in cancer: spouse caregivers. *Journal of Clinical Oncology, 25*, 4829–4834.

Breen, L. J., O'Connor, M., Hewitt, L. Y., et al. (2014). The 'specter' of cancer: Exploring secondary trauma for health professionals providing cancer support and counseling. *Psychological Services, 11*, 60–67.

Breitbart, W., & Cohen, K. (2000). Delirium in the terminally ill. In H. M. Chochinov, & W. Breitbart (Eds.), *Handbook of psychiatry in palliative medicine* (pp. 75–90). New York: Oxford University Press.

Burke, S., Utley, A., Belchamber, C., & McDowall, L. (2020). Physical activity in hospice care: A social ecological perspective to inform policy and practice. *Research Quarterly for Exercise and Sport, 91*(3), 500–513.

Butler, L. D., Koopman, C., Neri, E., et al. (2009). Effects of supportive-expressive group therapy on pain in women with metastatic breast cancer. *Health Psychology, 28*, 579–587.

Carty, J. L. (1997). Relaxation to reduce nausea, vomiting, and anxiety chemotherapy in Japanese patients. *Cancer Nursing, 20*, 342–349.

Chentsova-Dutton, Y., Shuchter, S., Hutchin, S., Strause, L., Burns, K., & Zisook, S. (2000). The psychological and physical health of hospice caregivers. *Annals of Clinical Psychiatry, 72*(1), 19–27.

Cheung, Y. L., Molassiotis, A., & Chang, A. M. (2003). The effect of progressive muscle relaxation training on anxiety and quality of life after stoma surgery in colorectal cancer patients. *Psychooncology, 12*, 254–266.

Chochinov, H. M., Hassard, T., McClement, S., et al. (2009). The landscape of distress in the terminally ill. *Journal of Pain and Symptom Management, 38*, 641–649.

Chochinov, H. M. (2004). Palliative care: An opportunity for mental health professionals. *Canadian Journal of Psychiatry, 49*, 347–349.

Choi, Y. K. (2010). The effect of music and progressive muscle relaxation on anxiety, fatigue and quality of life in family caregivers of hospice patients. *Journal of Music Therapy, XLVII*(1), 53–69.

Cooper, J. (1997). Occupational therapy in specific symptom control and dysfunction. In J. Cooper (Ed.), *Occupational therapy in oncology and palliative care* (pp. 59–86). London: Whurr Publishers.

Corà, A., Partinico, M., Munafò, M., & Palomba, D. (2012). Health risk factors in caregivers of terminal cancer patient: A pilot study. *Cancer Nursing, 35*(1), 38–47.

Corner, J., Plant, H., Hern, R. A., & Bailey, C. (1996). Non-pharmacological intervention for breathlessness in lung cancer. *Palliative Medicine, 10*, 299–305.

Decker, T. W., Cline-Elsen, J., & Gallagher, M. (1992). Relaxation therapy as an adjunct in radiation oncology. *Psychooncology, 12*, 254–266.

Department of Health (DOH). (2009). *NHS health and wellbeing review: Interim report.* London: DOH.

Dezutter, J., Luyckx, K., & Wachholtz, A. (2015). Meaning in life in chronic pain patients over time: Associations with pain experience and psychological well-being. *Journal of Behavioral Medicine, 38*, 384–396.

Duseck, J. A., Hibberd, P. I., Buczynski, B., et al. (2008). Stress management versus lifestyle modification on systolic hypertension and medication elimination: A randomised trial. *Journal of Alternative and Complementary Medicine, 14*, 129–138.

Eisenberger, N. I. (2012). Broken hearts and broken bones: A neural perspective on the similarities between social and physical pain. *Psychological Science, 21*(1), 42–47.

Etkind, S. N., Bone, A. E., Gomes, B., et al. (2017). How many people will need palliative care in 2040? Past trends, future projections and implications for services. *BMC Medicine, 15*, 102.

Eyigor, S., & Akdeniz, S. (2014). Is exercise ignored in palliative cancer patients? *World Journal of Clinical Oncology, 5*(3), 554–559.

Ewer-Smith, C., & Patterson, S. (2002). The use of an occupational therapy programme within a palliative care setting. *European Journal of Palliative Care, 9*, 30–33.

Ferrell, B., Connor, S. R., Cordes, A., et al. (2007). The national agenda for quality palliative care: The National Consensus Project and the National Quality Forum. *Journal of Pain and Symptom Management, 33*(6), 737–744.

Frankl, V. E. (2006). *Man's search for meaning.* Boston: Beacon Press.

Gold, J. I., Douglas, M. K., Thomas, M. L., et al. (2012). The relationship between posttraumatic stress disorder, mood states, functional status, and quality of life in oncology outpatients. *Journal of Pain and Symptom Management, 44*, 520–531.

Gomes, B., & Higginson, I. J. (2008). Where people die (1974–2030): Past trends, future projections and implications for care. *Palliative Medicine, 22*, 33–41.

Hanratty, J., & Higginson, I. (1994). *Palliative care in terminal illness*. Northampton, UK: EPL Publications.

Haley, W., LaMonde, L., Han, B., Narramore, S., & Schonwetter, R. (2001). Family caregiving in hospice: Effects on psychological and health functioning among spousal caregivers in hospice patients with lung cancer or dementia. *Hospice Journal*, 15(4), 118.

Hanks, G., Cherny, N. I., Christakis, N. A., Fallon, M., Kaasa, S., & Portenoy, R. K. (2010). *Oxford textbook of palliative medicine* (4th ed.). Oxford, UK: Oxford University Press.

Harding, R., List, S., Epiphaniou, E., et al. (2012). How can informal caregivers in cancer and palliative care be supported? An updated systematic literature review of interventions and their effectiveness. *Palliative Medicine*, 26, 7–22.

Hately, J., Laurence, V., Scott, A., Baker, R., & Thomas, P. (2003). Breathlessness clinics within specialist palliative care settings can improve the quality of life and functional capacity of patients with lung cancer. *Palliative Medicine*, 17(5), 410–417.

Hill, R. C., Dempster, M., Donnelly, M., & McCorry, N. K. (2016). Improving the wellbeing of staff who work in palliative care settings: A systematic review of psychosocial interventions. *Palliative Medicine*, 30(9), 825–833.

Hospice UK. (2015). *Rehabilitative palliative care: Enabling people to live fully until they die. A challenge for the 21st century*. London: Hospice UK. Retrieved March 2020 from file:///C:/Users/carol/Downloads/rehabilitative-palliative-care-enabling-people-to-live-fully-until-they-die.pdf.

Hospice UK. (2016). Hospice care in the UK 2016. Retrieved March 2020 from https://www.hospiceuk.org/what-we-offer/publications?kwrd=hospice%20care%20in%20the%20UK.

Hotopf, M., Chidgey, J., Addington-Hall, J., & Lan Ly, K. (2002). Depression in advanced disease: A systematic review. Part 1. Prevalence and case finding. *Palliative Medicine*, 16, 81–97.

Jacquart, J., Miller, K. M., Radossi, A., et al. (2014). The effectiveness of a community-based mind-body group for symptoms of depression and anxiety. *Advances in Mind-Body Medicine*, 4, 286–293.

Johannsen, M., Farver, I., Beck, N., et al. (2013). The efficacy of psychosocial intervention for pain in breast cancer patients and survivors: A systematic review and meta-analysis. *Breast Cancer Research and Treatment*, 138, 675–690.

Jaiswal, R., Alici, Y., & Breitbart, W. (2014). A comprehensive review of palliative care in patients with cancer. *International Review of Psychiatry*, 26, 87–101.

Kamau, C., Medisauskaite, A., & Lopes, B. (2014). Orientations can avert psychosocial risks to palliative staff. *Psychooncology*, 23, 716–718.

Kandasamy, A., Chaturvedi, S. K., & Desai, G. (2011). Spirituality, distress, depression, anxiety, and quality of life in patients with advanced cancer. *Indian Journal of Cancer*, 48(1), 55–59.

Kangas, M., Milross, C., Taylor, A., et al. (2013). A pilot randomized controlled trial of a brief early intervention for reducing post-traumatic stress disorder, anxiety and depressive symptoms in newly diagnosed head and neck cancer patients. *Psychooncology*, 22, 1665–1673.

Keefe, F. J., Ahles, T. A., Porter, L. S., et al. (2003). The self-efficacy of family caregivers for helping cancer patients manage pain at end-of-life. *Pain*, 103, 157162.

Keefe, F. J., Abernethy, A. P., & Campbell, C. (2005). Psychological approaches to understanding and treating disease-related pain. *Annual Review of Psychology*, 56, 601–630.

Kerney, M. K., Weininger, R. B., Vachon, M. S., Harrison, R. I., & Mount, B. M. (2009). Self-care of physicians caring for patients at the end of life: 'Being connected … a key to my survival'. *JAMA*, 301, 1155–1164.

Krasner, M. S., Epstein, R. M., Beckman, H., et al. (2009). Association of an educational program in mindful communication with burnout, empathy and attitudes among primary care physicians. *JAMA*, 302, 1284–1293.

Kumar, S. P., & Jim, A. (2010). Physical therapy in palliative care: From symptom control to quality of life: A critical review. *Indian Journal of Palliative Care*, 16(3), 138–146.

Laird, B., & Mitchell, J. (2005). The assessment and management of depression in the terminally ill. *European Journal of Palliative Care*, 12(3), 101–104.

Lawlor, P. G., Gagnon, B., Mancini, L., et al. (2000). Occurrence, causes, and outcome of delirium in patients with advanced cancer: A prospective study. *Archives of Internal Medicine*, 160(6), 786–794.

Lord, S., Mitchell, D., & Williams, P. (1993). Effect of water exercise on balance and related factors in older people. *Australian Physiotherapy*, 39, 217–222.

Lovejoy, L. C., Tabor, D., Matteis, M., & Lillis, P. (2000). Cancer related depression: Part 1—neurologic alterations and cognitive-behavioral therapy. *Oncology Nurses Forum*, 27(4), 667–680.

Lowe, S. S., Watanabe, S. M., & Courneya, K. S. (2009). Physical activity as a supportive care intervention in palliative cancer patients: A systematic review. *The Journal of Supportive Oncology*, 7(1), 27–34.

Leubbert, K., Dahme, B., & Hasenbring, M. (2001). The effectiveness of training in reducing treatment-related symptoms and improving emotional adjustment in acute non-surgical cancer treatment, a meta-analysis. *Psychooncology*, 10, 490–502.

Maben, J., Peccei, R., Adams, M., et al. (2012). *Exploring the relationship between patients' experience of care and the influence of staff motivation, affect and wellbeing: SDO report*. Southampton, UK: NIHR.

Malcolm, L., Mein, G., Jones, A., Talbot-Rice, H., Maddocks, M., & Bristowe, K. (2016). Strength in numbers: Patient experiences of group exercise within hospice palliative care. *BMC Palliative Care*, 15, 97.

McClement, S. E., & Chochinov, H. (2008). Hope in advanced cancer patients. *European Journal of Cancer*, 44, 1169–1174.

Mehta, D. H., Perez, G. K., Treger, L., et al. (2016). Building resiliency in a palliative care team: A pilot study. *Journal of Pain and Symptom Management*, 51(3), 604–608.

Mitchell, A. J., Chan, M., Bhatti, H., et al. (2011). Prevalence of depression, anxiety, and adjustment disorder in oncological, haematological, and palliative-care settings: A meta-analysis of 94 interview-based studies. *Lancet Oncology*, 12, 160–174.

Moody, L. E., & McMillan, S. (2003). Dyspnea and quality of life indicators in hospice patients and their caregivers. *Health and Quality of Life Outcomes*, 1, 1–13.

Moore, K., Talwar, V., & Moxley-Haegert, L. (2015). Definitional ceremonies: Narrative practices for psychologists to inform interdisciplinary teams' understanding of children's spirituality in pediatric settings. *Journal of Health Psychology, 20,* 259–272.

Moreno, P. I., & Stanton, A. L. (2013). Personal growth during the experience of advanced cancer: A systematic review. *Cancer Journal, 19*(5), 421–430.

Mundle, R. (2015). A narrative analysis of spiritual distress in geriatric physical rehabilitation. *Journal of Health Psychology, 20*(3), 273–285.

Murtagh, F., Bausewein, C., Verne, J., Groeneveld, E. I., Kaloki, Y. E., & Higginson, I. J. (2014). How many people need palliative care? A study developing and comparing methods for population-based estimates. *Palliative Medicine, 28*(1), 49–58.

National Coalition for Hospice and Palliative Care (NCHPC). (2018). *Clinical practice guidelines for quality palliative care* (4th ed.). London: NCHPC. Retrieved March 2020 from https://www.nationalcoalitionhpc.org/wp-content/uploads/2018/10/NCHPC-NCPGuidelines_4thED_web_FINAL.pdf.

National Council for Palliative Care (NCPC). (2013). In *Inside palliative care: End of life care at a tipping point – Highlights from NCPC's National Conference on Refreshing the Strategy* (Vol. 26). London: NCPC.

National Institute of Care and Clinical Excellence (NICE). (2005). *The diagnosis and treatment of lung cancer: Methods, evidence and guidance.* London: National Collaborating Centre for Acute Care.

O'Connor, M., White, K., Kristjanson, L. J., Cousins, K., & Wilke, S. L. (2010). The prevalence of anxiety and depression in palliative care patient with cancer in Western Australia and New South Wales. *Medical Journal of Australia, 193*(5), 44.

Oldervoll, L. M., Loge, J. H., Paltiel, H., et al. (2006). The effect of a physical exercise program in palliative care: A phase II study. *Journal of Pain and Symptom Management, 31*(5), 421–430.

O'Mahony, S., Goulet, J. L., & Payne, R. (2010). Psychosocial distress in patients treated for cancer pain: A prospective observational study. *Journal of Opioid Management, 6*(3), 211–222.

Osborn, R. L., Demoncada, A. C., & Feuerstein, M. (2006). Psychosocial interventions for depression, anxiety, and quality of life in cancer survivors: Meta-analyses. *International Journal of Psychiatry Medicine, 36,* 13–34.

Paice, J. (2002). Managing psychological conditions in palliative care: Dying need not mean enduring uncontrollable anxiety, depression or delirium. *American Journal of Nursing, 102*(11), 36–42.

Pan, C. X., Morrison, R. S., Ness, J., Fugh-Berman, A., & Leipzig, R. M. (2000). Complementary and alternative medicine in the management of pain, dyspnoea and nausea and vomiting near the end of life: A systematic review. *Journal of Pain and Symptom Management, 20*(5), 374–386.

Park, Y., Jeong, Y., Lee, J., et al. (2018). The influence of family adaptability and cohesion on anxiety and depression of terminally ill cancer patients. *Supportive Care in Cancer, 26,* 313–321.

Park, E. R., Traeger, I., Vranceanu, A. M., et al. (2013). The development of a patient-centred program based on the relaxation response: The relaxation response resiliency program (3RP). *Psychosomatics, 54,* 165–174.

Pereira, S. M., Fonesca, A. M., & Carvalho, A. S. (2011). Burnout in palliative care: A systematic review. *Nursing Ethics, 18,* 317–326.

Perez, G. K., Haime, V., Jackson, V., Chittenden, E., Mehta, D. H., & Park, E. R. (2015). Promoting resiliency among palliative care

clinicians: Stressors, coping strategies and training needs. *Journal of Palliative Medicine, 18,* 332–337.

Piko, B. F., & Brassai, L. (2016). A reason to eat healthy: The role of meaning in life in maintaining homeostasis in modern society. *Journal of Health Psychology, 3*(1). 2055102916634360.

Pipe, T. B., Buchda, V. I., Launder, S., et al. (2012). Building personal and professional resources of resilience and agility n the healthcare workplace. *Stress and Health, 28,* 11–22.

Porter, L. S., & Keefe, F. J. (2011). Psychosocial issues in cancer pain. *Current Pain and Headache Reports, 15,* 263270.

Potter, J., & Higginson, I. J. (2004). Pain experienced by lung cancer patients: A review of prevalence, causes and pathophysiology. *Lung Cancer, 43,* 247–257.

Price, A., Hotopf, M., Higginson, I. J., Monroe, B., & Henderson, M. (2006). Psychological services in hospices in the UK and Republic of Ireland. *Journal of the Royal Society of Medicine, 99*(12), 637–639.

Puchalski, C., Ferrell, B., Virani, R., et al. (2009). Improving the quality of spiritual care as a dimension of palliative care: The report of the Consensus Conference. *Journal of Palliative Medicine, 12*(10), 885–904.

Rabow, M. W., & Knish, S. J. (2015). Spiritual well-being among outpatients with cancer receiving concurrent oncologic and palliative care. *Supportive Care in Cancer, 23,* 919–923.

Rawdin, B., Evans, C., & Rabow, M. W. (2013). The relationships among hope, pain, psychological distress, and spiritual well-being in oncology outpatients. *Journal of Palliative Medicine, 16*(2), 167–172.

Reeve, J., Lloyd-Williams, M., & Dowrick, C. (2007). Depression in terminal illness: The need for primary care-specific research. *Family Practice, 24,* 263–268.

Rego, F., & Nunes, R. (2019). The interface between psychology and spirituality in palliative care. *Journal of Health Psychology, 24*(3), 279–287.

Rief, W., Bardwell, W. A., Dimsdale, J. E., et al. (2011). Long-term course of pain in breast cancer survivors: A 4-year longitudinal study. *Breast Cancer Research and Treatment, 130,* 579–586.

Robb, S. L. (2000). Music assisted progressive muscle relaxation, progressive muscle relaxation, music listening, and silence: A comparison of relaxation techniques. *Music Therapy, 37,* 2–21.

Robinson, J. A., & Crawford, G. B. (2005). Identifying palliative care patients with symptoms of depression: An algorithm. *Palliative Medicine, 19*(4), 278–287.

Rogind, H., Bibow-Nielsen, B., Jensen, B., Moller, H., Frimodt-Moller, H., & Bliddal, H. (1998). The effects of physical training programme on patients with osteoarthritis of the knees. *Archives of Physical Medicine and Rehabilitation, 79,* 1421–1427.

Rokach, A. (2005). Caring for those who care for the dying: Coping with the demands on palliative care workers. *Palliative Support Care, 3,* 325–332.

Ross, S., Mosher, C. E., Ronis-Tobin, V., Hermele, S., & Ostroff, J. S. (2010). Psychosocial adjustment of family caregivers of head and neck cancer survivors. *Supportive Care in Cancer, 18,* 171–178.

Roth, M. I., St Cyr, K., Harle, I., & Katz, J. D. (2013). Relationship between pain and post-traumatic stress symptoms in palliative care. *Journal of Pain and Symptom Management, 46* (2), 182–91.

Sanchez-Reilly, S., Morrison, I. J., Carey, E., et al. (2013). Caring for oneself to care for others: Physicians and their self-care. *Journal of Supportive Oncology, 11*, 75–81.

Saunders, C. (1959). Care of the dying. 3. Control of pain in terminal cancer. *Nursing Times*(October 23), 1031–1032.

Saunders, C. (1963). The treatment of intractable pain in terminal cancer. *Proceedings of the Royal Society of Medicine, 56*(3), 195–197.

Saunders, C. (1964). The symptomatic treatment of incurable malignant disease. *Prescribers Journal, 4*(4), 68–73.

Shen, J., Andersen, R., Albert, P. S., et al. (2002). Use of complementary/alternative therapies by women with advanced-stage breast cancer. *BMC Complementary and Alternative Medicine, 2*, 1–7.

Sheinfeld, G. S., Krebs, P., Badr, H., et al. (2012). Meta-analysis of psychosocial interventions to reduce pain in patients with cancer. *Journal of Clinical Oncology, 30*, 539–547.

Sloman, R. (2002). Relaxation and imagery for anxiety and depression control in community patients with advanced cancer. *Cancer Nursing, 25*(6), 432–435.

Smith, S. K., Zimmerman, S., Williams, C. S., et al. (2011). Posttraumatic stress symptoms in long-term non Hodgkin's lymphoma survivors: Does time heal? *Journal of Clinical Oncology, 29*, 4526–4533.

Stuber, M. L., Meeske, K. A., Krull, K. R., et al. (2010). Prevalence and predictors of posttraumatic stress disorder in adult survivors of childhood cancer. *Pediatrics, 125*, e1124–e1134.

Sulmasy, D. P. (2006). Spiritual issues in the care of dying patients: '… it's okay between me and god'. *JAMA, 296*(11), 1385–1392.

Syrjala, K., Donaldson, G., Davis, M., Kippes, M., & Carr, J. (1995). Relaxation and imagery and cognitive-behavioural training reduce pain during cancer treatment, a controlled clinical trial. *Pain, 63*, 489–498.

Syrjala, K. L., Jensen, M. P., Mendoza, E., Yi, J. C., Fisher, H. M., & Keefe, F. J. (2014). Psychological and Behavioural Approaches to Cancer Pain Management. *Journal of Clinical Oncology, 32*, 1703–1711.

Tatrow, K., & Montgomery, G. H. (2006). Cognitive behavioral therapy techniques for distress and pain in breast cancer patients: A meta-analysis. *Journal of Behavioral Medicine, 29*, 7–27.

Thomas, S., Bausewein, C., Higgiinson, I., & Booth, S. (2011). Breathlessness in cancer patients – Implications, management and challenges. *European Journal of Oncology Nursing, 15*, 459–469.

Thompson, G. N., & Chochinov, H. M. (2010). Reducing the potential for suffering in older adults with advanced cancer. *Palliative Support Care, 8*, 83–93.

Tsigaroppoulos, T., Mazaris, E., Chatzidarellis, E., et al. (2009). Problems faced by relatives caring for cancer patients at home. *International Journal of Nursing Practice, 15*, 1–6.

Turk, D. C. (2002). Remember the distinction between malignant and benign pain? Well, forget it. *Clinical Journal of Pain, 18*, 75–76.

Ullrich, A., Ascherfeld, L., Marx, G., Bokemeyer, C., Bergelt, C., & Oechsle, K. (2017). Quality of life, psychological burden, needs, and satisfaction during specialized inpatient palliative care in family caregivers of advanced cancer patient. *BMC Palliative Care, 16*, 31.

Uren, S., Graham, T. (2013). Subjective experiences of coping among caregivers in palliative care. Retrieved April 2020 from https://ojin.nursingworld.org/MainMenuCategories/ANAMarketplace/ANAPeriodicals/OJIN/TableofContents/Vol-18-2013/No2-May-2013/Articles-Previous-Topics/Subjective-Experiences-of-Coping-Among-Caregivers-in-Palliative-Care.html.

Vranceanu, A. M., Merker, V. I., Plotkin, S. R., & Park, E. R. (2014). The relaxation response resiliency program (3RP) in patients with neurofibromatosis 1, neurofibromatosis 2, and schwannomata: Results from a pilot study. *Journal of Neurooncology, 4*(120), 103–109.

Wachholtz, A. B., Fitch, C. E., Makowski, S., & Tjia, J. (2016). A comprehensive approach to the patient at end of life: Assessment of multidimensional suffering. *Southern Medical Journal, 109*(4), 200–206.

Walsh, S., & Schmidt, L. (2003). Telephone support for caregivers of hospice patients. *Cancer Nursing, 26*, 358–363.

West, C. P., Huschka, M. M., Novotny, P. J., et al. (2006). Association of perceived medical errors with resident distress and empathy: A prospective longitudinal study. *JAMA, 296*, 1071–1078.

White, K., Wilkes, L., Cooper, K., et al. (2004). The impact of unrelieved patient suffering on palliative care nurses. *International Journal of Palliative Nursing, 10*, 438–444.

Williams, M.A. (1994). *Exercise testing and training in elderly cardiac patients.* Current issues in cardiac rehabilitation. Monograph no 1. Champaign, IL: Human Kinetics.

Wilson, K. G., Lander, M., Chochinov, H., M. (2000). Diagnosis and management of depression in palliative care. In H. M. Chochinov, & W. Breitbart (Eds.), *Handbook of psychiatry in palliative medicine* (pp. 25–49). New York: Oxford University Press.

Wilson, K. G., Chochinov, H. M., Skirko, M. G., et al. (2007). Depression and anxiety disorders in palliative cancer care. *Journal of Pain and Symptom Management, 33*, 118–129.

Winkelman, W. D., Lauderdale, K., Balboni, M. J., et al. (2011). The relationship of spiritual concerns to the quality of life of advanced cancer patients: Preliminary findings. *Journal of Palliative Medicine, 14*(9), 1022–1028.

Wise, M. G., & Taylor, S. E. (1990). Anxiety and mood disorders in medically ill patients. *Journal of Clinical Psychiatry, 51*(Suppl.), 27–32.

World Health Organization (WHO) 1990. *Cancer pain relief and palliative care: Report of a WHO expert committee.* Technical Report Series 804. Geneva: WHO.

World Health Organization (WHO). (2020). WHO definition of palliative care. Retrieved April 2020 from https://www.who.int/cancer/palliative/definition/en/.

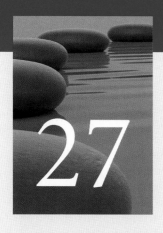

27

COVID-19

DR CAROLINE BELCHAMBER – CASE STUDIES
PROFESSOR TEENA CLOUSTON

CHAPTER CONTENTS

LEARNING OBJECTIVES

The aim of this chapter is to provide an understanding of the application of relaxation techniques for people after the outbreak of COVID-19.

By the end of this chapter you will be able to:

1. Recognize COVID-19's origin, signs and symptoms.

2. Understand how COVID-19 affects people's well-being from diverse environments.

3. Describe the physiological and psychological elements of COVID-19.

4. Acknowledge the mental health needs during and after COVID-19.

5. Identify psychological interventions and relaxation techniques which can improve well-being and quality of life of individuals during COVID-19 recovery and rehabilitation.

6. Know how digital technology may enhance psychological interventions in COVID-19 recovery and rehabilitation.

The chapter will conclude with key points and time for reflection, providing learning opportunities through case studies.

INTRODUCTION TO COVID-19

Coronavirus disease 2019 (COVID-19) is a pandemic that has rapidly spread across the world, placing our health care systems and resources under immense pressure. COVID-19 comes from a family of viruses known as coronaviruses (CoVs) that cause diseases ranging from mild infections to death and includes severe acute respiratory syndrome (SARS). SARS-CoV-2 was first detected in Wuhan, Hubei province of China in December 2019 and is now known as COVID-19 (Du et al 2020). The outbreak of COVID-19 has similarities to the 2003 outbreak of SARS, such as the cause of the infection, the epidemiological features of the disease, the pattern and speed of transmission and health care services being unprepared for the outbreak (Xiang et al 2020).

In the 21st century there has been an increase in the discovery of new coronaviruses, which include, SARS CoV, HCoV-NL63, HCoV-HKU1 and a number of others, such as the novel coronavirus (Zaki et al 2012), now known as the middle east respiratory syndrome coronavirus (MERS CO-V). With the number of coronaviruses emerging the World Health Organization (WHO) has warned that coronaviruses pose a serious threat to public health (WHO 2017). Thus COVID-19 is gaining intense attention nationally, internationally and globally. This has resulted in several measures urgently being put in place across the world to try to combat the spread. Measures include early identification and isolation of any diagnosed or suspected cases, as well as tracing and monitoring.

The coronavirus incubation period is between 2 to 14 days and contact amongst people who are infected with coronavirus in households, communities and health care facilities have contributed to the spread of the disease. Common physical symptoms include cough, temperature, fatigue, breathlessness and loss of smell and taste. Interestingly, a review of reported skin conditions in people with COVID-19 has found that although the coronavirus predominantly involves the epithelium (see Glossary) of the airways, evidence is growing that people are also presenting with several skin conditions. These symptoms have been observed in children and younger adults with a milder form of COVID-19, as well as in adults with a severe form of COVID-19. These findings may help early identification of the disease (Wollina et al 2020). However, the full psychological impact of COVID-19 on people recovering from the disease, those in lockdown, isolation and shielding, as well as health care professionals is unknown.

Psychological Effects of COVID-19

The 2003 SARS outbreak reported several mental health issues, including ongoing anxiety and depression, panic attacks, delirium, psychomotor excitement, psychotic symptoms, and suicidal thoughts (Liu et al 2003, Maunder et al 2003). Furthermore, anxiety and guilt around the effects of potential spread of the disease and stigma on families and friends was heightened by the public health responses of 14-day quarantine and mandatory contact tracing (Xiang et al 2020). During the COVID-19 quarantine in China, there were reports of psychological distress across the general population (Qiu et al 2020), reflecting the mental health issues seen in the SRAS outbreak (Chong et al 2004, Maunder et al 2003, McAlonan et al 2007).

To date the mental health and well-being of the general public and health care professionals, affected by the COVID-19 outbreak has been poorly addressed. The language used in the media, such as 'killer virus', has added to mental health issues by increasing people's fears and anxieties, leading to uncertainty and stress (Xiang et al 2020, Zhaokui 2020). For health care professionals the need for personal protective equipment (PPE), fears of potential infection from those they are treating and fears of transferring COVID-19 to their families is causing widespread anxiety and distress. These anxieties and fears, coupled with exhaustion as a result of the sheer number of people health care professionals are treating, is having a negative impact on their overall mental health and well-being.

In the 2003 SARS outbreak, health care professionals working in high-risk clinical settings, such as SARS units or those with family or friends with SARS, presented with higher levels of posttraumatic stress symptoms than those who have not experienced these situations (Wu et al 2009). Therefore health care professionals working in high-risk COVID-19 intensive care units are most vulnerable to mental health issues. This is confirmed by a rapid review and meta-analysis, which studied the occurrence, prevention, and management of the psychological effects of emerging virus outbreaks on health care professionals (Kisely et al 2020). This study described the psychological reactions of health care professionals from a variety of settings where there was an outbreak of an emerging virus, such as SARS, COVID-19, MERS, Ebola virus and influenza A virus. Psychological distress risk factors included being a parent of a dependent child or children, juniority or less experience, younger, with preexisting mental or physical health issues or having a member of the family with the virus. Other contributing factors included, length of quarantine, isolation, lack of practical support and stigma. However, psychological distress was seen to reduce if there was access to PPE, practical and psychological support, rest and clear communication systems. Studies also report that health care professionals working on the frontline during the COVID-19 outbreak are under moderate-to-severe stress and have increased levels of anxiety and depression (Du et al 2020, Kang et al 2020).

People with suspected or confirmed COVID-19 may also have fears of the outcome of the infection, because it is potentially fatal, whereas those in quarantine or shielding are reporting loneliness, boredom, and frustration. Anxiety, depression, anger, and despair have also been reported (Xiang et al 2020). In addition to this the adverse effects of medications for the common physical symptoms of cough, temperature and breathlessness can lead to insomnia compounding anxiety and mental distress in the general public (Xiang et al 2020). Thus in managing the COVID-19 outbreak, special attention needs to be made to both the public's mental health needs (Zandifar & Badrfam 2020), as well as health care professionals' mental health needs (Kisely et al 2020). In addition, understanding mental health needs will help health care professionals and the public prepare an appropriate response, as well as inform the quality and efficiency of future mental health interventions for such a crisis (Kang et al 2020, The King's Fund 2020).

MENTAL HEALTH NEEDS

It is thought that the effects of the COVID-19 pandemic on mental health will have profound and enduring consequences, but because of the lack of data it is unknown to what extent, duration or distribution (Pierce et al 2020). Even so, risk factors of long-term mental health issues have been identified as key predictors, which include posttrauma, social support and stressors experienced while recovering from COVID-19 (Ozer et al 2003). There are, therefore, three key challenges in meeting individual mental health needs (Campion 2019, WHO 2017):

1. To prevent an increase in COVID-19 related mental health issues and decrease in people's well-being across populations
2. To protect people with mental health issues from COVID-19 and related outcomes, due to their heightened vulnerability
3. To provide appropriate interventions for the public, health care professionals and carers

However, there is a lack of training for health care professionals in providing mental health care during and after COVID-19, which urgently needs to be addressed. As a consequence there is a lack of studies to guide clinical practice on mental health issues and psychiatric morbidity for people diagnosed or suspected to have COVID-19 (Xiang et al 2020).

Observations of psychological issues and measurements after the 2003 SARS outbreak may provide an understanding of the types of psychological interventions that would be beneficial to people in the current COVID-19 outbreak.

INTRODUCTION TO EVIDENCE

COVID-19 is a new disease and therefore there are limited data and a lack of comparisons from published international cohorts. Only a few studies have explored the course of the illness, patterns of practice, patient characteristics, utilization of resources, morbidity and mortality (Arentz et al 2020, Richardson et al 2020). However, there is some international research from Wuhan, China (Guan et al 2020, Huang et al 2020, Zhou et al 2020) and Lombardy, Italy (Grasselli et al 2020) which can be drawn upon, as well as previous research from other coronavirus outbreaks.

One study looked at the coping responses after the 2003 SARS outbreak and found that within a supportive health care environment, adaptive coping techniques were chosen by the health care professionals, whereas others chose humour or religion. It was concluded that psychological interventions to support health care professional must also address these preferences (Phua et al 2004). This would suggest that personalization is key and Dr Gail Stuart's stress adaptation model (Fig. 27.1) may be useful to apply in practice to support the COVID-19 recovery and rehabilitation.

There is evidence that digital interventions have a huge potential for public health (Campion 2019, Fairburn & Patel 2014, Munoz et al 2016) in the current COVID-19 crisis, supporting the mental health of carers and health care professionals and reducing social isolation with the ability to deliver education and training (Campion 2020). In addition, there are well-established digital interventions for anxiety and depression for issues such as insomnia (Andersson & Titov 2014). However, most digital interventions are for cognitive–behavioural therapy (Andersson & Titov 2014) and mindfulness interventions (Spijkerman et al 2016) with little evaluation of their effectiveness (Fairburn & Patel 2017). There

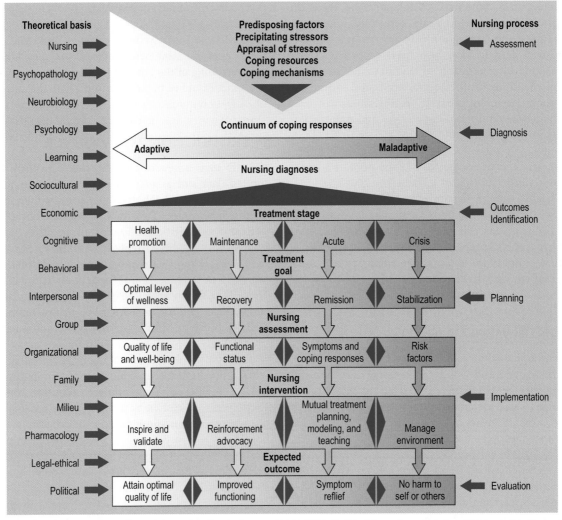

Fig. 27.1 ■ Stuart's stress adaptation model. (From Stuart, G. W. [2014]. *Principles and practice of psychiatric nursing.* St Louis, Missouri: Elsevier Mosby)

is also a lack of research on digital technology used to deliver relaxation techniques and psychological interventions during the COVID-19 pandemic. However, a systematic review of 49 studies using digital technology to disseminate psychological interventions where digital technology was used for training or education of health care professionals, treatment, diagnosis or management of mental health issues concluded that digital technology could increase workforce capacity, reach isolated groups of people and support younger people, empowering individuals and families to manage their own

care and support one another via online communities (Naslund et al 2017).

THEORIES BEHIND RELAXATION TECHNIQUES FOR COVID-19

The theory behind Stuart's stress adaptation model (see Fig. 27.1) is that it provides a framework of reference within which individuals, states of health, environments and care can be described, using a structure of observation, critical thinking and interpretation.

This model of health and well-being incorporates the biological, psychological, sociocultural, environmental and legal-ethical factors of health care, integrating care into a unified framework of practice (Stuart 2014). This model addresses the individual as part of a family as well as a group, community and society and includes three levels of prevention describing four key stages (Stuart 2014):

Stage 1: Crisis
Stage 2: Acute
Stage 3: Maintenance
Stage 4: Health promotion

These stages provide structure around which the COVID-19 crisis, recovery and rehabilitation needs may be met. Furthermore, delivery of psychological interventions via digital technology is thought to initiate positive behaviour change and improve emotional regulation (Jones et al 2014). For example, digital interaction is evidenced to enhance certain aspects of mindfulness training such as interactive breathing apps using colours to visualize the process of breathing. These apps improve mindful breathing training (Chittaro & Sioni 2014) through touching and swiping screens using animated ripples on the water accompanied by water sounds, which can enhance distancing and mindfulness (Chittaro & Vianello 2014).

COVID-19 Recovery and Rehabilitation

For the majority of the world's population, including health care professionals, behavioural and emotional responses can help individuals to adapt to the unprecedented levels of stress experienced during the COVID-19 outbreak. Therefore psychotherapeutic techniques based on Stuart's stress adaptation model (see Fig. 27.1) may be beneficial as a treatment intervention or framework (Folkman & Greer 2000, Maunder et al 2003) for COVID-19 survivors, health care professionals and people shielding and in quarantine. Furthermore, appropriate training in stress management, education around COVID-19, self-care, psychological support and relaxation techniques may be beneficial. These techniques along with strong family support can increase resilience to psychological symptoms and stress experienced in situations such as the COVID-19 outbreak (Du et al 2020).

ONLINE SUPPORT

As there are so many people isolated at home, through quarantine, shielding or advice from the government, new ways of working have developed to provide non-contact mental health interventions. As a consequence, there has been a growth in online mental health support using various different platforms for delivery such as websites, WeChat and apps. However, there is concern about the appropriateness of delivering these interventions to a collective target audience, such as health care professionals, the general public and those looking after people with COVID-19 or who are recovering from COVID-19 (Yao et al 2020). In the current situation with countries in isolation, online mental health interventions are better than having no mental health support at all and have been shown to relieve the pressure around mental health needs in a pandemic (Zhaokui 2020). Thus self-help through digital technology can be used to maximize existing resources. Examples of self-help resources can be found in Appendix 2. In addition, educational resources for health care professionals, students, volunteers and carers are available from e-Learning for Health (e-LfH), which have been developed by Health Education England (HEE) to increase knowledge around COVID-19 recovery and rehabilitation. Information on e-LfH can also be found in Appendix 2.

PRECAUTIONS AND CONSIDERATIONS

1. Internet literacy may be limited, requiring training and support.
2. Individuals may not have access to digital technology.
3. English maybe individuals' second language and therefore they may find it difficult to correctly and appropriately access online support and intervention.
4. Guidance regarding when and how to implement the intervention is paramount.
5. Awareness of the risk of excessive screen time needs to be addressed.
6. Recognition that there is a lack of regulatory procedures in place to ensure privacy and confidentiality of individuals' digital health data (Fairburn & Patel 2017).

KEY POINTS

1. Coronavirus disease 2019 (COVID-19) has reached pandemic levels, rapidly spreading across the world and placing our health care systems and resources under immense pressure.
2. The COVID-19 incubation period is between 2 to 14 days, and contact with people who are infected with coronavirus within households, communities and health care facilities have contributed to the spread of the disease.
3. The full psychological impact of COVID-19 on people recovering from the disease, those in lockdown, isolation and shielding and health care professionals is unknown.
4. Individuals in quarantine or shielding are reporting loneliness, boredom and frustration. Anxiety, depression, anger, posttraumatic distress and despair have also been reported.
5. The effects of the COVID-19 pandemic on mental health will have profound and enduring consequences, but it is unknown to what extent, duration or distribution.
6. For the majority of the world's population, including health care professionals, behavioural and emotional responses can help individuals to adapt to the unprecedented levels of stress experienced.
7. Self-help through digital technology can be used to maximize existing resources.

Reflection

Describe your understanding of COVID-19.

What changes will you make to your personal life and practice?

What is the main learning point you will take away from this chapter?

What is your future action plan in terms of using relaxation techniques/digital technology for COVID-19?

CASE STUDY LEARNING OPPORTUNITIES

The key points and reflection provide background and knowledge required in relation to the case studies, Audrey (Case Study 1) and Jonah (Case Study 2), to help deepen understanding of how relaxation techniques can help reduce psychological symptoms experienced through COVID-19.

CASE STUDY 1

Frontline Working Related Stress and Anxiety: *COVID-19 Outcomes for Audrey*

Audrey is 55 years old and is a nurse on the COVID-19 wards of the hospital she works for. She has been feeling very anxious and fearful about going into work. Audrey is aware that she is feeling threatened and vulnerable about catching COVID-19. She is also concerned about transmission to her family; this is fuelled not only by the risks associated with the job itself, but by her ethnic background, which reports have suggested put her, and therefore her family, at extra risk of not only catching, but dying from the coronavirus. Audrey has recognized this is affecting her ability to work and indeed her capacity to support her family in the way she would like. After reporting her concerns to occupational health, Audrey has been referred to you to seek support for her health and well-being. If possible, the hospital wants to sustain Audrey's ability to continuing working on

the COVID-19 wards, as staff rotas are already problematic because of people self-isolating or shielding.

After an initial assessment through a phone call, you virtually meet Audrey online via Zoom. Audrey explains to you that she does want to continue working on the COVID-19 wards if possible: it's her job and she cares deeply about the patients and does not want to let her colleagues down. Nonetheless, she feels insecure and afraid of the possible outcomes, and this is causing very stressful thoughts and fears. What if she contracts it herself? What if she takes it home? How will she live with the consequences? She is, after all, an 'at risk' category and no one is recognizing this or taking steps to address her concerns. Using simple cognitive–behavioural techniques, you explore the good points in the workplace and find there is good access to personal protective equipment, teamwork is excellent and communication channels are good. However, recognizing that much of Audrey's thinking is understandable, you decide that an adapted applied relaxation approach is likely to work best to support Audrey. You explain to Audrey how this works (see Chapter 9).

You begin by practicing a traditional tense–release relaxation cycle for the whole body to enable her to become aware of any tension held, either physically or emotionally. After completion, Audrey tells you that she recognized tension in her face, jaw, neck, and shoulders and had some success in releasing it. You the run through some simple deep breathing techniques, by inhaling through the nose, feeling the abdomen rise, and exhaling through the mouth three times. Returning to a normal but relaxed pattern of breathing, you explain to Audrey how this breathing technique can be used to help break cycles of anxiety or fear. Together you review a positive phrase or 'mantra' that Audrey can use when breathing out; she chooses 'I am calm'. You also ask her to think of an image or colour she associates with feeling calm, and she chooses the colour green. You then ask her to practice this deep breathing technique again, with the image of the colour and the word in her mind's eye. Returning to a normal pattern of breathing, you explain how the breathing techniques can be used in work and at home, whenever she feels tense or stressed. You ask Audrey to practice the tense–release cycle, along with the breathing techniques regularly over the next week and direct her to the online resources provided by occupational health that offer guided audio versions of to support her. You arrange a second Zoom meeting for the following week.

In the second session you compress the stages of applied relaxation further and run through a release only script. After discussion and feedback, you describe how scanning the body to pick up tension and relaxation can be used in any situation. You also practise the deep breathing along with the chosen cues – in this case, 'I am calm' and the colour green. You explore with Audrey situations that cause her stress in relation to work and she identifies thinking about work the day before a shift, driving into work and actually going onto the ward at specific points. Beginning with the one that feels least anxiety provoking, which for Audrey is worrying the night before work, you use a release-only script and a guided visualization of the situation asking Audrey to practice her cue word and colour to induce a more relaxed state when she begins to feel stressed. On completion, Audrey is able to see that this is a possible way to help her practise feeling calmer about her work situation. You ask Audrey to practise this technique and describe the process of graded exposure. Using this technique, the night before a shift Audrey can change the imagery to visualize herself getting into her car and driving, then entering the workplace. You advise Audrey to follow the online package provided by the workplace to support her with her ongoing journey.

CASE STUDY 2

Post–COVID-19 Recovery, Insomnia, Anxiety and Depression: *COVID-19 Outcomes for Jonah*

Jonah is 60 years old. He has a history of anxiety but was physically fit and well before contracting COVID-19. After a period of rehabilitation at one of the COVID-19 rehabilitation hospitals, he was discharged home with a package of techniques to support him in implementing the strategies he had learned during his rehabilitation. These comprised practical strategies for managing fatigue (pacing) in his everyday life, provided by an occupational therapist; a sitting and standing exercise regime from a physiotherapist; and breathing techniques to expand his lung function, including deep breathing and breath stacking techniques from a respiratory nurse specialist (see Chapter 4). Together, the package seems to be helping him get on with living reasonably well at home. However, he has been experiencing ongoing insomnia, anxiety and depression, which at times feels overwhelming. He feels that this is getting progressively worse and he is very emotional at times. After pressure from his wife, Jonah contacts his general practitioner, who prescribes antidepressants and refers him to you to consider whether relaxation techniques may assist. Your service is only providing online appointments at the moment, so you speak to Jonah via Skype.

On chatting to Jonah, it becomes clear that the anxiety and depression he is experiencing is affecting his quality of life. He reports how he has found 'the whole virus thing … you know lockdown and not being able to see the family' very distressing. He is also ruminating on his experience of having COVID-19 and worries about the future, both for himself and other members of his family. He is having difficulty getting off to sleep and is also frequently waking in the middle of the night; he is struggling to 'get back off' because he begins to ruminate and worry.

You direct Jonah to several online platforms providing psychological interventions developed to support people experiencing stress and anxiety in their everyday lives. These links offer a comprehensive package of techniques and options, including a tense–release script on YouTube, which you recommend to Jonah, explaining to him how this will help him recognize tension in his body. You explain that you want him to run through this a few times because it is a good step to build on for other techniques, like release-only and autogenic relaxation (see Chapter 20). The pamphlet you will email has links to sites that provide these options too, and you suggest he listens to this type of relaxation on his phone before going to bed and when he wakes up in the middle of the night. You also suggest a mindful breathing and mindful walking script (see Chapter 23) on the YouTube platform; you advise that the mindful walking can be used as a form of guided imagery, so he does not actually have to physically go out until he feels stronger. You agree a time for a follow-up call in 3 weeks' time.

When you meet Jonah for his review on Skype, he tells you that he has found the relaxation practice useful in helping him feel less 'wound up'. He did not like the tense–release type, though, because he felt it made him tenser. You explain that this is not unusual. He also reports that the mindful breathing and guided walking technique have been used very successfully both during the day and to help him sleep. His wife, Mariah, has also enjoyed these because she is self-isolating as a result underlying conditions and thus is not going out. They have walked their favourite walk together in their mind a few times now, and they can even hold hands when they are doing it.

ACTIVITY

For each of the case studies:

1. List key aspects used in COVID-19 rehabilitation.
2. Write down the impact post–COVID-19 rehabilitation is having from a psychological perspective.
3. Write down the impact post–COVID-19 rehabilitation is having from a physical perspective.
4. Write down the impact post–COVID-19 rehabilitation is having from an emotional perspective.
5. Consider the outcomes quality of life and overall well-being.

This chapter concludes Section 4 on application to practice. Chapter 28 will begin section 5, working towards best practice, commencing with measurement, to enable a decision on which outcome measures would best capture the person's response to relaxation techniques and psychosocial interventions.

REFERENCES

Andersson, G., & Titov, N. (2014). Advantages and limitations of internet-based interventions for common mental disorders. *World Psychiatry*, 13, 4–11.

Arentz, M., Yim, E., Klaff, L., et al. (2020). Characteristics and outcomes of 21 critically ill patients with COVID-19 in Washington State. *The Journal of the American Medical Association*, 323(16), 1612–1614.

Campion, J. (2019). *Public mental health: Evidence, practice and commissioning*. Retrieved June 2020 from https://www.rsph.org.uk/our-work/policy/wellbeing/public-mentalhealth-evidence-practice-and-commissioning.html.

Campion, J. (2020). *Public mental health*. MindEd e-Learning Programme (469-0001). DH e-Learning for Healthcare. Retrieved June 2020 from https://www.minded.org.uk/Component/Details/632895.

Chittaro, L., & Sioni, R. (2014). Evaluating mobile apps for breathing training: The effectiveness of visualization. *Computers in Human Behavior*, 40, 56–63.

Chittaro, L., & Vianello, A. (2014). Computer-supported mindfulness: Evaluation of a mobile thought distancing application on naive meditators. *International Journal of Human-Computer Studies*, 72(3), 337–348.

Chong, M. Y., Qang, W. C., Hsieh, W. C., et al. (2004). Psychological impact of severe acute respiratory syndrome on health workers in a tertiary hospital. *British Journal of Psychiatry, 185*, 127–133.

Du, J., Dong, L., Wang, T., et al. (2020). Psychological symptoms among frontline healthcare workers during COVID-19 outbreak in Wuhan. *General Hospital Psychiatry, 67*, 144–145.

Fairburn, C. G., & Patel, V. (2014). The global dissemination of psychological treatments: A road map for research and practice. *American Journal of Psychiatry, 171*, 495–498.

Fairburn, C. G., & Patel, V. (2017). The impact of digital technology on psychological treatments and their dissemination. *Behaviour Research and Therapy, 88*, 19–25.

Folkman, S., & Greer, S. (2000). Promoting psychological well-being in the face of serious illness: When theory, research and practice inform each other. *Psychooncology, 9*, 11–19.

Grasselli, G., Zangrillo, A., Zanella, A., et al. (2020). Baseline characteristics and outcomes of 1591 patients infected with SARS-CoV-2 admitted to ICUs of the Lombardy region. *The Journal of the American Medical Association, 323*(16), 1574–1581.

Guan, W. J., Ni, Z. Y., Hu, Y., et al. (2020). China Medical Treatment Expert Group for Covid-19. Clinical characteristics of coronavirus disease 2019 in China. *New England Journal of Medicine, 382*, 708–720.

Huang, C., Wang, Y., Li, X., et al. (2020). Clinical features of patients infected with 2019 novel coronavirus in Wuhan, China. *Lancet, 395*, 497–506.

Jones, C. M., Scholes, L., Johnson, D., Katsikitis, M., & Carras, M. C. (2014). Gaming well: Links between videogames and flourishing mental health. *Frontiers in Psychology, 5*, 260.

Kang, L., Li, Y., Shaohua, H., et al. (2020). The mental health of medical workers in Wuhan, China dealing with the 2019 novel coronavirus. *Lancet, 7*, E-14.

King's Fund, The. (2020). *What has Covid-19 taught us about supporting workforce mental health and wellbeing?* Retrieved June 2020 from https://www.kingsfund.org.uk/blog/2020/06/covid-19-supporting-workforce-mental-health.

Kisely, S., Warren, N., McMahon, L., Dalais, C., Henry, I., & Siskind, D. (2020). Occurrence, prevention, and management of the psychological effects of emerging virus outbreaks on healthcare workers: Rapid review and meta-analysis. *British Medical Journal, 369*, m1642.

Liu, T. B., Chen, X. Y., Miao, G. D., et al. (2003). Recommendations on diagnostic criteria and prevention of SARS-related mental disorders. *Journal of Clinical Psychological Medicine, 13*, 188–191 [in Chinese].

Maunder, R., Hunter, J., Vincent, L., et al. (2003). The immediate psychological and occupational impact of the 2003 SARS outbreak in a teaching hospital. *Canadian Medical Association Journal, 168*, 1245–1251.

McAlonan, G. M., Lee, A. M., Cheung, V., et al. (2007). Immediate and sustained psychological impact of an emerging infectious disease outbreak on healthcare workers. *Canadian Journal of Psychiatry, 52*(4), 241–247.

Munoz, R. F., Bunge, E. L., Chen, K., et al. (2016). Massive open online interventions: A novel model for delivering behavioural-health services worldwide. *Clinical Psychological Science, 4*, 194–205.

Naslund, J. A., Aschbrenner, K. A., Araya, R., et al. (2017). Digital technology for treating and preventing mental disorders in low-income and middle-income countries: A narrative review of the literature. *Lancet Psychiatry, 4*(6), 486–500.

Ozer, E. J., Best, S. R., Lipsey, T. L., & Weiss, D. S. (2003). Predictors of posttraumatic stress disorder and symptoms in adults: A meta-analysis. *Psychology Bulletin, 129*, 52–73.

Phua, D. H., Tang, H. K., & Tham, K. Y. (2004). Coping responses of emergency physicians and nurses to the 2003 severe acute respiratory syndrome outbreak. *Academy of Emergency Medicine, 12*(4), 322–328.

Pierce, M., McManus, S., Jessop, C., et al. (2020). Says who? The significance of sampling in mental health surveys during COVID-19. *Lancet Psychiatry, 7*(7), 567–568.

Qiu, J., Shen, B., Zhao, M., Wang, Z., Xie, B., & Xu, Y. (2020). A nationwide survey of psychological distress among Chinese people in the COVID-19 epidemic: Implications and policy recommendations. *General Psychiatry, 33*(2), e100213.

Richardson, S., Hirsch, J. S., Narasimhan, M., et al., and Northwell COVID-19 Research Consortium (2020). Presenting characteristics, comorbidities, and outcomes among 5700 patients hospitalized with Covid-19 in the New York City area. *The Journal of the American Medical Association, 323*(20), 2052–2059.

Spijkerman, M. P. J., Pots, W. T. M., & Bohlmeijer, E. T. (2016). Effectiveness of online mindfulness-based interventions in improving mental health: A review and meta-analysis of randomised controlled trials. *Clinical Psychology Review, 45*, 102–114.

Stuart, G. W. (2014). *Principles and practice of psychiatric nursing* (10th ed.). London: Elsevier Health Sciences.

Wollina, U., Karadag, A. S., Rowland-Payne, C., Chiriac, A., & Lotti, T. (2020). Cutaneous signs in COVID-19 patients: A review. *Dermatologic Therapy*, e13549.

World Health Organization (WHO). *Mental health atlas 2017*. Retrieved June 2020 from https://apps.who.int/iris/bitstream/handle/10665/272735/9789241514019-eng.pdf?ua=1.

Wu, P., Fang, Y., Guan, Z., et al. (2009). The psychological impact of the SARS epidemic on hospital employees in China: Exposure, risk perception, and altruistic acceptance of risk. *Canadian Journal of Psychiatry, 54*, 302–311.

Xiang, Y. T., Yang, Y., Li, W., et al. (2020). Timely mental health care for the 2019 novel coronavirus outbreak is urgently needed. *Lancet Psychiatry Comment, 7*, 228–229.

Yao, H., Chen, J. H., & Xu, Y. F. (2020). Rethinking online mental health services in China during the COVID-19 epidemic. *Asian Journal of Psychiatry, 50*, 102015.

Zaki, A. M., Van Boheemen, S., Bestebroer, T. M., Osterhause, A. D. M. E., & Fouchier, R. A. M. (2012). Isolation of a novel coronavirus from a man with pneumonia in Saudi Arabia. *New England Journal of Medicine, 367*, 1814–1820.

Zandifar, A., & Badrfam, R. (2020). Iranian mental health during the COVID-19 epidemic. *Asian Journal of Psychiatry, 51*, 101990.

Zhaokui, D. (2020). China adopts non-contact free consultation to help the public cope with the psychological pressure caused by new coronavirus pneumonia. *Asian Journal of Psychiatry, 52*, 102093.

Zhou, F., Yu, T., Du, R., et al. (2020). Clinical course and risk factors for mortality of adult inpatients with COVID-19 in Wuhan, China: A retrospective cohort study. *Lancet, 395*, 1054–1062.

Section 5

WORKING TOWARDS BEST PRACTICE

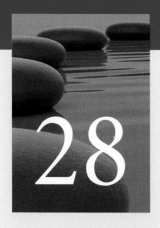

28

MEASUREMENT

DR CAROLINE BELCHAMBER

LEARNING OBJECTIVES

The aim of this chapter is to understand the importance of measuring the outcome of relaxation techniques.

By the end of this chapter you will be able to:

1. Understand the importance of validity and reliability of measurement tools.

2. Appreciate the need to choose an appropriate measurement tool.

3. Ascertain the importance of patient assessment.

4. Recognize key aspects of relaxation training assessment.

5. Acknowledge the different tools used in psychological and physiological assessments.

6. Identify the differences and similarities between research, service evaluation and audit.

This chapter will conclude with key points and time for reflection, providing learning opportunities through a case study.

INTRODUCTION TO MEASUREMENT

This chapter is devoted to the topic of measurement and includes discussion on the evidence of validity and reliability of measurement tools, patient assessment and clinical audit. Measurement, in this context, is the process of observing and recording the outcomes resulting from treatment intervention. Measurement, however, is not finite; errors and uncertainties can arise, undermining accuracy. To minimize this effect, assessment tools need to be reliable and valid.

Selecting the most appropriate tool can be challenging because there are many kinds of measuring tools, including questionnaires, self-assessment inventories, sweat sensors, heart rate monitors and biofeedback monitors. Before deciding on the measuring tool, some basic questions should be considered, such as: What is likely to change as a result of applying the treatment intervention? What is it I am trying to measure?

Is there a validated tool that I can use? Is it applicable for this population, with regard to age, gender, culture and condition? Do I need training to be able to use it? Is it freely available or do I need to purchase it? How often should I use it?

Knowledge and experience of the topic may help to suggest a suitable measurement tool. If not, the World Confederation of Physical Therapy provides links to a wide range of evidence-based centres and organizations. Box 28.1 contains contact information about this and other sources of information. As some tools are designed for particular diseases or certain population groups (such as children or older people), it is therefore necessary to check that the selected measurement tool is an appropriate one. Introduction to the evidence will explore some of the key measurement tools that can be used to measure anxiety, depression and mental health, which will provide further information on this topic. Other measurement tools available will briefly be discussed further on in the chapter.

INTRODUCTION TO EVIDENCE

Audit as a measuring tool is not supported by robust evidence (Benjamin 2008); however, a number of studies have explored the validity and reliability of measurement tools.

Two major reviews of the Hospital Anxiety and Depression Scale (HADS) (Herrmann 1997, Bjelland et al 2002) reinforced its two-dimensional structure of anxiety and depression, construct validity, internal consistency and test-retest reliability. However, Martin's (2005) review of HADS challenged its content validity, concluding that it is a three-dimensional rather than a two-dimensional measure, which means it is not a reliable and valid measure of anxiety and depression. However, a more recent systematic review and meta-analysis of HADS was used to determine the screening efficacy for depression and mental health disorders in cancer patients. The results from the 28 studies reviewed indicated that HADS diagnostic accuracy varied widely even though it is an extensively validated screening tool for emotional distress. The study concluded that HADS is consistently superior for screening depression than it is for mental health disorders (Vodermaier & Millman 2011). HADS reliability as a tool for screening depression is reinforced by Yuan and colleagues (2019), who assessed the reliability and criterion validity of the Patient Health Questionnaire-9 (PHQ-9) versus HADS – Depression (HADS-D) as a screening tool for people with acute coronary syndrome. There were 782 people who participated in the study, completing the PHQ-9 and HADS-D questionnaires. The International Neuropsychiatric Interview (MINI) was used to assess validity. The study concluded that both PHQ-9 and HADS-D are reliable and valid screening tools for major depressive disorders.

A major review of the Beck Depression Inventory (BDI) demonstrated internal consistency and test-retest reliability (Richter et al 1998). However, Boyle (1985) states that high internal consistency may indicate item redundancy and stability of scores may be due to insensitivity to variations in depression. Another study found evidence of instability due to the order of the answer options, which may have a carryover effect when the measurement is repeated (Demyttenaere & de Fruyt 2003). Furthermore, two studies concluded that the format of the response is not suitable for telephone use (Arnau et al 2001, Williams et al 2002). Content validity was also challenged in relation to depression, due to the number of items used. Therefore people with different backgrounds and treatment requirements could potentially end up with the same end score (Demyttenaere & de Fruyt 2003). In addition, BDI's ability to distinguish between depression and anxiety has been questioned (Enns et al 1998, Richter et al 1998); however, BDI is able to differentiate between people with depression and those without (Fitzpatrick et al 2009).

Dunstan and colleagues (2017) re-examined the characteristics of Zung's Self-Rating Depression Scale

(SDS) and Self-Rating Anxiety Scale (SAS). They compared the self-report measures with the Depression Anxiety Stress Scale (DASS) in relation to their ability to predict a clinical diagnosis of anxiety and depression against the Patient Health Questionnaire (PHQ). Participants consisted of 376 adults, with 87 participants reporting that they were receiving psychological treatment at the time. Results indicated that the DASS was a slightly stronger predictor of PHQ diagnosis of anxiety and depression. Even so, the Zung indices performance was seen to be a very acceptable comparison. The study also found that DASS performed higher on specificity, whereas the Zung scales performed higher on sensitivity. The researchers suggest having more conservative cut-offs to enable similar numbers of 'misses' and 'false positives' to those acquired with DASS, but further research was required to find the optimum cut-off levels.

A systematic review of goal setting and goal attainment scaling investigated the reliability, validity and sensitivity of the measurement tools as outcome measures in people of working age and older. A literature search was carried out over a 36-year period from the introduction of the theory of goal setting. Key findings demonstrated strong evidence of reliability, validity and sensitivity of goal attainment scaling. There was, however, limited sensitivity and reliability in goal setting, but evidence was found to support validity in this measurement tool (Hurn et al 2006).

To understand this evidence further, the theory behind measurement tool characteristics will be discussed.

THEORIES BEHIND MEASUREMENT TOOLS

The process of measurement enables the researcher to establish if and in what quantity a characteristic is present and ensures the right conclusions are reached. The characteristics of a measure, therefore, needs to be precise, reliable and valid (Davis 2004, Waltz et al 2004) to provide credibility to the research study. Precision means that the measure needs to be reproducible – that is, it repeatedly produces a consistent and accurate value each time it is used, providing confidence that it is measuring the differences between individuals rather than differences in the measurement tool.

Physiological measurement tools need to be calibrated to ensure they generate identical values and minimize measurement error. In contrast, psychological measurement tools depend on reliability and validity as they cannot be calibrated. In physiological measurement tools, internal reliability provides a way to calculate the amount of measurement error (Houser 2008). In psychological measurement tools, an item-total correlation is used, which represents the consistency of a person's performance on a single item with the person's overall performance across all items. Interreliability is an additional measure which measures the stability amongst raters, with stability over time measured by a test-retest correlation coefficient (Sim & Wright 2005).

A measurement tool can be consistent and precise, but that doesn't mean that it is measuring what is required. A measurement tool therefore is only valid if it accurately represents what is being measured. This involves assessing content validity, which is a subjective judgement on the measurement tool with regards to what it is measuring – for example, experts in the topic area have verified that the correct concepts are incorporated into the measurement tool. Construct validity then indicates whether the measurement tool captures the conceptual basis for the variable (Houser 2008). Criterion-related validity correlates the measurement tool to an external appearance of the characteristic. Two other forms of validity are also considered: predictive validity, which indicates that a measurement tool can predict future performance; and discriminate validity, where the measurement tool has the ability to differentiate between individuals who have a characteristic from individuals who do not.

Thus the psychometric characteristics of a measurement tool include its precision, reliability and validity. These characteristics are taken into account when a measurement tool is tested and must attain an appropriate level of reliability and validity to be accepted for a research study or used as part of patient assessment.

The reader will now be taken through the process of assessment and provided with a few examples of assessment / measurement tools which could be used in the context of relaxation. A section on measuring exercise intensity is also included to illustrate how assessment can be applied to physical activity (see Chapter 15).

PATIENT ASSESSMENT

Assessment means 'deciding' or 'judging' the 'amount, value, or importance of something' (McIntosh 2013), in this case deciding on the degree of stress, anxiety or relaxation present in an individual. Two types of information are found during assessment: objective and subjective. *Objective* information is factual and measurable. *Subjective* information relates to the personal experience of the individual, their interpretation of events and other thoughts and feelings. Both areas of information are equally important in gaining an understanding of the problem (Table 28.1). Assessment is ongoing and the health care professional will constantly monitor, reassess and update the information gathered.

Assessment Tools

The most commonly used tool for initial assessment is the clinical interview. In the course of this and in a relatively short time, relevant information will emerge. This will refer to previous medical history, current signs and symptoms, reason for referral and information specific to the person's sense of current well-being. The findings from this interview will be written up in case notes. Other assessments may also be undertaken at this time or on subsequent visits.

The data collected can be broadly grouped into three categories: nominal, functional and attitudinal. *Nominal* data describe people by their ethnic origin, place of residence and the type of work they do. Such data give some idea of the person's identity and allows the health care professional to make a few assumptions such as the ability to attend weekly classes. They may also provide some clues about stress levels.

Functional data are items of information which reflect the overall functional ability of the individual, such as their inclination to learn from and apply knowledge, their ability to cope with general tasks or demands and their willingness to discuss health and well-being. Functional data include the readiness of the person to take part in relaxation, exercise or other physical activity, a feature which is highlighted by the World Health Organization's International Classification of Functioning (ICF) checklist (WHO 2003).

Attitudinal data are gathered by taking account of the people's opinions, mindset and cultural beliefs. By asking questions, the health care professional can elicit information which will be helpful when analyzing the data and in selecting an appropriate intervention.

Assessment findings should be reviewed with the person, checking that they understand the findings and giving them time to ask questions. The proposed intervention is then discussed with the individual, together with its likely timescale. It is important to gain the person's consent before proceeding any further. Where function is limited, measurement is accompanied by a standardized assessment. This is a tool with a clearly defined scope, designed to identify a particular aspect of a condition. It has typically been through a process to check its reliability and validity. Such standard measures usually carry instructions regarding method of scoring and interpretation of results (Burlingame & Blaschko 2002). They will also indicate the type of professional for whom they are designed.

Relaxation Training Assessment

Relaxation training, assessment is required to do the following:

1. Obtain a profile of the individual's problems as they are observed and expressed by the individual and communicated to the health care professional. It is likely that the relaxation training will be part of a wider programme of anxiety management, in which case the activities of the relevant professionals will need to be integrated.

TABLE 28.1	
Examples of Objective and Subjective Information	
Objective Information	**Subjective Information**
Blood pressure	People's interpretation of their stress
Pulse	
Respiration rate	How well (or unwell) they feel
Temperature	Degree to which they like
Distance that can be walked in a given time	a particular relaxation technique
Ability to follow relaxation instruction	Their belief in the usefulness of relaxation and or exercise as an intervention for stress
Ability to complete exercise diary	Types of physical activity they find most satisfying
Quality of sleep – ability to record hours of sleep	

2. Measure existing indicators of stress: for example, heart rate, blood pressure, anxiety levels. One or more of these measures can provide a baseline when evaluating progress. The assessment should be carried out after a short period of rest to allow for the relaxation effects which occur, in the absence of any relaxation technique, as part of the process of adapting to a restful environment.

3. Inform decisions regarding the selection of interventions: for example, where there are high levels of worrying intrusive thoughts, cognitive–behavioural approaches may be recommended.

4. Measure the benefits of the relaxation training in terms of key outcomes over time. A key outcome could be muscle tension, heart rate, mood state or sense of well-being. This can be assessed before and immediately after a relaxation session and/or 1 week and up to 6 months following relaxation training. Alternatively, assessment may focus on symptoms such as tension headache or hypertension and the degree to which these have been relieved by the relaxation training.

5. Evaluate the success of the intervention and provide feedback to both the health care professional and the participant. Positive feedback acts as a reinforcer, negative feedback indicates the need for corrective action.

6. Gather quantifiable data for the purpose of retrospective research or where data are being collected as part of an intervention study, for example, measuring the effectiveness of relaxation in reducing tension headaches.

Although assessment is time-consuming, it is an essential process with clear benefits.

For those who wish to manage their own stress and anxiety, and who are using this book as a self-help guide, self-monitoring is also important. (See next for ways in which the reader can measure their own progress.)

Ways of Measuring Relaxation

Relaxation has psychological, physiological and behavioural components, so a test which is restricted to only one of these cannot claim to be comprehensive.

To give an accurate measure of the degree of relaxation present, standardized assessment should cover all three components. Only an assessment which takes account of these multiple dimensions can reflect the complexity of the relaxation state.

Since there is no test which covers all three, the components must be measured separately.

PSYCHOLOGICAL ASSESSMENT

Measurement covers a wide range of psychosocial factors including mood state, anxiety and depression, mental health and quality of life. This type of assessment is generally undertaken by questionnaires and self-rating scales. Two key examples of self-rating scales for depression and anxiety are Zung's SDS and SAS (Dunstan et al 2017). Where questionnaires and self-rating scales indicate moderate-to-severe depression or anxiety, referral to the general practitioner or other specialist within the health care team should be considered. Previous medical history is also an important factor.

Questionnaires

A questionnaire is a list of questions requiring 'yes/no' or similar answers, which can be converted into numerical scores. Its purpose is to obtain information about a specific topic. A standardized questionnaire is the instrument of choice as it will have been tested on different groups of people and average scores will have been established, against which the individual's scores can be compared. As a validated assessment tool, this kind of questionnaire is the only kind that can be used for quantitative assessment and research. In the case of relaxation, such a questionnaire could be used to obtain information both at the start and at the end of a course of treatment, in order to see how people progress and to compare them with groups diagnosed as 'anxious' or 'normal', for example.

The advantages of questionnaires are that they are quick, cheap and easy to complete. It is also easy to collate the results. Their disadvantages include the possibility of inaccuracy if the questions are misunderstood or if information is missed out, if forcing responses into 'yes/no' categories should fail to express the complexity of a person's position.

1	2	3	4
Not at all	Somewhat	Moderately so	Very much so

			1	2	3	4
A	I feel at ease		1	2	3	4
B	I feel upset		1	2	3	4

(A)

1	2	3	4
Almost never	Sometimes	Often	Almost always

			1	2	3	4
A	I am a steady person		1	2	3	4
B	I lack self-confidence		1	2	3	4

(B)

Fig. 28.1 ■ (A) The State Anxiety Scale consists of 20 statements that evaluate how respondents feel 'right now, at this moment'. (B) The Trait Anxiety Scale consists of 20 statements that assess how respondents feel 'generally'.

The Interview Schedule

An alternative and more sensitive approach is to use an interview schedule. Here, the interviewer guides the individual through the questions, making sure those questions have been understood and drawing fuller answers than are possible in a questionnaire. Thus the interview schedule provides more detailed and more complete information than the questionnaire. Quantifying the additional information, however, is more difficult and the interview schedule is subject to variability between interviewers, each of whom may have different ways of interviewing people. The value of the interview depends to a great extent on the clinical experience and judgement of the interviewer.

Examples of Questionnaires

There is a wide range of standardized questionnaires available, each designed to measure specific or generic aspects of mental distress. The following are examples of questionnaires that may be considered for measuring anxiety, depression and mental health.

- *State Trait Anxiety Inventory Y (STAI Y)* (Spielberger 1980). This contains 40 questions in two 20-item scales with a range of four possible responses to each. They measure differentiates between the temporary condition of 'state anxiety' and the more general and long-standing 'trait anxiety'. The scale measures feelings of apprehension, tension and nervousness. It is the most widely used instrument for measuring anxiety and is available in 40 languages. The inventory takes 10 minutes to complete. This tool has been found to be sensitive to measuring change in state anxiety following relaxation training. An example of the questions is provided in Fig. 28.1.

- *The Hospital Anxiety and Depression Scale (HAD)* (Zigmond & Snaith 1983). This contains 14 items, 7 relating to anxiety and seven to depression. The score gives an indication of the degree to which the individual is suffering from either condition. The scale is also able to pick up alterations over time.

■ *The Short Form 36 (SF-36)* (Ware & Sherbourne 1992). This measure consists of 36 questions and is designed to provide information regarding a person's current physical and emotional health, including the ability to participate in daily activities and work. The questions were designed to be easy to understand and relevant to most people's lives. It was originally developed in the United States and is now one of the most commonly used measures of quality of life. It has been translated into many languages and has been used as an outcome measure in more than 2000 studies.

■ *The Beck Depression Inventory* (Beck 1988, Beck et al 1961). Measures of the level of depression can be obtained from this questionnaire which can be used at different stages of illness and recovery.

■ *The Cognitive Anxiety Questionnaire* (Lindsay & Hood 1982). This contains 12 items and reflects some of the most common thoughts associated with anxiety. It measures the tendency of the individual to engage in such thoughts.

These are all simple screening devices for use with individuals. The results, when obtained at the beginning and end of a training course, give an indication of change over time in the individual concerned. The results can also be used to assess the effectiveness of relaxation training on groups of people and can be used in clinical trials under controlled conditions.

HADS (Fig. 28.2) has been picked as an example because of its widespread use and general applicability. Questions 1, 4, 5, 8, 9, 12 and 13 relate to anxiety, and questions 2, 3, 6, 7, 10, 11 and 14 relate to depression. Scoring instructions are attached to the assessment sheet but not included here. A score of 8 to 10 in either section indicates a mild degree of the condition, whereas a score of 11 or higher suggests the advisability of referral to a specialist agency. Although the scale is seen as a screening tool, it is, in the present context, used primarily to measure tendencies to states of distress which may change over the period in which relaxation is practised. Any resulting change should not, however, be totally attributed to relaxation, because other factors such as changing environmental circumstances may be contributing to alterations in scores.

Tests show that the HAD possesses a considerable degree of validity and reliability although, as with most scales, further testing is required before confident judgements on its performance can be made. The scale is also easy to understand and has been found acceptable to patients, taking only 5 minutes to complete (Bowling 2017).

Some of these tools, such as the State Trait Anxiety Inventory, need to be purchased. Others, like HADS, are freely available. Bowling (2017) provides a comprehensive overview of subjective health, well-being and quality of life measurement scales and includes new measurement tools such as the World Health Organization quality of life (WHOQOL) measurement tools and the Warwick-Edinburgh Well-Being Scale (WEWBS).

Self-Rating

Related to the questionnaire is the self-rating scale – that is, the rating an individual gives themselves. It often takes the form of a visual analogue. Though it is a highly subjective assessment, it nevertheless has value since relaxation is an internal state with a strong subjective component. The self-rating scale is particularly useful for recording levels of pain and anxiety. Two forms are described here.

■ A rating scale in the form of a line calibrated from 0 to 10 where 0 represents total relaxation and 10 represents maximum tension. The intervening numbers refer to intermediate states. The participant rings the appropriate number.

■ A rating scale which consists of numbered descriptors signifying different degrees of relaxation and tension, as in Poppen's (1998) self-rating scale (see Chapter 10). Again, the participant rings the appropriate number.

These may be used before and after the relaxation session. Marking scales in this way gives a measure of the effect of the treatment.

Another form of self-monitoring is the diary, seen as a useful way of logging feelings of tension and situations of high anxiety. The diary can be used to record immediate change after a relaxation session and also change over a longer period. It provides feedback and can act as an extrinsic motivator, helping to ensure that practice is carried out.

A record sheet is another way of logging the occurrence and intensity of anxious feelings. Fig. 9.2

SECTION 1

NAME: DATE: AGE:

This section is designed to help identify how you feel. Read each item and place a tick in the box opposite the reply which comes closest to how you have been feeling in the past few weeks. Don't take too long over your replies: your immediate reaction to each item will probably be more accurate than a long thought-out response.

Tick only one box in each section

(1) I feel tense or 'wound up':
   Most of the time
   A lot of the time
   Time to time. Occasionally
   Not at all

(2) I feel as if I am slowed down:
   Nearly all the time
   Very often
   Sometimes
   Not at all

(3) I still enjoy the things I used to enjoy:
   Definitely as much
   Not quite so much
   Only a little
   Hardly at all

(4) I get a sort of frightened feeling like 'butterflies' in the stomach:
   Not at all
   Occasionally
   Quite often
   Very often

(5) I get a sort of frightened feeling as if something awful is about to happen:
   Very definitely and quite badly
   Yes, but not too badly
   A little, but it doesn't worry me
   Not at all

(6) I have lost interest in my appearance:
   Definitely
   I don't take so much care as I should
   I may not take quite as much care
   I take just as much care as ever

(7) I can laugh and see the funny side of things:
   As much as I always could
   Not quite so much now
   Definitely not so much now
   Not at all

(8) I feel restless as if I have to be on the move:
   Very much indeed
   Quite a lot
   Not very much
   Not at all

(9) Worrying thoughts go through my mind:
   A great deal of the time
   A lot of the time
   From time to time but not too often
   Only occasionally

(10) I look forward with enjoyment to things:
   As much as ever I did
   Rather less than I used to
   Definitely less than I used to
   Hardly at all

(11) I feel cheerful:
   Not at all
   Not often
   Sometimes
   Most of the time

(12) I get sudden feelings of panic:
   Very often indeed
   Quite often
   Not very often
   Not at all

(13) I can sit at ease and feel relaxed:
   Definitely
   Usually
   Not often
   Not at all

(14) I can enjoy a good book or radio or TV programme:
   Often
   Sometimes
   Not often
   Very seldom

Fig. 28.2 ■ The Hospital Anxiety and Depression Scale. (Adapted from Zigmond & Snaith 1983 with permission from the authors. Reproduced from Powell and Enright 1990, Fig. 3.3, with permission from Routledge, Taylor & Francis Books Ltd.)

illustrates this approach and contains a numbered scale relating to feelings, together with details of the particular coping strategy adopted.

Homework can be recorded on a form such as that in Fig. 9.3. This is a useful method of ensuring that practice is carried out, as well as providing an indication of the degree of benefit obtained.

Written self-reports have the advantage of being quick, easy, cheap and non-threatening to the participant. They are an essential part of the process in dealing with varying levels of stress and anxiety. Monitoring relaxation sessions, that is, writing down feelings and behaviours immediately before and after the session and then at other key points throughout the day, provides an element of control over situations of stress/anxiety, where feelings of helplessness or limited control might otherwise prevail.

The value of self-rating lies particularly on an individual level, where it helps the person to check their own progress. It is less useful in research, where two or more groups are being compared and where a validated questionnaire would be the tool of choice. A range of self-report measures can be found in Johnstone et al (1995) and Holbrook (2011).

PHYSIOLOGICAL ASSESSMENT

Assessing the effect of relaxation training on body systems provides an objective measurement. A variety of indicators are in current use, including pulse rate, blood pressure, respiratory rate, muscle tension, peripheral blood flow, palmar sweating and electrical activity in the brain. Most of these can easily be measured and machines are available for the purpose. The results show the level of physiological arousal in an individual, and the test or tests are carried out before and after relaxation sessions. The baseline is established before training begins and, in common with all pretreatment measures, should be recorded after a short period of rest.

It might be supposed that this approach offered the perfect solution. The field of physiological assessment, however, it is not as straightforward as it appears. Keable (1997) discusses certain points.

■ Physiological measures can be distorted by circumstances. The individual may have eaten before a relaxation session, which would result in artificially low arousal scores; the person may have taken exercise immediately before, which would raise their scores; emotional distress would also raise them and drugs would distort them. Tests therefore need to be conducted under controlled conditions.

■ Because the physiological response of individuals is to some extent idiosyncratic, a single measure may not include relevant information. To gain an accurate picture, therefore, a system which provides multiple measurements is needed.

Poppen (1998) adds the following point.

■ Even in the case of specific symptoms, it is not always clear how their measurement should be approached. In tension headache, for example, it might be thought that electromyography of the surrounding muscles would be appropriate; however, exactly which muscles should be measured is less clear. Or again, instead of measuring the electrical activity, it might be more constructive to measure the blood flow through the surrounding muscles (Olton & Noonberg 1980). Researchers hold different views.

Furthermore, while measurement of the pulse and breathing rate are simple procedures, most other physiological measures require equipment and expertise, neither of which may be available. In spite of these difficulties, however, physiological measurement is an important part of general assessment.

MEASURING CHANGE THROUGH GOAL SETTING

All stress-reducing programmes have a goal. It may be getting to the supermarket without experiencing feelings of panic; it may be facing an audience without shaking with fright. These goals can seem insurmountable to the individual who has high levels of stress. One solution is to break them down into short-term goals as these will appear more manageable than the main goal while yet leading in the desired direction (see Fig. 19.1). The concept of a goal can be compared with a staircase where the main goal is to reach the landing above; the easiest way of doing this is by travelling through the intervening steps. Goal setting is a useful way of measuring behaviour change with Goal Attainment Scaling (GAS) adopted by many human and rehabilitation services (Calsyn & Davidson 1978, Williams & Steig 1987, Rockwood et al 1993).

Long-Term and Short-Term Goals

Goals that produce a desired outcome are called long-term goals, such as reducing the number of panic attacks. Short-term goals are daily actions which lead to the long-term goal and include, for example, attending a weekly relaxation class and keeping a diary. Both activities focus on specific targets which can be documented, such as the number of relaxation sessions attended, the level of anxiety experienced, or the type of benefit obtained. Feedback for the individual is thereby provided and, for the health care professional, a means of reviewing progress.

Goal setting is jointly decided between the person and the health care professional, which means that the person retains ownership of the goal. Consequently they are more likely to give it priority status.

Setting Goals

A useful acronym relating to goal setting, SMART, is explained in Box 28.2, which lists ways in which the goals can be made more powerful, and itemizes the following.

Specific: a defined target such as 'I want to attend a weekly class and learn how to relax' is easier to follow than a vague aspiration such as 'I'd like to be more relaxed'. Specific short-term goals can be set up, and these are effective because they enable people to know

---

BOX 28.2
SMART GOALS

A useful way of making goals more powerful is to use the SMART mnemonic. SMART, in this context, stands for:
  S Specific
  M Measurable
  A Attainable
  R Relevant
  T Time bound.
  A long-term goal, such as 'I want to stop having panic attacks when I go shopping', is less powerful than 'In 6 months' time I want to have stopped having panic attacks every time I go shopping'. The second statement requires that a number of short-term goals are successfully completed.

---

whether they are moving in the right direction; if they are not, those goals can be adjusted. The process provides a continuous assessment. Where goals have not been met, a commentary on the supposed reason should be included in the report.

Measurable: it is important that goals should be measurable. This is made possible by careful record keeping with the use of diaries and/or tabulated sheets which reflect the work done at home. Reading back entries provides the person with feedback which helps maintain motivation. It also enables the health care professional to review progress or chart setbacks.

Attainable: all goals must be realistic. The possibility of achievement must exist in the mind of both the individual and the health care professional; otherwise the goals are doomed to failure and loss of confidence. Information gathered in the clinical interview will enable the health care professional to judge whether or not the person's goal is attainable.

Relevant: any goal must relate to the individual's life as they wish to lead it. It is for this reason that the goals are set jointly.

Time bound: effective treatment in the domain of relaxation training needs to be limited by a time span. It helps the person to focus on the process. A time-restricted treatment scheme should be agreed at the start.

The Importance of Goal Setting

Stress and anxiety can prevent people from fulfilling their hopes. Goal setting can help to reduce that stress by offering a step-by-step approach in the form of short-term goals. As each one is achieved, the possibility of reaching the desired outcome increases. Thus, by setting a goal and defining the steps needed to reach it, a difficult challenge is transformed into a series of routine daily behaviours. Advice on setting up the goals can be provided by health care professionals; however, the success of the programme depends largely on the strength of the individual's personal desire and their determination to work for the outcome of their choice.

Measuring Progress in the Self-Help Context

For people using this book as a self-help approach, progress can be monitored by setting short- and long-term goals following the SMART principles. Keeping a diary to monitor feelings of tension and mood change allows the individual to track their own progress. Printed forms, as illustrated in Fig. 9.2 and 9.3, can also be used for this purpose. The measurement of physiological outcomes is relatively easy: pulse rate and blood pressure can be monitored using one of the electronic devices available from a local pharmacy. Electronic heart rate monitors are also widely available at retail outlets and consist of a simple device worn as a chest strap, plus a wristwatch.

The Placebo Effect

The belief in a treatment and the benefit felt to be derived from that treatment is important for a positive outcome. Faith in the remedy will aid recovery (Kaptchuk et al 2008). This is called the placebo effect and it is separate from the procedure's intrinsic value. Simply believing in the treatment creates benefit, and this contributes to the total effect. The placebo response, however, is not the same as spontaneous improvement. It may produce the same result but whereas spontaneous improvement is unrelated to treatment, the placebo response is an essential feature of treatment. Research on the placebo effect and the relaxation response support these phenomena as physical processes that can be used to improve patient care (Stefano et al 2001). Therefore, when conducting randomized controlled trials to investigate the efficacy of a relaxation intervention, it is necessary to have a placebo control as well as a waiting list control.

Since recovery, to a large extent, depends on the person's belief in the efficacy of the intervention, without it, recovery may be delayed or hindered and; harm may even arise. This is called the nocebo effect (Benson & Stark 1996). To reduce the likelihood of the nocebo effect, it is important that individuals are involved in the choice of appropriate relaxation techniques. This is important as belief in a relaxation technique as a treatment, may stimulate physiological processes, augmenting naturally occurring 'healthy' processes by increasing their level of performance (Stefano et al 2001, Micozzi 2018).

TOOLS FOR MEASURING EXERCISE INTENSITY

A standard measure of exercise intensity is the percentage of maximum oxygen uptake (O_2max). This requires skills and apparatus which may not always be available. Simpler to measure is the percentage of maximum heart rate (HRmax) and since the two scales bear a linear relationship to each other, the HRmax is the method commonly employed (Smeaton 1995).

HRmax is estimated by subtracting the person's age from the figure 220. In the case of a 40-year-old individual this would be 180, representing their hypothetical maximum. If the programme requires a 60% to 65% HRmax level of intensity, then the pulse rate for this individual should be kept within the range of 108 to 117 during exercise.

This figure is appropriate for healthy individuals. People who are less fit, however, can take the figure of 200 instead of 220 as their starting point, and those under medical supervision should seek the advice of their doctor.

Criticisms of this method include the possibility of error within the age categories and difficulty in palpating the pulse for those unfamiliar with the practice (Birk & Birk 1987). An alternative method for determining exercise intensity has been developed by Borg (1970, 1998). This researcher considers that the single best indicator of physical strain is the individual's own perception of exertion. This entails the integration of signals from all parts of the body including muscles, joints, pulmonary and cardiac organs and the central nervous system. For the novice, this means concentrating on what Morgan (1981) has called the 'total inner feeling of exertion'.

Borg, a psychologist from Stockholm, devised a scale for rating this perceived exertion. It consists of descriptive phrases indicating the subjective response to different levels of exercise intensity (Fig. 28.3). The perceived exertion rating of 13 to 14 is seen as corresponding to 70% HRmax and the rating of 10 to 11 as corresponding to 60% HRmax. Thus a glance at the scale helps the exerciser to judge the degree of effort required. Its sheer simplicity makes the scale attractive. Validity has been repeatedly demonstrated and high coefficients obtained (Borg 1998). Burke and Collins (1984) have found that the scale correlates strongly with oxygen consumption. Reliability has also been shown but although coefficients have often been high, Bowling (2001) considers that more work still needs to be done. Negative criticisms include the possibility of discrepancies between subjective reports and physiological effects.

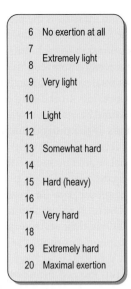

6	No exertion at all
7	
8	Extremely light
9	Very light
10	
11	Light
12	
13	Somewhat hard
14	
15	Hard (heavy)
16	
17	Very hard
18	
19	Extremely hard
20	Maximal exertion

Fig. 28.3 ■ The Borg Scale.

Regarding targets of distance and energy expenditure, electronic devices can be purchased. For example, a device which counts steps and converts them into calorific values can be used to monitor progress in walking. Measures can be taken before and after physical activity to estimate immediate effect, on the one hand, and longer term (over periods up to 6 months) on the other.

RESEARCH, SERVICE EVALUATION AND AUDIT

As well as research, measurement tools can be used for service evaluations and audits, the main differences being the scope and intent of the project (Twycross & Shorten 2014). There are however, a number of similarities. All three start with key questions that are answered by collecting appropriate data, using a rigorous design and a methodical approach (Wade 2005). Service evaluation looks at the effect of relaxation techniques on the person's experiences and outcomes and whether the service provided is achieving its intended aims. In other words a service evaluation is designed and delivered with the main aim of defining or judging the current service, the results of which can then inform local decision making (NRES 2013, Twycross & Shorten 2014).

Clinical audit on the other hand consists of the systematic analysis of procedures used for diagnosis, care and treatment (NICE 2002; Department of Health 2004). It poses questions such as:

- To what extent do these procedures benefit the patient?
- Do these procedures make the best use of resources?
- Can this service be improved?

Clinical audit was introduced into the NHS in the early 1990s and it has continued to be developed since that time. A practical handbook on clinical audit, published by the NHS and accessible on line, provides useful guidance for health care professionals (Copeland 2005). The handbook aims to provide guidance through the processes and structures necessary to deliver clinical audit.

Audit assesses the effectiveness of a particular intervention in a particular context or location and acts as a guide in the planning of services. Interventions result in outcomes of different kinds: they may be measures of access to care (e.g., time to first appointment) or results of care (blood pressure reduction in response to a relaxation programme). The audit can be undertaken either retrospectively (involving the analysis of data such as medical case notes) or prospectively. One advantage of prospective audit is that it can be planned with regard to the selection of an appropriate timescale and outcome measure(s). In addition, prospective audit allows time for health care professional to be allocated in a more fruitful way (Copeland 2005).

As well as measuring the effects of clinical practice, audit is concerned with issues such as resource allocation and may be used to highlight a need for departmental funding. This distinguishes it from research which aims to generate new knowledge or to test old knowledge and methods of treatment, seeking to identify the most effective intervention. Put another way, audit examines existing practice and looks for examples of good practice while research defines best practice (Sealey 1999, Twycross & Shorten 2014). However, there is an interaction between audit and research in that the standards by which clinical practice is measured are established mainly from the research literature (Barnard & Hartigan 1998, Bury & Mead 1998,

Benjamin 2008). This relationship underlies the principles of evidence-based practice.

If the set standards are not met by current practice, changes are discussed and introduced, followed by further evaluation to assess the quality of the changes. The result of this process is called the outcome, which has been defined as 'that part of the output of a process which can be attributed to the process' (Long et al 1993). In the context of health care, outcome can be seen as change in the health of an individual which is likely to be due to the therapeutic intervention.

Outcome is measured by an instrument, which might be a questionnaire or other measuring tool, and the results then undergo analysis to determine the degree to which the intervention was responsible for any change in the health status of the individual.

Outcome measures can be objective or subjective. Objective measures include quantifiable factors such as blood pressure; subjective measures include, on the one hand, the level of pain experienced by the person and on the other, observational judgements made by the health care professional (Barnard & Hartigan 1998, Benjamin 2008). Tools for measuring outcome are designed for different purposes. They may also vary in their range of concern, that is, be multidimensional or condition specific. An example of a multidimensional outcome measure is the Short Form 36 (Ware & Sherbourne 1992); an example of a condition-specific outcome measure is the BDI (Beck 1988) which focuses on one particular area of mental health. Since a treatment outcome can have several aspects, the question can be answered more fully if a variety of measures are used.

It can be seen that the same devices may be used for assessing the person's progress as for auditing the service or conducting research. For example, an instrument such as the BDI can be useful in all three contexts. To make outcome measurement as accurate as possible, certain criteria must be fulfilled (Donaghy 2001). The measuring device should be:

- Appropriate, i.e., suitable for the purpose and contain relevant items
- Valid, i.e., shown to be measuring what it claims to measure
- Reliable, i.e., capable of providing the same answer when the test is repeated by other health

care professionals or by the same health care professional on different occasions
- Responsive, i.e., sensitive to change, able to detect small variations over time and sensitive to individual differences
- Specific, i.e., able to isolate particular characteristics, for example, to focus on depressive symptoms as opposed to general symptoms of ill health
- Acceptable, i.e., presented in such a way that the clients feel comfortable with the questions and fully understand what is being asked
- Feasible, in the sense of the equipment being available and within budget costs.

Clinical audit is thus concerned with the ability to demonstrate effectiveness, which, together with efficiency, form the basis of Cochrane's philosophy (Cochrane 1972). It's essential feature is measurement, as it is in patient assessment. However, in seeking to make therapeutic care more effective for everyone, audit goes beyond the treatment outcome of the individual person to encompass wider issues.

National clinical audit topics are published and regularly reviewed. Their selection at a local level should be informed by the usual service criteria of high volume, high risk, high profile and high cost; that is to say, high levels of those factors indicate areas to be focused on. Clinical audit should include as many members of the multidisciplinary team delivering care as possible. Copeland (2005) recommends that, as a minimum, 10% of audits should be across service providers, 30% of audit should be multiservice and 50% should be multiprofessional.

Further discussion of audit is beyond the scope of this book, but the interested reader is referred to the works of Copeland (2005).

KEY POINTS

1. Measurement is an essential part of monitoring outcomes from treatment interventions.
2. Measurement tools need to be reliable, valid and appropriate for the selected outcome.
3. Assessment of relaxation interventions covers physiological, psychological and behavioural outcomes.

4. The clinical assessment should include nominal, functional and attitudinal data.

5. Goals should be agreed, recorded and regularly reviewed.

6. Personal activity goals should be developed using SMART principles.

7. The placebo effect should be considered in relaxation training and in the design of clinical trials.

8. Clinical audit is integral to the improvement of patient care.

Reflection

Describe your understanding of key aspects of measurement.

What measurement tools have you used?

How did you select the measurement tool (s)?

What is the main learning point you will take away from this chapter?

What is your future action plan in terms of measuring the progress of relaxation techniques?

CASE STUDY LEARNING OPPORTUNITY

The key points and reflection provide background and knowledge required in relation to the case study, relaxation programme for stress and anxiety, to help deepen understanding of the application of a measurement tools in practice.

CASE STUDY

Relaxation Programme for Stress and Anxiety: *Measurement Outcomes for the Group*

A group relaxation programme was set up within a rehabilitation setting for people experiencing stress and anxiety. The relaxation programme consisted of eight appointments covering education on stress and anxiety and how it affects the way individuals feel, think and act – an understanding of relaxation and introducing different relaxation techniques to discover individual preferences to self-manage stress and anxiety. As part of the relaxation programme individuals were asked to practice the relaxation techniques between sessions. A recording was provided to support this element of the relaxation programme.

Each participant was asked to complete self-rating scales and goal setting at the start and end of the relaxation programme. The measurement tools were selected to identify any changes in symptoms and to evaluate the overall usefulness of the relaxation programme. Measurement tools included the Hospital Anxiety and Depression Scale (HADS), Goal Attainment Scale (GAS) and self-rating scale in the form of a line calibrated from 0 to 10, where 0 was no stress/anxiety and 10 indicated extreme stress/anxiety. The facilitator reviewed the self-rating outcomes after each relaxation session, and if there were positive changes, the individual was encouraged to

continue the relaxation technique. If there were no changes, this was explored with the individual to understand any issues or reasons contributing to this outcome. All relaxation techniques were explored with the individual on a one to one basis, with preferred relaxation techniques ascertained at the end of the relaxation programme. HADS and GAS were also revisited with the individual at this point and advice given or referral made if the individual required further support in managing their symptoms.

ACTIVITY

For the case study:

1. List key aspects used to measure relaxation techniques.

2. How may this relaxation programme support people with stress and anxiety?

3. Write down the impact measuring relaxation is having from a psychological perspective.

4. Write down the impact measuring relaxation is having from a physical perspective.

5. Consider the outcomes on quality of life and overall well-being for the participants.

Chapter 29 will focus on evidence from research to understand the importance of measuring the outcome of relaxation techniques.

REFERENCES

Arnau, R. C., Meagher, M. W., Norris, M. P., & Bramson, R. (2001). Psychometric evaluation of the Beck Depression Inventory-II with primary care medical patients. *Health Psychology, 20*(2), 112–119.

Barnard, S., & Hartigan, G. (1998). *Clinical audit in physiotherapy: From theory into practice.* Oxford, UK: Butterworth-Heinemann.

Beck, A. T. (1988). *The Beck Depression Inventory.* Sidcup, UK: Psychological Corporation.

Beck, A. T., Ward, C. H., Mendelson, M., Mock, J. E., & Erbaugh, J. K. (1961). An inventory for measuring depression. *Archives of General Psychiatry, 4,* 53–63.

Benjamin, A. (2008). Audit: how to do it in practice. *British Medical Journal (BMJ), 336,* 1241–1245.

Benson, H., & Stark, M. (1996). *Timeless healing: The power and biology of belief.* New York: Scribner.

Birk, T. J., & Birk, C. A. (1987). Use of ratings of perceived exertion for exercise prescription. *Sports Medicine, 4,* 1–8.

Bjelland, I., Dahl, A. A., Haug, T. T., & Neckelmann, D. (2002). The validity of the Hospital Anxiety and Depression Scale. An updated literature review. *Journal of Psychosomatic Research, 52*(2), 69–77.

Borg, G. A. V. (1970). Perceived exertion as an indicator of somatic stress. *Scandinavian Journal of Rehabilitation Medicine, 2,* 92–98.

Borg, G. A. V. (1998). *Borg's perceived exertion and pain scales.* Champaign, IL: Human Kinetics.

Bowling, A. (2017). *Measuring health: A review of subjective health, well-being and quality of life measurement scales* (4th ed.). London: Open University Press.

Bowling, A. (2001). *Measuring disease: A review of disease-specific quality of life measurement scales* (2nd ed.). Buckingham, UK: Open University Press.

Boyle, G. J. (1985). Self-report measures of depression: some psychometric considerations. *British Journal of Clinical Psychology, 24*(Pt 1), 45–49.

Burke, E. J., & Collins, M. S. (1984). Using perceived exertion for the prescription of exercise in healthy adults. In R. C. Cantu (Ed.), *Clinical sports medicine.* Lexington, VA: Collamore Press.

Burlingame, J., & Blaschko, T. (2002). *Assessment tools for recreational therapy and related fields* (third ed.). USA: Idyll Arbor.

Bury, T. J., & Mead, J. M. (Eds.). (1998). *Evidence-based health care: A practical guide for therapists.* Oxford, UK: Butterworth-Heinemann.

Calsyn, R. J., & Davidson, W. S. (1978). Do we really want a program evaluation strategy based solely on individualized goals? A critique of goal attainment scaling. *Community Mental Health Journal, 14,* 300–308.

Cochrane, A. L. (1972). Effectiveness and Efficiency: Random Reflections on Health Services. Nuffield Provincial Hospitals Trust, London.

Copeland, G. (2005). A practical handbook for clinical audit. NHS Clinical Governance Support Team, Leicester. Retrieved from www.cgsupport.nhs.uk/downloads/practical. [Accessed April 2020]

Davis, D. W. (2004). Reliability and validity: Part 11. *Neonatal Network, 23*(3), 74–76.

Demyttenaere, K., & De Fruyt, J. (2003). Getting what you ask for: on the selectivity of depression rating scales. *Psychotherapy & Psychosomatics, 72*(2), 61–70.

Department of Health (DOH). (2004). *At least five a week: Evidence on the impact of physical activity and its relationship to health. A report from the Chief Medical Officer.* London: HMSO.

Donaghy, M. E. (2001). *A critical approach to physiotherapy in mental health. Workshop pack.* Edinburgh: Queen Margaret University College.

Dunstan, D. A., Scott, N., & Todd, A. K. (2017). Screening for anxiety and depression: Reassessing the utility of the Zung scales. *BMC Psychiatry, 17*(329), 2–8.

Enns, M. W., Cox, B. J., Parker, J. D., & Guertin, J. E. (1998). Confirmatory factor analysis of the Beck Anxiety and Depression Inventories in patients with major depression. *Journal of Affective Disorders, 47*(1–3), 195–200.

Fitzpatrick, R., Gibbons, E., & Mackintosh, A. (2009). *An overview of patient-reported outcome measures for people with anxiety and depression.* Oxford, UK: Department of Public Health, University of Oxford.

Herrmann, C. (1997). International experiences with the Hospital Anxiety and Depression Scale: A review of validation data and clinical results. *Journal of Psychosomatic Research, 42*(1), 17–41.

Holbrook, A. (2011). Self-reported measure. *Encyclopedia of survey research methods.* Thousand Oaks, CA: Sage Publications.

Houser, J. (2008). Precision, reliability, and validity: Essential elements of measurement in nursing research. Scientific inquiry. *JSPN, 13*(4), 297–299.

Hurn, J., Kneebone, I., & Cropley, M. (2006). Goal setting as an outcome measure: A systematic review. *Clinical Rehabilitation, 20*(9), 756–772.

Johnstone, M., Wright, S., & Weinman, J. (1995). Stress, emotion and life events. *Measures in health psychology: A user's portfolio.* Windsor, UK: NFER-Nelson.

Kaptchuk, T. J., Kelley, J. M., Conboy, L. A., et al. (2008). Components of the placebo effect: A randomized controlled trial in patients with irritable bowel syndrome. *BMJ: British Medical Journal, 336,* 999–1003.

Keable, D. (1997). *The management of anxiety: A manual for therapists* (2nd ed). Churchill Livingstone.

Lindsay, W. R., & Hood, E. H. (1982). *A cognitive anxiety questionnaire. [Unpublished].* Edinburgh: University of Sheffield.

Long, A. F., Dixon, P., Hall, R., Carr-Hill, R. A., & Seldon, T. A. (1993). The outcomes agenda: contribution of the UK clearing house on health outcomes. *Quality Health Care, 2,* 49–52.

Martin, C. R. (2005). What does the Hospital Anxiety and Depression Scale (HADS) really measure in liaison psychiatry settings? *Current Psychiatry Reviews, 1*(1), 69–73.

McIntosh, C. (2013). *Cambridge advanced learner's dictionary* (4th ed.). Cambridge, UK: Cambridge University Press.

Micozzi, M. S. (2018). Mind-body physiology and placebo effects *Fundamentals of complementary, alternative and integrative medicine.* (6th ed.). St. Louis, MO: Elsevier.

Morgan, W. P. (1981). Psychophysiology of self-awareness during vigorous physical activity. *Research Quarterly for Exercise and Sports, 52,* 385–427.

National Institute for Clinical Excellence (NICE). (2002). *Principles for best practice in clinical audit.* Oxon, UK: Radcliffe Medical Press Ltd.

Olton, D. S., & Noonberg, A. R. (1980). *Biofeedback: Clinical applications in behavioural medicine.* Englewood Cliffs, NJ: Prentice-Hall.

Poppen, R. (1998). *Behavioural relaxation training and assessment* (2nd ed.). Thousand Oaks, CA: Sage.

Richter, P., Werne, J., Heerlein, A., Kraus, A., & Sauer, H. (1998). On the validity of the Beck Depression Inventory. A review. *Psychopathology, 31*(3), 160–168.

Rockwood, K., Stolee, P., & Fox, R. A. (1993). Use of goal attainment scaling in measuring clinically important change in the frail elderly. *Journal of Clinical Epidemiology, 46,* 1113–1118.

Sealey, C. (1999). Two common pitfalls in clinical audit: Failing to complete the audit cycle and confusing audit with research. *British Journal of Occupational Therapy, 62*(6), 238–243.

Smeaton, J. (1995). Exercise and mental health. In T. Everett, M. Dennis, & E. Ricketts (Eds.), *Physiotherapy in mental health.* Oxford, UK: Butterworth-Heinemann.

Sim, J., & Wright, C. (2005). The kappa statistic in reliability studies: Use, interpretation and sample size requirements. *Physical Therapy, 85*(3), 257–268.

Spielberger, C. D. (1980). *Manual for the State–Trait Anxiety Inventory.* Palo Alto, CA: Consulting Psychologists Press.

Stefano, G. B., Fricchione, G. L., Slingsby, B. T., & Benson, H. (2001). The placebo effect and relaxation response: neural processes and their coupling to constitutive nitric oxide. *Brain Research Reviews, 35,* 1–19.

Twycross, A., & Shorten, A. (2014). Service evaluation, audit and research: What is the difference? *Evidence Based Nursing, 17*(3), 65–66.

Vodermaier, A., & Millman, R. D. (2011). Accuracy of the Hospital Anxiety and Depression Scale as a screening tool in cancer patients: A systematic review and meta-analysis. *Supportive Care in Cancer, 19*(12), 1899–1908.

Wade, D. (2005). Ethics, audit, and research: All shades of grey. *BMJ: British Medical Journal, 330,* 468.

Waltz, C., Strickland, O., & Lenz, E. (2004). *Measurement in nursing and health research.* New York: Springer.

Ware, J. E., & Sherbourne, C. D. (1992). The MOS 36–item short form health survey (SF–36) 1. Conceptual framework and item selection. *Medical Care, 30,* 473–483.

Williams, R. C., & Steig, R. L. (1987). Validity and therapeutic efficacy of individual patient goal attainment procedures in a chronic pain treatment centre. *Clinical Journal of Pain, 2,* 219–228.

Williams, J. W. J., Pignone, M., Ramirez, G., & Perez-Stellato, C. (2002). Identifying depression in primary care: A literature synthesis of case-finding instruments. *General Hospital Psychiatry, 24*(4), 225–237.

World Health Organization (WHO). (2003). ICF checklist: version 2: 1a clinician form for international classification of functioning, disability and health. Retrieved from https://www.who.int/classifications/icf/icfchecklist.pdf?ua=1. [Accessed April 2020]

Yuan, J., Ding, R., Wang, L., Sheng, L., Li., J., & Hu, D. (2019). Screening for depression in acute coronary syndrome patients: A comparison of patient health questionnaire-9 versus Hospital Anxiety and Depression scale-depression. *Journal of Psychosomatic Research, 121,* 24–28.

Zigmond, A. S., & Snaith, R. P. (1983). The Hospital Anxiety and Depression Scale. *Acta Psychiatrica Scandinavica, 67,* 361–370.

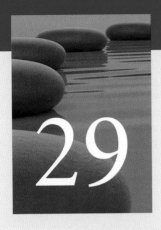

29

EVIDENCE FROM RESEARCH

DR CAROLINE BELCHAMBER

CHAPTER CONTENTS

LEARNING OBJECTIVES

The aim of this chapter is to bring together evidence from research covering 37 specified conditions.

By the end of this chapter you will be able to:

1. Understand the necessity of demonstrating effectiveness and validity of relaxation techniques.

2. Appreciate the evidence of effectiveness of relaxation techniques in the context of 37 specified conditions.

3. Recognize different types of research supporting the evidence of effectiveness in the use of relaxation techniques.

4. Identify when a study is methodologically flawed.

5. Acknowledge that randomized research trials are not always ethical and appropriate to use.

This chapter will conclude with key points and time for reflection, providing learning opportunities through a case study.

INTRODUCTION TO EVIDENCE FROM RESEARCH

There is a pressing need for health care professionals to demonstrate the effectiveness of their treatments, not only to treat people in the best way, but also to validate their work. Carefully designed and rigorously executed studies, repeated many times, help to build a robust foundation of effective treatments which contribute to current best practice.

Much work has been done to measure the effect of different methods or to weigh up relaxation techniques against other approaches such as cognitive interventions, exercise or pharmacology. This work is, however, beset by frequent methodological shortcomings; moreover, the diversity of methodologies makes it difficult to compare one study with another (Donaghy & Morss 2000). Therefore this chapter draws on systematic reviews and clinical studies. It explores the effectiveness of relaxation techniques in the context of 37 specified conditions, the majority of which are long-term conditions. The list does, however, also include other short-term conditions or naturally occurring conditions such as childbirth. The range of conditions discussed is by no means comprehensive. Many other conditions, including long-term conditions have been investigated which are not included. The chapter simply offers a selection to give the reader a glimpse of the kind of work that is being carried out in the field of relaxation techniques. A table suggesting applications for the various relaxation techniques may be found in Appendix 1.

In some cases relaxation techniques are provided in isolation or as a monotherapy; in others it is used adjunctively, alongside other approaches such as pharmacology or exercise, according to the requirements of the condition (see Chapter 30).

Although the choice of relaxation technique is based on information from research, it is intended only as a guide for the following 37 specified conditions discussed in this chapter:

- Addiction – illicit drugs
- Alcohol dependence
- Anxiety
- Arthritis
- Asthma
- Athletic injury
- Cancer
- Cardiovascular disease (CVD)
- Childbirth
- Chronic fatigue syndrome (CFS)
- Chronic obstructive pulmonary disease (COPD)
- Dementia
- Depression
- Diabetes
- Dysmenorrhoea
- Eating disorders
- Fibromyalgia
- Headache disorders
- HIV/AIDS
- Hypertension
- Inflammatory bowel disease (IBD)
- Irritable bowel syndrome (IBS)
- Low back pain (LBP)
- Menopause
- Multiple sclerosis (MS)
- Musculoskeletal problems
- Obsessive compulsive disorder (OCD)
- Occupational stress
- Pain
- Panic
- Parkinson's disease (PD)
- Posttraumatic stress disorder (PTSD)
- Peri- and postoperative states
- Psoriasis
- Schizophrenia
- Sleep disorders
- Tinnitus

The conditions listed will now be explored with regard to the evidence supporting a variety of relaxation techniques.

INTRODUCTION TO EVIDENCE

Relaxation techniques, such as progressive muscular relaxation (PMR), applied relaxation (AR), autogenic training (AT), meditation and mindfulness have received the most scientific attention and validation (Pagnini et al 2013). Furthermore research into mindfulness as a relaxation technique to manage, hypertension, pain, inflammatory bowel disease, myocardial ischaemia, substance misuse and human immunodeficiency virus has been supported by the National Institute of Health (Ludwig & Kabat-Zinn 2008). There has been increasing attention and empirical study in cognitive–behavioural therapy (CBT) (see Chapter 16) for the treatment of anxiety disorders (Norton 2012). These techniques will now be reviewed in relation to the 37 conditions.

Addiction – Illicit Drugs

The use of illegal drugs for recreational purposes has increased over the last two decades. Substance misuse is becoming one of the most prevalent psychiatric disorders in modern society, with addiction to opiates, crack cocaine, heroin and tranquillizers creating problems of addiction worldwide. Addictions are linked to multifactorial psychosocial and cultural factors. According to data from the Vinland National Centre in Minnesota, 71% of adults with substance misuse have brain injury with the second most common disability being mental health illnesses (Gary 2012); however, in some situations drugs may be taken to reduce stress. Cannabis smoking is the most common recreational drug used in the UK.

Hoppes (2006) reviewed the evidence regarding the use of mindfulness-based CBT in addictive disorders. He discussed the theory underpinning it and the effectiveness of its application and proposed that prolonged use of addictive substances impairs the brain pathways which help to control the emotions and offered a structured protocol for the treatment of co-occurring addictive and mood disorders (see Chapter 23). Further research has confirmed that the core clinical symptoms of addiction, which include craving, impulsiveness, negative mood, increased stress and diminished self-control, are due to impaired networks in the anterior cingulate cortex (ACC) and adjacent prefrontal cortex (PFC) of the brain (Rudebeck et al 2008, Tang et al 2016).

Of the many treatments which have been applied to drug addiction, CBT has often been found to be successful (Denis et al 2006). In their systematic review these researchers found extended individual CBT to be more effective than brief individual motivational therapy. A controlled trial in 2008 investigated the efficacy of behavioural therapy versus structured relaxation. Thirty-eight participants who were methadone maintained opiate dependent with a depressive disorder were randomly assigned to either behavioural therapy or structured relaxation technique for sessions over 24 weeks. Data were collected pre- and posttreatment using the Hamilton Depression Scale. The results indicated that both behavioural and relaxation-based techniques demonstrated promise for managing comorbid depression in substance misuse populations (Carpenter et al 2008). However, Tang and colleagues' 2016 study using brief mindfulness meditation in a series of randomized controlled trials tested whether improving the ACC and PFC was linked to improved self-control, regulation of emotion and response to stress in addicted and non-addicted populations. They measured emotion regulation, salivary cortisol and stress response. Results indicated improved self-control in emotion regulation and stress reduction, which was linked to increased ACC and PFC activity.

A randomized controlled trial (RCT) investigating acupuncture and relaxation response against usual care in the treatment of substance misuse disorders found that the relaxation response group had greater improvements in mental health and spiritual dimensions of quality of life (QOL), with significant reductions in anxiety levels compared with usual care. There was also no significant difference between the two intervention groups (Chang et al 2010).

Participation in structured exercise programmes can also bring benefits. Six studies published between 1991 and 2002 provide some support for the use of a structured programme of exercise for people in drug rehabilitation. Such a programme may be useful in reducing withdrawal symptoms; it could also increase physical fitness levels and self-esteem (Donaghy & Ussher 2005).

Smith (2006) undertook a multiple baseline design study with 21 participants in a 10-week structured exercise programme. Although adherence to the programme was a problem, qualitative data gathered in the study indicated that it helped participants to feel fitter and improved their feelings of mental well-being. Biddle and Mutrie (2008) suggest that for those who find it difficult to maintain regular exercise class attendance, home-based exercise, through a video or DVD, may be useful, backed up by regular phone call support.

A randomized controlled interventional study of Indian men with substance misuse disorders, where stress, anxiety and depression are common, explored biofeedback as an adjunct to relaxation techniques to ascertain its effectiveness (Ghadse et al 2019). Sixty male inpatients aged between 18 and 55 participated in the study. Half were randomly allocated to the control group and half to the biofeedback-assisted relaxation techniques group. Depression Anxiety Stress Scale (DASS) data were recorded pre and post 30 days of 30-minute relaxation sessions for each group. Results demonstrated significant differences in stress, anxiety and depression in the biofeedback-assisted relaxation technique group compared with the control group.

Alcohol Dependence

There is a substantial body of evidence to support the use of cognitive–behavioural approaches as a treatment in alcohol dependency (Donaghy 2008a). These approaches are primarily effective in developing new coping strategies for dealing with addictive inclinations; for example, social skills training may help to strengthen the person's motivation to abstain or cut down. Practising these skills helps develop self-efficacy, which leads to greater confidence, whereas the cognitive restructuring helps people to see themselves in a new light. However, an RCT building on a previous pilot study investigated CBT compared with relaxation training control (RTC) for individuals with alcohol-dependent depressive symptoms (Brown et al 2011). Participants were selected using the Beck Depression Inventory (BDI), those who obtained a score of more than 15 were randomly assigned to either eight individual sessions of CBT or RTC. For all participants there were significant improvements in depression and alcohol use, with CBT having significantly lower levels of depression at the 6-week follow-up using the BDI. Even so, this study found inconsistencies because no differences were identified in the modified Hamilton Rating Scale for depression at the 6-week follow-up or any other follow-up. There were also no significant differences between group alcohol use outcomes.

Alcohol dependence is a condition which is often accompanied by high levels of depression and anxiety, where exercise is shown to have more to offer than relaxation. Exercise regimens lead to improved aerobic fitness and strength which help people to view themselves more favourably. Such links with self-esteem help to increase people's confidence in their capacity to change

their behaviour. Exercise is thus a useful adjunct to other treatments (Donaghy & Ussher 2005). However, a systematic review investigating the relationship between physical activity behaviour of people with an alcohol use disorder found that lack of participation was due to a variety of complex factors, such as anxiety, depression, lower self-efficacy, functional impairments, distress, increased smoking rates, and obesity (Vancampfort et al 2015). This work therefore supports the need to combine treatments for a successful outcome.

Anxiety

Most diseases and conditions are accompanied by some degree of fear: fear of pain, fear of deterioration and doubts about recovery. The notion of relaxation as a useful intervention would therefore be logical. Anxiety conditions themselves have been found to respond to this training. Manzoni et al (2008a) carried out a systematic review investigating the effects of relaxation in the context of different forms of anxiety. Results indicated an efficacy which was both consistent and significant although the component trials were not tested for their rigour (see Chapter 2). Conrad and Roth (2007) studied the efficacy of muscular relaxation techniques in this context but found their work hampered by inadequate evidence and were unable to support a theory which suggested that decreased physiological activation took place when people reported feeling less anxious. Self-reporting of muscle tension does not always match that of the physiological recording.

Generalized anxiety disorder (GAD) is common, affecting 7% of the general population. In a systematic review of this condition, Hunot and colleagues (2007) found that symptoms were alleviated by cognitive–behavioural approaches and that these were more effective than usual treatment. Other systematic reviews suggest that both AR and CBT are effective in the treatment of GAD (Gorman 2003, Siev & Chambless 2007). These approaches were often effective whether used as monotherapies or adjunctive therapies. A meta-analysis of CBT in adults with anxiety disorders supports the finding that CBT is the most efficacious and effective intervention (Hofmann & Smits 2008), which is reinforced by an RCT that compared CBT with AR for people with GAD. This study concluded that the two relaxation techniques were comparable; nevertheless, the results indicated greater support in CBT efficacy than AR (Dugas et al 2010). However, there is a lack of research around CBT for people with GAD in relation to interpersonal issues (Newman et al 2015, Newman & Fisher 2013). A study looking at participants with GAD whose interpersonal issues were dominant and intrusive investigated how they responded to relaxation-based behavioural therapy compared with cognitive therapy or CBT. The researchers concluded that relaxation-based behavioural therapy had better outcomes for this group of people than cognitive interventions (Newman et al 2017).

Social anxiety disorder, another commonly reported condition, has been shown to benefit from CBT in a number of investigations. For example, Clark et al (2006) conducted an RCT which compared CBT with a combination of AR and exposure in the context of public speaking. Their conclusions pointed to a greater effectiveness of CBT over AR and exposure. CBT has also been shown to provide benefit in most systematic reviews of psychotherapeutic approaches to anxiety disorders (Gorman 2003, Hambrick et al 2003, Hunot et al 2007, Rodebaugh et al 2004, Siev & Chambless 2007). Many researchers find it the treatment of choice, with exercise and relaxation valuable contributions often used as part of CBT interventions to reduce anxiety (Ralston 2008). Other researchers have concentrated on children and adolescents with anxiety disorders and found CBT more effective than waiting list or attention control (James et al 2005). This finding applied to more than half the participants. Conclusions drawn from systematic reviews can vary according to not only the results of their component trials but also the quality of the research. This is particularly so where evidence is sparse. Some reviews have focused on different age groups. For example, Ayers et al (2007) studied the effect of relaxation training and CBT in different forms of late-life anxiety. Here, CBT was found to be particularly effective. An earlier work had produced a similar finding, while also indicating the benefit of relaxation training for subjective anxiety symptoms (Wetherell et al 2005).

Transcendental meditation has been shown to reduce anxiety, but its effect was no greater than that of other relaxation techniques, including yoga (Krisanaprakornkit et al 2006). Mindfulness meditation produced results which were equivocal when applied to anxiety and mood symptoms (Toneatto &

Nguyen 2007); however, the authors in this case found the results had low reliability because adherence to the programme in the trials was not always assessed. In the case of exercise, Jorm et al (2004) found that, together with relaxation training, it was an effective procedure for treating GAD. However, the paucity of evidence suggested to Larun et al (2006) that the effect of exercise might be quite modest.

An abbreviated form of grounded theory was carried out to explore retrospectively perceived changes in anxiety associated with AT (Yurdakul et al 2009). Participants included 12 self-selected women who had received group AT for anxiety (see Chapter 20). This research provided a preliminary model of change, where theoretical generalizations were made regarding the process of change. The researchers concluded that the recorded cognitive changes have implications in the treatment of anxiety. Results of a brief literature review of relaxation techniques for anxiety disorders across community and clinical populations supported the efficacy of relaxation techniques, either as independent or combined treatment programmes (Pagnini et al 2013). The researchers concluded that relaxation techniques should be used more widely in clinical practice. The use of combined relaxation techniques is supported by more recent research using guided respiration mindfulness therapy, a combination of respiration, mindfulness and relaxation techniques. This uncontrolled clinical trial of 42 participants diagnosed with anxiety or depression using standard outcomes found significant clinical reductions in participant symptoms with reduced anxiety sensitivity and increased overall well-being (Lalande et al 2017).

Arthritis: Rheumatoid and Osteo

Psychological interventions such as relaxation training and CBT have been investigated for their effectiveness in the pain management of rheumatoid arthritis (Astin et al 2002). These authors suggest that such interventions are useful as adjunctive therapies alongside medical management of the condition, adding that efficacy is likely to be greater in the early stages of the disease. A randomized trial assessed and compared CBT, relaxation response training and arthritis education to explore pain, role impairment and psychological distress in people with rheumatoid arthritis (Barsky et al 2010). The researchers concluded that all three interventions benefitted the participants over and above medical management of the disease.

Bagheri-Nesami et al (2006) conducted a study to investigate the effect of Benson's relaxation technique on rheumatoid arthritis. Their results suggested that the approach might help to slow down the disease process (see Chapter 22).

For people with osteoarthritis research has demonstrated that psychological and behavioural self-management interventions can improve physical as well as psychological well-being (Astin 2004, Bradley & Alberts 1999).

Osteoarthritis has been shown to benefit from a programme of combined progressive relaxation and guided imagery in a longitudinal randomized controlled study (Baird & Sands 2004). Twenty-eight older women with osteoarthritis participated. At the end of the course they reported significantly reduced pain and a significant reduction in difficulties associated with mobility. No differences in pain or mobility were reported in the control group. A more recent longitudinal randomized experimental study (Baird et al 2010) looked at the efficacy of guided imagery with relaxation to reduce pain, medication use and improve mobility in 30 adults with osteoarthritis. Participants who completed the guided imagery relaxation showed significant reduction in pain, improvement in mobility and reduction in medication compared with the sham intervention (see Glossary).

Asthma

Breathing retraining has received considerable attention from researchers as a way of helping to relieve symptoms of asthma. A systematic review was set up to assess the value of breathing exercises in this area. However, the authors, Holloway and Ram (2004), were unable to draw conclusions because treatment interventions and outcome measurements varied so much. On the whole, studies looking into relaxation techniques for asthma find a lack of evidence for their efficacy. The systematic review of Huntley and colleagues (2002), hampered by poor methodology and the problems inherent in this field, did, however, find some evidence that PMR might improve lung function in an adjunctive role. This benefit was not observed with other relaxation techniques. In a paper discussing the effectiveness of PMR in adult asthma, Ritz (2001)

suggests a possible mechanism for its effects. Contrary to popular belief, he proposes that the tensing component is the one which might be useful in relieving asthma because tensing is associated with excitation of the sympathetic nervous system, one of whose functions is to open the airways. By contrast, the release component is associated with parasympathetic dominance and a relative constriction of the airways. However, there is a lack of independent interventional studies supporting the efficacy of PMR for asthma symptoms (Nickel et al 2005, 2006).

It is believed that some asthma is triggered by psychological factors; however, on the basis of the current literature, this hypothesis cannot be supported. Yorke et al (2005) reviewed the role of psychological factors as they affect children and concluded that, although they might play an important part in the aetiology of asthma, the evidence to support their involvement in subsequent attacks was lacking.

Mental imagery has also been put forward as a possible means of relieving symptoms of asthma. Epstein et al (2004) explored this idea but were unable to draw conclusions regarding efficacy.

It is suggested that asthma is associated with over-breathing. The theory underpinning the claim suggests that asthma is exacerbated by hyperventilation with resulting hypocapnia and bronchoconstriction. Two approaches are based on this assumption: the Buteyko and the Papworth methods. Evidence for these techniques are reported in Chapter 4. However, a 2019 RCT that looked at the effectiveness of the Papworth method of relaxation training (Pourdowlat et al 2019) is discussed here. Thirty participants with asthma aged between 20 to 45 years were randomly allocated to either the Papworth group or the control group. Two questionnaires were used, Spielberger Anxiety Questionnaire (STAI) for anxiety and the 36-Item Short Form Health Survey (SF-36) (see Chapter 28) to measure QOL. Data were collected before and after six sessions. Findings showed that the group receiving the Papworth method had significant reductions in anxiety levels and improved QOL compared with the control group. The researchers concluded that the Papworth method helped people with asthma to manage stressful situations and prevent further asthma attacks. They suggested that the Papworth method was a helpful adjunct to the treatment of asthma.

An RCT looked at the effect of stress management using biofeedback-assisted relaxation breathing and PMR for people with asthma. Data were collected before and after 8 weeks of treatment. Participants (n = 23) in the stress management groups had significantly less perceived stress and improved QOL, reporting increased control of asthma symptoms and higher frequency of physical activity than participants (n = 19) in the control group. However, the researchers concluded that the trustworthiness of the findings was reduced as a result of numerous limitations encountered and further research was required (Georga et al 2019).

Athletic Injury

Athletic injury carries with it a number of stresses. In addition to the fear of pain and the fear of non-recovery, there is the fear of reinjury when play is resumed. Cupal and Brewer (2001) studied the effects of muscular relaxation and guided imagery in 30 participants undergoing rehabilitation after anterior cruciate ligament reconstruction. Among the positive effects demonstrated at 6-month follow-up was a significantly reduced level of reinjury anxiety and a decreased level of pain.

Long-term injuries are known to lower the mood of injured athletes. In an attempt to find a way of raising that mood, Johnson (2000) studied the effect of different short-term interventions such as stress management, goal setting and relaxation training with guided imagery. Of the three interventions, the only one to show statistical differences of benefit was relaxation training with guided imagery. In a further study Johnson et al (2005) found that psychologically based intervention programmes significantly reduced the number of injuries, critical incidents and stress among 32 soccer players. The interventions employed were somatic and cognitive relaxation, stress management, goal setting training, attribution and self-confidence training. This work was supported by that of Maddison and Prapavessis (2005) who, in a controlled study of 48 rugby players, found that psychological interventions resulted in less time lost in recovery from injuries than in control conditions.

Donaghy (2008b) reviewed the sports literature on the use of relaxation techniques (within stress management packages) to reduce risk of injury but found the evidence for efficacy of prevention limited by the small number of RCTs, most of which had methodological weaknesses. Evidence which supported the use of stress management techniques in the mental preparation of athletes for competition was more convincing.

Imagery is widely used in sport and particularly by athletes in training and competition. Sordoni et al (2002) defined three kinds of imagery: motivational, cognitive and healing. All three types are used by athletes, whether in recreational or competitive situations; however, competitive athletes use more cognitive imagery than do their recreational counterparts. When athletes are injured, they also use healing imagery which has been found to be associated with a variety of benefits such as decreased pain, anxiety and distress, accelerated healing and improved immune responses. Healing imagery is also related to self-efficacy; that is to say, athletes with a strong sense of self-efficacy tend to use more healing imagery than those with a weaker sense (see Chapter 19). In addition, relaxation techniques as a whole are reported as an effective intervention strategy in sport psychology literature (Bois et al 2009, D'Arripe-Longuevill et al 2009, Thelwell et al 2010).

A 2018 systematic review of imagery in athletic injury rehabilitation found a limited number of studies despite employing a wide inclusion criteria. In addition to this, the quality of the studies identified were diverse and sample size small, suggesting the need for high-quality studies in the future. However, the systematic review did find a number of studies recording benefits of imagery on a variety of muscle groups, but reduction in pain was varied (Multhaupt & Beuth 2018).

Cancer

There is a large body of research focusing on the pain and distress associated with different forms of cancer. Patients with cancer often develop anxiety and depression for which psychological treatments are prescribed. Sloman (2002) measured the effects of PMR and guided imagery on the psychological health of 56 people with advanced cancer and accompanying anxiety and depression and found that, whereas there were significant positive changes for depression, no significant improvement occurred for anxiety. Guided imagery is a psychological technique commonly used with cancer patients. Roffe and Schmidt (2005) conducted a systematic review to test its effectiveness as a sole adjuvant cancer therapy but found it had little to offer in the relief of nausea and vomiting associated with chemotherapy. However, there were indications that it might help to increase comfort and provide psychological support.

Mindfulness meditation has been found to be supportive to patients experiencing cancer care. In their systematic review, Smith et al (2005) found improvements in mood, reduction in stress and better sleep quality after a course of mindfulness-based stress reduction although a number of the included studies had methodological defects. The authors concluded that mindfulness-based stress reduction may have clinically valuable potential. As a further advantage, it could be self-administered. A meditation programme designed for patients with cancer was proposed in an article by Tacon (2003).

Negative thought intrusions can add to the pain experienced by cancer sufferers. Antoni et al (2006) set up a stress reduction programme consisting of relaxation training, cognitive restructuring and coping skills in a controlled trial of 200 women newly treated for stage 0 to stage 3 breast cancer. Significant benefit was derived in the form of reduced thought intrusion and reduced anxiety and distress over the year after recruitment. The conclusion drawn from this trial was that group-based cognitive–behavioural stress management was a helpful adjunct to medical treatment in this context.

Ernst et al (2006) conducted a systematic review of RCTs investigating the effect of psychological interventions for breast cancer. Among the mind–body techniques tested were CBT, group support and a combination of PMR and imagery. However, the authors were unable to draw conclusions on account of the poor quality of much of the methodology.

The value of increased activity for people with cancer has been emerging over the last decade and is linked to survival rates. Benefits of this increased activity include a measure of relief in their symptoms of nausea and fatigue (Stricker et al 2004). Research looking at breast cancer survivors has indicated that those who are regularly active have a 50% reduction in mortality compared with those who are inactive (Holmes et al 2005). A large study by Mutrie and colleagues

(2007), looking at women with breast cancer who participated in a 12-week exercise programme, found they had significant improvements in functional and psychological outcomes compared with women who received care as usual. These benefits, alongside the findings that women with breast cancer who exercise have an improvement in QOL up to 1 year after their cancer treatment (Daley et al 2004, 2007), make this an area worthy of promotion in cancer treatment programmes. Knols and colleagues (2005), in a systematic review of exercise trials with cancer patients, conclude that benefit may be derived from exercise, particularly where patients are ambulant and their limitations allow it. There are special considerations for this population related to muscle weakness after chemotherapy and the time required to recover from surgery and chemotherapy. There may also be embarrassment because of obvious signs of treatment such as hair loss or scarring after surgical intervention.

A 2016 systematic review and meta-analysis looked at the efficacy of psychological interventions for women after breast cancer surgery. Results indicated that CBT was the most beneficial technique for improving, anxiety, depression and QOL. However, the study did acknowledge that there were some methodological weaknesses in existing studies reviewed, such as the length of follow-up and small sample size, which limited the generalizability of the findings (Matthews et al 2016). A longitudinal randomized trial in women with breast cancer looked at the efficacy of mindfulness-based stress reduction (MBSR) on mood disorders. The MBSR programme included self-instructed sessions over an 8-week period with or without a trainer. The programme was delivered weekly in group sessions or no intervention. Outcome measures included the Hospital Anxiety and Depression Scale (HADS), the SF-36, and a number of other outcome measures over a 5-year period. Results indicated a significant improvement in depression scores, psychological and physical measurement and the ability to cope. Significant improvements were also found in scores for mental health, symptom burden, immune response and distress (Kenne et al 2017).

A review article of clinical trial data demonstrating the benefits of mindfulness in different areas of cancer management, including techniques commonly used in practice, concluded that mindfulness-based relaxation techniques are increasingly being applied in cancer management. The majority of evidence presented demonstrates that mindfulness is beneficial in reducing toxicity and stress in people with cancer (Mehta et al 2019).

Cardiovascular Disease

Cardiovascular disease (CVD) is an umbrella term which covers disorders of the heart and blood vessels (WHO 2017) – for example, ischaemic heart disease and cardiac failure. In their systematic review and meta-analysis, van Dixhoorn and White (2005) studied the effects of muscular relaxation therapy on recovery from a cardiac ischaemic event. Various forms of progressive relaxation were employed. Findings included a reduction in resting heart rate, improved exercise tolerance and increased high-density lipoprotein cholesterol. There was no effect on low-density cholesterol or blood pressure. State anxiety and depression were reduced, attacks of angina became less frequent and arrhythmia and exercise-induced ischaemia less of a problem. Cardiac events and death became less frequent. These effects, however, tended to be quite small in those studies which used abbreviated methods of relaxation. The authors concluded that intensive supervised muscular relaxation practice can play a valuable role in the rehabilitation of people recovering from an ischaemic heart event, making an important contribution to secondary prevention. This approach is best combined with a programme of appropriate exercise.

Secondary prevention was an area of concern to Walton et al (2002) in their review of RCTs exploring the effectiveness of transcendental meditation in the area of cardiovascular disease. Earlier work had shown that this approach might help to reduce risk factors and slow down the pathological changes which lead to or exacerbate this disease. However, they found that transcendental meditation had similar effects to those of conventional practices. A further review in 2004 resulted in a strengthening of these views (Walton et al 2004).

Results from a Cochrane meta-analysis of psychological interventions, which included cognitive–behavioural strategies, relaxation techniques and the use of cognitive techniques demonstrated a small-to-moderate reduction in anxiety and depression. The findings also stated that these interventions can reduce cardiac mortality in people with coronary heart disease (Whalley et al 2011).

Childbirth

Relaxation training has long been associated with childbirth and studies have included meditation, mindfulness, hypnotherapy (guided and imagery), diaphragmatic breathing and muscle relaxation with positive results in reducing stress, perceived stress as well as improving mood and well-being (Teixeira et al 2005, Tragea et al 2014, Urech et al 2010, Vieten & Astin 2008). Research has also demonstrated that relaxation techniques reduce the probability of premature or delayed births, caesarean sections, birth interventions and improvements in the infant's body weight (Bastani et al 2005, Nickel et al 2006, Teixeira et al 2005).

Simkin and Boulding (2004) conducted a review of non-pharmacological methods of pain relief and found evidence in favour of continuous support in labour, maternal movement and positioning, baths, and nerve blocks. Other methods may confer similar benefit but require further study before conclusions can be drawn. User satisfaction, however, was high among all methods. A 2019 study conducted a narrative review on the effectiveness of patterned breathing techniques to manage labour pain, demonstrating a positive reduction in pain using this technique (Qumer & Ghosh 2019).

The psychological and emotional benefits of physical activity during pregnancy are emerging. In a well-controlled study, Rankin (2002) assigned 157 women to antenatal classes with and without exercise. They were assessed at early and late stages of pregnancy and after childbirth. The study found that adding exercise to routine antenatal care prevented a decline in the women's perceptions of their well-being, which is often seen during pregnancy. These findings led to local service changes, with exercise being included in antenatal classes and training provided for leaders of these classes. In addition, a 2018 study identified 76 systematic reviews and meta-analyses published between 2006 and 2018 on the effects of physical activity in maternal health during pregnancy and after childbirth. Robust evidence indicated that physical activity of moderate intensity decreased the risk of weight gain, diabetes and depression after childbirth. However, there was limited evidence to suggest an inverse link between physical activity and the risk of antenatal anxiety and depression, gestational hypertension and preeclampsia. Furthermore, because of a lack of evidence it was difficult to determine the effect of physical activity on weight loss and anxiety after childbirth and whether these links were affected by prepregnancy weight, race and ethnicity, socioeconomic status or age (Dipietro et al 2018).

Chronic Fatigue Syndrome

Chronic fatigue syndrome (CFS) (also known as myalgic encephalomyelitis) is a condition in which the predominating symptom is tiredness in the absence of previous exertion. Dysfunction is present in the neurological, endocrine and immune systems and this gives rise to a wide range of symptoms in addition to fatigue. The aetiology is unknown. Tested therapies include graded exercise therapy (GET), activity pacing, CBT (Pemberton & Cox 2014, Price et al 2008), relaxation techniques and more recently mindfulness-based approaches (Fjorback et al 2011, Rimes & Wingrove 2013).

GET, carried out in a flexible manner to suit the person's capacity, has been shown in an audit to result in significant improvements (White & Naish 2001). Walking, swimming, cycling and tai chi were the activities featured in a programme where exercise was gentle and individually tailored. These interventions are all variants of physical activity programmes, with the aim to manage symptoms and improve functional ability (Larun et al 2017). Activity pacing enables people to be active within their own physical and mental limits (Goudsmit et al 2012). An RCT evaluated the effectiveness of activity pacing as a self-management strategy for 33 women living with CFS and the effect it had on performing activities of daily living (ADLs). Results indicated a significant difference in the pacing activity group compared with the control group in optimizing participation in ADLs. However, because of a small sample size it was concluded that a long-term follow-up was required (Kos et al 2015).

The long-term outcome of CBT versus relaxation therapy was explored in a 5-year follow-up study of 53 people with CFS. Of the 25 who received CBT, 68% reported improvements in their symptoms and of the 28 who received relaxation therapy 36% reported improvements in their symptoms. In total 80% of participants still used CBT with positive evaluation at the end

of the follow-up (Deale et al 2001). The value of this approach was endorsed in an RCT published in 2005. Its authors, Stulemeijer et al (2005), gave 10 sessions of activity (appropriate to the participant's condition) to 71 adolescent patients in a cognitive–behavioural framework. The results indicated a significantly greater decrease in fatigue severity as reported by the intervention group than was reported by the controls. This echoed the findings of Price and Couper (2003), whose systematic review of adults had previously found cognitive techniques to be not only effective but significantly more effective than orthodox medical management. Cognitive techniques were also shown to be more effective than relaxation.

Chronic Obstructive Pulmonary Disease

Chronic obstructive pulmonary disease (COPD) is a chronic lung condition sometimes referred to as chronic bronchitis and emphysema. It is a condition which causes the airways to become inflamed, leading to irreversible destruction of the lung tissue and breathlessness. As the disease progresses breathlessness and perceived breathlessness escalates, often with an increased prevalence of anxiety and depression. Mindfulness-based interventions and relaxation have been reported as effective in reducing anxiety and depression. Other benefits include improved exercise capacity, fatigue levels, lung function and perception of breathlessness (Faver-Vestergaard et al 2015).

A systematic review and meta-analysis investigated the efficacy of psychologically based interventions to improve anxiety, depression and QOL in people with COPD (Baraniak & Sheffield 2011). In this research nine studies were reviewed, eight evaluating a CBT intervention or psychotherapeutically orientated intervention and one evaluating recorded PMR. Results indicated only a small improvement in anxiety, but not in depression or QOL. However, there were limitations noted in this research because not all the studies reported all three areas of interest, with nine studies reporting anxiety, seven studies reporting depression and five studies addressing QOL. The outcome measures were also diverse, and there were variations in the quality of the methodology. A similar issue was found in a Cochrane review, carried out in 2017, which evaluated the efficacy of psychological interventions for the management of anxiety in people with COPD. Three prospective RCTs evaluating CBT were included in the review. Evidence indicated minor improvements in anxiety over a 3- to 12-month period, but because of small sample sizes and significant differences in the studies, the studies were deemed of low quality. This Cochrane review was, however, limited by the fact that the participant's recruited in all three studies had anxiety and depression and not just anxiety, which may have had an overall effect on the results (Usmani et al 2017).

In more recent research, an RCT investigated the use of CBT to reduce symptoms of anxiety in people with COPD. A total of 279 participants were randomly allocated into either the CBT group or a control group, which provided self-help leaflets. Baseline measurements included, anxiety, depression and QOL, with data collected at 3, 6 and 12 months. Results indicated that the CBT group had better outcomes than the control group at 3 months, with significant reduction in hospital admissions and visits to emergency departments at 12 months (Heslop-Marshall et al 2018).

Dementia

Dementia is a neurocognitive disorder which interferes with the individual's ability to carry out normal activities of daily living. Across the world dementia affects about 50 million people and is projected to increase to 152 million by 2050 (WHO 2017). Anxiety and depression are common symptoms in people with dementia. In addition, people caring for an individual with dementia have reported deterioration in their physical and mental health, including perceived anxiety and depression proportional to the severity of the individual with dementia (Ferrara et al 2008). Therefore appropriate interventions are required to manage both anxiety and depression in people with dementia as well as their caregivers (see Chapter 26).

A systematic review of interventions to manage anxiety in caregivers of individuals with dementia reviewed 24 studies that met the inclusion criteria. The authors concluded that CBT and other relaxation techniques developed to treat depression did not treat anxiety effectively. However, there were limitations to the review such as the diversity of the interventions used and similarities between some of the groups. Furthermore, CBT and the other interventions targeted depression rather than anxiety and consequently the evidence for the efficacy of managing anxiety was absent. The

study concluded that future studies need to include robust RCTs that specifically target anxiety (Cooper et al 2007). A 2019 systematic review and meta-analysis investigated CBT for anxiety, depression and stress in caregivers of individuals with dementia. Of the 25 studies included, depression and stress were shown to significantly reduce after CBT; however, anxiety did not, which supports the findings of the earlier systematic review. The study concluded that group CBT offers a small but significant benefit in improving depression and stress in caregivers (Hopkinson et al 2019).

A systematic review of CBT use in managing anxiety and depression in individuals with dementia identified 11 studies with 116 older adults in total. Findings indicated that CBT can be effective in decreasing anxiety and depression in people with dementia. The study concluded that the findings provided a promising foundation to carry out a major RCT with a larger sample size (Tay et al 2019).

Mindfulness-based intervention (MBI) for stress reduction in caregivers of individuals with dementia was investigated in a systematic review and meta-analysis. Of the five RCTs identified that met the inclusion criteria, 144 participants qualified for the meta-analysis. The analysis demonstrated a significant reduction in stress levels in the caregivers immediately after MBI, but this was not sustained. Even so, this study was limited by the small sample size and concluded that multi-centre RCTs were required with a larger sample size to make a well-founded conclusion (Kor et al 2018).

A systematic review and meta-analysis investigating the effects of long-term exercise (12 months or longer) in relation to prevention of dementia, mild cognitive impairment and decline in older adults included five RCTs. The study found no significant effects of exercise in lowering the risk of dementia, cognitive impairment or cognitive decline. However, the evidence from the RCTs was limited and therefore more long-term exercise RCTs are required to be able to draw any firm conclusions (de Souto Barreto et al 2018).

Depression

Depression is characterized by a lack of interest and a loss of pleasure in usual concerns. It is described as clinical when symptoms become marked enough to interfere with normal activities and to persist for 2 weeks or longer (Peveler et al 2002). Depression can be a primary disorder, as in the case of major depression, or it may be secondary to the experience of an already existing disorder such as cancer (Craft & Landers 1998).

A Cochrane review suggests that relaxation techniques may make a useful first-line psychological treatment for people with depression (Jorm et al 2008). The study is reported in Chapter 2. CBT has also been found to be effective in the treatment of depression either as a non-pharmacological sole treatment or as an adjunct to medication (Davidson 2008). In a review of exercise and mental health, Donaghy (2007) highlights the efficacy of structured exercise for reducing symptoms of clinical depression as well as for mild-to-moderate depression, where exercise is advocated either as a treatment in its own right or as an adjunct to other forms (see Chapter 15). Most research has focused on adults. However, a few studies have been on children. Larun et al (2006) systematically reviewed these studies to determine the effect of exercise on children and adolescents who were depressed. However, the authors found the evidence base too small to draw conclusions. Furthermore, a paucity of good-quality evidence precludes the drawing of conclusions in the field of postpartum depression. A wide variety of non-biological methods (relaxation training, CBT, psychotherapy, counselling, massage, maternal exercise) have been tested, only to find no difference between them in terms of efficacy (Dennis 2004).

More recently a study exploring mindful breathing (Burg & Michalak 2011) found that the intensity and duration of guided self-regulated breathing may reduce mind wandering and rumination, an activity associated with depression (Nolan-Hocksema et al 2008). As a consequence mindful breathing may improve the outcome of relaxation techniques. This is supported by a study using mindfulness breathing in a combined relaxation programme with results demonstrating clinically significant reductions in depressive symptoms in the group of participants diagnosed with depression (Norton 2012). Other relaxation techniques such as meditation with self-regulated breathing have also shown promise in the treatment of depression (Streeter et al 2017).

Diabetes Mellitus Types 1 and 2

Physical activity forms part of the treatment of diabetes mellitus, along with medication, dietary control and monitoring of glucose levels. This holds for both type 1 (insulin dependent) and type 2 (non–insulin dependent) diabetes and is now well established. The benefits of physical activity in controlling glucose levels has been reported in a systematic review and meta-analysis of physical activity in young people with type 1 diabetes (MacMillan et al 2014). In addition, the National Institute for Health and Care Excellence (NICE) has recommended exercise in children and young people with diabetes to prevent cardiovascular disease (NICE 2015). A position statement of the American Diabetes Association also provides comprehensive evidence-based recommendations for physical activity and exercise in a range of people with diabetes (Colberg et al 2016). People with type 1 diabetes need to maintain a critical balance between insulin control, glucose levels and exercise (its amount and timing). It is essential that individuals are guided to monitor blood glucose before and after exercise and are helped by an appropriate health care professional in making decisions about frequency, duration and intensity of exercise.

Type 2 diabetes is spreading, particularly in the developing world, and is linked to lifestyles. Changes in diet and activity have contributed to its prevalence. People with type 2 diabetes have needs which are different from those in type 1 and which may be linked to motivation and obesity. The work of Marsden and Kirk (Kirk et al 2007, Marsden & Kirk 2005) provides a comprehensive guide for health care professionals and exercise consultants when constructing exercise regimens for people in both type 1 and type 2 diabetes categories.

Although the role of exercise is now established, there is also an indication that relaxation can provide benefits. One study found that relaxation was as useful as exercise in controlling blood glucose levels. van Rooijen et al (2004) conducted a randomized trial to compare the effect of exercise with that of relaxation, using glycated haemoglobin (HbA_1c) as the outcome measure (a high reading indicates an uncontrolled diabetes). These two groups consisted of South African women with type 2 diabetes mellitus. The trial ran for 12 weeks after which time significant improvement was seen in both groups but with no significant difference between them. A 2019 study compared mindfulness-based meditation and progressive relaxation in older women with diabetes who had chronic peripheral neuropathic pain, one of the most common complications of diabetes. The study was conducted over 12 weeks and it reported significant improvements in pain levels in both groups compared with the control group (Hussain & Said 2019).

Dysmenorrhoea

As menstrual pain is related to uterine cramps (primary dysmenorrhoea) usually in the lower abdomen before or after menstruation it has been suggested that relaxation techniques may help to relieve it. Secondary dysmenorrhoea on the other hand is associated with an underlying pathological condition and would require further investigations. Proctor et al (2007) reviewed behavioural interventions for primary dysmenorrhoea. The reviewers found some evidence to suggest that progressive relaxation with or without imagery may be a useful strategy for relieving cramping pain; however, methodological deficiencies in some of the component studies made it necessary to view these results with caution. More recently, a randomized clinical trial compared Laura Mitchell's physiological relaxation technique versus Jacobson's progressive relaxation technique on women aged between 18 and 22 years with primary dysmenorrhoea. Results indicated a significant reduction in pain using Laura Mitchell's physiological relaxation technique compared with Jacobson's progressive relaxation technique and significant improvements in QOL were reported in Jacobson's progressive relaxation technique compared with Laura Mitchell's physiological relaxation technique (Ganesh et al, 2017).

Another study screened 207 female students for primary dysmenorrhoea of which 60 students were identified and split equally into a control group and experimental group. The control group received deep breathing relaxation therapy and the experimental group received muscle relaxation therapy. Results indicated that muscle relaxation therapy effectively reduced the intensity of pain compared with the deep breathing relaxation with significant changes in breathing measurements and pulse (Dwi Kustriyanti & Boediarsih 2017).

Eating Disorders

Eating disorders are common in Western society and include anorexia nervosa, binge eating disorders (emotional disorders) and bulimia nervosa. These disorders involve distorted body image associated with eating or weight loss behaviours, which cause severe distress, impaired physical health, psychosocial functioning and depression, consequently decreasing QOL (Treasure et al 2010, Winkler et al 2014). Binge eating disorders and bulimia nervosa are disorders characterized by loss of control over eating behaviours where binging takes place. In bulimia nervosa this loss of control is followed by self-induced vomiting, laxatives or use of diet pills, excessive exercise or starvation. Hay et al (2004) carried out a systematic review of psychotherapies for bulimia nervosa but found that the sample sizes were generally small and the quality of the research variable, making it difficult to have confidence in the results. From the more rigorous of the studies, however, it emerged that benefit could be gained from cognitive–behavioural approaches which were found to be significantly better than no treatment and more effective than other strategies at reducing binge eating. However, evidence for the efficacy of CBT as a form of treatment for binge eating disorders is growing (Hay et al 2009, Moffitt et al 2015, Vocks et al 2010). In addition, three RCTs demonstrated promise for the efficacy of physical activity therapy as a treatment for binge eating disorders (Vancampfort et al 2014). However, CBT combined with exercise is deemed more effective in improving depressive symptoms and body mass index (BMI) (Soundy et al 2016).

The reverse disorder, anorexia nervosa is associated with hyperactivity and excessive dieting with a pathological fear of weight gain, leading to severe weight loss which can be life threatening and requires specialist treatment not covered in this work.

Stress and negative emotions can induce binge eating; therefore psychological and behavioural interventions for plus size individuals should include techniques for stress management. In plus size individuals who have emotional eating disorders, food-related anxiety may be reduced through relaxation techniques (Manzoni et al 2008b), which has shown to improve with virtual reality, producing long-term effects (Manzoni et al 2009). However, CBT as recommended for binge eating disorders is the favoured intervention for plus size individuals. Even so this is a complex condition involving multifactorial factors such as, familial, biological, genetic, behavioural, social, environmental, psychological and cultural aspects. Therefore evidence indicates a number of integrated psychological and relaxation interventions are required to improve and maintain weight loss and reduce related conditions, such as cancer, cardiovascular disease, type 2 diabetes and osteoarthritis (Castelnuovo et al 2017).

Fibromyalgia

Fibromyalgia is a chronic condition which displays a variety of symptoms. Pain is the most evident but there is a degree of chronic fatigue and long-term functional impairment. Stress seems to play a part. The defining criteria, however, reflect medical opinion rather than hard science (Skelly 2008), so it is best seen as a syndrome, not a disease. In many respects it resembles CFS, with which it is often confused.

Research into fibromyalgia has been systematically reviewed by Sim and Adams (2002). The review indicates an absence of strong evidence for any single non-pharmacological intervention in the treatment of this condition, although there was some preliminary support for moderate aerobic exercise. King et al (2002a) compared aerobic exercise and education as combined therapies versus individual interventions, concluding that the combined group gained the most benefit. Williams (2003) also suggests that greatest benefit is derived from a combined approach, in this case exercise and CBT used adjunctively with medical treatment. More recent studies have demonstrated brief CBT as an effective way to reduce emotional distress (Vázquez-Rivera et al 2009) and a systematic review and meta-analysis of RCTs demonstrated that CBT improved the person's ability to cope with pain through decreasing depression and improving health care–seeking behaviours (Bernardy et al 2010). Evidence is therefore growing to support a combination of educational programmes (Luciano et al 2011), relaxation techniques, stress management and meditation (Grossman et al 2007, Khan & Khan 2011) to provide immediate or sustained benefits in the management of fibromyalgia.

Guided imagery has also been investigated as a therapeutic intervention in the RCT of Fors and colleagues (2002), in which it was suggested that fibromyalgia pain could be reduced by pleasant visualizations. A further study investigated the treatment of fibromyalgia pain, stress, anxiety and depression comparing the effectiveness of relaxation training and stress management. Both techniques were found to be significantly effective in the management of all four symptoms, with significant improvements in the treatment groups compared with the control group. However, there were no significant differences between the two treatment groups (Roshan et al 2017). Mindfulness meditation is also starting to show promise for treating fibromyalgia especially in combination with other techniques, such as exercise and CBT (Adler-Neal & Zeidan 2017).

Headache Disorders

The International Headache Society (IHS 2013) classifies headaches into two groups, primary and secondary. Secondary headache disorders require specialist treatment and are therefore not included in this work. Tension-type headaches and migraine, which are primary headaches, are included. These are disorders in which psychological treatments are widely used in a variety of populations ranging from children to the elderly. Tension-type headaches are characterized by pain on both sides of the head and a feeling of pressure as if a tight band is encircling the head, and can last for hours or days. This type of headache can also be associated with neck pain (IHS 2013). In contrast to tension-type headaches, migraine is characterized by one-sided throbbing pain which results from spasm and overdilation of certain arteries. It is sometimes preceded by visual disturbance described as an aura. Nausea and vomiting are often experienced. These symptoms are known to be caused by a combination of physiological, psychological and neurological factors and is acknowledged as a common recurrent neurological disorder (Gasparini et al 2013).

In the case of schoolchildren, Eccleston and colleagues (2003) report that there is good evidence for the effectiveness of relaxation and cognitive–behaviour training in children and adolescents with chronic headache; both severity and frequency of attack have been shown to fall. Other researchers working in this context, however, have pointed out methodological deficiencies which reduce the confidence that can be placed in these results (Verhagen et al 2005). Rains and colleagues' (2005) overview indicates that behavioural interventions produce benefit which is significantly greater than that provided by control conditions. This benefit has been shown to vary in magnitude between

35% and 55%. Among the behavioural interventions employed were relaxation training, CBT and stress management training. Larsson et al (2005) found, however, that relaxation techniques were more effective when administered by a trained therapist rather than an untrained adult or the people themselves.

It has also been suggested that AT is effective in preventing tension-type headaches. Kanji and colleagues (2006) conducted a systematic review to determine its efficacy, but they found no consistent evidence that AT was superior to other psychological or behavioural interventions. Loder and Rizzoli (2008), in their evaluation of treatment for tension-type headache, found evidence for the effectiveness of a combination of amitriptyline and biofeedback-assisted relaxation training and in a literature review of RCTs, cohort studies and case-control studies investigating the management of headaches associated with neck pain established exercise as a beneficial factor. In addition, stress coping strategies and relaxation training were found to be beneficial for managing chronic tension headaches (Varatharajan et al 2016).

Much of the investigatory work on migraine has been done with children and adolescents, where it has focused on prophylaxis. A systematic review of non-pharmacological trials suggested that relaxation was effective in this area. It also found evidence to suggest that relaxation plus behaviour therapy was more effective than placebo or waiting list controls (Damen et al 2006).

Many treatments for this disorder consist of multiple approaches. To determine which component of treatment was responsible for the effects, Kaushik and colleagues (2005) carried out a randomized test to compare the effects of relaxation with those of propranolol. Results showed that the relaxation training had a long-term prophylactic effect that significantly exceeded that of the drug. The relaxation techniques used in the study were diaphragmatic breathing and muscular relaxation accompanied by daily home practice for 6 months.

PMR is routinely used in migraine prevention (Buse & Andrasik 2009) and has been shown to have positive effects in the prevention of migraine attacks (D'Souza et al 2008, Varkey et al 2011). A recent quasi-RCT investigated PMR and its effect on cortical levels. Results indicated a significant reduction in the frequency of migraine confirming clinical efficacy of progressive muscle relaxation as a prophylaxis for migraine. It also concluded that PMR had an effect on changes in cortical information processing (Meyer et al 2016).

HIV/AIDS

The human immunodeficiency virus (HIV) that causes acquired immunodeficiency syndrome (AIDS) has gradually shifted from a fatal to a chronic disease. This is due to advances in medical science, clinical care, public health advice and pharmacology. Alongside pharmacological approaches, mind–body techniques such as mindfulness have been associated with improved management of the stress which accompanies this long-term condition (Logsdon-Conradsen 2002). Stressors may include stigma, pressure to be compliant to medication, perceived loss of control over health, anticipatory grief and major behavioural changes, especially sexual behaviour (Howland et al 2000, Khatoon 2016). Symptoms of anxiety and depression have also been associated with HIV/AIDS–related outcomes and health predictors (Hunter-Jones et al 2019, Paulus et al 2020). Ampunsiriratana et al (2005) combined mindfulness meditation with Watson's caring theory in an 8-week programme to develop a model for self-care. Sixteen selected patients took part. Researchers found that participants were able to cultivate self-healing in a number of physical and psychological dimensions of pain. This programme was found to be particularly helpful during the later stages of the disease.

Mindfulness is seen by some researchers as the antithesis of impulsivity: a state of mind which promotes action without thought as to its consequences. Impulsive behaviour, in the case of AIDS, carries risks of interpersonal contamination and tendencies to seek intoxication. Lower levels of impulsivity are likely to lead to reduced risky behaviour and drug use.

In a randomized clinical trial with a sample of 38 HIV-positive drug users, the effects of mindfulness were compared with those of standard care. Patients' reports showed that greater reductions in impulsivity and intoxicant use were found among the mindfulness group than in the standard care group. The authors, Margolin et al (2007), regard this work as a first step in the examination of the role of mindfulness in this context. A systematic review of mindfulness-based interventions concluded that it was a cost-effective and simple way of reducing stress and improving QOL in people living with HIV/AIDS. However, further research was required to determine optimal implementation strategies in community and clinical settings (Bhochhibhoya et al 2018). Another systematic review and meta-analysis of mindfulness-based interventions on psychological symptoms, stress and disease biomarkers also found it to be a promising approach for improving QOL and psychological symptoms, but larger sample sizes, longer follow-ups and more robust research designs were required to confirm potential benefits of this intervention (Scott-Sheldon et al 2019).

Cognitive–behavioural interventions are sometimes used in the treatment of HIV/AIDS. Brown and Carlos (2003) used a psychoeducational module as a means of reducing the symptoms of anxiety and depression in people testing positive for HIV/AIDS. The intervention did not, however, result in a statistically significant outcome. However, a mindfulness-based cognitive therapy intervention in a qualitative study of African American women with HIV has been shown to be efficacious in reducing anxiety and depression (Hunter-Jones et al 2019). In addition, a study examining treatment-related changes in anxiety sensitivity and changes related to anxiety, depression and overall QOL receiving CBT demonstrated reductions in anxiety sensitivity significantly related to changes in anxiety, depression and QOL (Paulus et al 2020).

Hypertension

The World Health Organization Technical Report (WHO 1983) recommends the use of non-pharmacological interventions for the treatment of hypertension (high blood pressure). Non-pharmacological methods, for example, relaxation training, have been extensively studied with respect to their effectiveness in reducing blood pressure. Much of this work has supported the use of relaxation techniques. Muscular techniques, AT and meditation have repeatedly been associated with a lowering of blood pressure (both systolic and diastolic) in hypertensive patients, often by a significant margin (Stefano & Esch 2005). This is supported by a recent experimental study which found significant differences in systolic and diastolic blood pressure as well as heart rate 30 minutes after Jacobsnon's PMR,

concluding that PMR could be used in addition to other treatments for immediate control of hypertension (Shinde et al 2013). Furthermore, a study examining the effect of PMR combined with deep breathing technique on 40 people with essential hypertension (no identifiable cause) immediately after aerobic exercise found significant reductions in systolic and diastolic blood pressure, which was deemed impossible with medication alone (Gupta 2014).

There is an increasing evidence base to support associations between mind-body interventions and reduction in blood pressure as well as reducing levels of anxiety and depression in people with hypertension (Blom et al 2014, Hughes et al 2013). Also a review by King and colleagues (2002b) looked at the research on transcendental meditation in the treatment of hypertension and coronary heart disease. In their conclusions they found an association between transcendental meditation and lowered blood pressure, together with indications that the method showed promise as a preventative strategy. As the strongest risk factor in hypertension is age, it would be useful to know how effective behavioural interventions can be for this group of people. Schneider and colleagues (2005) reviewed RCTs in which transcendental meditation and other stress-reducing interventions had been employed. Results indicated that transcendental meditation may well contribute to a decrease in mortality in older people with systemic hypertension.

In the management of essential hypertension, it has been shown that the risk factor with the strongest and most consistent correlation (apart from age) is being overweight (Anand 1999). A cognitive–behavioural approach with an exercise component would seem an appropriate way to address this problem. Although a wealth of research supports the use of exercise in helping to reduce blood pressure, previous studies have chiefly focused on aerobic exercise with resistance training having conventionally been avoided. However, Cornelissen and Fagard (2005) conducted a meta-analysis of nine RCTs in which resistance training was the sole intervention and concluded that moderate resistance training should not be contraindicated. More recent meta-analysis studies demonstrated that both aerobic and resistance training in isolation can reduce blood pressure for acute and chronic hypertension (Carpio-Rivera et al 2016, Cornelissen & Smart 2013).

The combination of both aerobic and resistance training was also effective in reducing blood pressure for older people with hypertension in a meta-analysis of 28 RCT; however, there was a lack of information on the delivery of resistance training (Corso et al 2016). Even so, a blind controlled randomized clinical trial looked at the effects of resistance training and aerobic training in older people and concluded that the combined exercises reduced blood pressure and increased cardiorespiratory fitness and upper limb muscle strength (de Oliveira et al 2020).

Lifestyle has attracted the attention of many researchers working in the field of hypertension. Dickinson et al (2006) carried out a systematic review of RCT on lifestyle interventions which were believed to reduce blood pressure. The most effective approaches were found to be weight reduction, regular exercise, restricted alcohol and reduced salt intake (see Chapter 15 for role of exercise). There was less support for stress reduction. Relaxation therapy had a significant effect when compared with non-intervention controls but this was not as great as that provided by lifestyle changes. NICE support and recommend these lifestyle changes (NICE 2019).

Inflammatory Bowel Disease

Inflammatory bowel disease (IBD) is a chronic disorder with inflammatory and immune activation relapses which includes Crohn's disease and ulcerative colitis. Recent evidence, however, suggests that IBD also presents with microbial changes in the gut and can affect the person's psychological well-being, which are characteristics of irritable bowel syndrome (IBS) (Rani et al 2016). In addition there are a few studies which link an increased risk of IBD in people with symptoms of IBS (García Rodríguez et al 2000; Molodecky et al 2012; Porter et al 2008, 2012).

Levy and colleagues (2007) reviewed work in respect of the illness behaviour associated with IBD. They found that people's reactions became more positive after psychological therapies, such as relaxation training, CBT and social learning. Benefit was also shown to occur from body awareness therapy (see Glossary). In addition, a prospective, RCT, investigated guided imagery and relaxation techniques for anxiety and QOL in people with IBD, demonstrating significant improvement in the relaxation training group for symptoms of pain, stress and anxiety and an overall improvement in mood (Mizrahi et al 2012).

Irritable Bowel Syndrome

IBS causes abdominal pain and changes in bowel habits, which can affect psychological status and QOL (Frank et al 2002). Traumatic events, stress and emotional avoidance as well as physiological arousal are known to cause or increase IBS (Blomhoff et al 2000, Porcelli et al 2014).

A number of behavioural and psychological interventions for IBS have been studied including PMR, guided imagery and relaxed breathing. These relaxation techniques have been shown to directly reduce negative emotions and physiological arousal in people with IBS (Ford et al 2014, Laird et al 2016). As well as relaxation training being a common part of stress management it has also been shown to be as effective as a standalone intervention (Blanchard et al 1993, van der Veck et al 2007). However, one study which compared the effects of relaxation training with those of CBT, using a control of standard care found that improvement occurred in all three groups in equal measure, suggesting that participants were not gaining added benefit from the psychological treatments and that the standard care was adequate (Boyce et al 2003).

In an RCT, emotional awareness and expression training as well as relaxation training both demonstrated improvements in anxiety, depression and QOL in people with IBS (Thakur et al 2017). Holmes and colleagues (2018) secondary analysis of Thakur's data investigating possible facilitators of treatment outcomes concluded that people with tendencies to avoid emotional disclosure and expression might find relaxation training of benefit, with emotional awareness and expression training being more beneficial to a wider range of people with IBS.

Low Back Pain

Pain is a complex phenomenon with biological, psychological and cultural dimensions. In recent years, these strands have come together to inform the treatment of chronic low back pain (LBP). From a wide array of approaches, the most commonly used is CBT – that is, the modification of the patient's cognitive processes and environmental contingencies. It is administered either in place of or in combination with usual treatment, such as physiotherapy, back education and medical treatment (Martin & McLeod 2008).

Multidisciplinary group rehabilitation for women with chronic LBP was evaluated in a randomized trial to determine whether this approach was more effective than individual physiotherapy. The group work consisted of back school, physical training, relaxation training, workplace interventions and cognitive–behavioural stress management. The individual physiotherapy consisted of physical exercise and mobilization. In both interventions the before-and-after measurements showed favourable effects which were maintained at 2-year follow-up. No statistically significant differences were found between the two treatment approaches and the authors concluded that multidisciplinary group rehabilitation and individual physiotherapy seemed equally effective in the treatment of women with chronic LBP (Kaapa et al 2006).

Chou and Huffman (2007) conducted a systematic review of non-pharmacological therapies for acute and chronic LBP. They found that, for chronic LBP, the use of CBT, exercise, spinal manipulation and interdisciplinary rehabilitation was supported by good evidence of moderate efficacy. For acute LBP, superficial heat was the only intervention that was effective. However, the evidence from systematic reviews is not consistent. Ostelo and colleagues (2005), reviewing 21 studies, found that when CBT with a progressive relaxation component was compared with usual treatment, no significant differences were found. There was some benefit when compared with a waiting list control but this was not maintained. Thus it is suggested that cognitive–behavioural approaches may be no more effective than usual treatment. This was confirmed in an RCT where internet-delivered CBT had no additional benefits to physical treatments (Petrozzi et al 2019). Factors which may reduce the effectiveness of CBT are thought to be psychiatric comorbidities, sleep disturbances, overuse of medication, stress and poor coping strategies (Theadom et al 2015). Studies have therefore started to investigate the immediate effect of guided imagery and mindfulness of breathing in the management of non-specific chronic LBP, concluding that these relaxation techniques are a beneficial adjunct to pain relieving treatments (Khan & Khatri 2016). Another study examined Jacobson's PMR compared with usual care in a randomized controlled crossover

study and found higher reductions in pain relief in the PMR group compared with the control group (Mateu et al 2018).

Menopause

Peri- and postmenopausal women experience a number of physical and psychological changes are a result of reduction in oestrogen levels (Celik & Pasinlioglu 2014). The three most common changes experienced are vasomotor (hot flushes and night sweats), fatigue and insomnia (sleep disturbances) (Ameratunga et al 2012, Lai et al 2006). A decrease in oestrogen levels has also been shown to increase the risk of cardiovascular disease and osteoporosis (Wellons et al 2012).

A brief version of AR technique was compared with AR in an RCT for the management of two of these symptoms, vasomotor and insomnia. The study concluded that the brief version of AR was equally if not more effective than AR. However, the sample size was small and would warrant further research to confirm the findings (Saensak et al 2013). Another RCT was carried out to investigate the effect of PMR and sleep hygiene training compared with routine health care in 161 postmenopausal women experiencing insomnia. The PMR and sleep hygiene training (81 women) was delivered once a week over an 8-week period with significant improvements in insomnia compared with the control group (80 women) suggesting that teaching these techniques would be beneficial (Duman & Tashan 2018).

Hypnotic relaxation therapy has been demonstrated as beneficial in reducing vasomotor symptoms in postmenopausal women (Elkins et al 2013). It is thought that the effect may be due to an altered physiological response to psychological stress. Using cortisol as a biomarker of stress a study examined the effect of hypnotic relaxation using changes in cortisol levels in 62 postmenopausal women. Results indicated significant decreases in cortisol levels in evening saliva, however the effect of hypnotic relaxation therapy on changes in salivary cortisol levels was insignificant. Therefore further research is required to understand the factors in which hypnotic relaxation therapy reduces vasomotor symptoms to establish effective treatments (Kendrick et al 2015).

In a 2017 systematic review to investigate the efficacy of a variety of relaxation techniques (yoga, hypnosis, mindfulness, relaxation, paced breathing, reflexology and CBT) for vasomotor symptoms, out of the 26 RCTs that met the inclusion criteria for the study it was concluded that CBT and relaxation therapy were consistent in improving vasomotor symptoms. For the other relaxation techniques findings were mixed and supporting evidence weak as a result of methodological differences. Therefore large, robust studies are required to establish the effectiveness of these interventions, how they work and the long-term outcomes (Stefanopoulou & Grunfeld 2017).

A review of non-pharmacological treatments for the adverse symptoms of menopause was carried out by McKee and Warber (2005). They found that exercise and a range of relaxation techniques (progressive relaxation and abdominal slow breathing) may help some women to reduce these symptoms. The evidence to support the benefits of regular physical activity to alleviate symptoms other than bone loss has mostly been gathered from surveys.

In a large UK survey, Daley et al (2007) reported better health-related QOL scores for women who were physically active, suggesting that menopausal women who participated in regular physical activity benefited psychologically. The psychological benefits of physical activity, however, extend to women at all stages of life. This includes the elderly. A study in a large cohort of Australian women in their 70s across a 3-year period demonstrated an association between physical activity and emotional well-being (Lee & Russell 2003). Furthermore, a recent systematic review and meta-analysis of 17 RCTs investigated exercise as an intervention for menopausal women in relation to cardiovascular risk, body composition and bone mineral density found that exercise has significant benefits on triglyceride level, body fat, waist circumference and bone mineral density of the lumbar spine, with aerobic exercise specifically improving body fat in menopausal women (Yeh et al 2018).

Multiple Sclerosis

Multiple sclerosis (MS) is a chronic disease of the nervous system, a condition which causes damage to the myelin sheath (protective cover) of neurones (nerve fibres) in the brain, optic nerve and spinal cord. The damage causes neurological issues as a result of the slowing down or caseation of nerve impulses. This

can lead to balance and mobility impairments often with reduced trunk stability (postural control). The diagnosis can cause significant emotional and psychological problems such as anxiety, depression and decreased QOL (Byatt et al 2011, Moore et al 2012).

Psychological interventions include the process of helping people with MS to adjust to and cope with their condition. The systematic review of Thomas and colleagues (2006) has suggested that cognitive–behavioural approaches can go some way towards achieving a better adjustment. CBT has also been shown to alleviate anxiety and depression. These findings have been confirmed in a 2016 systematic review and meta-analysis (Fiest et al 2016), which demonstrated that CBT had a moderate effect on depression. MS studies using mindfulness techniques to manage psychological stress and QOL in people with MS have also shown positive results. Trait mindfulness demonstrates significant decreases in psychological stress improving QOL, resilience and coping strategies (Senders et al 2014). Further research has verified these findings, emphasizing that the reduction in the person's inability to control their emotional response could be significant, linking mindfulness and QOL, particularly for those with higher levels of depression (Schirda et al 2015). Two other systematic reviews corroborate these findings, as well as demonstrating improvements in levels of fatigue (Levin et al 2014, Simpson et al 2014). However, limitations include a lack of control group, a need for larger sample size and more robust methodologies.

Other studies have investigated PMR in relation to stress management for people with MS. One such study, an RCT, involved PMR activities carried out on a daily basis over an 8-week period. Results indicated a significant reduction in perceived levels of stress after PMR. However, the sample size was small and cortisol levels were not monitored (Novais et al 2016). As well as stress, trigeminal neuralgia can cause distress and pain in people with MS. A woman with MS reporting trigeminal neuralgia reported pain relief from hypnosis and self-hypnosis in a case study of hypnosis as an additional method for pain relief (McCall 2016).

Research is starting to explore exercises such as Pilates to improve balance and mobility in people with MS who are mobile. For example, a multicentre, assessor-blinded, RCT compared 12 weeks of Pilates exercises with relaxation and then compared standard exercises with relaxation, followed by the comparison of Pilates exercises with standardized exercises. Home exercises were monitored 1 month after the face-to-face interventions. Statistical and clinical improvements were recorded for balance and mobility in the standardized exercise group compared with the relaxation group, with results maintained 1 month after the intervention. Standardized exercises were deemed more beneficial than Pilates exercises in this study. However, the study was limited by standardized exercises which could have influenced the outcomes of the study as well as outcome measures used, which may have been less sensitive to changes (Fox et al 2016).

Musculoskeletal Disorders

Certain occupations give rise to repetitive strain injuries (RSIs). RSIs, also referred to as work-related musculoskeletal disorders, mainly occur in the upper limb regions, such as the shoulder girdle and neck region (Andersen & Gaardboe 1993, Pun et al 2004). These can be very painful and can interfere with output. A form of rehabilitation which takes account of the patients's social and psychological life is believed to augment the benefits of a physical approach. Karjalainen and colleagues (2007) reviewed the research in biopsychosocial rehabilitation for upper limb RSI in working-age adults but were unable to form any conclusion owing to a lack of high-quality trials in this field. A recent study investigated physical activity programmes for work-related musculoskeletal disorders and pain experienced by garment workers. The programme included, 15-minute sessions of stretching exercises, group dynamics, muscular endurance, self-massage relaxation and massage techniques. Results indicated significant reductions in pain experienced in the neck and wrists. There was also a reduction in the intensity of pain in the shoulders, arms, fingers and wrist. However, this study was limited by a small sample size (Pereira et al 2013).

Psychosocial aspects of musculoskeletal disorders are particularly relevant in the world of the performing arts. de Greef and colleagues (2003) reported on a programme addressed to professional musicians in situations where there was a high rate of absenteeism owing to musculoskeletal disorders. Its aim was to change the playing habits of the musicians and reduce the effects of physical overload, which interferes with perceived physical competence. The programme consisted of relaxation procedures, postural exercises for the shoulder, neck and lower back and exercises to cope with mental stress. Researchers found that the programme significantly decreased playing-related musculoskeletal disorders. At the same time, it increased perceived physical competence.

Obsessive Compulsive Disorder

Obsessive compulsive disorder (OCD) is characterized by compulsive rituals and intrusive obsessive thoughts and is associated with high levels of impairment in social functioning and QOL (Eisen et al 2006, Stengler-Wenzke et al 2006). NICE recommends the use of CBT and exposure and response prevention (ERP) (see Glossary) in the treatment of this condition (NICE 2006). O'Kearney and colleagues (2006), in their systematic review, evaluated the effects of cognitive–behavioural approaches in the treatment of OCD. Findings showed that CBT had favourable effects in the treatment of this condition. There is no evidence to suggest that the psychological approach is better than medication, or medication better than the psychological approach, but when the two treatments are combined the outcome is better than when medication is administered on its own. Their combined effect is not, however, any different from the effect of CBT on its own. These findings suggest that CBT has potential value in the treatment of OCD and might serve as a useful adjunct to conventional treatment. A case study combining six sessions of relaxation training (deep muscle relaxation, breathing control and autogenic relaxation) were integrated to standard CBT to enhance motivation, which was deemed a contributing component for the treatment of OCD and therefore more research is required in this area. However, the research does confirm previous research findings (Okumus et al 2019).

There is limited research on the efficacy of mindfulness-based therapy for the management of OCD, but a few studies have demonstrated the importance of mindfulness-based therapies in relation to thought action and thought suppression (see Glossary) (Hannan & Tolin 2005, Fairfax 2008, Orsillo et al 2005). Following on from this research a case series design was used to investigate whether mindfulness-based therapy might benefit people with OCD who express obsessive intrusive thoughts by addressing thought action fusion and thought suppression. Mindfulness skills such as observation, awareness and acceptance were reported as beneficial; however, a larger sample size is required to establish the full effect of this approach (Wilkinson-Tough et al 2010).

Occupational Stress

In the workplace stress may arise for a variety of reasons including high expectations, time constraints, inadequate work skills and ineffective social support (see Chapter 1). Prolonged exposure to workplace stressors can lead to burnout; therefore workplaces are increasingly offering mindfulness, meditation and other relaxation techniques to improve overall mental health well-being.

A systematic review found that both person-directed and work-directed interventions could be effective in relieving work stress. Cognitive–behavioural approaches with relaxation techniques were found to ease the situation for individuals while visible management modifications were found useful for organizations. Benefits derived from well-designed stress reduction programmes were found to survive long after closure of the programme – that is, for 6 to 24 months. However, results should be interpreted with caution owing to a mixed quality of research evidence (Marine et al 2006). A meta-analysis has since been carried out to reappraise the existing evidence base on relaxation techniques for the management of psychological distress in employees. Results indicate that overall relaxation techniques are effective in decreasing stress in employees, with small to moderate effects maintained at follow-up. However, there was evidence of publication bias, more apparent in uncontrolled singe-sample studies than large RCT studies, which may have inflated effects reported. Even so the meta-analysis supports the effectiveness of relaxation techniques in decreasing occupational distress (Slemp et al 2019).

A meta-analysis investigating the effectiveness of relaxation techniques in employee burnout, included peer-reviewed journals and key studies identified in previous reviews. The study concluded that relaxation techniques provided modest but lasting effects (up to 6 months) in their ability to decrease burnout, with CBT and relaxation interventions significantly decreasing emotional exhaustion. However, to increase the effects of relaxation techniques on reducing burnout, new personalized strategies are required to tackle issues of depersonalization and personal accomplishment (Maricutoiu et al 2016).

Pain

A widely adopted view sees the perception of pain as governed by a neural 'gate' in the spinal cord (Melzack & Wall 1965). When this gate is open it allows signals from the pain receptors on the skin to pass to the brain, exposing the individual to the full experience of the pain. However, signals sent down from the cortex can help to 'close' the gate, thereby reducing the perceived intensity of the pain. For example, if you are enjoying a film you will be less inclined to notice body irritations that might otherwise claim your attention. Most non-pharmacological pain relief can be explained by the gate theory.

There exists a body of research relating to non-pharmacological methods which are said to 'close' the gate. Their effectiveness has been the subject of several literature reviews. Kwekkeboom and Gretarsdottir (2006) systematically reviewed randomized trials of relaxation interventions for pain in adults. Findings showed support for these interventions in 8 out of 15 studies. PMR stood out as the most commonly supported technique, particularly for arthritis, but jaw relaxation and PMR were found effective for the relief of postoperative pain. There was little support for AT and none for rhythmic breathing. Researchers call for more well-designed trials to test all relaxation techniques.

Kessler et al (2003) reviewed work featuring relaxation and hypnosis, both of which were found to significantly reduce different indices of pain. Of the two interventions, the evidence for hypnosis is stronger, being effective in acute and chronic pain. In the case of relaxation, the evidence is modest for acute pain, although more convincing for chronic. The authors add that neither hypnosis nor relaxation was found to be consistently more effective than other self-regulation methods. They suggest that these approaches might form useful adjunctive therapies in various conditions of pain.

Evidence for mind–body therapies has also been reviewed by Astin (2004). He looked at muscular relaxation, meditation, imagery and CBT in the treatment of pain. Based on his findings, he made the following recommendations.

1. *Low back pain*: this may respond favourably to a combination of relaxation training, coping skills, stress management and cognitive restructuring.
2. *Arthritis, rheumatoid and osteo*: these seemed to benefit from a combination of CBT and education administered adjunctively to conventional treatment.
3. *Tension headache*: this appeared to benefit from relaxation and muscle biofeedback, whereas migraine seemed to respond to relaxation training and thermal biofeedback.
4. *Perioperative states*: postoperative recovery time may be reduced when techniques are taught preoperatively. Suggested methods include muscular relaxation, imagery and hypnosis.
5. *Invasive medical procedures*: the pain that accompanies some of these procedures can be ameliorated by mind–body approaches used adjunctively.

Schaffer and Yucha (2004) investigated the role of Benson's relaxation response in the management of chronic and acute pain (see Chapter 22) and Weydert (2006) reported on the effects of imagery in children with abdominal pain (see Chapter 18). A number of relaxation techniques have also been shown to be effective in decreasing acute and chronic pain in children and young people with a variety of pain conditions, such as fibromyalgia, abdominal pain and headaches (Birrie et al 2014, Chambers et al 2009, Palermo et al 2010).

Panic Disorder

Panic disorder is related to fear and anxiety that manifests in panic attacks that can occur on a daily basis or may occur weeks or months apart. CBT stands out as being the treatment of choice for panic disorder (Carlbring et al 2003, Siev & Chambless 2007, Wetherell et al 2005) and is effective in treating panic attacks in panic disorder (Butler et al 2006). Studies in the area of anxiety and panic disorder tend to show specific treatment effects; for example, relaxation training and cognitive therapy show equivalent effects in GAD, whereas for panic disorder, cognitive therapy

provides greater benefit (Siev & Chambless 2007). Or again, in a review of psychological interventions, relaxation training showed particular effectiveness in cases of subjective anxiety, whereas for GAD and panic, the treatment of choice was CBT (Wetherell et al 2005). However, a study comparing the effectiveness of relaxation techniques and cognitive interventions, which included breathing training, muscle relaxation and CBT to find out the core element of these therapies, found that they reduced the expectation of a panic attack and therefore disrupted the vicious circle of fearing fear. The study concluded that this might be a key element for treating panic and therefore interventions should be evaluated by encouraging positive thinking or by nurturing non-expectancy (Roth 2010).

Many people with panic disorder also experience agoraphobia, which makes it difficult for them to travel to treatment locations. A solution has been created in the form of internet-administered self-help whose effectiveness was tested by Carlbring et al (2003, 2007). These studies are reported in Chapter 9.

Parkinson's Disease

Parkinson's disease (PD) is a neurodegenerative disease of unknown origin which progresses over time, causing motor and cognitive changes. The three main symptoms are rigidity, slowness and tremor (which can exacerbate during stress), with postural instability developing towards the later stages of the disease. Anxiety and depression often occur in PD, increasing the severity of the symptoms and reducing overall QOL (Weisskopf et al 2003). Therefore treatment is aimed at reducing the severity of symptoms and improving QOL. Relaxation techniques have been recommended for people with PD who are experiencing anxiety (Marsh 2000). Lundervold and colleagues (2009) carried out a multiple-baseline, cross-behaviours experimental design to evaluate the effect of multicomponent behavioural interventions for anxiety in a 67-year-old man with PD. The Clinical Anxiety Scale (CAS), Subjective Unit of Discomfort (SUD) ratings and the Behavioural Relaxation Scale was used to collect data before and after behavioural relaxation training. The researchers concluded that behavioural relaxation training had a beneficial outcome in reducing anxiety above that achieved from medication alone.

Stallibrass et al (2002) conducted an RCT to investigate whether the Alexander technique benefited people with idiopathic PD. They found that motor symptoms in the Alexander group improved significantly compared with no treatment (see Chapter 12).

A study investigated relaxation guided imagery (RGI), self-relaxation and relaxing music to determine their effect on PD tremor. A small cohort of 20 participants with moderate-to-severe tremor were included in the study. Each participant's tremor was recorded using an accelerometer. Results indicated a dramatic decrease in tremor in all the participants. RGI completely reduced PD tremor in 15 of the participants, with average PD tremor remaining significantly reduced 15 to 30 minutes after RGI and results were maintained for 1 to 14 hours. The relaxing music also significantly reduced the PD tremor but not to the degree achieved with RGI. There was no significant effect in self-relaxation. The study concluded that RGI could support pharmacological treatment for the management of PD tremor as best practice (Schlesinger et al 2009).

A multicentre RCT investigated mental practice within standard physiotherapy compared with relaxation within standard physiotherapy on their effect on mobility tasks in 47 people with PD living in the community. The interventions were delivered in two separate groups, relaxation (n = 22) and mental practice (n = 25) over a 6-week period. Outcome measures were recorded at 6 weeks and 3 months. This study did not find any significant differences between the group's outcomes, concluding that both mental practice and relaxation had beneficial effects on mobility tasks. This may be due to lack of contrast between the two interventions or a sample size too small to detect possible effects (Braun et al 2011).

Posttraumatic Stress Disorder

Traumatic events can give rise to posttraumatic stress disorder (PTSD) with accompanying distress and reduced functioning. Psychological interventions are therefore commonly employed in the treatment of this disorder. Bisson and Andrew (2007) conducted a systematic review to determine their effectiveness. Results showed that individual trauma-focused CBT and eye movement desensitization and reprocessing (see Glossary) offer significant benefit. Stress management

and group trauma-focused CBT are also useful. Trauma-focused approaches were more effective than non–trauma-focused ones and treatment was best started within 3 months of the event. Drug treatment was second line.

PTSD may occur in childhood where a single incident has been experienced (Adler-Nevo & Manassis 2005). In this review, the same forms of treatment as just described were in use, with the addition of play therapy. Most of the studies showed statistically significant improvement. However, the methodology was not always sound enough for conclusions about best treatment to be drawn.

A recent study reviewed the efficacy of CBT to determine the key elements for clinical improvement in PTSD. The study also included CBT and exposure therapy (see Glossary) and compared them to other well-known treatments, such as counselling and supportive therapy or assessment only conditions. The study replicated a previous literature review (Mendes et al 2008) to update the findings, including 29 RCTs which met the inclusion criteria. Findings indicated that all three interventions were beneficial compared with the assessment only conditions and there was no difference found between the interventions. The study concluded that CBT and its key elements are equally beneficial in improving the diagnosis and symptoms of PTSD; however, further research was needed to understand the long-term effects and benefits of the other interventions (Mello et al 2013).

Recent literature reviews infer that there is inadequate evidence to recommend mindfulness as a standard intervention for PTSD; however, it may be helpful (Scarlet & Lang 2014). Several meta-analyses on the efficacy of mindfulness-based interventions for the management of PTSD symptoms have reported medium benefits for anxiety, depression and chronic pain (Oded 2018).

Peri- and Postoperative States

There is often a lack of appropriate pain control in perioperative states, which can cause negative outcomes for the person's surgery and overall satisfaction. If this is not addressed, it can lead to physiological changes and consequently chronic pain with loss of health and QOL (Miranda et al 2011, Rico et al 2013).

In postoperative states, pain is categorized as acute, developing from a mixture of tissue injury, anxiety and pain and can be influenced by psychological factors such as culture and previous illnesses. It can also be influenced by physical factors such as place and type of incision, extent of the trauma during surgery and the skill and competence of the surgeon (Darnall 2016, Miranda et al 2011).

Relaxation and guided imagery are reported as effective interventions for people admitted to hospital for various types of surgery (Hansen 2015), encouraging self-efficacy and active participation in the recovery process (Alam et al 2016, Glickman-Simon & Tessier 2014). Furthermore, it has been stated that relaxation and hypnosis should be considered in addition to standard analgesia to manage perioperative pain (Payati & Tong 2007), but there is a lack of research in this area.

A programme of mixed relaxation techniques was carried out in an RCT on 102 adults after abdominal surgery in a large hospital in Thailand. It resulted in reports of decreased pain sensation and distress in the intervention group compared with the control. State anxiety reduction did not quite reach significance, but the trend was noticeably in that direction. Most participants reported that their pain had been reduced by the intervention and fewer participants asked for opioids. They also liked the sense of control that the relaxation techniques had offered them (Roykulcharoen & Good 2004).

Laurion and Fetzer (2003) tested the effect of guided imagery and music on gynaecological laparoscopy outcomes such as pain levels. Results showed a significant reduction of reported pain among the intervention participants compared with controls. The mechanism is unclear, but the authors suggest that the distraction inherent in the treatment reduces the reporting of negative outcomes. A 2019 literature review to identify the evidence base for the use of relaxation therapy with guided imagery for postoperative pain management selected 8 out of 291 articles. The knowledge gathered from this integrative review concluded that relaxation therapy with guided imagery could be used as an adjunct to pharmacological approaches to effectively manage postoperative pain. However, the use of relaxation therapy with guided imagery is minimal and would warrant new RCTs to gain further understanding and strengthen the evidence base (Felix et al 2019).

Psoriasis

Psoriasis is a chronic inflammatory skin disorder estimated to affect 2% to 4% of the world population and is linked to extensive psychological illness (Gelfand et al 2005, Stern et al 2004), such as depression (Patel et al 2017), affecting QOL. It is characterized by a proliferation of the epidermal layers of the skin creating red raised patches covered with white scales. In plaque psoriasis, these appear typically on the knees, elbows and scalp. The condition is commonly treated with ultraviolet light which promotes clearing of the lesions; however, stress is recognized as a trigger as well as a cause of exacerbation of psoriasis.

The role of stress has been tested by Picardi et al (2005). These researchers investigated the relationship between stress, perceived social support, emotional awareness and diffuse plaque psoriasis. Stress was assessed by the impact of negative life events experienced by the individual, using Paykel's Interview for Recent Life Events (Paykel 1997). The researchers found a correlation between psychological distress and the length of time it took for phototherapy to clear the plaque. They also found that a mindfulness-based approach significantly reduced the healing time. In their conclusions they suggested that increased emotional awareness and greater social support might help to reduce susceptibility to exacerbations of psoriasis.

Life events as a measure of perceived stress was employed by Payne et al (1985) in a controlled study which compared the effect of such events on plaque psoriasis with their effect on three other skin disorders: viral warts, fungal infections and new growths. Thirty-two patients with varying degrees of plaque psoriasis participated in a matched pair design. However, in this small study no significant difference among the groups was found and results suggested that exacerbations of psoriasis were no more affected by life events than were warts, fungal infections and new growths.

A literature review evaluated the effectiveness of psychological interventions, such as hypnosis and meditation, as additions to standard skin treatments for the management of psoriasis. The study concluded that these psychological interventions demonstrated a potential benefit and could be used as an addition to standard skin treatments. However, the literature review was limited by non-validated or lack of outcome measures, small number of trials and sample sizes, high attrition rates and potential reporting of bias (Tran & Koo 2014).

Schizophrenia

Schizophrenia is a severe chronic mental disorder that mainly consists of positive, negative and cognitive symptoms, with reduced life expectancy (Vancampfort et al 2012), presenting with high levels of disability, compromised social functioning and internalized stigma (Krupchanka & Katliar 2016). Therefore for some years now the suggested psychological treatment for schizophrenia has been CBT. This approach addresses the problem by linking feelings with thinking patterns. In their systematic review of the effectiveness of CBT, Jones and colleagues (2004) found that this treatment holds promise, particularly in the short term. NICE guidelines continue to recommend individual CBT for people diagnosed with schizophrenia (NICE 2014).

Hallucinations experienced by people with schizophrenia are often treated with distraction techniques. As a coping strategy within a cognitive–behavioural framework, these techniques are applied adjunctively. Crawford-Walker and colleagues (2005) systematically reviewed studies in this area but no clear effect emerged owing partly to a paucity of good evidence. Thomas and colleagues (2014) have since reviewed research findings on psychological therapies for auditory hallucinations (voices). The researchers concluded that psychological therapies have an overall beneficial effect with positive symptoms, but further research was required to understand the specific use of psychological therapies to voices.

Exercise has been shown in a review to have potential benefits, both in reducing negative symptoms and as a coping strategy for the positive symptoms of schizophrenia (Faulkner & Biddle 1999). These findings are supported in a study investigating the patient experience: people with schizophrenia who participated in a 3-month programme of exercise in a community care setting in Melbourne indicated through focus groups that they enjoyed the graduated, individualized programme and took pleasure in feeling fitter.

They also enjoyed participating in group exercise and they all indicated their intention to continue with the exercise programme (Fogarty & Happel 2005). A systematic review of 10 RCTs has been carried out since to investigate the effectiveness of physical therapy for people with schizophrenia. Out of the 10 studies reviewed, 6 investigated aerobic and strengthening exercises and 4 of the studies investigated PMR. Aerobic and strengthening exercises were seen to reduce psychiatric symptoms, psychological distress and anxiety and improve health-related QOL. Aerobic exercise was also seen to improve short-term memory and PMR decreased psychological distress and state anxiety. However, the results are limited by the small sample sizes of the studies as well as the diversity of the interventions used (Vancampfort et al 2012).

A 2019 literature review of 13 RCTs included studies on mindfulness interventions, yoga, tai chi, and relaxation techniques. These interventions were found to have medium to large benefits on improving anxiety, stress, insight, well-being and social functioning reducing admittance to hospital. However, several of the studies reviewed had small sample sizes, so findings should be interpreted with caution (Wang et al 2019).

Sleep Disorders

Without sleep, we can hardly be said to enjoy psychological well-being. Interventions for the relief of insomnia have typically been pharmacological. However, a wide range of non-pharmacological treatments exist in the form of sleep health techniques, stimulus control instruction, sleep restriction, relaxation therapy, cognitive therapy, paradoxical intention and others. These approaches are popular with people who fear the possibility of drug side effects and dependency which can occur with many pharmacological remedies. Side effects include daytime sedation, increased risk of motor accidents, falls, and cognitive impairment.

A review of these treatments was authorized by the American Academy of Sleep Medicine. Reporting on its findings, Morgenthaler and colleagues (2006) showed that psychological and behavioural interventions were effective in the treatment of both primary and secondary insomnia. The most effective treatments for chronic insomnia were stimulus control therapy, relaxation training and CBT.

Insomnia accompanies many conditions, one of which is PTSD. A critical review sees CBT as a promising treatment option (Lamarche & de Koninck 2007). However, health care professionals faced with this condition are advised to collaborate with mental health professionals or sleep medicine specialists.

Sleep problems often increase with age, but because of the high risk of falls in older age groups, there has been a need to search for effective alternatives to drug treatment. A review conducted by Montgomery and Dennis (2003) focused on cognitive–behavioural interventions among adults older than age 60 years. Sleep quality and duration were examined. However, in the absence of an adequate research base, the authors could not draw conclusions beyond suggesting a mild benefit derived from CBT.

A meta-analysis of behavioural interventions for insomnia was carried out by Irwin and colleagues (2006). They were looking at the effect of relaxation training, behavioural interventions and CBT on quality, latency and duration of sleep for people in the second half of life. All three methods showed robust and similar improvement for middle-aged and older participants. These results suggest that mature adults with insomnia benefit from a wide range of non-pharmacological treatments. Other work has focused on the combination of pharmacological and non-pharmacological therapies for insomnia. The author (Mendelson 2007) considered the way in which these two approaches might interact with each other and decided there was a possibility of the one potentiating the other. However, he found the research base too small to draw firm conclusions. Since then relaxation training has been indicated as an effective treatment to reduce insomnia, especially when used in support or in combination with other intervention forms, both pharmacological and psychotherapeutic (Langford et al 2012). Moreover, the use of relaxation techniques proved to be useful in the treatment of nightmare disorders (Aurora et al 2010).

A systematic review and meta-analysis investigated poor sleep health in otherwise healthy adults to investigate the efficacy of a number of relaxation techniques in this group of people. Eleven studies were evaluated after screening for inclusion criteria. Findings indicated that overall there was a medium effect on sleep quality, with stress management, relaxation techniques, sleep hygiene, exercise and stimulus control being used the most (Murawski et al 2018).

Tinnitus

Tinnitus is a condition characterized by ringing or buzzing in the ears, in the absence of external acoustic stimulation. In recent years it has been treated with CBT, which has included AR, distraction, imagery, restructuring of beliefs and thoughts and management of sleep. Andersson (2002), in his overview, found that CBT showed promise of being effective, but at present there is no specific therapy that suits everyone.

In a review by Martinez-Devesa and colleagues (2007), the researchers looked for differences between the subjective loudness of the tinnitus before CBT and its perceived loudness after treatment. They found no significant difference between the two. Neither was there any difference in the degree of associated depression experienced by the person before and after treatment. However, the researchers did find a significant improvement in the reported QOL, and this was important because it suggested that people found it easier to cope with the tinnitus after a course of CBT.

Some authors have suggested that tinnitus is associated with psychophysiological overactivation of the head and shoulder muscles. Rief et al (2005) conducted an RCT to test this hypothesis. Psychological outcome measures were self-ratings, questionnaires and diary data, and physiological outcome measures were muscle activity of the head and shoulders and electrodermal activity. After seven treatment sessions, participants in the intervention group had improved significantly more than their counterparts on the waiting list. The authors concluded that these results appeared to support the hypothesis that tinnitus is associated with overactive head and shoulder muscles.

A review investigated potential interventions (invasive and non-invasive) to manage chronic tinnitus. Study sample included research representing a sample of different interventions used to manage tinnitus. A meta-analysis was not possible because of the diversity of the studies reviewed. Findings indicated a lack of evidence for invasive treatments, with the majority being ineffective and therefore should be avoided, as a result of the increased risk to the person. Non-invasive treatments that were found to be beneficial included acoustic therapy, CBT, hypnosis, relaxation training, biofeedback and counselling (Folmer et al 2014). A 10-year retrospective outcome analysis of 268 people on the efficacy of treating tinnitus with CBT found significant reductions in tinnitus, hyperacusis (see Glossary), depression and distress (Nolan et al 2017).

THEORIES BEHIND THE EVIDENCE

Although research is not the only source of evidence for the value of relaxation training, it is the principal one, enabling the health care professional to provide the best treatment. Other sources include clinical experience, expert consensus, reflective practice, individual assessment and preferences (Bury & Mead 1998).

Evidence of effectiveness is most valued in the form of the review, which collects and scrutinizes relevant studies. Reviews may vary in terms of scientific rigour, the most respected one being the Cochrane systematic review. Here, strict criteria are laid down; for instance, the databases employed must be cited, the years which relate to the search stated, the number and quality of papers involved recorded, the basis on which the selection was made stated and the key words listed. Meta-analysis is another way of presenting reviewed work: here, the data from the studies included in the review are reanalysed using statistical techniques; this allows the pooling of a number of studies to obtain an effect size which can be stated as an overall conclusion.

A critical review is also a useful document. It is often described as a narrative review and tends to express the opinion of the researcher. Critical reviews can vary in quality. Another type of review is the overview which is a description of key findings.

Individual studies can also be classified in terms of scientific rigour. Here, the most highly respected form is the RCT. A hypothesis is first formulated and tested, then the data are analysed for statistical significance. A well-designed RCT will fulfil the following criteria. It will:

- contain a control group which does not receive the intervention and acts as a baseline;
- adopt a randomized process, both for the selection of participants and their assignment to particular groups;

- allow for blinding of study participants and, where appropriate, also the researcher;
- be designed so that the results can be statistically analyzed;
- consist of a sample large enough to have a chance of reaching statistical significance;
- carry a precise description of the intervention so that the study can be replicated;
- be free of bias and order effects which may confound the results;
- follow intention-to-treat analysis of data.

When these criteria are not met the study is said to be methodologically flawed, which means that the results lose some of their credibility. However, it is not always ethical or appropriate to use the RCT as a design and in these situations other forms of trial may be adopted such as non-randomized controlled studies and single-system studies.

The experiment, however, is not the only way to answer a question in research: a qualitative approach, in which descriptive data are collected, can also provide useful information and may be the method of choice where the function of research is one of exploration (Sim 1999). Interviews can be employed here.

Wherever subtleties in the therapeutic situation are being studied, the qualitative approach has much to offer. It reflects the lived experience of individuals (Gibson & Martin 2003). Qualitative methods can also be used to complement the findings of experimental work, thereby building up a more complete picture.

BEST PRACTICE

Scientific evidence therefore supports the efficacy of relaxation techniques, promoting QOL and overall well-being across a number of conditions. Results indicate that relaxation techniques are effective in reducing anxiety and depression across a wide range of people, whether they are adult, ageing, young, male, female, with or without physical or psychological conditions.

Research indicates that over time, relaxation techniques have demonstrated effectiveness in managing a number of conditions both physical and psychological. This evidence base therefore confirms that relaxation techniques should be promoted as a valuable option and best practice within the clinical setting.

KEY POINTS

1. Most stress-related conditions seem to benefit in some degree from relaxation techniques.
2. CBT and exercise therapy have also been shown to play a part in the relief of stress.
3. In some instances relaxation is presented as sole treatment; in others, the relaxation forms part of a wider approach.
4. Results of scientific investigation indicate to the therapist which technique is likely to bring benefit in a particular condition.
5. Therapists should seek out guidelines where they are available. These may be obtained from organizations such as NICE and the Scottish Intercollegiate Guidelines Network (SIGN) which have used panels of reviewers to provide evidence statements and best practice guidance. As new evidence emerges, the health care professional may be directed to different approaches.
6. Although relaxation has been around for many years, the research base is relatively small. For this reason, findings may need to be interpreted with caution. This leaves many questions unanswered.

Reflection

Describe the key aspects of research and RCTs.
What research have you undertaken if any?
How did you decide on your research method?
Did you need to refine your research question and why?
What is the main learning point you will take away from this chapter?
What is your further action plan in terms of researching?

CASE STUDY LEARNING OPPORTUNITY

The key points and reflection provide background and knowledge required in relation to the case study, evidence into practice, to help deepen understanding of how evidence from research can be implemented into practice.

CASE STUDY

Evidence into Practice: Research Outcomes for Cancer Patients With Anxiety

It was noted during assessment by health care professionals that a number of their patients with cancer were experiencing anxiety. In many cases anxiety was reducing their ability to engage with treatments, such as physical activity. The thought of having some treatments was also causing nausea and vomiting. In addition to this, family and social life was affected by the emotional roller coaster some patients were experiencing. Further assessments were carried out to understand individual concerns, which highlighted fears of treatment, fear of reoccurrence, changes in physical functioning and worries about the future. This triggered discussions between the health care professionals to discern what evidence-based interventions there were to improve the outcomes for their patients. After initial talks the health care professionals decided to form a project team to review the current literature on the management of anxiety. From this review the group concluded that there was robust evidence around psychosocial and psychoeducational interventions that were recommended for their area of practice. An implementation plan was then developed to transfer and embed this new knowledge into practice. This included identification of outcome measures to assess the enhanced service delivery at baseline and post 12-week pilot.

Screening for anxiety was instigated and psychosocial issues were addressed as part of routine care. Therapeutic support was offered, which included support groups, relaxation techniques and CBT. Education was also offered to both the patient and their families around cancer and its treatment. Furthermore, symptom management and self-care strategies were promoted. Where more specialized input was required, such as referral to the clinical psychologist, a referral system was put in place.

This small service evaluation and quality improvement initiative demonstrated improvements in the patients overall well-being increasing patient satisfaction and QOL. Fears or treatment and reoccurrence diminished. Patients started to engage in physical activity improving their overall physical functioning, well-being and QOL. It also triggered a desire by the health care professionals to take this project forward as a piece of research to add to the evidence base.

ACTIVITY

For the case study:

1. List physical and psychological symptoms noted in patients with cancer.
2. List key aspects used in the enhanced service.
3. Write down the impact the enhanced service is having from a psychological perspective.
4. Write down the impact the enhanced service is having from a physical perspective.
5. Write down the impact the enhanced service is having from an emotional perspective.
6. Consider the outcomes on quality of life and overall well-being and how this has been improved by implementing evidence into practice.

Chapter 30 will focus on combined relaxation techniques, building on the knowledge gained from this chapter on evidence from research to enable best practice.

REFERENCES

Adler-Neal, A. L., & Zeidan, F. (2017). Mindfulness meditation for fibromyalgia: Mechanistic and clinical considerations. *Current Rheumatology Report, 19*, 59.

Adler-Nevo, G., & Manassis, K. (2005). Psychological treatment of pediatric post-traumatic stress disorder: The neglected field of single-incident trauma. *Depression & Anxiety, 22*(4), 177–189.

Alam, M., Roongpisuthipong, W., Kim, N. A., et al. (2016). Utility of recorded guided imagery and relaxing music in reducing patient pain and anxiety and surgeon anxiety, during cutaneous surgical procedures: A single-blinded randomized controlled trial. *Journal of the American Academy of Dermatology, 75*, 585–589.

Ampunsiriratana, A., Triamchaisri, S., Nontasorn, T., et al. (2005). A palliated-suffering model for HIV infected patients: A combination of the foundations of mindfulness meditation and Watson's Caring. *Thailand Journal of Nursing Research, 9*(4), 268–280.

Ameratunga, D., Goldin, J., & Hickey, M. (2012). Sleep disturbance in menopause. *Climacteric, 42*, 742–747.

Andersen, J. H., & Gaardboe, O. (1993). Musculoskeletal disorders of the neck and upper limb among sewing machine operators: A clinical investigation. *American Journal of Industrial Medicine, 24*(6), 689–700.

Andersson, G. (2002). Psychological aspects of tinnitus and the application of cognitive-behavioural therapy. *Clinical Psychology Review, 22*(7), 977–990.

Anand, M. P. (1999). Non-pharmacological management of essential hypertension. *Journal of the Indian Medical Association, 97*(6), 220–225.

Astin, J. A. (2004). Mind-body therapies for the management of pain. *Clinical Journal of Pain, 20*(1), 27–32.

Astin, J. A., Beckner, W., Soeken, K., et al. (2002). Psychological interventions for rheumatoid arthritis: A meta-analysis of randomized controlled trials. *Arthritis & Rheumatology, 47*(3), 291–302.

Antoni, M. H., Wimberly, S. R., Lechner, S. C., et al. (2006). Reduction of cancer-specific thought intrusions and anxiety symptoms with a stress management intervention among women undergoing treatment for breast cancer. *American Journal of Psychiatry, 163*(10), 1791–1797.

Aurora, R., Zak, R. S., Auerbach, S. H., et al. (2010). *Journal of Clinical Sleep Medicine, 6*(4), 389–401.

Ayers, C. R., Sorrell, J. T., Thorp, S. R., et al. (2007). Evidence-based psychological treatments for late-life anxiety. *Psychology and Aging, 22*(1), 8–17.

Bagheri-Nesami, M., Mohseni-Bandpei, M. A., & Shayesteh-Azar, M. (2006). The effect of Benson's relaxation technique on rheumatoid arthritis patients: Extended report. *International Journal of Nursing Practice, 12*(4), 214–219.

Baird, C. L., & Sands, L. (2004). A pilot study of the effectiveness of guided imagery with progressive muscle relaxation to reduce chronic pain and mobility difficulties of osteoarthritis. *Pain Management Nursing, 5*(3), 97–104.

Baird, C. L., Murawski, M. M., & Wu, J. (2010). Efficacy of guided imagery with relaxation for osteoarthritis symptoms and medication intake. *Pain Management Nursing, 11*(1), 56–65.

Baraniak, A., & Sheffield, D. (2011). The efficacy of psychologically based interventions to improve anxiety, depression and quality of life in COPD: A systematic review and meta-analysis. *Patient Education and Counselling, 83*, 29–36.

Barsky, A. J., Ahern, D. L., Orav, J. E., et al. (2010). A randomized trial of three psychosocial treatments for the symptoms of rheumatoid arthritis. *Seminars in Arthritis and Rheumatism, 40*(3), 222–232.

Bastani, F., Hidarnia, A., Kaxemnejad, A., Vafaei, M., & Kashanian, M. (2005). A randomized controlled trial of the effects of applied relaxation training on reducing anxiety and perceived stress in pregnant women. *Journal of Midwifery and Women's Health, 50*, 36–40.

Bernardy, K., Füber, N., Köllner, V., & Häuser, W. (2010). Efficacy of cognitive-behavioral therapies in fibromyalgia syndrome: A systematic review and meta-analysis of randomized controlled trials. *Rheumatology, 37*(10), 1991–2005.

Bhochhibhoya, A., Stone, B., & Xiaoming, L. (2018). Mindfulness-based intervention among people living with HIV/AIDS: A systematic review. *Complementary Therapies in Clinical Practice, 33*, 12–19.

Biddle, S. J. H., & Mutrie, N. (2008). *Psychology of physical activity: Determinants, well-being and interventions* (2nd ed.). New York: Routledge.

Birrie, K. A., Noel, M., Parker, J. A., et al. (2014). Systematic review and meta-analysis of distraction and hypnosis for needle-related pain and distress in children and adolescents. *Journal of Pediatric Psychology*, 39, 783–808.

Bisson, J., & Andrew, M. (2007). Psychological treatment of post-traumatic stress disorder (update). *Cochrane Database of Systematic Reviews*, 3, CD003388.

Blanchard, E. B., Greene, B., Scharff, I., & Schwarz-McMorris, S. P. (1993). Relaxation training as a treatment for irritable bowel syndrome. *Biofeedback Self-regulation*, 18(3), 125–132.

Blom, K., Baker, B., How, M., et al. (2014). Hypertension analysis of stress reduction using mindfulness meditation and yoga: Results from the HARMONY randomized controlled trial. *American Journal of Hypertension*, 27, 122–129.

Blomhoff, S., Spetalen, S., Jacobsen, M. B., Vatn, M., & Malt, U. F. (2000). Intestinal reactivity to words with emotional content and brain information processing in irritable bowel syndrome. *Digestive Disease and Science*, 45(6), 1160–1165.

Bois, J., Sarraxin, P., Southon, J., & Boiche, J. (2009). Psychological characteristics and their relation to performance in professional golfers. *Sport Psychology*, 23, 252–270.

Boyce, P. M., Telley, N. J., Balaam, B., et al. (2003). A randomized controlled trial of cognitive behaviour therapy, relaxation training and routine clinical care for the irritable bowel syndrome. *American Journal of Gastroenterology*, 98(10), 2209–2218.

Bradley, L. A., & Alberts, K. R. (1999). Psychological and behavioural approaches to pain management for patients with rheumatic disease. *Rheumatic Diseases Clinics of North America*, 25(1), 215–232.

Braun, S., Beurskens, A., Kleynen, M., Schols, J., & Wade, D. (2011). Rehabilitation with mental practice has similar effects on mobility as rehabilitation with relaxation in people with Parkinson's disease: A multicentre randomised trial. *Journal of Physiotherapy*, 57, 27–34.

Brown, W. H., & Carlos, A. (2003). A cognitive behavioural intervention to decrease symptoms of depression, anxiety and somatic complaints in adults diagnosed with human immunodeficiency virus (HIV) and acquired immunodeficiency syndrome (AIDS). *Dissertation Abstracts International: The Sciences and Engineering*, 64(5B), 2412.

Brown, R. A., Ramsey, S. E., Kahler, C. W., et al. (2011). A randomised controlled trial of cognitive-behavioural treatment for depression versus relaxation training for alcohol-dependent individuals with elevated depressive symptoms. *Journal of Studies on Alcohol and Drugs*, 72(2), 286–296.

Burg, J. M., & Michalak, J. (2011). The healthy quality of mindful PMR: Associations with ruination and depression. *Cognitive Therapy and Research*, 35(2), 179–185.

Bury, T. J., & Mead, J. M. (Eds.). (1998). *Evidence-based health care: A practical guide for therapists*. Oxford, UK: Butterworth-Heinemann.

Buse, D. C., & Andrasik, F. (2009). Behavioral medicine for migraine. *Neurolig Clinics*, 27(2), 445–465.

Butler, A. C., Chapmen, J. E., & Forman, E. M. et al., (2006). The empirical status of cognitive-behavioural therapy: a review of meta-analyses. *Clin. Psychol. Rev*, Ch 26, 17–31.

Byatt, N., Rothschild, A. J., Riskind, P., Ionete, C., & Hunt, A. T. (2011). Relationships between multiple sclerosis and depression. *Journal of Neuropsychiatry and Clinical Neurosciences*, 23, 198–200.

Carlbring, P., Ekselius, L., & Andersson, G. (2003). Treatment of panic disorder via the Internet: A randomized controlled trial of cognitive behavioural therapy versus applied relaxation. *Journal of Behavior Therapy and Experimental Psychiatry*, 34(2), 129–140.

Carlbring, P., Gunnarsdóttir, M., Hedensjö, L., Andersson, G., Ekselius, L., & Furmark, T. (2007). Treatment of social phobia: Randomised trial of internet-delivered cognitive-behavioural therapy with telephone support. *British Journal of Psychiatry*, 190, 123–128.

Carpenter, K. M., Smith, J. L., Aharonovich, E., & Nunes, E. V. (2008). Developing therapies for depression in drug dependence: Results of a Stage 1 therapy study. *The American Journal of Drug and Alcohol Abuse*, 34, 642–652.

Carpio-Rivera, E., Moncada-Jiménez, J., Salazar-Rojas, W., & Solera-Herrera, A. (2016). Acute effects of exercise on blood pressure: A meta-analytic investigation. *Arquivos Brasileiros De Cardiologia*, 106(5), 422–433.

Castelnuovo, G., Pietrabissa, G., Manzoni, G.M., Cattivelli, R., Rossi, A., Novelli, M. (2017). Cognitive behavioural therapy to aid weight loss in obese patients: Current perspectives. *Psychology Research and Behaviour Management*, 10, 165+ Gale Academic OneFile. Retrieved April 2020 from https://link.gale.com/apps/doc/A534235472/GPS?u=bu_uk&sid=GPS&xid=ec08d9c4.

Çelik, A, Pasinlioğlu, T. Women's menopausal sypmtoms and factors affecting it during climacteric period. *Hacettepe University Journal of Nursing Faculty*. 2014;1:16–29.

Chambers, C. T., Taddio, A., Uman, L. S., & McMurty, M. (2009). Psychological interventions for reducing pain and distress in routine childhood immunizations: A systematic review. *Clinical Therapy*, 31, S77–S103.

Chang, B., Sommers, E., & Herz, L. (2010). Acupuncture and relaxation response for substance use disorder recovery. *Journal of Substance Use*, 15(6), 390–401.

Chou, R., & Huffman, L. H. (2007). Non-pharmacologic therapies for acute and chronic low back pain: A review of the evidence for an American Pain Society/American College of Physicians' clinical practice guideline. *Annals of Internal Medicine*, 147(7), 492–504.

Clark, D. M., Ehlers, A., Hackmann, A., et al. (2006). Cognitive therapy versus exposure and applied relaxation in social phobia: A randomized controlled trial. *Journal of Consulting and Clinical Psychology*, 74(3), 568–578.

Colberg, S. R., Sigal, R. J., Yardley, J. E., et al. (2016). Physical activity/exercise and diabetes: A position statement of the American Diabetes Association. *Diabetes Care*, 39, 2065–2079.

Conrad, A., & Roth, W. T. (2007). Muscle relaxation therapy for anxiety disorders: It works, but how? *Journal of Anxiety Disorders*, 21(3), 243–264.

Cooper, C., Balamurali, T. B. S., Selwood, A., & Livingston, G. (2007). A systematic review of intervention studies about anxiety in caregivers of people with dementia. *International Journal of Geriatric Psychiatry*, 22, 181–188.

Cornelissen, V. A., & Fagard, R. H. (2005). Effect of resistance training on resting blood pressure: A meta-analysis of randomized controlled trials. *Journal of Hypertension*, 23(2), 251–259.

Cornelissen, V. A., & Smart, N. A. (2013). Exercise training for blood pressure: A systematic review and meta-analysis. *Journal of the American Heart Association*, 2(1).

Corso, L. M. L., Macdonald, H. V., Johnson, B. T., et al. (2016). Is concurrent training efficacious antihypertensive therapy? A meta-analysis. *Medicine & Science in Sports & Exercise*, 48(12), 2398–2406.

Craft, L. L., & Landers, D. M. (1998). The effect of exercise on clinical depression and depression resulting from mental illness: A meta-analysis. *Journal of Sports and Excercise Psychology*, 20, 357–399.

Crawford-Walker, C. J., King, A., & Chan, S. (2005). Distraction techniques for schizophrenia. *Cochrane Database of Systematic Reviews*, CD004717.

Cupal, D. D., & Brewer, B. W. (2001). Effects of relaxation and guided imagery on knee strength, reinjury anxiety and pain following anterior cruciate ligament reconstruction. *Rehabilitation Psychology*, 46(1), 28–43.

Daley, A. J., Mutrie, N., Crank, H., Coleman, R., & Saxton, J. (2004). Exercise therapy in women who have had breast cancer: Design of the Sheffield women's exercise and well-being project. *Health Education Research*, 19(6), 686–697.

Daley, A. J., Crank, H., Saxton, J., Mutrie, N., Coleman, R., & Roalfe, A. (2007). A randomized trial of exercise therapy in women treated for breast cancer. *Journal of Clinical Oncology*, 25(13), 1713–1721.

Damen, L., Bruijen, J., Koes, B. W., et al. (2006). Prophylactic treatment of migraine in children. Part 1: A systematic review of non-pharmacological trials. *Cephalalgia*, 26(4), 373–383.

Darnall, B. D. (2016). Pain psychology and pain catastrophizing in the perioperative setting: A review of impacts, interventions and unmet needs. *Hand Clinics*, 32, 33–39.

Davidson, K. (2008). Cognitive-behavioural therapy: Origins and developments. In M. Donaghy, M. Nicol, & K. Davidson (Eds.), *Cognitive-behavioural interventions in physiotherapy and occupational therapy* (pp. 3–18). Edinburgh: Butterworth-Heinemann.

D'Arripe-Longuevill, F., Hars, Debois, N., & Calmels, C. (2009). Perceived development of psychological characteristics in male and female elite gymnasts. *Internaltional Journal of Sport Psychology*, 40, 424–455.

Deale, A., Husain, K., Chalder, T., & Wessely, S. (2001). Long-term outcome of cognitive behaviour therapy verus relaxation therapy for chronic fatigue syndrome: A 5-year follow-up study. *American Journal of Psychiatry*, 158, 2038–2042.

de Greef, M., van Wijck, R., Reynders, K., et al. (2003). Impact of the Groningen Exercise Therapy for Symphony Orchestra Musicians program on perceived physical competence and playing-related musculoskeletal disorders of professional musicians. *Medical Problems of Performing Artists*, 18(4), 156–160.

De Oliveira, S. N., Moro, A. R. P., Polito, M. D., de Jesus, J. H., & de Souza Bezerra, E. (2020). Effects of concurrent training with elastic tubes in hypertensive patients: A blind controlled randomized clinical trial. *Experimental Aging Research*, 46(1), 68–82.

De Souto, B., Demougeot, L., Vellas, B., & Rolland, Y. (2018). Exercise training for preventing dementia, mild cognitive impairment, and clinically meaningful cognitive decline: A systematic review and meta-analysis. *The Journals of Gerontology: Series A*, 73(11), 1504–1511.

Dennis, C. L. (2004). Treatment of postpartum depression part 2: A critical review of non-biological interventions. *Journal of Clinical Psychiatry*, 65(9), 1252–1265.

Denis, C., Lavie, E., Fatseas, M., & Auriacombe, M. (2006). Psychotherapeutic interventions for cannabis abuse and/or dependence in outpatient settings. *Cochrane Database of Systematic Reviews*, 3, CD005336.

Dickinson, H. O., Mason, J. M., Nicolson, D. J., et al. (2006). Lifestyle interventions to reduce raised blood pressure: A systematic review of randomized controlled trials. *Journal of Hypertension*, 24(2), 215–233.

Dipietro, L., Evenson, K. R., Bloodgood, B., et al. (2018). Benefits of physical activity during pregnancy and postpartum: An umbrella review. *Medicine and Science in Sports and Exercise*, 51(6), 1292–1302.

Donaghy, M. E., & Morss, K. (2000). Guided reflection: A framework to facilitate and assess reflective practice within the discipline of physiotherapy. *Physiotherapy: Theory and Practice*, 16, 3–14.

Donaghy, M. E., & Ussher, M. (2005). Exercise interventions in drug and alcohol rehabilitation. In G. Faulkner, & A. H. Taylor (Eds.), *Exercise health and mental health: Emerging relationships* (pp. 46–89). London: Routledge.

Donaghy, M. E. (2007). Exercise can seriously improve your mental health: Fact or fiction? *Advances in Physiotherapy*, 9(2), 76–89.

Donaghy, M. E. (2008a). Cognitive-behavioural approaches in the treatment of alcohol addiction. In M. Donaghy, M. Nicol, & K. Davidson (Eds.), *Cognitive-behavioural interventions in physiotherapy and occupational therapy* (pp. 105–120). Edinburgh: Butterworth-Heimemann Elsevier.

Donaghy, M.E. (2008b). *The importance of psychological preparation in injury prevention*. The 13th European Conference in Sports Science, Estoril. Portugal, European College of Sports Science.

D'Souza, P. J., Lumley, M. A., Kraft, C. A., & Dooley JA (2008). Relaxation training and written emotional disclosure for tension or migraine headaches: A randomized, controlled trial. *Annals of Behavioral Medicine*, 36(1), 21–32.

Dugas, M. J., Brillon, P., Savard, P., et al. (2010). A randomised clinical trial of cognitive-behavioural therapy and applied relaxation for adults with generalised anxiety disorder. *Behaviour Therapy*, 41, 46–58.

Duman, M., & Tashan, S. T. (2018). The effect of sleep hygiene education and relaxation exercises on insomnia among postmenopausal women: A randomized clinical trial. *International Journal of Nursing Practice*, 24, e12650.

Dwi Kustriyanti, B. (2017). Muscle relaxation therapy for dysmenorrhea. Health Notions: Humanistic Network for Science and Technology. Retrieved April 2020 from http://www.heanoti.com/index.php/hn/article/view/64.

Eccleston, C., Yorke, L., Morley, S., Williams, A. C. deC., & Mastroyannopoulou, K. (2003). Psychological therapies for the management of chronic and recurrent pain in children and adolescents. *Cochrane Database of Systematic Reviews, 1*, CD003968.

Eisen, J., Mancebo, M., Pinto, A., et al. (2006). Impact of obsessive compulsive disorder on quality of life. *Comprehensive Psychiatry, 47*, 270–275.

Elkins, G. R., Fisher, W. I., Johnson, A. K., Carpenter, J. S., & Keith, T. Z. (2013). Clinical hypnosis in the treatment of postmenopausal hot flashes: A randomized controlled trial. *Menopause, 20*, 291–298.

Epstein, G. N., Halper, J. P., & Barret, E. A. M. (2004). A pilot study of mind–body changes in adults with asthma who practise mental imagery. *Alternative Therapies in Health and Medicine, 10*(4), 66–71.

Ernst, E., Schmidt, K., & Baum, M. (2006). Complementary/alternative therapies for the treatment of breast cancer: A systematic review of randomized clinical trials and a critique of current terminology. *Breast Journal, 12*(6), 526–530.

Fairfax, H. (2008). The use of mindfulness in obsessive compulsive disorder: Suggestions for its application and integration into existing treatment. *Clinical Psychology and Psychotherapy, 15*, 53–59.

Faulkner, G., & Biddle, S. (1999). Exercise as an adjunct treatment for schizophrenia: A review of the literature. *Journal of Mental Health, 8*(5), 441–457.

Faver-Vestergaard, I., Jacobsen, D., & Zachariae, R. (2015). Efficacy of psychosocial interventions on psychological and physical health outcomes in chronic obstructive pulmonary disease: A systematic review and meta-analysis. *Psychotherapy and Psychosomatics, 84*(1), 37–50.

Felix, M. M. S., Ferreira, M. B. G., & Barbosa, M. H. (2019). Relaxation therapy with guided imagery for postoperative pain management: An integrative review. *Pain Management Nursing, 20*, 3–9.

Ferrara, M., Langiano, E., Di Brango, T., Di Cioccio, L., Bauco, C., & De Vito, E. (2008). Prevalence of stress, anxiety and depression in with Alzheimer caregivers. *Health and Quality of Life Outcomes, 6*(1), 93.

Fiest, K. M., Walker, J. R., Bernstein, C. N., et al. (2016). Systematic review and meta-analysis of interventions for depression and anxiety in persons with multiple sclerosis. *Multiple Sclerosis and Related Disorders, 5*, 12–26.

Fjorback, L. O., Arendt, M., Ornbol, E., Fink, P., & Walach, H. (2011). Mindfulness-based stress reduction and mindfulness-based cognitive therapy: A systematic review of randomized controlled trials. *Acta Psychiatrica Scandinavica, 124*(2), 102–119.

Fogarty, M., & Happel, B. (2005). Exploring the benefits of an exercise programme for people with schizophrenia: A qualitative study. *Issues in Mental Health Nursing, 26*, 341–351.

Folmer, R. L., Theodoroff, S. M., Martin, W. H., & Shi, Y. (2014). Experimental, controversial and futuristic treatments for chronic tinnitus. *Journal of the American Academy of Audiology, 25*, 106–125.

Ford, A. C., Quigley, E. M., Lacy, B. E., et al. (2014). Effect of antidepressants and psychological therapies, including hypnotherapy, in irritable bowel syndrome: systematic review and meta-analysis. *American Journal of Gastroenterology, 109*, 1350–1365.

Fors, E. A., Sexton, H., & Gotestam, K. G. (2002). The effect of guided imagery and amitriptyline on daily fibromyalgic pain: A

prospective randomized controlled trial. *Journal of Psychiatric Research, 36*(3), 179–187.

Fox, E. E., Hough, A. D., Creanor, S., Gear, M., & Freeeman, J. A. (2016). Effects of pilates-based core stability training in ambulant people with multiple sclerosis: Multicentre, assessor-blinded, randomized controlled trial. *Physical Therapy, 96*(8), 1170–1178.

Frank, I., Kleinman, I., Rentz, A., Ciesla, G., Kim, J. J., & Zacker, C. (2002). Health-related quality of life associated with irritable bowel syndrome: Comparison with other chronic diseases. *Clinical Therapy, 24*(4), 675–689.

Ganesh, B., Chodankar, A., Parvatkar, B. (2017) Comparative Study of Laura Mitchell's Physiological Relaxation Technique Versus Jacobson's Progressive Relaxation Technique on Severity of Pain And Quality of Life in Primary Dysmenorrhea: Randomized Clinical Trial. Journal of Medical Science and Clinical Research, 5 (7), 25379-25387.

García Rodríguez, L. A., Ruigómez, A., Wallander, M. A., Johansson, S., & Olbe, L. (2000). Detection of colorectal tumor and inflammatory bowel disease during follow-up of patients with initial diagnosis of irritable bowel syndrome. *Scandinavian Journal of Gastroenterology, 35*, 306–311.

Gary, A.E. (2012). Multiple disabilities, multiple strategies: Assisting the cognitively impaired client requires patience from the clinical team. Addiction Professional: Vendome Grup LLC. Retrieved January 2020 from www.addictionpro.com.

Gasparini, C. F., Sutherland, H. G., & Griffiths, L. R. (2013). Studies on the pathophysiology and genetic biasis of migraine. *Current Genomics, 14*(5), 300–315.

Gelfand, J. M., Weinstein, R., Porter, S. B., et al. (2005). Prevalence and treatment of psoriasis in the United Kingdom: A population-based study. *Archives in Dermatology, 141*(12), 1537–1541.

Ghadse, A. M., Ranjan, L. K., & Gupta, P. R. (2019). Biofeedback as an adjunct to conventional stress management and relaxation techniques in substance abuse disorders: A randomized controlled interventional study. *The Indian Journal of Occupational Therapy, 51*(1), 26–30.

Gibson, B. E., & Martin, D. K. (2003). Qualitative research and evidence-based physiotherapy practice. *Physiotherapy, 89*(6), 350–358.

Gorman, J. M. (2003). Treating generalized anxiety disorder. *Journal of Clinical Psychiatry, 64*(Suppl. 2), 24–29.

Georga, G., Chrousos, G., Artemiadis, A., Panagiotis, P. P., Bakakos, P., & Darviri, C. (2019). The effect of stress management incorporating progressive muscle relaxation and biofeedback-assisted relaxation breathing on patients with asthma: A randomized controlled trial. *Advances in Integrative Medicine, 6*, 73–77.

Glickman-Simon, R., & Tessier, J. (2014). Guided imagery for postoperative pain, energy healing for quality of life, probiotics for acute diarrhea in children, acupuncture for postoperative nausea and vomiting and animal-assisted therapy for mental disorders. Explore. *The Journal of Science and Healing, 10*, 326–329.

Goudsmit, E. M., Nijs, J., Jason, L. A., & Wallman, K. E. (2012). Pacing as a strategy to improve energy management in myalgic encephalomyelitis/chronic fatigue syndrome: A consensus document. *Disability and Rehabilitation, 34*, 1140–1147.

Grossman, P., Tiefenthaler-Gilmer, U., Raysz, U., & Kesper, U. (2007). Mindfulness training as an intervention for fibromyalgia:

Evidence of postintervention and 3-year follow-up benefits in well-being. *Psychotherapy and Psychosomatics, 76*(4), 226–233.

Gupta, S. S. (2014). Effect of progressive muscle relaxation combined with deep breathing technique immediately after aerobic exercises on essential hypertension. *Indian Journal of Physiotherapy and Occupatonal Therapy, 8*(1), 227–231.

Hambrick, J. P., Weeks, J. W., Harb, G. C., et al. (2003). Cognitive-behavioral therapy for social anxiety disorder: Supporting evidence and future directions. *CNS Spectrums, 8*(5), 373–381.

Hannan, S. E., & Tolin, D. F. (2005). Acceptance and mindfulness-based behaviour therapy for obsessive–compulsive disorder. In S. M. Orsillo, & L. Roemer (Eds.), *Acceptance and mindfulness-based approaches to anxiety: Conceptualisation and treatment* (pp. 271–299). New York: Springer.

Hansen, M. M. (2015). A feasibility pilot study on the use of complementary therapies delivered via mobile technologies on Icelandic surgical patients' reports of anxiety, pain and self-efficacy in healing. *BMC Complementary and Alternative Medicine, 15*, 92.

Hay, P. J., Bacaltchuk, J., & Stefano, S. (2004). Psychotherapy for bulimia nervosa and binging. *Cochrane Database of Systematic Reviews, 3*, CD000562.

Hay, P. P., Bacaltchuk, J., Stefano, S., & Kashyap, P. (2009). Psychological treatments for bulimia nervosa and binging. *Cochrane Database of Systematic Review, 4*, CD000562.

Heslop-Marshall, K., Baker, C., Carrick-Sen, D., et al. (2018). Randomised controlled trial of cognitive behavioural therapy in COPD. *ERJ Open Research, 4*, 00094–2018.

Hofmann, S. G., & Smits, J. A. J. (2008). Cognitive-behavioural therapy for adult anxiety disorders: A meta-analysis of randomized placebo-controlled trials. *Journal of Clinical Psychiatry, 69*, 621–632.

Hopkinson, M. D., Reavell, J., Lane, D. A., & Mallikarjun, P. (2019). Cognitive behavioral therapy for depression, anxiety, and stress in caregivers of dementia patients: A systematic review and meta-analysis. *The Gerontologist, 59*(4), e343–e362.

Hoppes, K. (2006). The application of mindfulness-based cognitive interventions in the treatment of co-occurring addictive and mood disorders. *CNS Spectrums, 11*(11), 829–851.

Holloway, E. A., & Ram, F. S. F. (2004). Breathing exercises for asthma. In *Cochrane Database of Systematic Reviews* (1). Chichester, UK: John Wiley.

Holmes, M. D., Chen, W. Y., Feskanich, D., Kroenke, C. H., & Colditz, G. A. (2005). Physical activity and survival after breast cancer diagnosis. *JAMA, 293*, 2479–2486.

Holmes, H. J., Thakur, E. R., Carty, J. N., et al. (2018). Ambivalence over emotional expression and perceived social constraints as moderators of relaxation training and emotional awareness and expression training for irritable bowel syndrome. *General Hospital Psychiatry, 53*, 38–43.

Howland, K. C., Ausubel, I. J., London, C. A., & Abbas, A. K. (2000). The roles of CD28 and CD40 ligand in T cell activation and tolerance. *Journal of Immunology, 164*(9), 4465–4470.

Hughes, J. W., Fresco, D. M., Myerscough, R., et al. (2013). Randomized controlled trial of mindfulness-based stress reduction for prehypertension. *Psychosomatic Medicine, 75*, 721–728.

Hunot, V., Churchill, R., Teixeira, & Silva da Lima, M. (2007). Psychological therapies for generalized anxiety disorder. *Cochrane Database of Systematic Reviews, 1*, CD001848.

Hunter-Jones, J. J., Gilliam, S. M., Carswell, A. L., & Hansen, N. B. (2019). Assessing the acceptability of a mindfulness-based cognitive therapy intervention for African-American women living with HIV/AIDS. *Journal of Racial and Ethnic Health Disparities, 6*, 1157–1166.

Huntley, A., White, A. R., & Ernst, E. (2002). Relaxation therapies for asthma: A systematic review. *Thorax, 57*(2), 127–131.

Hussain, N., & Said, A. S. A. (2019). Mindfulness-based meditation versus progressive relaxation meditation: Impact on chronic pain in older female patients with diabetic neuropathy. *Journal of Evidence-Based Integrative Medicine, 24*, 1–8.

International Headache Society (IHS). (2013). *The International Classification of Headache Disorders* (3rd ed., beta version). Retrieved April 2020 from https://journals.sagepub.com/doi/pdf/10.1177/0333102413485658.

Irwin, M. R., Cole, J. C., & Nicassio, P. M. (2006). Comparative meta-analysis of behavioral interventions for insomnia and their efficacy in middle-aged adults and in older adults 55+ years of age. *Health Psychology, 25*(1), 3–14.

Jorm, A. F., Christensen, H., Griffiths, K. M., et al. (2004). Effectiveness of complementary and self-help treatments for anxiety disorders. *Medical Journal of Australia, 181*(Suppl. 7), S29–S46.

Jorm, A. F., Morgan, A. J., & Hetrick, S. E. (2008). Relaxation for depression. *Cochrane Database of Systematic Reviews, 4*, CD007142.

James, A., Soler, A., & Weatherall, R. (2005). Cognitive behavioural therapy for anxiety disorders in children and adolescents. *Cochrane Database of Systematic Reviews, 4*, CD004690.

Johnson, U. (2000). Short-term psychological intervention: A study of long-term injured competitive athletes. *Journal of Sport Rehabilitation, 9*(3), 207–218.

Johnson, U., Ekengren, J., & Andersen, M. B. (2005). Injury prevention in Sweden: Helping soccer players at risk. *Journal of Sports and Excercise Psychology, 1*, 32–38.

Jones, C., Cormac, I., Silveiro da Mota Neto, J. I., et al. (2004). Cognitive behaviour therapy for schizophrenia. *Cochrane Database of Systematic Reviews, 4*, CD00054.

Kaapa, E. H., Frantsi, K., Sarna, S., et al. (2006). Multidisciplinary group rehabilitation versus individual physiotherapy for chronic non-specific low back pain: A randomized trial. *Spine, 31*(4), 371–376.

Kanji, N., White, A. R., & Ernst, E. (2006). Autogenic training for tension-type headaches: A systematic review of controlled trials. *Complementary Therapies in Medicine, 14*(2), 144–150.

Karjalainen, K., Malmivaara, A., & van Tulder, M. (2007). Biopsychosocial rehabilitation for upper limb repetitive strain injuries in working age adults. Cochrane Database Systematic. Review. Issue 3.

Kaushik, R., Kaushik, R. M., Mahajan, S. K., et al. (2005). Biofeedback-assisted diaphragmatic breathing and systematic relaxation versus propranolol in long-term prophylaxis of migraine. *Complementary Therapies in Medicine, 13*(3), 165–174.

Kendrick, C., Johnson, A. K., Sliwinski, J., Patterson, V., Fisher, W. I., & Elkins, G. R. (2015). Hypnotic relaxation therapy for reduction of hot flashes in postmenopausal women: Examination of cortisol as a potential mediator. *International Journal of Clinical and Experimental Hypnosis*, 63(1), 76–91.

Kenne, S. E., Mårtensson, L. B., Andersson, B. A., Karlsson, P., & Bergh, I. (2017). Mindfulness and its efficacy for psychological and biological responses in women with breast cancer. *Cancer Medicine*, 6, 1108–1122.

Kessler, R. S., Patterson, D. R., & Dane, J. (2003). Hypnosis and relaxation with pain patients: Evidence for effectiveness. *Seminars in Pain Medicine*, 1(2), 67–78.

Khan Niazi, A., & Khan Niazi, S. (2011). Mindfulness-based stress reduction: A non-pharmacological approach for chronic illnesses. *North American Journal of Medicine & Science*, 3(1), 20–23.

Khan, N., & Khatri, S. M. (2016). Immediate effectiveness of relaxation in management of chronic low back pain. *Revista Romana de Kinetoterapie*, 22(37), 23–29.

Khatoon, F. (2016). Identifying spiritual coping strategies in persons living with HIV/AIDS. *Indian Journal of Health and Wellbeing*, 7(10), 1004.

King, S. J., Wessel, J., Bhambhani, Y., Sholter, D., & Maksymowyc, W. (2002a). The effects of exercise and education, individually or combined, in women with fibromyalgia. *Rheumatology*, 29(12), 2620–2627.

King, M. S., Carr, T., & D'Cruz, C. (2002b). Transcendental meditation, hypertension and heart disease: A review. *Australian Family Physician*, 31(2), 164–168.

Kirk, A., Barnett, J., & Mutrie, N. (2007). Physical activity consultation for people with type 2 diabetes: Evidence and guidelines. *Diabetes Medicine*, 24(8), 809–816.

Knols, R., Aaronson, N. K., Uebelhart, D., et al. (2005). Physical exercise in cancer patients during and after medical treatment: A systematic review of randomized and controlled clinical trials. *Journal of Clinical Oncology*, 23(16), 3830–3842.

Kor, P. P. K., Chien, W. T., Liu, J. Y. W., & Lai, C. K. Y. (2018). Mindfulness-based intervention for stress reduction of family caregivers of people with dementia. *Cochrane Database of Systematic Reviews*, 9, 7–22.

Kos, D., van Eupen, I., Meirte, J., et al. (2015). Activity pacing self-management in chronic fatigue syndrome: A randomized controlled trial. *The American Journal of Occupational Therapy*, 69(5), 1–11.

Krisanaprakornkit, T., Krisanaprakornkit, W., Piyavhatkul, N., et al. (2006). Meditation therapy for anxiety disorders. *Cochrane Database of Systematic Reviews*, 1, CD004998.

Krupchanka, D., & Katliar, M. (2016). The role of insight in moderating the association between depressive symptoms in people with schizophrenia and stigma among their nearest relatives: A pilot study. *Schizophrenia Bulletin*, 42(3), 600–607.

Kwekkeboom, K. L., & Gretarsdottir, E. (2006). Systematic review of relaxation interventions for pain. *Journal of School Nursing*, 38(3), 269–277.

Lai, J. N., Chen, H. J., Chen, C. M., Chen, P. C., & Wang, J. D. (2006). Quality of life and climacteric complaints amongst women seeking medical advice in Taiwan. Assessment using the WHOQOL-BREF questionnaire. *Climcteric*, 9, 119–128.

Laird, K. T., Tanner-Smith, E. E., Russell, A. C., Hollon, S. D., & Walker, L. S. (2016). Short-term and long-term efficacy of psychological therapies for irritable bowel syndrome: A systematic review and meta-analysis. *Clinical Gastroenterology and Hepatology*, 4(7), 937–947.

Lalande, L., Kind, R., Bambling, M., & Schweltzer, R. D. (2017). An uncontrolled clinical trial of guided reparation mindfulness therapy (GRMT) in the treatment of depression and anxiety. *Journal of Contemporary Psychotherapy*, 47, 251–258.

Lamarche, L. J., & de Koninck, J. (2007). Sleep disturbance in adults with post-traumatic stress disorder: A review. *Journal of Clinical Psychiatry*, 68(8), 1257–1270.

Langford, D. J., Lee, K., & Miaskowski, C. (2012). Sleep disturbance interventions in oncology patients and family caregivers: A comprehensive review and meta-analysis. *Sleep Medicine Reviews*, 16(5), 397–414.

Larsson, B., Carlsson, J., Fichtel, A., et al. (2005). Relaxation treatment of adolescent headache sufferers: Results from a school-based replication series. *Headache*, 45(6), 692–704.

Larun, L., Nordheim, L. V., Ekeland, E., Hagen, K. B., & Heian, F. (2006). Exercise in prevention and treatment of anxiety and depression among children and young people. *Cochrane Database of Systematic Reviews*, 3, CD004691.

Larun, L., Brurberg, K. G., Odgaard-Jensen, J., & Price, J. R. (2017). Exercise therapy for chronic fatigue syndrome. *Cochrane Database of Systematic Reviews*, 4, CD003200.

Laurion, S., & Fetzer, S. J. (2003). The effect of two nursing interventions on the postoperative outcomes of gynecologic laparoscopic patients. *Journal of PeriAnesthesia Nursing*, 18(4), 254–261.

Lee, C., & Russell, A. (2003). Effects of physical activity on emotional well-being among older Australian women: cross-sectional and longitudinal analyses. *Journal of Psychosomatic Research*, 54(2), 155–160.

Levin, A. B., Hadgkiss, E. J., Weiland, T. J., & Jelinek, G. A. (2014). Meditation as an adjunct to the management of multiple sclerosis. *Neurology Research International*, 704691.

Levy, R. L., Langer, S. L., & Whitehead, W. E. (2007). Social learning contributions to the etiology and treatment of functional abdominal pain and inflammatory bowel disease. *World Journal of Gastroenterology*, 13(17), 2397–2403.

Logsdon-Conradsen, S. (2002). Using mindfulness meditation to promote holistic health in individuals with HIV/AIDS. *Cognitive and Behavioral Practice*, 9(1), 67–71.

Loder, E., & Rizzoli, P. (2008). Tension-type Headache. *British Medical Journal*, 336, 88–92.

Luciano, J. V., Martínez, N., Peñarrubia-María, M. T., et al. (2011). Effectiveness of a psychoeducational treatment program implemented in general practice for fibromyalgia patients: A randomized controlled trial. *Clinical Journal of Pain*, 27(5), 383–391.

Lundervold, D. A., Pahwa, R., & Lyons, K. E. (2009). Effect of behavioural intervention on comorbid general anxiety disorder and Parkinson's disease. *Clinical Gerontologist*, 32, 104–117.

Ludwig, D. S., & Kabat-Zinn, J. (2008). Mindfulness in medicine. *JAMA*, 300(11), 1350–1352.

MacMillan, F., Kirk, A., Mutrie, N., et al. (2014). A systematic review of physical activity and sedentary behavior intervention studies in youth with type 1 diabetes: Study characteristics, intervention design, and efficacy. *Pediatric Diabetes*, 15, 175–189.

Maddison, R., & Prapavessis, H. (2005). A psychological approach to the prediction and prevention of athletic injury. *Journal of Sports and Excercise Psychology, 27*, 289–310.

Manzoni, G. M., Pagnini, F., Castelnuovo, G., & Molinari, E. (2008a). Relaxation training for anxiety: A ten years' systematic review with meta-analysis. *BMC Psychiatry, 8*, 41.

Manzoni, G. M., Gorini, A., Pagnini, F., Riva, G., Castelnuovo, G., & Molinari, E. (2008b). New technology and relaxation: An explorative study on obese patients with emotional eating. *Journal of Cybertherapy and Rehabilitation, 1*(2), 182–192.

Manzoni, G. M., Pagnini, F., Gorini, A., Riva, G., Castelnuovo, G., & Molinari, E. (2009). Can relaxation training reduce emotional eating in obese females? An explorative study with three months follow-up. *Journal of the American Dietetic Association, 109*(8), 1427–1432.

Margolin, A., Schuman-Oliver, Z., Beitel, M., et al. (2007). A preliminary study of spiritual self-schema (3-S+) therapy for reducing impulsivity in HIV positive drug users. *Journal of Clinical Psychology, 63*(10), 979–999.

Maricutoiu, L. P., Sava, F. A., & Butta, O. (2016). The effectiveness of controlled interventions on employee's burnout: A meta-analysis. *Journal of Occupational and Organizational Psychology, 89*, 1–27.

Marine, A., Ruotsalainen, J. H., Serra, C., & Verbeek, J.H., (2006_. Preventing occupational stress in healthcare workers. Cochrane Database Syst. Rev. Issue 4. Art. No.: CD002892. DOI: 10.1002/14651858. CD002892.pub2.

Marsden, E., & Kirk, A. (2005). Becoming and staying physically active. In D. Nagi (Ed.), *Exercise and sport in diabetes* (pp. 161–192). London: Wiley.

Marsh, L. (2000). Anxiety disorders in Parkinson's disease. *International Review of Psychiatry, 12*, 307–318.

Martin, D., & McLeod, L. (2008). Chronic pain. In M. Donaghy, M. Nicol, & K. Davidson (Eds.), *Cognitive-behavioural interventions in physiotherapy and occupational therapy* (pp. 121–134). Edinburgh: Butterworth-Heinemann Elsevier.

Mateu, M., Olga, A., Inda, M., et al. (2018). Randomized, controlled, crossover study of self-administered Jacobson relaxation in chronic, nonspecific, low-back pain. *Alternative Therapies, 24*(6), 22–30.

Martinez-Devesa, P., Waddell, A., Perera, R., & Theodoulou, M. (2007). Cognitive behavioural therapy for tinnitus. *Cochrane Database of Systematic Reviews, 1*, CD005233.

Masterman, D., Desalles, A., Baloh, R. W., et al. (2006). Preventing occupational stress in healthcare workers. *Cochrane Database of Systematic Reviews, 4*, CD002892.

Matthews, H., Grundfeld, E. A., & Turner, A. (2016). The efficacy of interventions to improve psychosocial outcomes following surgical treatment for breast cancer: A systematic review and meta-analysis. *Psycho-Oncology, 26*, 593–607.

McCall, L. (2016). Hypnosis for adjunctive pain relief in a patient with multiple sclerosis related trigeminal neuralgia. *Australian Journal of Clinical and Experimental Hypnosis, 41*(2), 174–181.

McKee, J., & Warber, S. L. (2005). Integrative therapies for menopause. *Southern Medical Journal, 98*(3), 319–326.

Mehta, R., Sharma, K., Potters, L., Wernicke, A. G., & Parshar, B. (2019). Evidence for the role of mindfulness in cancer: Benefits and techniques. *Cureus, 11*(5), e4629.

Mello, P. G., Silva, G. R., Donat, J. C., & Kristensen, C. H. (2013). An update on the efficacy of cognitive-behavioural therapy, cognitive therapy and exposure therapy for posttraumatic stress disorder. *International Journal Psychiarty in Medicine, 46*(4), 339–357.

Melzack, R., & Wall, P. D. (1965). Pain mechanisms: A new theory. *Science, 150*, 971–979.

Mendelson, W. B. (2007). Combining pharmacologic and nonpharmacologic therapies for insomnia. *Journal of Clinical Psychiatry, 68*(Suppl. 5), 19–23.

Mendes, D. D., Mello, M. F., Ventura, P., Passarela, C. M., & Mari, J. J. (2008). A systematic review on the effectiveness of cognitive behavioral therapy for posttraumatic stress disorder. *Psychiatry in Medicine, 38*, 241–259.

Meyer, B., Keller, A., Wohlbier, H., Overath, C. H., Muller, B., & Kropp, P. (2016). Progressive muscle relaxation reduces migraine frequency and normalizes amplitudes of contingent negative variation (CNV). *The Journal of Headache and Pain, 17*(37).

Miranda, A. F., Silva, L. F., Caetano, J. A., Sousa, A. C., & Almeida, P. C. (2011). Evaluation of pain intensity and vital signs in the cardiac surgery postoperative period. *Revista da Escola de Enfermagem da USP, 45*, 327–333.

Mizrahi, M. C., Reicher-Atir, R., Levy, S. l., Haramati, S., Wengrower, D., Israeli, E., & Goldin, E. (2012). Effects of guided imagery with relaxation training on anxiety and quality of life among patients with inflammatory bowel disease. *Psychology and Health, 27*(12), 1463–1479.

Molodecky, N. A., Soon, I. S., Rabi, D. M., et al. (2012). Increasing incidence and prevalence of the inflammatory bowel diseases with time, based on systematic review. *Gastroenterology, 142*, 46–54e42.

Moffitt, R., Haynes, A., & Mohr, P. (2015). Treatment beliefs and preferences for psychological therapies for weight management. *Journal of Clinical Psychology, 71*(6), 584–596.

Montgomery, P., & Dennis, J. A. (2003). Cognitive behavioural interventions for sleep problems in adults aged 60+. *Cochrane Database of Systematic Reviews, 1*, CD003161.

Moore, P., Hirst, C., Harding, K. E., Clarkson, H., Pickersgill, T. P., & Robertson, N. P. (2012). Multiple sclerosis relapses and depression. *Journal of Psychosomatic Research, 73*, 272–276.

Morgenthaler, T., Kramer, M., Alessi, C., et al. (2006). Practice parameters for the psychological and behavioral treatment of insomnia: An update. An American Academy of Sleep report. *Sleep, 29*(11), 1415–1419.

Multhaupt, G., & Beuth, J. (2018). The use of imagery in athletic injury rehabilitation: A systematic review. *Deutsche Zeitschrift für Sportmedizin, 69*, 57-64.

Murawski, B., Wade, L., Plotnikoff, R. C., Lubans, D. R., & Duncan, M. J. (2018). A systematic review and meta-analysis of cognitive and behavioural interventions to improve sleep health in adults without sleep disorders. *Sleep Medicine Reviews, 40*, 160–169.

Mutrie, N., Campbell, A. M., Whyte, F., et al. (2007). Benefits of supervised group exercise for women being treated for early stage breast cancer: A pragmatic randomized controlled trial. *British Medical Journal, 334*(7592), 517–520B.

National Institute of Health and Care Excellence (NICE). (2006). Obsessive compulsive disorder: Core interventions in the treatment of obsessive compulsive disorder and body dysmorphic disorder [NG31]. London: NICE. Retrieved April 2020 from https://www. nice.org.uk/guidance/cg31/evidence/cg31-obsessivecompulsive-disorder-full-guideline2.

National Institute of Health and Care Excellence (NICE). (2014). Psychosis and schizophrenia in adults: Prevention and management [CG 178]. Retrieved April 2020 from https://www.nice.org. uk/guidance/cg178.

National Institute of Health and Care Excellence (NICE). (2015). Diabetes (type 1 and type 2) in children and young people: Diagnosis and management [CG18]. Retrieved April 2020 from https://www.nice.org.uk/guidance/ng18.

National Institute of Health and Care Excellence (NICE). (2019). Hypertension in adults: Diagnosis and management, NICE guideline [NG136]. Retrieved April 2020 from https://www.nice.org. uk/guidance/ng136/chapter/Recommendations#treating-and-monitoring-hypertension.

Newman, M. G., Castonguay, L. G., Jacobson, N. C., & Moore, G. A. (2015). Adult attachment as a moderator of treatment outcome for generalized anxiety disorder: Comparison between cognitive-behavioural therapy (CBT) plus supportive listening and CBT plus interpersonal and emotional processing therapy. *Journal of Consulting and Clinical Psychology*, 83, 915–925.

Newman, M. G., & Fisher, A. J. (2013). Mediated moderation in combined cognitive behavioural therapy versus component treatments for generalized anxiety disorder. *Journal of Consulting and Clinical Psychology*, 81, 405–414.

Newman, M. G., Jacobson, N. C., Erickson, T. M., & Fisher, A. J. (2017). Interpersonal problems predict differential response to cognitive versus behavioural treatment in a randomized controlled trial. *Behaviour Therapy*, 48, 56–68.

Nickel, C., Kettler, C., Muehlbacher, et al. (2005). Effect of progressive muscle relaxation in adolescent female bronchial asthma patients: A randomized, double-blind, controlled study. *Journal of Psychosomatic Research*, 59(6), 393–398.

Nickel, C., Lahmann, C., Muehlbacher, M., et al. (2006). Pregnant women with bronchial asthma benefit from progressive muscle relaxation: A randomized, prospective, controlled trial. *Psychotherapy and Psychosomatics*, 75(4), 237–243.

Nolan, D. R., Schneeberger, A. R., Huber, C. G., & Gupta, R. (2017). Efficacy of treatment for tinnitus based on cognitive behavioural therapy in an inpatient setting: A 10 year retrospective outcome analysis. *Journal of Hearing Science*, 7(2), 41, 155.

Nolan-Hocksema, S., Wisco, B. E., & Lyubomirsky, S. (2008). Rethinking rumination. *Perspectives on Psychological Science*, 3(5), 400–424.

Norton, P. J. (2012). A randomized clinical trial of transdiagnostic cognitive-behavioural treatments for anxiety disorder by comparison to relaxation training. *Behaviour Therapy*, 43, 506–517.

Novais, P. G. N., de Melo Batista, K., da Silva Grazziano, E., & Costa Amorim, M. H. (2016). The effects of progressive muscular relaxation as a nursing procedure used for those who suffer from stress due to multiple sclerosis. *Revista Latino-Americana de Enfermagem*, 24, e2789.

Oded, Y. (2018). Integrating mindfulness and biofeedback in the treatment of posttraumatic stress disorder. *Biofeedback*, 46(2), 37–47.

O'Kearney, R. T., Anstey, K. J., & von Sanden, C. (2006). Behavioural and cognitive behavioural therapy for irritable bowel syndrome in children and adolescents. *Cochrane Database of Systematic Reviews*, 4, CD004856.

Okumus, F. E. E., Berk, O. S., & Yucel, B. (2019). Obsesif kompulsif bozuklukta gevseme egitimi ve bilissel davranisci tekniklerin uygulanmasi: Vaka Ornegi. *Journal of Cognitive and Behavioral Psychotherapies*, 8(1), 63–68.

Orsillo, S. M, Romer, L., Block-Lerner, J., et al. (Eds.) (2005). A practical guide to acceptance and commitment therapy (pp. 103-132). New York: Springer.

Ostelo, R. W. J. G., van Tulder, M. W., Vlaeyen, J. W. S., Linton, S. J., Morley, S., & Assendelft, W. J. J. (2005). Behavioural treatment for chronic low-back pain. *Cochrane Database of Systematic Reviews*, 1, CD002014.

Pagnini, F., Manzoni, G. M., Castelnovo, G., & Molinari, E. (2013). A brief literature review about relaxation therapy and anxiety. *Body, Movement and Dance in Psychotherapy*, 8(2), 71–81.

Palermo, T. M., Eccleston, C., Lewandowski, A. S., et al. (2010). Randomized controlled trials of psychological therapies for management of chronic pain in children and adolescents: An updated meta-analytic review. *Pain*, 148, 387–397.

Patel, N., Nadkarni, A., Cardwell, L. A., et al. (2017). Psoriasis, depression, and inflammatory overlap: A review. *American Journal of Clinical Dermatology*, 18, 613–620.

Paulus, D., Brandt, C. P., Lemaire, C., & Zvolensky, M. J. (2020). Trajectory of change in anxiety sensitivity in relation to anxiety, depression and quality of life among persons living with HIV/AIDS following transdiagnostic cognitive-behavioural therapy. *Cognitive Behaviour Therapy*, 29(2), 149–163.

Payati, S., & Tong, J. G. (2007). Perioperative pain management. *CNS Drugs*, 21(3), 185–211.

Paykel, E. S. (1997). The interview for recent life events. *Psychological Medicine*, 27(2), 301–310.

Payne, R. A., Rowland Payne, C. M. E., & Marks, R. (1985). Stress does not worsen psoriasis. A controlled study of 32 patients. *Clinical and Experimental Dermatology*, 10, 239–245.

Pemberton, S., & Cox, D. L. (2014). Experiences of daily activity in chronic fatigue syndrome/myalgic encephalomyelitis (CFS/ME) and their implications for rehabilitation programmes. *Disability and Rehabilitation*, 36, 1790–1797.

Pereira, C. C. D. A., Lopez, R. F. A., & Vilarta, R. (2013). Effects of physical activity programmes n the workplace (PAPW) on the perception and intensity of musculoskeletal pain experienced by garment workers. *Work*, 44, 415–421.

Petrozzi, M. J., Leaver, A., Ferreira, P. H., Rubinstein, S. M., Jones, M. K., & Mackey, M. G. (2019). Addition of MoodGYM to physical treatments for chronic low back pain: A randomized controlled trial. *Chiropratic and Manual Therapies*, 27(54), 1–12.

Peveler, R., Carson, A., & Rodin, G. (2002). Depression in medical patients. *British Medical Journal*, 325, 149–152.

Picardi, A., Mazzotti, E., Gaetano, P., et al. (2005). Stress, social support, emotional regulation and exacerbation of diffuse plaque psoriasis. *Psychosomatics*, 46, 556–564.

Porcelli, P., De Carne, M., & Leandro, G. (2014). Alexithymia and gastrointestinal-specific anxiety in moderate to severe irritable bowel syndrome. *Comprehensive Psychiatry*, 55, 1647–1653.

Porter, C. K., Cash, B. D., Pimentel, M., Akinseye, A., & Riddle, M. S. (2012). Risk of inflammatory bowel disease following a diagnosis of irritable bowel syndrome. *BMC Gastroenterology*, *12*, 55.

Porter, C. K., Tribble, D. R., Aliaga, P. A., Halvorson, H. A., & Riddle, M. S. (2008). Infectious gastroenteritis and risk of developing inflammatory bowel disease. *Gastroenterology*, *135*, 781–786.

Pourdowlat, G., Hejrati, R., & Lookzadeh, S. (2019). The effectiveness of relaxation training in the quality of life and anxiety of patients with asthma. *Advances in Respiratory Medicine*, *87*, 146–151.

Price, J. R., & Couper, J. (2003). Cognitive-behaviour therapy for chronic fatigue syndrome in adults (Cochrane Review). In *The Cochrane Library* (4). Chichester, UK: John Wiley.

Price, J. R., Mitchell, E., Tidy, E., & Hunot, V. (2008). Cognitive behaviour therapy for chronic fatigue syndrome in adults. *Cochrane Database of Systematic Reviews*, *3*, CD001027.

Proctor, M. L., Murphy, P. A., Pattison, H. M., et al. (2007). Behavioural interventions for primary and secondary dysmenorrhoea. *Cochrane Database of Systematic Reviews*, *3*, CD002248.

Pun, J. C., Burgel, B. J., Chan, J., & Lashuay, N. (2004). Education of garment workers: Prevention of work related musculoskeletal disorders. *AAOHN Journal*, *52*(8), 338–343.

Qumer, S., & Ghosh, D. (2019). Effectiveness of patterned breathing technique on pain during first stage of labour – a narrative review. *International Journal of Nursing Education*, *11*(3), 60–62.

Ralston, G. E. (2008). Cognitive behavioural therapy for anxiety. In M. Donaghy, M. Nicol, & K. Davidson (Eds.), *Cognitive behavioural interventions in physiotherapy and occupational therapy* (pp. 75–90). Edinburgh: Butterworth-Heinemann Elsevier.

Rains, J. C., Penzien, D. B., McCrory, D. C., et al. (2005). Behavioural headache treatment: history, review of the empirical literature and methodological critique. *Headache*, *45*(Suppl. 2), S92–S109.

Rani, A. R., Raja Ali, R. A., & Lee, Y. Y. (2016). Irritable bowel syndrome and inflammatory bowel disease overlap syndrome: Pieces of the puzzle are falling into place. *Intestinal Research*, *14*(4), 297–304.

Rankin, J. (2002). *Effects of antenatal exercise on psychological wellbeing in pregnancy and birth outcomes*. London: Whurr.

Rico, P. M. A., Veitl, V. S., Buchuck, G. D., et al. (2013). Evaluacion de un programa de dolar agudo: Effacacia, segurdad y percepcion de la atencion por parte de los pacientes. Experiencia clinica Alemana, Santiago-Chile. *Revista Chillena de Anestesia*, *42*, 145–156.

Rief, W., Weise, C., Kley, N., et al. (2005). Psychophysiologic treatment of chronic tinnitus: A randomized clinical trial. *Psychosomatic Medicine*, *67*(5), 833–838.

Rimes, K. A., & Wingrove, J. (2013). Mindfulness-based cognitive therapy for people with chronic fatigue syndrome still experiencing excessive fatigue after cognitive behaviour therapy: A pilot randomized study. *Clinical Psychology and Psychotherapy*, *20*(2), 107–117.

Ritz, T. (2001). Relaxation therapy in adult asthma: Is there new evidence for its effectiveness? *Behavior Modification*, *25*(4), 640–666.

Rodebaugh, T. L., Holaway, R. M., & Heimberg, R. G. (2004). The treatment of social anxiety disorder. *Clinical Psychology Review*, *24*(7), 883–908.

Roffe, L., Schmidt, K., & Ernst, E. (2005). A systematic review of guided imagery as an adjuvant cancer therapy. *Psychooncology*, *14*(8), 607–617.

Roshan, R., Tavoli, A., Sedighimornani, N., Goljani, Z., & Shariatpanahi, S. S. (2017). Effects of relaxatio and stress management training on fibromyalgia symptoms in women. *Rheumatology Research*, *2*(4), 119–126.

Roth, W. T. (2010). Diversity of effective treatments of panic attacks: What do they have in common? *Depression and Anxiety*, *27*, 5–11.

Roykulcharoen, V., & Good, M. (2004). Systematic relaxation to relieve post-operative pain. *Journal of Advanced Nursing*, *48*(2), 140–148.

Rudebeck, P. H., Bannerman, D. M., & Rushworth, F. (2008). The contribution of distinct subregions of the ventromedial frontal cortex to emotion, social behaviour, and decision making. *Cognitive, Affective, Behavioral Neuroscience*, *8*, 485–497.

Saensak, S., Vutyavanich, T., Somboonporn, W., & Srisurapanont, M. (2013). Effectiveness of a modified version of the applied relaxation technique in treatment of perimenopausal and postmenopausal symptoms. *International Journal of Women's Health*, *5*, 765–771.

Scarlet, J., & Lang, A. J. (2014). Incorporating complementary and alternative practices into treatment of PTSD. In C. R. Martin, V. R. Preedy, & V. P. Patel (Eds.), *Comprehensive guide to post-traumatic stress disorder* (pp. 1979–1995). New York: Springer.

Schaffer, S. D., & Yucha, C. B. (2004). Relaxation and pain management: The relaxation response can play a role in managing chronic and acute pain. *American Journal of Nursing*, *104*(8), 75–76. 78-79, 81-82.

Schlesinger, I., Benyakov, O., Erikh, I., Suraiya, S., & Schiller, Y. (2009). Parkinson's Disease tremor is diminished with relaxation guided imagery. *Movement Disorders*, *24*(14), 2059–2062.

Schirda, B., Nicholas, J. A., & Prakash, R. S. (2015). Examining trait mindfulness, emotion dysregulation, and quality of life in multiple sclerosis. *Health Psychology*, *34*, 1107–1115.

Shinde, N., Shinde, K. J., Khatri, S. M., & Hande, D. (2013). Immediate effect of Jacobson's progressive muscular relaxation in hypertension. *Indian Journal of Physiotherapy, and Occupational Therapy*, *7*(3), 234–237.

Schneider, R. H., Alexander, C. N., Staggers, F., et al. (2005). Long-term effects of stress reduction on mortality in persons ≥55 years of age with systematic hypertension. *American Journal of Cardiology*, *95*(9), 1060–1064.

Scott-Sheldon, L. A. J., Belletto, B. L., Donahue, M. L., et al. (2019). Mindfulness-Based Interventions for Adults Living with HIV/AIDS: A Systematic Review and Meta-analaysis *AIDS and Behaviour*, *23*, 60–75.

Senders, A., Bourdette, D., Hanes, D., Yadav, V., & Shinto, L. (2014). Perceived stress in multiple sclerosis: The potential role of mindfulness in health and wellbeing. *Journal of Evidence-Based Complementary and Alternative Medicine*, *19*, 104–111.

Siev, J., & Chambless, D. L. (2007). Specificity of treatment effects: Cognitive therapy and relaxation for generalized anxiety and panic disorders. *Journal of Consulting and Clinical Psychology*, *75*(4), 513–522.

Sim, J. (1999). Randomized controlled trials. In *Frontline. Clinical effectiveness supplement* (pp. 12–13). London: Chartered Society of Physiotherapy.

Sim, J., & Adams, N. (2002). Systematic review of randomized controlled trials of non-pharmacological interventions for fibromyalgia. *Clinical Journal of Pain, 18*, 324–336.

Simkin, P., & Bolding, A. (2004). Update on non-pharmacologic approaches to relieve labor pain and prevent suffering. *Journal of Midwifery and Women's Health, 49*(6), 489–504.

Simpson, R., Booth, J., Lawrence, M., Byrne, S., & Mair, F. (2014). Mercer S. Mindfulness based interventions in multiple sclerosis—a systematic review. *BMC Neurology, 14*, 15.

Skelly, M. (2008). Fibromyalgia management using cognitive-behaviour principles: A practical approach for therapists. In M. Donaghy, M. Nicol, & K. Davidson (Eds.), *Cognitive-behavioural interventions in physiotherapy and occupational therapy*. Edinburgh: Butterworth-Heinemann.

Slemp, G. R., Jach, H. K., Chia, A., Loton, D. J., & Kern, M. L. (2019). Contemplative interventions and employee distress: A meta-analysis. *Stress and Health, 35*, 227–255.

Sloman, R. (2002). Relaxation and guided imagery for anxiety and depression control in community patients with advanced cancer. *Cancer Nursing, 25*(6), 432–435.

Smith, J. E., Richardson, J., Hoffman, C., et al. (2005). Mindfulness-based stress reduction as supportive therapy in cancer care: A systematic review. *Journal of Advanced Nursing, 52*(3), 315–327.

Smith, J.F. (2006). *Is exercise beneficial in the rehabilitation of drug users?* MPhil dissertation, University of Strathclyde, Glasgow.

Sordoni, C., Hall, C., & Forwell, L. (2002). The use of imagery in athletic injury rehabilitation and its relationship to self-efficacy. *Physiotherapy Canada, 54*(3), 177–185.

Soundy, A., Stubbs, B., Probst, M., et al. (2016). Considering the role of physical therapists within the treatment and rehabilitation of individuals with eating disorders: An international survey of expert clinicians. *Physiotherapy Research, 21*, 237–246.

Stallibrass, C., Sissons, P., & Chalmers, C. (2002). Randomized controlled trial of the Alexander technique for idiopathic Parkinson's disease. *Clinical Rehabilitation, 16*, 705–718.

Stefano, G. B., & Esch, T. (2005). Integrative medical therapy: Examination of meditation's therapeutic and global medicinal outcomes via nitric oxide. *International Journal of Molecular Medicine, 16*(4), 621–630.

Stefanopoulou, E., & Grunfeld, E. A. (2017). Mind-body interventions for vasomotor symptoms in health menopausal women and breast cancer survivors. A systematic review. *Journal of Psychosomatic Obstetrics and Gynecology, 38*(3), 210–225.

Stengler-Wenzke, K., Kroll, M., Matschinger, H., & Angermeyer, M. C. (2006). Subjective quality of life of patients with obsessive-compulsive disorder. *Social Psychiatry and Psychiatric Epidemiology, 41*, 662–668.

Stern, R. S., Nijsten, T., Feldman, S. R., Margolist, D. J., & Rolstad, T. (2004). Psoriasis is common, carries a substantial burden even when not extensive, and is associated with widespread treatment dissatisfaction. *Journal of Investigative Dermatology Symposium Proceedings, 9*(2), 136–139.

Streeter, C., Gerberg, P. I., Whitfield, T., et al. (2017). Treatment of major depressive disorder with Iyengar yoga and coherent breathing: A randomised controlled dosing study. *Journal of Alternative and Complementary Medicine, 23*(3), 201–207.

Stricker, C., Drake, D., Hoyer, K., & Mock, V. (2004). Evidence-based practice for fatigue management in adults with cancer: Exercise as an intervention. *Oncology Nursing Forum, 31*(5), 963–976.

Stulemeijer, M., de Jong, L. W. A. M., Fiselier, T. J. W., Hoogveld, S. W. B., & Bleijenberg, G. (2005). Cognitive behaviour therapy for adolescents with chronic fatigue syndrome: Randomized controlled trial. *British Medical Journal, 330*, 14–17.

Tacon, A. M. (2003). Meditation as a complementary therapy in cancer. *Family and Community Health, 26*(1), 64–73.

Tang, Y., Tang, R., & Posner, M. I. (2016). Mindfulness meditation improves emotion regulation and reduces drug abuse. *Drug and Alcohol Dependence, 163*, S13–S18.

Tay, K., Subramaniam, P., & Oei, T. P. (2019). Cognitive behavioural therapy can be effective in treating anxiety and depression in persons with dementia: A systematic review. *Psychogeriatrics, 19*, 264–275.

Teixeira, J. M., Martin, D., Prendiville, O., & Glover, V. (2005). The effects of acute relaxation on indices of anxiety during pregnancy. *Journal of Psychosomatic Obstetrics and Gynaecology, 26*, 271–276.

Thakur, E. R., Holmes, H. J., Lockhart, N. A., et al. (2017). Emotional awareness and expression training improves irritable bowel syndrome: A randomized controlled trial. *Neurogastroenterology and Motility, 29*. doi: 10.1111/nmo.13143.

Theadom, A., Cropley, M., Smith, H. E., Feigin, V. L., & McPherson, K. (2015). Mind and body therapy for fibromyalgia. *Cochrane Database of Systematic Reviews, 4*, CD001980.

Thelwell, R., Greenlees, I., & Weston, N. (2010). Examining the use of psychological skills throughout soccer performance. *Journal of Sport Behavior, 33*, 109–127.

Thomas, P. W., Thomas, S., Hillier, C., et al. (2006). Psychological interventions for multiple sclerosis. *Cochrane Database of Systematic Reviews, 1*, CD004431.

Thomas, N., Hayward, M., Peter, E., et al. (2014). Psychological therapies for auditory hallucinations (voices), current status and key directions for future research. *Schizophrenia Bulletin, 40*(4), S202–S212.

Toneatto, T., & Nguyen, L. (2007). Does mindfulness meditation improve anxiety and mood symptoms? A review of the controlled research. *Canadian Journal of Psychiatry, 52*(4), 260–266.

Tragea, C., Chrousos, G. P., Alexopoulos, E. C., & Darviri, C. (2014). A randomized controlled trial of the effects of a stress management programme during pregnancy. *Complementary Therapies in Medicine, 22*, 203–211.

Tran, A. N., & Koo, J. Y. (2014). Evaluating the effectiveness of psychological interventions in patients with psoriasis: A review. *Journal of Dermatology, 41*, 775–778.

Treasure, J., Claudion, A. M., & Zucker, N. (2010). Eating disorders. *Lancet, 375*, 583–593.

Urech, C., Flink, N. S., Hoeslie, I., Wilhelm, F. H., Bitzer, J., & Alder, J. (2010). Effects of relaxation on psychobiological wellbeing during pregnancy: A randomized controlled trial. *Psyshoneuroendocrinology, 8*, 1781.

Usmani, Z. A., Carson, K. V., Heslop, K., Esterman, A. J., De Soyza, A., & Smith, B. J. (2017). *Psychological therapies for the treatment of anxiety disorders in chronic obstructive pulmonary disease. The Cochrane Collaboration, Issue 3.* Chichester, UK: John Wiley & Sons.

Vancampfort, D., Probst, M., & Skjaerven, L. H. (2012). Systematic review of the benefits of physical therapy within a multidisciplinary care approach for people with. *Schizophrenia. Physical Therapy, 92*(1), 11–23.

Vancampfort, D., Vanderlinden, J., Stubbs, B., Soundy, A., Pieters, G., & De Hert, M. (2014). Physicalactivitycorrelates inpersons with binge eating disorder: Asystematic review. *European Eating Disorders Review, 22*(0), 1e8.

Vancampfort, D., De Hert, M., Stubbs, B., Soundy, A., De Herdt, A., & Detraux, J. (2015). Correlates of physical activity among individuals with alcohol use disorders: A systematic review of the literature. *Archives of Psychiatric Nursing, 29*(4), 196–201.

Van der Veck, P., Van Rood, Y., & Masclee, A. A. (2007). Clinical trial: Short and long-term benefit of relaxation training for irritable bowel syndrome. *Alimentary Pharmacology & Therapeutics, 26*(6), 943–952.

van Dixhoorn, J., & White, A. (2005). Relaxation therapy for rehabilitation and prevention in ischaemic heart disease: A systematic review and meta-analysis. *European Journal of Cardiovascular Prevention & Rehabilitation, 12*(3), 193–202.

van Rooijen, A. J., Rheeder, P., Eales, C. J., et al. (2004). Effect of exercise versus relaxation on haemoglobin A1C in black females with type 2 diabetes mellitus. *Queensland Journal of Medicine, 97*(6), 343–351.

Varatharajan, S., Ferguson, B., Chrobak, K., et al. (2016). Are non-invasive interventions effective for the management of headaches associated with neck pain? An update of the bone and joint deade task force on neck pain and its associated disorders by the Ontario protocol for traffic injury management (OPTIMa) collaboration. *European Spine Journal, 25*, 1971–1999.

Varkey, E., Cider, A., Carlsson, J., & Linde, M. (2011). Exercise as migraine prophylaxis: A randomized study using relaxation and topiramate as controls. *Cephalalgia, 31*(14), 1428–1438.

Vázquez-Rivera, S., González-Blanch, C., Rodríguez-Moya, L., Morón, D., González-Vives, S., & Carrascom, J. L. (2009). Brief cognitive-behavioral therapy with fibromyalgia patients in routine care. *Comprehensive Psychiatry, 50*, 517–525.

Verhagen, A. P., Damen, L., Berger, M. Y., et al. (2005). Conservative treatments of children with episodic tension-type headache. A systematic review. *Journal of Neurology, 252*(10), 1147–1154.

Vieten, C., & Astin, J. (2008). Effects of a mindfulness-based intervention during pregnancy on prenatal stress and mood: Results of a pilot study. *Archives of Women's Mental Health, 11*, 67–74.

Vocks, S., Tuschen-Caffier, B., Pietrowsky, R., Rustenbach, S. J., Kersting, A., & Herpertz, S. (2010). Meta-analysis of the effectiveness of psychological and pharmacological treatments for binge eating disorder. *International Journal of Eating Disorders, 43*, 205–217.

Walton, K. G., Schneider, R. H., Nidich, S., et al. (2002). Psychosocial stress and cardiovascular disease, part 2: Effectiveness of the transcendental meditation programme in treatment and prevention. *Behavioral Medicine, 28*(3), 106–123.

Walton, K. G., Schneider, R. H., & Nidich, S. (2004). Review of controlled research on the transcendental meditation program and cardiovascular disease. Risk factors, morbidity and mortality. *Cardiology Review, 12*(5), 262–266.

Wang, X., Beauchemin, J., Liu, C., & Lee, M. Y. (2019). Integrative body-mind-spirit (I-BMS) practices for Schizophrenia: An outcome literature review on randomized controlled trials. *Community Mental Health Journal, 55*, 1135–1146.

Weisskopf, M. G., Chen, H., Schwarzschild, M. A., Kawachi, I., & Ascherio, A. (2003). Prospective study of phobic anxiety and risk of Parkinson's disease. *Movement Disorders, 18*, 646–651.

Wellons, M., Ouyang, P., Schreiner, P. J., Herrington, D. M., & Vaidya, D. (2012). Early menopause predicts future coronary heart disease and stroke: The multi-ethnic study of atherosclerosis. *Menopause, 19*(10), 1081–1087.

Wetherell, J. L., Sorrell, J. T., Thorp, S. R., et al. (2005). Psychological interventions for late-life anxiety: A review and early lessons from the CALM study. *Journal of Geriatroc Psychiatry and Neurology, 18*(2), 72–82.

Weydert, J. A. (2006). Evaluation of guided imagery as treatment for recurrent abdominal pain in children: A randomized controlled trial. *BMC Pediatrics, 6*, 29.

Whalley, B., Rees, K., Davies, P., et al. (2011). Psychological interventions for coronary heart disease. *Cochrane Database of Systematic Reviews, 8*, CD002902.

White, P., & Naish, V. (2001). Graded exercise therapy for chronic fatigue syndrome: An audit. *Physiotherapy, 87*(6), 285–288.

Wilkinson-Tough, M., Bocci, L., Thorne, K., & Herlihy, J. (2010). Is mindfulness-based therapy an effective intervention for obsessive-intrusive thoughts: A case series. *Clinical Psychology ad Psychotherapy, 17*, 250–268.

Williams, D. A. (2003). Psychological and behavioural therapies in fibromyalgia and related syndromes. *Best Practice & Research: Clinical Rheumatology, 17*(4), 649–665.

Winkler, L. A., Christiansen, E., Lichtenstein, M. B., Hansen, N. B., Bilenberg, N., & Stoving, R. K. (2014). Quality of life in eating disorders: A meta-analysis. *Psychiatry Research, 219*, 1–9.

World Health Organization (WHO). (1983). Primary prevention of essential hypertension. World Health Organization Technical Report Series 686. Geneva: World Health Organization. Retrieved April 2020 from https://www.worldcat.org/title/primary-prevention-of-essential-hypertension-report-of-a-who-scientific-group/oclc/11366397/editions?referer=di&editionsView=true.

World Health Organization (WHO). (2017). Cardiovascular diseases (CVDs). Retrieved April 2020 from https://www.who.int/news-room/fact-sheets/detail/cardiovascular-diseases-(cvds).

World Health Organization (WHO). (2017). Dementia. Retrieved April 2020 from https://www.who.int/news-room/fact-sheets/detail/dementia.

Yeh, M., Liao, R., Hsu, C., Chung, Y., & Lin, J. (2018). Exercises improve body composition, cardiovascular risk factors and bone mineral density for menopausal women: A systematic review and meta-analysis of randomized controlled trials. *Applied Nursing Research, 40*, 90–98.

Yorke, J., Fleming, S., & Shuldam, C. (2005). Psychological interventions for children with asthma. *Cochrane Database of Systematic Reviews, 4*, CD003272.

Yurdakul, L., Holttum, S., & Bowden, A. (2009). Perceived changes associated with autoenic training for anxiety: A grounded theory study. *Psychology and Psychotherapy: Theory Research and Practice, 82*, 403–419.

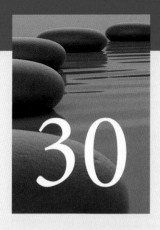

30

COMBINED RELAXATION TECHNIQUES

DR CAROLINE BELCHAMBER

LEARNING OBJECTIVES

The aim of this chapter is to understand how relaxation techniques can be successfully combined.

By the end of this chapter you will be able to:

1. Understand similarities among relaxation technique approaches.

2. Appreciate how relaxation techniques can be combined.

3. Identify key relaxation techniques that can be effectively combined.

4. Acknowledge the evidence behind combining relaxation techniques.

5. Recognize the theory behind combining relaxation techniques.

6. Know how different relaxation techniques can be worked into a single passage.

This chapter will conclude with key points and time for reflection, providing learning opportunities through a case study. Final concluding comments will bring the book to a close.

INTRODUCTION TO COMBINED RELAXATION TECHNIQUES

In an enterprise such as relaxation training where many approaches all lead to the same goal, there are likely to be wide areas of overlap; for example, dwelling on the breath (as in meditation), reciting phrases (as in autogenic training) and concentrating on muscle sensations (as in progressive relaxation) are activities which resemble one another in that they all involve attention focusing and the reduction of motor activity. Moreover, all three approaches are characterized by a monotonous, repetitive stimulus equivalent to the mantra. Thus the differences between the approaches might be more apparent than real, their similarities concealed by their terminology. This might help to explain why the different approaches are so often shown to be equally effective when compared with each other. Hence, it is not suggested in this book that attention should be systematically given to each of the relaxation techniques in turn. Health care professionals may take up any approach that they feel comfortable with. They may, however, wish to take up more than one approach and present them in a single training episode. This can have advantages. Combinations of different relaxation and stress reduction techniques seem to be more effective than single techniques (Davis et al 2000).

Ways of combining techniques may be found in *The Relaxation and Stress Reduction Workbook* (Davis et al 2000), from which the following two combinations are drawn. The first is for mental stress, the second is for physical tension.

1. 'Changing channels':
   a. Thought-stopping (see Chapter 24)
   b. Guided imagery (see Chapter 18)
   c. Coping mantra, such as 'I am at peace' (see Chapter 21).
2. 'Stretch and relax':
   a. Stretching (see Chapter 14)
   b. Abdominal breathing (see Chapter 4)
   c. Mitchell method (see Chapter 13).

For groups of people with varied kinds of stress, more general combined programmes can be constructed. A few examples taken from previous chapters are presented here:

1. Abdominal breathing (see Chapter 4), tense–release (see Chapter 7) and guided imagery (see Chapter 18).
2. Passive muscular relaxation (see Chapter 8), goal-directed visualizations using receptive and programmed components (see Chapter 19) and self-statements (see Chapter 19).
3. Abdominal breathing (see Chapter 4), warmth and heaviness phrases (see Chapter 20) and differential relaxation (see Chapter 11).
4. Passive muscular relaxation (see Chapter 8), Benson's relaxation technique (see Chapter 22) and self-awareness exercises (see Chapter 17).
5. Behavioural relaxation training (see Chapter 10), breathing meditation (see Chapter 4) and guided imagery (see Chapter 18).
6. Breathing pouch (see Chapter 4), eye and tongue muscle work (see Chapter 5) and meditation on a visual object (see Chapter 21).

Set patterns will not suit everyone because the needs and preferences of each individual are different. Davis et al (2000) urge people to construct their own combination of techniques.

Although individual preferences cannot be predicted, it is clear that they exist (Davis et al 2000, Payne 1989)

and that they may be important (McPherson 2009). Rosemary Payne in her experience found that it was useful to ask the person which relaxation technique best suited the person's needs. Involving the individual in the choice of relaxation technique, as in other aspects of therapy, enriches the treatment. All this, of course, means that health care professionals may need to learn several approaches if they are to respond to the person's needs and achieve the desired outcomes.

INTRODUCTION TO EVIDENCE

Not all researchers support the notion of combining relaxation techniques. For example, Manzoni et al (2008), in their systematic review and meta-analysis, suggest that some people may find it easier to respond to a programme involving a single approach rather than one which involves a variety of approaches. However, other researchers have found that combining relaxation techniques, such as progressive muscle relaxation techniques and visual imagery, can be successful when used to improve people's compliance to physical therapy in the treatment of burns (Jong et al 2006, Khanolkar et al 2013). Progressive muscle relaxation and visual imagery have also been shown to support rehabilitation progress from a physical and emotional perspective. It has been found to be particularly effective in managing pain and reducing anxiety and depression, while enabling tolerance to physical therapy and improved functional outcomes (Khanolkar et al 2013). In addition, progressive relaxation techniques and transcendental meditation, combined with other relaxation techniques, such as abdominal breathing, have been shown to improve outcomes in the treatment of hypertension (Kisner & Colby 2002, Rainforth 2007, Schneider et al 1995).

The theories behind how these combined relaxation techniques work is discussed in the next section.

THEORIES BEHIND COMBINED RELAXATION TECHNIQUES

Research has demonstrated that anxiety and pain are interconnected and that people's level of anxiety directly influences their perception of pain (Arntz et al 1994, Atchison & Osgood 1991). Furthermore, anxiety and depression can affect the person's sensation of pain as well as their behaviour (Khanolkar et al 2013). Hence, a strong psychological component to the perception of pain means that the application of relaxation techniques such as progressive muscle relaxation and visual imagery are effective interventions (Kwekkeboom et al 2008). Research also indicates that anxiety levels are affected indirectly by promoting parasympathetic dominance through relaxation techniques such a meditation (see Chapter 21) and progressive muscle relaxation can help to release muscle tension (see Chapter 6). Consequently, blood pressure can be reduced by lowering peripheral vascular resistance (Gupta 2014), with abdominal breathing reducing systolic and diastolic blood pressure (Lee et al 2003).

To aid understanding of how to combine relaxation techniques an example script is presented.

Example of a Script Containing a Variety of Relaxation Techniques

As well as grouping different relaxation techniques together, several relaxation techniques can be worked into a single passage, as shown here.

Please lie down. Get yourself comfortable. Allow your eyelids to grow heavy and eventually to close.

Feel the rest of your body also growing heavy … feel it sinking into the rug or the upholstery … compressing the fibres … sinking down so that more body area comes in contact with it … let your weight flow out … feel your body totally freed from its responsibility to hold you up …

Turn your attention to your breathing … without attempting to alter its rhythm, become aware of the movement of your chest and abdomen … notice the passage of the air … the coolness of the air entering your nostrils … travelling through your nose and down the back of your throat … notice also the warm, moist air being exhaled … next time you breathe out, think the word 'relax' … continue slowly …

Now, I'd like you to scan your muscle groups one by one, checking them for tension … adjust your position if you are uncomfortable … starting with the feet, notice how they rest heavily on the floor … heavy as lead … now your legs, imagine them too heavy to lift … your hips too are lying heavily …

and your shoulders, feel how they are dropped down … with your arms resting heavily by your sides …

Now, your head, let it sink back, giving its weight to the pillow, making a dent in it … feel your brow smoothed and your jaw relaxed … feel your whole body heavy, warm and relaxed … if tension returns, just let it go … let it flow out through your fingertips and toes …

Transfer yourself in your mind's eye to a sandy beach … see yourself lying in the soft sand … run your fingers through the dry grains … smell the sea air … feel the hot sun on your skin … listen to the waves breaking on the shore … enjoy the peace … if disturbing thoughts intrude, accept that they exist … then let them drift away like clouds passing across the sky … you'll attend to them later …

When you are ready, let the scene fade … gradually bring your attention back to the room in which you are lying … count one … two … three … and slowly open your eyes … then give your arms and legs a gentle stretch …

KEY POINTS

1. Where many approaches all lead to the same goal, there are likely to be wide areas of overlap.
2. It is not suggested in this book that attention should be systematically given to each of the relaxation techniques in turn.
3. Combinations of different relaxation and stress reduction techniques seem to be more effective than single techniques.
4. For groups of people with varied kinds of stress, more general combined programmes can be constructed.
5. Set patterns will not suit everyone because the needs and preferences of each individual are different.
6. Several relaxation techniques can be worked into a single passage.

Reflection

Describe your understanding of why the combination of different relaxation techniques is beneficial.

What is the common goal of the different approaches?

How does the combination of relaxation techniques work?

Which relaxation techniques can you combine and why?

What is the main learning point you will take away from this chapter?

What is your future action plan after this learning?

CASE STUDY LEARNING OPPORTUNITY

The key points and reflection provide background and knowledge required in relation to the case study, Bill, to help deepen understanding of the application of combined relaxation techniques.

CASE STUDY

Primary Hypertension: Combined Relaxation Technique Outcomes for Bill

Bill was diagnosed with high blood pressure with unknown secondary cause. Based on Bill's history the likely reason for his high blood pressure was environmental factors, such as stress and lack of exercise. This led to a number of symptoms including, severe headaches, fatigue, chest pain and difficulty breathing.

Before a course of medication Bill consented to try a closely monitored programme of aerobic exercise, progressive muscle relaxation and abdominal breathing to manage his symptoms and overall condition. The programme consisted of a warmup, aerobic exercise and cool down, followed by progressive muscle relaxation and abdominal breathing techniques. Bill's systolic and diastolic blood pressure was taken before and after his aerobic exercise and after carrying out progressive muscle relaxation and abdominal breathing techniques.

The blood pressure readings indicated that there was a significant reduction in Bill's blood pressure after carrying out progressive muscle relaxation and abdominal breathing after exertion. Bill therefore continued with this programme to manage his high blood pressure. Over time Bill's headaches diminished, he found more energy and no longer had chest pain and difficulty breathing. The programme was so successful that Bill no longer required medication to control his high blood pressure.

ACTIVITY

For the case study:

1. List physical and psychological symptoms of Bill's high blood pressure.
2. Write down the key aspects of the combined relaxation techniques used in Bill's monitored programme.
3. Write down the impact that combined relaxation techniques are having from a psychological perspective.
4. Write down the impact that combined relaxation techniques are having from a physical perspective.
5. Write down the impact that combined relaxation techniques are having from an emotional perspective.
6. Consider the outcomes of on quality of life and overall well-being for Bill.

CONCLUDING COMMENTS

Relaxation training is part of the growing trend to view health in terms of the whole person. Its techniques are designed to have a global effect whether they are targeting the healthy individual with difficulty 'switching off' or the person with a chronic condition trying to self-manage their disease.

The book is not comprehensive; many relaxation techniques are not included. The reader will find only a selected range in these chapters (see Introduction, p4) but they are presented with enough detail to be used by someone previously unfamiliar with them. Such a work can be regarded as a toolkit, a collection of relaxation techniques from which the health care professional can choose whatever seems appropriate for the task in hand. The book does not profess to turn people into experts. Training courses exist for that purpose. Perhaps the book is best described as a professional starter.

After reading Chapter 29, the reader may feel the evidence to support the use of relaxation techniques is not compelling. Such an impression may be gained because relaxation therapy is a new science with a comparatively small research base. Many of its studies contain methodological flaws. Moreover, scientific investigation in this area is beset by intrinsic problems which means it is not easy to draw conclusions. No clear picture regarding the effectiveness of the different approaches has yet emerged. Relaxation techniques where research is currently prominent include mindfulness, cognitive-behavioural therapy and physical activity; however, more research is needed before we can confidently present best relaxation techniques, which are themselves likely to vary with each condition. Much also depends on psychosocial aspects of the person's life. Lack of evidence, however, is not the same as lack of effect and findings do paint a general picture of benefit.

Health care professionals are well placed to deliver relaxation techniques since the topic features in their own training. It is one of the areas where they share common ground, where resources can be pooled to create a functioning interdisciplinary service.

Training courses are widely available for health care professionals who wish to extend their knowledge (see Appendix 2). The author suggests that health care professionals consider including relaxation training among their professional skills. Readers of this book may themselves derive benefit from the regular use of relaxation techniques, as part of a healthy lifestyle.

This chapter concludes Section 5, working towards best practice. In Section 6 you will find the appendices, glossary and index.

REFERENCES

Arntz, A., Dreessen, L., & De Jong, P. (1994). The influence of anxiety on pain: Attentional and attributional mediators. *Pain, 56*(3), 307–314.

Atchison, N. E., & Osgood, P. F. (1991). Pain during burn dressing change in children: Relationship to burn area, depth and analgesic regimens. *Pain, 47*(1), 41–45.

Davis, M., Shellman, E., & McKay, M. (2000). *The relaxation and stress reduction workbook* (5th ed.). Oakland, CA: New Harbinger.

Gupta, S. S. (2014). Effect of progressive muscle relaxation combined with deep breathing technique immediately after aerobic exercises on essential hypertension. *Indian Journal of Physiotherapy and Occupational Therapy, 8*(1), 227.

Jong, A. E., & Gamel, C. (2006). The effect of PMR & visual imagery on anxiety and pain during range of motion. *Journal of Advance Nursing, 54*(6), 710–721.

Khanolkar, T. S., Metgud, S., & Verma, C. (2013). A study on combined effects of progressive muscle relaxation and visual imagery technique on perceived pain, levels of anxiety and depression in patients with burns. *Indian Journal of Physiotherapy and Occupational Therapy, 7*(2), 225–228.

Kisner, C., & Colby, L. A. (2002). Therapeutic exercise: Foundations and techniques (4th ed.). Philadelphia: FA Davis Company; pp. 154–163, 749–751.

Kwekkeboom, K., Wanta, B., & Bompus, M. (2008). Individual difference variables and effects of progressive muscle relaxation and analgesic imagery interventions on cancer pain. *Journal of Pain and Symptom Management, 36*(6), 604–615.

Lee, J. S., Lee, M. S., Lee, J. Y., Cornélissen, G., Otsuka, K., & Halberg, F. (2003). Effects of diaphragmatic breathing on ambulatory blood pressure and heart rate. *Biomedical Pharmacotherapy, 57*(Suppl. l), 87s–91s.

Manzoni, G. M., Pagnini, F., Castelnuovo, G., & Molinari, E. (2008). Relaxation training for anxiety: A ten years' systematic review with meta-analysis. *BMC Psychiatry, 8*, 41.

McPherson, K. (2009). Do patients' preferences matter? Editorial. *British Medical Journal, 338*, 59–60.

Payne, R. A. (1989). Glad to be yourself: A course of practical relaxation and health education talks. *Physiotherapy, 75*, 8–9.

Rainforth, M. V., Schneider, R. H., Sandford, I. N., Gaylord-King, C., Salerno, J. W., & Anderson, J. W. (2007). Stress Reduction programs in Patients with Elevated Blood Pressure: A Systematic Review and Meta-analysis. *Current Hypertension Reports, 9*(6), 520–528.

Schneider, R. H., Staggers, F., Alexander, C. N., Sheppard, W., Rainforth, M., Kondwani, K., Smith, S., & Gaylort-King, C. (1995). A randomized controlled trial of stress reduction for hypertension in older African Americans. *Hypertension, 26*(5), 820–828.

Section 6

APPENDICES, GLOSSARY AND INDEX

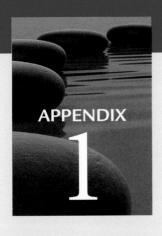

TABLE OF METHODS, MAJOR PRINCIPLES AND SUGGESTED APPLICATIONS WITH SUMMARY AND KEY POINTS

Method	Major principles	Suggested applications	Relevant chapters
Breathing	■ based on physiological principles which link the method to the autonomic nervous system ■ slow breathing is associated with parasympathetic dominance ■ a cognitive feature is represented by the imagery which accompanies some breathing sequences	asthma, childbirth, coronary heart disease, depression, hypertension, panic attacks, chronic pain, occupational stress used in combination with other techniques such as progressive muscular relaxation and mindfulness for migraines, irritable bowel syndrome and low back pain	Chapters 4, 29
Progressive relaxation	■ relaxed musculature is reflected in a relaxed mind ■ underpinned by unitary theory ■ physiological principles predominate but there are cognitive elements	anxiety, psychiatric conditions, hypertension, tension headache, asthma, insomnia, chronic pain, ulcerative colitis, before and after surgery, epilepsy, athletic injury, HIV/AIDS, chronic obstructive pulmonary disease, panic attacks, migraine, irritable bowel syndrome, multiple sclerosis	Chapters 5, 29
Progressive relaxation training	■ similar to progressive relaxation except that the cognitive element is stronger because of the use of suggestion	similar to progressive relaxation	Chapters 6, 29
Applied relaxation	■ built around a core technique of progressive relaxation ■ addresses the concept of anxiety from cognitive and behavioural as well as physiological standpoints	anxiety, panic attacks, phobia, headache, tinnitus, epilepsy, chronic pain	Chapters 9, 29
Behavioural relaxation training	■ underpinned by behaviourist principles of reinforcement and corrective adjustment ■ contains physical and cognitive elements	learning difficulties, ataxic tremor	Chapters 10, 29
Alexander technique	■ underpinned by principles of body positioning ■ is atheoretical	performance stress, motor problems, Parkinson's disease	Chapters 12, 29
Mitchell Method	■ based on physiological principles of reciprocal inhibition ■ has a weak cognitive element	childbirth, hypertension, rheumatoid arthritis	Chapters 13, 29
Stretching	■ these link into physiological principles ■ the process of stretching entails a relaxation of the muscles being stretched	physical and psychological stress, generalized anxiety, chronic neck tension, musculoskeletal disorders	Chapters 14, 29

Method	Major principles	Suggested applications	Relevant chapters
Physical activity	▪ essentially a physical approach to relaxation ▪ linked to neurobiological changes, it is underpinned by physiological principles	cardiovascular problems, osteopenia, osteoporosis, depression, chronic fatigue syndrome, drug and alcohol dependence, eating disorders, low self-esteem, childbirth, diabetes, menopause	Chapters 15, 29
Cognitive behavioural approaches	▪ these use a variety of techniques drawn from cognitive principles on the one hand and behavioural principles on the other ▪ the client is encouraged to adopt a collaborative role in the management of his or her condition	anxiety, depression, eating disorders, panic attack, drug and alcohol dependence, hypertension, chronic fatigue syndrome, insomnia, HIV/AIDS, psychiatric disorders, chronic pain, cancer, dementia	Chapters 16, 29
Self-awareness	▪ a cognitive approach concerned with the thoughts one has about the self	low self-esteem	Chapters 17, 29
Imagery	▪ cognitive principles underlie this approach ▪ image making is thought to be governed by the right cerebral hemisphere	chronic pain, anxiety, before and after surgery, athletic injury, arthritis, cancer, occupational stress	Chapters 18, 29
Goal-directed visualizations	▪ a cognitive approach which uses techniques of imagery and self-suggestion ▪ based on the belief that the body cannot distinguish between the event as imagined and the event as experienced	performance stress, alcohol and substance misuse, eating disorders, smoking abstinence, chronic pain, sport and athletics, phobia and panic attack	Chapters 19, 29
Autogenic training	▪ based on principles of suggestion, which create a light trance ▪ primarily a cognitive approach, although the sensations of warmth generated by the phrases provide a physiological element ▪ is atheoretical	anxiety, depression, insomnia, drug and alcohol misuse, eating disorders, tension headache, hypertension, coronary heart disease, injury rehabilitation, asthma, HIV/AIDS, different kinds of pain	Chapters 20, 29
Meditation	▪ a cognitive activity involving what is considered to be a shift in cerebral hemispherical dominance from left to right	hypertension, coronary heart disease, menopausal symptoms, insomnia, occupational stress, HIV/AIDS	Chapters 21, 29
Benson's method	▪ underpinned by unitary theory ▪ cognitive principles predominate in the focusing of attention on the mantra ▪ in diminishing the activity in the sympathetic nervous system, it draws on physiological principles	hypertension, coronary heart disease, psychological stress, irritable bowel syndrome, menopausal problems	Chapters 22, 29
Mindfulness meditation	▪ based on principles of meditation with an emphasis on the moment, accepting it as it occurs without judgement or criticism	cancer, chronic pain, fibromyalgia, smoking cessation, addictive practices, stress, depression	Chapters 23, 29

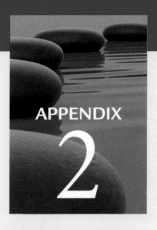

TRAINING COURSES AND CONTACT INFORMATION

The author is not in a position to endorse all the following training courses but includes them for information. The training courses mentioned here are all in the UK. People reading this book in other countries should consult their in-country register which is available on the Internet. However, the contact information for the International Committee on Autogenic Training (ICAT) has been added to this edition.

ICAT
C/O Dr Luis de Rivera
Calle Islas Filipinas
Madrid
28003
Spain

British Autogenic Society, Ltd
International House
24 Holborn Viaduct
Holborn
London
EC1A 2BN
Telephone: 07714247809
Website: www.autogenic-therapy.org.uk
Email: Admin@autogenic-therapy.org.uk
Training in this approach is offered to those who already hold a qualification in the field of medical, psychological, nursing, therapy or counselling professions.

Research Council for Complementary Medicine (RCCM)
C/O Dr John Huges
Royal London Hospital for Integrated Medicine
60 Great Ormond Street
London
WC1N 3HR
Website: www.rccm.org.uk
Email: info@rccm.org.uk

This organization provides information on university courses that offer training in complementary and alternative medicine to health care professionals.

Alexander technique
The Alexander Teacher Training School (ATTS)
3rd Floor
Danceworks
16 Balderton Street
London
W1K 6TN
Telephone: 020 7629 1808
Website: www.alexanderteacher.co.uk
Email: info@alexanderteacher.co.uk

This is one of the registered schools which offers training in the technique.

British Association for Behavioural and Cognitive Psychotherapies (BABCP)
Minerva House
Hornby street
Bury
Lancashire
BL9 5BN
Telephone: 0330 320 0851
Website: www.babcp.com
Email: babcp@babcp.com
BABCP can provide information regarding cognitive–behavioural courses run by universities and other educational establishments. The Internet is a useful source of information. Students are advised to contact the course providers to determine their entry requirements.

Breathworks CIC/Foundation
16–20 Turner Street
Manchester
M4 1DZ
Telephone: 0161 834 1110
Website: www.breathworks-mindfulness.org.uk
Email: info@breathworks.co.uk

This organization runs courses in mindfulness meditation for health care professionals who wish to become trainers.

e-Learning for Healthcare
Health Education England
Second Floor
Stewart House
32, Russell Square
London
WC1B 5DN
Website: https://www.e-lfh.org.uk/
Email: enquiries@e-lfh.org.uk

Health Education England e-Learning for Healthcare (HEE e-LfH) works in partnership with the NHS, third sector and professional bodies to support patient care by providing e-learning to educate and train the health and care workforce.

Online relaxation techniques
Professor Teena Clouston
Reader: Occupational Therapy
School of Healthcare Sciences
Cardiff University
Email: cloustontj@cardiff.ac.uk

This YouTube channel has guided mindfulness meditations, mindful waking and a variety of relaxation sessions you can listen to and use when needed or for regular practice: https://www.youtube.com/channel/UCoNpYN3mYrIgI458hpbhXFQ

Living life in balance website: https://teenaclouston.wordpress.com/

This website developed by Professor Teena Clouston provides a selection of resources around mindfulness and relaxation including practical techniques and theory. There is an interesting blog on the use of mindfulness during the COVID-19 crisis, which you can find here: https://teenaclouston.wordpress.com/2020/03/31/mindfulness-for-wellbeing-in-strange-covid-times/

Iona Mind
35, Lodge Avenue,
Romford,
RM2 5AB
E-mail: hello@ionamind.com
Website: www.Ionamind.com
Iona Mind builds technologies that digitise evidence-based tools and exercise from the CBT and mindfulness literature. The Iona app can be used to accompany therapy or as a standalone app and guides users through CBT and mindfulness-based practices. It was developed in collaboration with clinicians to help reinforce concepts and exercises in between therapy sessions and is currently used around the world in over 70 countries.

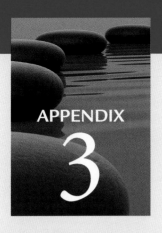

APPENDIX 3

EVENTS AND 1995 LIFE CHANGE UNIT (LCU) VALUES FOR THE RECENT LIFE CHANGES QUESTIONNAIRE ALL CORECT

Life change event	LCU
Health	
An injury or illness which:	
Kept you in bed a week or more, or sent you to the hospital	74
Was less serious than above	44
Major dental work	26
Major change in eating habits	27
Major change in sleeping habits	26
Major change in your usual type and/or amount of recreation	28
Work	
Change to a new type of work	51
Change in your work hours or conditions	35
Change in your responsibilities at work:	
More responsibilities	29
Fewer responsibilities	21
Promotion	31
Demotion	42
Transfer	32
Troubles at work:	
With your boss	29
With co-workers	35
With persons under your supervision	35
Other work troubles	28
Major business adjustment	60
Retirement	52

Life change event	LCU
Loss of job:	
Laid off from work	68
Fired from work	79
Correspondence course to help you in your work	18
Home and family	
Major change in living conditions	42
Change in residence:	
Move within the same town or city	25
Move to a different town, city or state	47
Change in family get-togethers	25
Major change in health or behaviour of family member	55
Marriage	50
Pregnancy	67
Miscarriage or abortion	65
Gain of a new family member:	
Birth of a child	66
Adoption of a child	65
A relative moving in with you	59
Spouse beginning or ending work	46
Child leaving home:	
To attend college	41
Due to marriage	41
For other reasons	45
Change in arguments with spouse	50

Life change event	LCU
In-law problems	38
Change in the marital status of your parents:	
Divorce	59
Remarriage	50
Separation from spouse:	
Due to work	53
Due to marital problems	76
Divorce	96
Birth of grandchild	43
Death of spouse	119
Death of other family member:	
Child	123
Brother or sister	102
Parent	100

Personal and social

Life change event	LCU
Change in personal habits	26
Beginning or ending school or college	38
Change of school or college	35
Change in political beliefs	24
Change in religious beliefs	29
Change in social activities	27

Life change event	LCU
Vacation	24
New, close, personal relationship	37
Engagement to marry	45
Girlfriend or boyfriend problems	39
Sexual difficulties	44
'Falling out' of a close personal relationship	47
An accident	48
Minor violation of the law	20
Being held in jail	75
Death of a close friend	70
Major decision regarding your immediate future	51
Major personal achievement	36

Financial

Life change event	LCU
Major change in finances:	
Increased income	38
Decreased income	60
Investment and/or credit difficulties	56
Loss or damage of personal property	43
Moderate purchase	20
Major purchase	37
Foreclosure on a mortgage or loan	58

From Miller, M. A., & Rahe, R. H. (1997). Life changes scaling for the 1990s. *Journal of Psychosomatic Research, 43*(3), 291–292, with permission from Elsevier.

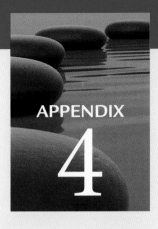

PAR-Q PHYSICAL ACTIVITY READINESS QUESTIONNAIRE

▪ ▪ ▪ ▪ ▪ ▪ ▪ ▪ ▪ ▪ ▪ ▪ ▪ ▪ ▪ ▪ ▪ ▪ ▪

Physical Activity Readiness
Questionnaire – PAR-Q
(revised 2002)

PAR-Q & YOU

(A Questionnaire for People Aged 15 to 69)

Regular physical activity is fun and healthy, and increasingly more people are starting to become more active every day. Being more active is very safe for most people. However, some people should check with their doctor before they start becoming much more physically active.

If you are planning to become much more physically active than you are now, start by answering the seven questions in the box below. If you are between the ages of 15 and 69, the PAR-Q will tell you if you should check with your doctor before you start. If you are over 69 years of age, and you are not used to being very active, check with your doctor.

Common sense is your best guide when you answer these questions. Please read the questions carefully and answer each one honestly: check YES or NO.

YES	NO	
☐	☐	**1. Has your doctor ever said that you have a heart condition <u>and</u> that you should only do physical activity recommended by a doctor?**
☐	☐	**2. Do you feel pain in your chest when you do physical activity?**
☐	☐	**3. In the past month, have you had chest pain when you were not doing physical activity?**
☐	☐	**4. Do you lose your balance because of dizziness or do you ever lose consciousness?**
☐	☐	**5. Do you have a bone or joint problem (for example, back, knee or hip) that could be made worse by a change in your physical activity?**
☐	☐	**6. Is your doctor currently prescribing drugs (for example, water pills) for your blood pressure or heart condition?**
☐	☐	**7. Do you know of <u>any other reason</u> why you should not do physical activity?**

If

you

answered

YES to one or more questions

Talk with your doctor by phone or in person BEFORE you start becoming much more physically active or BEFORE you have a fitness appraisal. Tell your doctor about the PAR-Q and which questions you answered YES.

- You may be able to do any activity you want – as long as you start slowly and build up gradually. Or, you may need to restrict your activities to those which are safe for you. Talk with your doctor about the kinds of activities you wish to participate in and follow his/her advice.
- Find out which community programs are safe and helpful for you.

NO to all questions

If you answered NO honestly to <u>all</u> PAR-Q questions, you can be reasonably sure that you can:
- start becoming much more physically active – begin slowly and build up gradually. This is the safest and easiest way to go.
- take part in a fitness appraisal – this is an excellent way to determine your basic fitness so that you can plan the best way for you to live actively. It is also highly recommended that you have your blood pressure evaluated. If your reading is over 144/94, talk with your doctor before you start becoming much more physically active.

→

DELAY BECOMING MUCH MORE ACTIVE:
- if you are not feeling well because of a temporary illness such as a cold or a fever – wait until you feel better; or
- if you are or may be pregnant – talk to your doctor before you start becoming more active.

PLEASE NOTE: If your health changes so that you then answer YES to any of the above questions, tell your fitness or health professional. Ask whether you should change your physical activity plan.

(From Physical Activity Readiness Questionnaire (PAR-Q) © 2002. Used with permission from the Canadian Society for Exercise Physiology www.csep.ca.)

GLOSSARY

Aerobic exercise: Sustained, rhythmic activity. It involves large muscle groups contracting in a repetitive manner at low-to-moderate levels of energy expenditure for long periods. Examples include walking, jogging, distance running, swimming, dancing and cycling.

Biopsychosocial: This approach gives weight to psychosocial aspects as well as biological ones.

Blinding: This is a condition built into the study design whereby participants are kept in ignorance of the group they are in: experimental or control. When the researchers are also in ignorance of this fact, the situation is called double blind. Single and double blinding are techniques for reducing the risk of bias in the results.

Body awareness therapy: A therapy based on the notion that human movement has a psychological dimension. Movements carried out by the body are recognized as part of the self and therefore part of a person's identity.

Catecholamines: These include adrenaline, noradrenaline and dopamine. They play an important role as neurotransmitters in the functioning of the autonomic and central nervous systems.

Catharsis: In psychoanalytic theory, this refers to the release of tension which occurs when repressed thoughts are brought into consciousness.

Centring: Refers to the focusing of attention on the interior of the self. To achieve this state all external stimuli must be disregarded. The purpose is to find and make contact with the essence of the self.

Clinical depression: Diagnosed by a cluster of symptoms that persist for weeks or months. Symptoms include feelings of hopelessness, sadness, guilt. They are accompanied by physical symptoms such as loss of energy, appetite, sleeplessness and a lack of concentration. Diagnosis of depression is usually undertaken by clinical interview. In research studies depression may be measured by using standardized screening devices such as the Beck Depression Inventory in which the severity of the condition can be classified into mild, medium and severe.

Cognitive–behavioural therapy: An approach concerned with helping the patient to identify and correct faulty patterns of thinking. It can lead to improved clinical outcomes. Patient and therapist are engaged in a collaborative effort to address and solve or alleviate the patient's problem. The therapy is of predetermined and short duration and is focused on the patient's current circumstances.

Cognitive restructuring: This involves a re-evaluation of a person's perception of danger or vulnerability and a questioning of the beliefs which underlie it. The technique consists of three stages: identifying negative thoughts, challenging their accuracy and replacing them with constructive alternatives based upon new judgements about the degree of risk.

Confidence interval: The distance between an upper and a lower point between which the true value lies with a probability of 95%. Presented in this way, the result assumes a range of possibilities. A narrow range will indicate a more precise result than a wide one.

Control group: The basic scientific study consists of two groups, resembling each other in as many ways as possible. One of these groups is the experimental group, which receives the intervention; the other group is the control, which does not receive the intervention. The control thus provides a baseline against which to measure the effects of the intervention.

Effect size: Refers either to the strength of the association or to the effect of the intervention and is expressed as a percentage of the total possible effect.

Epidemiology: The study of diseases in populations and concerned with the cause of the disease and the way the disease is distributed within a given population.

Evidence-based practice: Practice informed by research findings. It consists of procedures which current evidence shows to be the most effective. Thus it may be referred to as best practice.

Exposure techniques: Introduced to help individuals face situations which they find stress inducing such as, for example, public speaking. Exposure generally involves a hierarchy of low- to high-threat versions of this event. Individuals are first presented with the item of lowest threat. With the help of a relaxation technique, they work to overcome their fear at that level. When they succeed, they move on to the next level of threat, dealing with it in the same way.

Eye movement desensitization and reprocessing: A type of therapy that is used to manage trauma symptoms. The aim of this treatment is to aid the brain to process distressing memories and reduce their negative effect on everyday activities, enabling individuals to develop strategies to move forward with their lives. This is a treatment employed in posttraumatic stress disorder: the client focuses on the traumatic event while receiving bilateral stimulation, usually in the form of eye movements.

Fear avoidance: Behaviour which the individual adopts to avoid situations which give rise to fear. However, by avoiding the situation, the fear attached to it mounts. Avoidance may result in an immediate sense of relief but creates an increase in anxiety levels on the next occasion of threat. The solution is to face the feared situation.

Generalized anxiety disorder: Characterized by excessive worry, overly tense muscles and impairment of function, all of which have persisted for at least 6 months and are not confined to any specific circumstances.

Homeostasis: The process whereby a balanced state is maintained in body systems throughout varying external conditions. An example can be found in the regulation of body temperature during extreme heat and cold.

Hyperacusis: Refers to noise sensitivity. For example, when everyday noise is perceived by the individual to be much louder than normal.

Hypothesis: A statement which acts as a provisional explanation. In science a hypothesis must undergo a test, the findings of which will tell the researcher whether the hypothesis has been supported or whether it should be rejected. The conclusion reached, however, will only apply within the context of the particular piece of research.

Locus of control: Refers to the source of control of the behaviour of individuals. If they tend to take responsibility for their actions, they are said to have an internal locus; if they tend to attribute events to chance effects or external factors, they are said to have an external locus. In practice, people tend to display both forms; this places the individual's locus of control on a continuum, where it exhibits varying levels, internal and external, at different times.

Meta-analysis: A statistical technique which collates and analyses the findings of many different studies and identifies trends in outcome.

Mind–body approaches: Defined by the National Institutes of Health as 'interventions designed to facilitate the mind's capacity to affect bodily function and symptoms'. In a word, holistic.

Mindfulness: Refers to awareness and acceptance of the moment as it occurs; cherishing it, whatever we happen to be doing.

Motor skill: Refers to a skill which involves physical movement.

Number needed to treat (NNT): The number of people who would need to receive the intervention before one specific outcome occurred or one specific adverse outcome was avoided. For example, in an experimental group of elderly women wearing hip protectors, the NNT is an estimate of how many participants would be necessary before one hip fracture was prevented. The NNT is a way of presenting the usefulness of a treatment.

Outcome measures: The products of measurement used to determine the results of interventions. A range of tools are specifically designed for this purpose.

Pacing: Refers to the way a learning programme is structured to allow for the varying level of skill in the performer. New material is introduced in a gradual and controlled way, alternating with periods of rest.

Preexperimental studies: Here, a single system such as a cohort is studied to explore an idea. The exercise helps in formulating a hypothesis which may later be tested.

Psychogenic: This adjective is applied to symptoms which are brought about by faulty patterns of thinking or overemotional reactions.

Psychosocial: Encompasses both psychological and social aspects of a person's life. The 'psychological' includes a person's beliefs and attitudes, whereas the 'social' refers to environmental influences, including the influence of other people.

Quasi-experimental studies: These bear some characteristics of a true experiment but lack the full requirements of a randomized controlled trial. They feature, for example, in research where randomization is not possible.

Randomization: A process by which researchers allocate people into different groups. An example of this process is the use of numbered sealed envelopes; computer-aided lists are another. Randomization allows all study participants to have an equal chance of being selected for the active experimental intervention. The process helps to ensure that the groups are similar at the start of the study.

Randomized controlled trials: Studies which carry the full rigour of a scientific experiment. Participants are selected by a random process and divided into two or more groups, one of which receives the intervention. The presence of a control is essential, but it can take different forms.

Reflective practice: Refers to thinking about knowledge gained from one's experience in the past and the creative application of it in unfamiliar situations.

Reinforcement: Positive reinforcement refers to action which increases the likelihood of a certain behaviour; for example, giving a dog a biscuit every time it brings back a ball makes it more likely the dog will bring back the ball next time it is thrown.

Reliability: Refers to the consistency of results when the test is repeated, either by the same researcher on different occasions or by different researchers on the same occasion.

Repression: A psychoanalytical concept in which anxiety-inducing thoughts are prevented from reaching conscious awareness.

Reviews: Scientific reviews collate the results of all studies in a particular field. They are the result of extensive literature searches and provide the health care professional with the kind of information needed to form a view of the best treatment.

Schizophrenia: A condition characterized by symptoms such as hallucinations and thought disturbances. It may also be accompanied by social withdrawal, low self-esteem, reduced motivation, emotional and attentional deficits and other symptoms of depression.

Self-efficacy: The ability of individuals to predict their success in achieving a particular task in a given situation. Efficacy is effectiveness; self-efficacy is the belief in one's effectiveness.

Sham intervention: Also known as a placebo intervention, which is used in medical trials by researchers to determine the effectiveness of a treatment, intervention or drug. For example, the control group will receive a sham intervention where the actions of the intervention are carried out but without actually being given the intervention.

Skill: Enables a person to achieve a goal with a high level of certainty and an economy of time and energy.

Somatization: Said to occur when an individual complains of symptoms, such as pain, which cannot be explained in terms of organic disease. It differs from hypochondriasis, where the individual is constantly in fear of developing a disease.

States of altered consciousness: States of mental functioning which are different from the ordinary pattern. Examples are dreaming, drug-induced states, hypnotism, meditation, daydreaming, deep relaxation, guided imagery.

Statistical significance: Means that there is a 95% likelihood that the result of the experiment is due to the manipulations of the experimenter and not to chance factors. Expressed another way, the result achieved in the experiment could only have occurred by chance in fewer than 5 out of 100 cases.

Stimulus-control behaviour: Behaviour triggered and maintained by environmental stimuli.

Thought action: When an individual believes that just thinking about an action is the same as actually performing that action.

Thought suppression: When a person is motivated to consciously stop a specific thought to trigger memory inhibition.

Trait anxiety: An inherent tendency to interpret circumstances as more dangerous than they are and to respond with a disproportionate degree of anxiety. It contrasts with *state anxiety* which reflects the normal level of anxiety attached to particular events and situations perceived as threatening.

Validity: A test is valid when it measures what it claims to measure. It has internal validity when it is devoid of bias, and external validity when its results can be generalized to other situations. It has content validity when its components are representative of the item to be measured and face validity when it *seems* valid after superficial appraisal.

INDEX

Note: Page numbers followed by "*b*", "*f*", and "*t*" refer to boxes, figures, and tables, respectively.